INTRODUCTION TO

Health Care

Dakota Mitchell
Lee Haroun

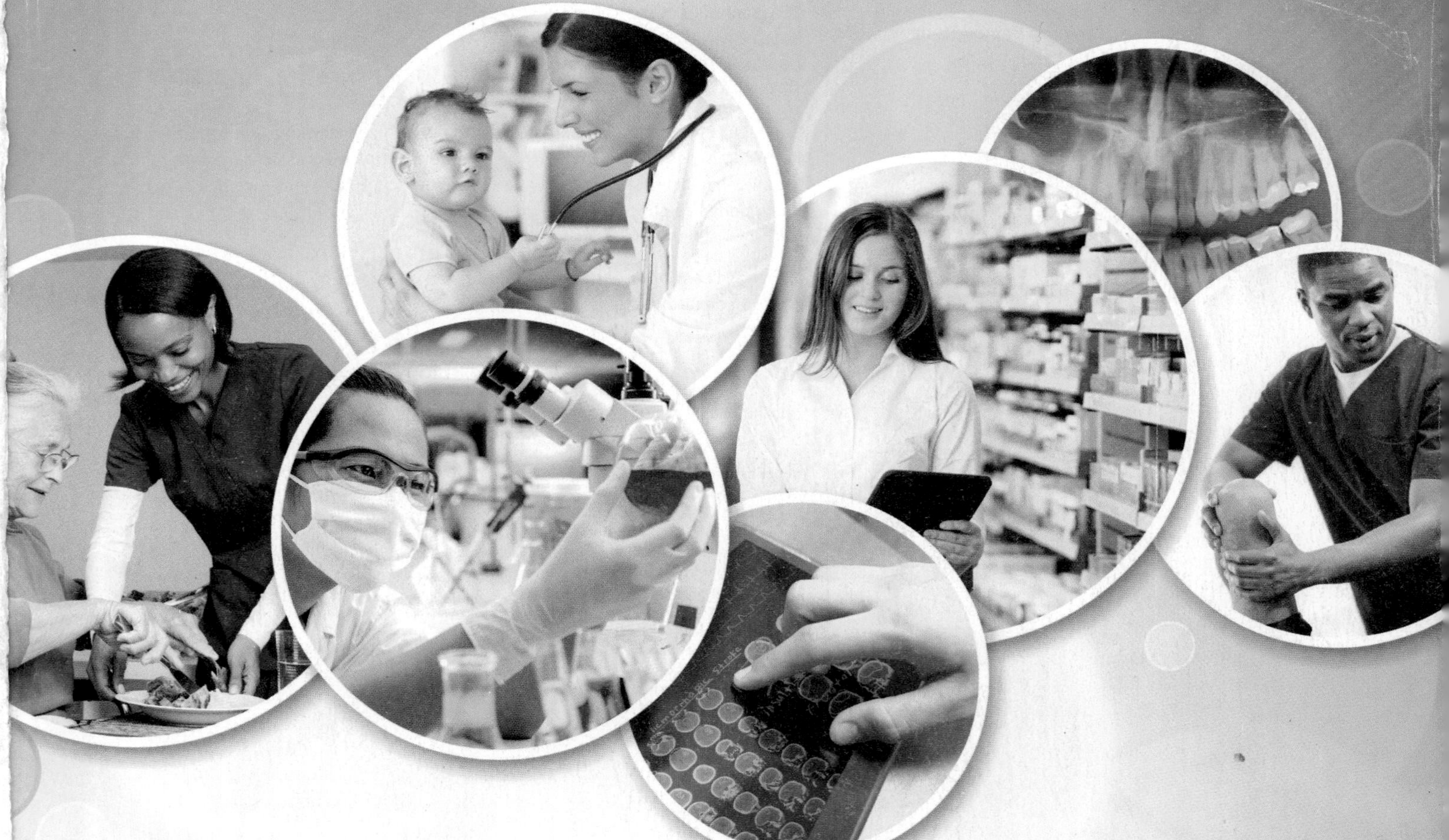

FOURTH EDITION

CENGAGE Learning

Australia • Brazil • Mexico • Singapore • United Kingdom • United States

CENGAGE Learning

Introduction to Health Care, Fourth Edition

Dakota Mitchell and Lee Haroun

SVP, GM Skills & Global Product Management: Dawn Gerrain

Product Director: Matthew Seeley

Senior Director, Development: Marah Bellegarde

Senior Product Development Manager: Juliet Steiner

Product Manager: Laura Stewart

Senior Content Developer: Debra M. Myette-Flis

Product Assistant: Deborah Handy

Vice President, Marketing Services: Jennifer Ann Baker

Marketing Manager: Cassie Cloutier

Marketing Coordinator: Courtney Cozzy

Senior Production Director: Wendy Troeger

Production Director: Andrew Crouth

Senior Content Project Manager: Kenneth McGrath

Managing Art Director: Jack Pendleton

Cover image(s): © iStock.com/zokara, © iStock.com/jonya, © iStock.com/svetkid, © iStock.com/Christopher Futcher, © iStock.com/sudok1, © Shutterstock/Tyler Olsen, © Shutterstock/Bullstar

Library of Congress Control Number: 2015955717

ISBN: 978-1-3055-7477-9

Cengage Learning
20 Channel Center Street
Boston, MA 02210
USA

Printed in the United States of America
Print Number: 01 Print Year: 2015

CONTENTS

Preface x
Dedication xviii
About the Authors xix
Acknowledgments xx
About this Book xxi

Unit 1: Health Care Today

Chapter 1
Your Career in Health Care 3
Your Future in Health Care 4
- Essential Qualities of Health Care Professionals 5

Standards for Health Care Professionals 6
Occupational Profiles 7
- Therapeutic and Treatment Occupations 8
- Diagnostic Occupations 23
- Health Information Management Occupations 25
- Environmental Occupations 27

Getting Off to a Good Start 28
- Learning for Mastery 28
- Getting the Most from Your Studies 29
- Returning Adult Learners 30
- Establishing Good Work Habits 30
- Learning to Think Like a Health Care Professional 31

Chapter 2
Current Health Care Systems and Trends 37
The Health Care Industry Today 38
- Technological Advancements 38
- Specialization 46
- Aging Population 46
- Increasing Costs 47

Health Care Facilities and Services 48
- Hospitals 48
- Ambulatory Services 50
- Long-Term Care Facilities 50
- Home Health Care Providers 50
- Hospice 52
- Consolidation of Health Care Services 52
- New Types of Health Care Facilities 52
- Government Health Services 53

Trends in Health Care 54
- Wellness 54
- Complementary, Alternative, and Integrative Health 54

Challenges in Health Care Today 58
- Providing Affordable Health Care 58
- Providing Long-Term Care 59
- Improving Social Conditions 59
- Maintaining the Quality of Care 60
- Treating Alzheimer's and Other Forms of Dementia 61
- Addressing Public Health Concerns 61
- Encouraging Medication Adherence 62
- Preventing Prescription Drug Overuse 62
- Preventing Antibiotic Resistance 62
- Encouraging Personal Responsibility for Health 62

Implications for Health Care Professionals 63

Chapter 3
Ethical and Legal Responsibilities 65
The Purpose of Ethics 66
Ethics and the Law 66
Ethics and Health Care 67
- Professional Codes of Ethics 69
- Personal Values 69

Guiding Principles of Health Care Ethics 70
- Preserve Life 72
- Do Good 74
- Respect Autonomy 74
- Uphold Justice 77
- Be Honest 79
- Be Discreet 79

Keep Promises 82
Do No Harm 83
Handling Ethical Dilemmas 84
Who Decides? 84

Unit 2: The Language of Health Care

Chapter 4
Medical Terminology 89
Importance of Medical Terminology 90
The Building Blocks of Medical Language 90
Word Roots and Combining Forms 90
Suffixes 91
Prefixes 92
Deciphering Medical Terms 95
Spelling and Pronunciation 97
Medical Abbreviations and Symbols 98
Medical Dictionary 99
Mastering Medical Terminology 101

Chapter 5
Medical Math 105
Importance of Math in Health Care 106
Math Anxiety 106
Basic Calculations 107
Whole Numbers 108
Decimals 109
Fractions 109
Percentages 112
Ratios 112
Converting Decimals, Fractions, Percentages, and Ratios 112
Rounding Numbers 112
Solving Problems with Proportions 113
Estimating 115
Military Time 115
Roman Numerals 117
Angles 117
Systems of Measurement 118
Household System 118
Metric System 120
Apothecary System 121
Converting Systems of Measurement 122
Medication Safety 123
Temperature Conversion 123

Unit 3: The Human Body

Chapter 6
Organization of the Human Body 129
The Basis of Life 130
Cells 132
Tissues 132
Describing the Body 134
Body Planes 134
Directional Terms 134
The Body Cavities 134
Abdominal Descriptions 136

Chapter 7
Structure and Function of the Human Body 141
The Importance of Anatomy and Physiology 142
Genetics 143
The Systems of The Body 143
Systems for Movement and Protection 143
Systems for Providing Energy and Removing Waste 155
Systems for Sensing, Coordinating, and Controlling 169
Systems for Producing New Life 182

Chapter 8
Growth and Development 189
Knowing Your Patient 190
Life Stages 191
Prenatal 192
Infancy 194
Toddler 194
Preschooler 195
School-Age Child 195
Adolescence 196
Young Adulthood 196
Middle Adulthood 197
Later Adulthood 197

Care Considerations 198
Other Developmental Theories 200
Jean Piaget 200
Lawrence Kohlberg 201
Carol Gilligan 202
Future Trends 202
Death and Dying 203

Unit 4: Personal and Workplace Safety

Chapter 9
Body Mechanics 211
The Importance of Prevention 212
General Guidelines 212
Back Belts 216
Computers and Ergonomics 218
Use of a Mouse as Pointing Device 218
Visual Problems 220

Chapter 10
Infection Control 223
Importance of Infection Control in Health Care 224
Microbiology 225
Types of Microbes 226
Chain of Infection 229
Scope of the Problem 230
Regulatory Agencies 231
Prevention Through Asepsis 231
Breaking the Chain of Infection 231
Standard Precautions 232
Transmission Precautions 242
Neutropenic Precautions 246
Antiseptics, Disinfectants, and Sterilization 247
Surgical Asepsis 247
The Risks 249
Hepatitis B 251
Human Immunodeficiency Virus 255
Tuberculosis 256
Other Infectious Organisms 258
Drug-Resistant Organisms 258
Reporting Accidental Exposure 263

Chapter 11
Environmental Safety 267
Importance of Environmental Safety in Health Care 268
General Safety Guidelines 268
Moving Safely 268
Dressing for Safety 268
Working Safely with Patients 269
Protecting Yourself and Others 271
Reporting for Safety 271
Workplace Violence 272
Fire and Electrical Hazards 273
Chemical Hazards 277
Radiation Hazards 278
Infectious Waste 278
Oxygen Hazards 278
Bioterrorism 279
Emergency Code System 279
Emergency Preparedness Plan 280
Triage 281

Unit 5: Behaviors for Success

Chapter 12
Lifestyle Management 285
Importance of a Healthy Lifestyle 286
Habits and Health 286
Diet and Nutrition 287
Types of Diets 289
Food Labels 290
Organic Foods 291
Improving Eating Habits 291
Maintaining a Normal Weight 292
Eating Disorders 294
Physical Activity 294
Sleep 295
Preventive Measures 295
Stress in Modern Life 296
External and Internal Stressors 297
Dealing with Stress 297
Minimizing Health Risks 301
Smoking 301

Substance Abuse 301
Occupational Hazards 302
Safe Sex 302
Burnout 303
Helping Patients Develop Healthy Lifestyles 304

Chapter 13
Professionalism 307
The Meaning of Professionalism 308
Professional Attitude 308
Professional Behaviors 309
Professional Health Care Skills 309
Professional Appearance 310
Professional Distance 311
Handling Difficult Situations Professionally 311
Professional Acceptance of Criticism 311
Professional Organizations 312
Professional Leadership 313

Chapter 14
Lifelong Learning 315
Importance of Lifelong Learning 316
Keeping Up with Changes in Health Care 316
Continuing Education Units 318
Ways to Earn CEUs 318
Self-Directed Learning 319

Unit 6: Communication in the Health Care Setting

Chapter 15
The Patient as an Individual 325
Patients as Individuals 326
Philosophy of Individual Worth 326
Dealing with Prejudice 327
The Meaning of Culture 327
Individuals and Culture 327
Dominant Culture 329
Health Care Beliefs 332
Religious Beliefs and Health 333
Harmony and Health 333
Herbs and Plant Medicines 334
Maslow's Hierarchy of Human Needs 335
Patient Needs 336
Physiological Needs 337
Safety and Security Needs 337
Love and Affection Needs 337
Self-Esteem Needs 338
Self-Actualization Needs 338
Defense Mechanisms 339
Dealing with Loss 339
Determining Individual Needs 341

Chapter 16
The Communication Process 345
Importance of Communication in Health Care 346
Communication and Patient Well-Being 347
The Communication Process 347
The Six Steps of the Communication Process 348
Overcoming Communication Barriers 356
Patients Who Are Terminally Ill 356
Patients Who Are in Pain, Medicated, Confused, or Disoriented 357
Patients with Alzheimer's Disease 358
Patients Who Are Depressed 358
Patients Who Are Anxious 358
Patients Who Have Hearing Impairments 358
Patients Who Have Visual Impairments 359
Patients Who Have Speech Impairments 360
Patients Who Are Angry 360
Patients Who Do Not Speak English 361
Special Applications of Communication Skills 361
Telephone Communication 361
Patient Education 362
Presentations to Groups 363
Gossip and Patient Privacy 364

Chapter 17
Written Communication 367
Written Communication: A Vital Link in Health Care 368
The Components of Good Writing 369
Organizing Content 369
Spell Your Way to Success 371
Grammar at a Glance 374
Business Letters 376
Using Form Letters 377
Writing Effective Letters 377
Business Letter Formats 377
Preparing Letters for Mailing 377
Memos 377
Meeting Agendas 382
Minutes of Meetings 383
Patient Education Materials 383
Confidentiality of Written Materials 384
Proofreading Written Work 384

Chapter 18
Computers and Technology in Health Care 387
Computers in Health Care 388
Information Management 389
Electronic Health Records 391
Creation of Documents 394
Spreadsheets 394
Diagnostics 396
Treatment 398
Patient Monitoring 400
Research 401
Education 401
Communication 402
Telemedicine 405
Telepharmacies 405
Virtual Communities 406
Computer Basics 406
Computer Hardware 406
Storing Information 407
Computer Software 407
Using Computers Effectively 408
Computer Security 409
Maintaining the Human Touch 409
Learning More about Computers 410

Chapter 19
Documentation and Medical Records 413
HIPAA 414
Medical Documentation 415
Purposes of Medical Documentation 415
Characteristics of Good Medical Documentation 416
Making Corrections on Medical Documentation 417
Contents of the Medical Record 418
Progress Notes 419
Electronic Health Records 421
Personal Health Record 422

Unit 7: Health Care Skills
Chapter 20
Physical Assessment 427
General Assessment 428
Noting Variances from Normal 429
General Survey 429
Psychosocial Observations 430
Physical Observations 430
Pain Evaluation 433
ADL Evaluation 433
Vital Signs 434
Temperature 434
Pulse 438
Respirations 443
Blood Pressure 444
Height and Weight 449

Chapter 21
Emergency Procedures 455
Emergency Situations 456
When an Emergency Occurs 457
Cardiopulmonary Resuscitation (CPR) 458

First Aid Procedures 458
Allergic Reactions 459
Bleeding and Wounds 461
Bone, Joint, and Muscle Injuries 462
Injuries to Facial Structures 470
Burns 470
Drug Abuse 476
Poisoning 476
Temperature-Related Illness 477
Other Conditions 481
Bandaging 481

Unit 8: Business of Caring

Chapter 22
Controlling Health Care Costs 499
The Rising Costs of Health Care 500
Health Care Institutions 500
History of Health Care Reimbursement 500
Health Care Payment Methods 501
Government Programs 501
Government Involvement in Health Care 502
Managed Care 502
Prepaid Plans 503
Negotiated Fees 503
Primary Care Providers 503
Review of Services 503
National Health Care Coverage 504
Controlling Organizational Costs 505
Health Care Professionals' Impact on Costs 506
Personal Efficiency 507
Acting with Thought 508

Chapter 23
Performance Improvement and Customer Service 511
Quality of Care 512
Approaches to Measuring Quality of Care 512
Quality Improvement 513
Internal Monitoring 513
Customer Service 515
Taking Responsibility for Quality 517
Customer Satisfaction 517
Internal Customers 518

Unit 9: Securing and Maintaining Employment

Chapter 24
Job Leads and the Resume 525
Overview of the Job Search 526
What Do You Have to Offer? 526
What Are Your Expectations? 527
Organizing Your Time 527
Organizing Your Space 528
Projecting a Professional Image 528
Finding Job Leads 528
Career Service Center 529
Community Career Centers 529
Networking 529
Clinical Experience 530
Cold Calls and Visits 531
Job Fairs and Orientations 531
Internet 531
Printed Ads for Job Openings 533
Telephone Joblines 533
The Resume 533
Resume Contents 533
Formatting the Resume 536
Important Resume Guidelines 536
Recent Resume Trends 539
Cover Letters 539
Writing Good Cover Letters 542

Chapter 25
Interview, Portfolio, and Application 545
The Job Interview 546
The Importance of Proper Preparation 546
Starting Off on the Right Foot 553
After the Interview 555
Accepting the Job 555
Declining the Job 557

Dealing with Rejection 557
Filling Out Applications 557

Chapter 26
Successful Employment Strategies 563
Getting Off to a Good Start 564
Learning about the Job 564
Policies and Procedures 564
Probationary Period 565
Guidelines for Workplace Success 566
Act with Integrity 566
Demonstrate Loyalty 566
Observe the Chain of Command 567
Give a Full Day's Work 567
Become Part of the Team 568
Go Beyond the Minimum 569
Learn from Role Models and Mentors 570
Employment Laws 570
Grievances 572
Sexual Harassment 572
Tracking Your Progress 572
Moving on 574
If You are Fired 574
Professional Development 576

Appendix 1
Health Care Professional Organizations 579
Therapeutic and Treating Occupations 579
Dental Occupations 579
Emergency Medical Occupations 579
Home-Care and Long-Term Care Occupations 579
Massage Therapy Occupations 579
Medical Office Occupations 579
Mental Health Occupations 580
Nursing Occupations 580
Occupational Therapy Occupations 580
Pharmacy Occupations 580
Physical Therapy Occupations 580
Respiratory Therapy Occupations 580
Surgical Occupations 581
Veterinary Occupations 581
Vision Care Occupations 581
Diagnostic Occupations 581
Diagnostic Imaging Occupations 581
Medical Laboratory Occupations 582
Health Information Management Occupations 582
Environmental Occupations 582
Dietary Services Occupations 582
Biomedical Engineering Occupations 582

Appendix 2
Useful Spanish Expressions for Health Care Professionals 583

Glossary 585

References 597

Index 603

PREFACE

Introduction to Health Care, Fourth Edition, is designed as an introductory text for learners who are entering college-level health care programs or for those who believe they may be interested in pursuing a career in health care. The fundamentals common to all health care professions are presented in this full-color text to create a foundation on which learners can build when they take their specific professional courses. The topics included are appropriate for professions that involve direct patient care, such as nursing and dental assisting, as well as those that provide support services, such as health information technology and pharmacy technician. The goal of the text is to present a broad base of health care essentials. Therefore, skills and procedures that apply only to specific professions are not included.

The text is written in easy-to-understand language. A variety of learning exercises are included in each chapter. These exercises are designed to appeal to the different ways that learners comprehend material, including visual, auditory, and kinesthetic. The text can be used by learners as a reference book after completion of their introductory courses.

Content for Today's Health Care Professional

Introduction to Health Care, Fourth Edition, includes topics essential for today's learner and tomorrow's health care professional. The basic concepts that create the foundation for health care education have been expanded beyond those usually included in an introductory text. The following topics have been included in response to the current needs of health care educators and employers.

- Thinking skills
- Learning styles and study techniques
- Complementary and alternative medicine
- Prevention and wellness strategies
- Lifelong learning and continuing education
- Documentation
- Cost-control measures
- Performance improvement
- Personal efficiency
- Customer service

Emphasis on Thinking Skills

The dramatic growth of the health care industry promises to provide increasing numbers of employment opportunities for graduates of health care programs. At the same time, today's graduates face new challenges. Changes in health care are rapid and continuous. Professionals at all levels are being given additional responsibilities. Efficiency and flexibility, combined with competency, are vital to workplace success. To be competent and successful in this ever-changing environment, health care professionals must be able to think for themselves and learn and adapt as necessary to meet current employment demands.

The authors recognize the need of health care educators for materials that can assist them in preparing students to assess new situations, determine appropriate action, and apply on the job what they learned in the classroom. This text is designed to help meet this need. Learners are introduced to the concept of thinking like a health care professional in Chapter 1. The specific skills that make up applied thinking are explained in everyday language. A five-step problem-solving model is clearly described to help learners systematically approach new situations. Every chapter includes exercises called "Thinking It Through" that require learners to apply the concepts presented in the text to typical on-the-job scenarios. Each chapter then concludes with two application exercises and one problem-solving exercise that provide opportunities to summarize and apply the chapter content. For a detailed review of the features in this book, see *About This Book* on page xxi.

Organization of the Text

Introduction to Health Care, Fourth Edition, is divided into nine units that contain between two and five chapters of related topics. The following overview highlights many of the major concepts included in the text.

Unit 1: Health Care Today

- Characteristics and trends of modern health care, including changing patient demographics and complementary and alternative medicine
- Descriptions of many health occupations, organized by type of work performed
- Explanation of how to think like a health care professional
- Legal and ethical responsibilities required of all health care professionals

Unit 2: The Language of Health Care

- Introduction to basic concepts of medical terminology
- Examples of common word elements
- Suggested ways to approach the study of terminology and to learn it systematically
- Review of math skills necessary for health care applications
- Tips for dealing with math anxiety

Unit 3: The Human Body

- Brief overview of the basic organization, structure, and functions of the body systems, intended as an introduction rather than a complete anatomy and physiology course
- Examples of diseases and conditions related to each body system
- Preventive measures for each system, including lifestyle management tips
- Physical and mental milestones of growth and development over the life span and the implications when providing health care

Unit 4: Personal and Workplace Safety

- Basic skills and habits needed to protect both health care professionals and patients
- Explanations of body mechanics and infection control
- Hands-on skills, such as using a fire extinguisher

Unit 5: Behaviors for Success

- Self-care practices important for health care professionals, including dealing with stress
- Characteristics of professionalism essential for career success
- Lifelong learning and continuing education strategies

Unit 6: Communication in the Health Care Setting

- Patients as individuals
- Basic human needs
- Acknowledging diversity while avoiding cultural stereotypes
- Using questions and observations to assess specific patient needs
- Basic oral and written communication techniques
- Overview of computer applications in health care
- Basics of health care documentation and medical records

Unit 7: Health Care Skills

- Basic assessment skills
- Hands-on skills, such as taking vital signs and measuring height and weight
- Normal ranges and significant changes
- Step-by-step instructions for performing basic emergency procedures (Cardiopulmonary resuscitation is not included because certification is often required of health care learners and the course is taught by certified instructors who use annually updated, written materials instead of a textbook.)

Unit 8: Business of Caring

- Health care as a business
- Improving care while controlling costs
- Working efficiently
- Customer service

Unit 9: Securing and Maintaining Employment

- Application of job search skills to health care employment
- Tips for remaining successfully employed
- Behaviors for job success, including teamwork and leadership skills
- Employment legalities

Major Changes to the Fourth Edition

Book Chapter	Description of Changes
Frontmatter	• Added "Infection Control Content at a Glance" for easy reference • Added a list of vital signs procedures to assist learners in locating this material quickly • Added a list of first aid procedures as an easy reference for students
Chapter 1	• Information updated for all careers: education, credentialing, state licensing requirements, job growth projections, etc. • All health care industry facts and figures updated • Added table listing occupations with largest numerical increases • Revised explanation of career categories and how they overlap • Added list of health care–related occupations such as art therapist and medical librarian • Added material on patient care technician and home health aide occupations • Reordered material in "Getting Off to a Good Start" section to be more logical • Moved "Learning to Think Like a Health Care Professional" to the end of the chapter for better order; narrative now presents information about being a student, followed by information about being a health care professional, and ending with problem solving, which is a theme woven throughout the text

Chapter 2	• Updated health care industry statistics
	• Expanded list of advancements in medicine and health care
	• Added information about incidence and the effects of Alzheimer's and other forms of dementia on costs of providing health care; effects on families and society
	• Chronic diseases and conditions and their effects
	  ○ Obesity
	  ○ Type 2 diabetes
	• Increase in use of pharmaceuticals and their costs
	  ○ Advertising of pharmaceuticals to the public: pros and cons
	• Patient Protection and Affordable Care Act (explained more fully in Chapter 22)
	• Challenges
	  ○ Access to health care in terms of number of providers and facilities
	  ○ Patients learning to use the health care system
	• Expanded on social conditions that affect health care
	• Public health concerns:
	  ○ Antivaccine movement and current incidence of measles
	  ○ Globalization
	  ○ Ebola, other
	  ○ Food safety

Chapter 3	• Updated to reflect changes in the law • Revised examples of ethical issues based on current issues
Chapter 5	• Added section on medication safety as reported by the Institute for Safe Medication Practices
Chapter 7	• Moved Table 7–1 (Organ Systems of the Body) toward front of chapter for easier referral by students
Chapter 8	• Added developmental theories by Piaget, Kohlberg, and Gilligan
Chapter 9	• Added ergonomics of using a mobile and adjustable computer station
Chapter 10	• All infectious diseases updated and Ebola virus added • Drug-resistant infections expanded to include *Clostridium difficile (C. difficile).*

(continued)

Book Chapter	Description of Changes
Chapter 11	• Updated information on emergency preparedness plans • Added information and a sample of an emergency code system as a way health care facilities might communicate with staff without distressing patients and visitors
Chapter 12	• Updated statistics for: ○ Leading causes of death in the United States ○ Prevalence of overweight and obesity ○ Deaths due to smoking and secondhand smoke ○ Incidence and deaths from substance abuse ○ Cases of HIV • Added information about the link between eating habits and health • Added material on processed foods and their contents (sodium, trans fats, etc.) • Updated USDA guidelines: Choose My Plate • Added explanations of confusing terms: organic, free-range, hormone-free, etc. • Expanded information and included example on calculating BMI • Added explanation of maximum heart rate during exercise • Added flu vaccine recommendation • Added list of conditions that may be helped by practicing meditation • Expanded information about abuse of prescription drugs • Added list of common STDs
Chapter 13	• Under section on appearance, added item: avoid long, painted fingernails
Chapter 14	• Added items to Table 14–1 (Changes that Affect Health Care): ○ Increase in incidence of Alzheimer's disease ○ Mandatory electronic records ○ Increase of drug-resistant bacteria ○ Implementation of Patient Protection and Affordable Care Act • Updated examples of how to earn CEUs
Chapter 15	• Updated population statistics • Corrected information on Native Americans (i.e., text now refers to medicine men and women, not shamans) • Added levels to Maslow's hierarchy per his revisions of original work • Expanded the section "Determining Individual Needs" and moved it to end of chapter to pull together all the aspects that make up the individual
Chapter 16	• Added examples of communication encounters
Chapter 17	• Reorganized punctuation and grammar rules into table form to improve readability • Added material on writing emails and email etiquette
Chapter 18	• Updated information and examples on use of technology in health care • Updated and expanded information on electronic health records (government requirements, security, etc.)
Chapter 19	• Expanded information about electronic health records (EHR), personal health records (PHR), and HIPAA (Health Insurance Portability and Accountability Act of 1996)
Chapter 20	• Clarification added, noting the distinction made in using *assessment* versus *observation* and *data collection*

(continued)

Book Chapter	Description of Changes
Chapter 22	• Added factors that are causing increased health care costs, types of funding for health care institutions, and types of payment methods • Added section on national health care coverage and passage of Patient Protection and Affordable Care Act (PPACA) in 2010, commonly called the Affordable Care Act (ACA) or "Obamacare"
Chapter 23	• Expanded approaches to measuring quality of care • Added section on "Taking Responsibility for Quality" by serving as an advocate
Chapter 24	• Expanded information on using the Internet in the job search • Added recommendation to avoid a career objective as first item in the resumé; instead, job seekers should state what they have to offer an employer
Chapter 25	• Increased emphasis on sending thank-you note after an interview (based on survey indicating one in five managers won't hire a candidate who fails to send a thank-you note) • Added recent trends in interviewing: ○ Group ○ Video ○ Peculiar questions ○ Psychometric tests
All chapters	• Added a Media Link feature that directs learners to animations and videos on the Student Companion website

Student Resources

Workbook

The workbook was created to provide additional practice in learning the material in the text, including review questions, vocabulary review, image labeling, critical thinking scenarios, and skill assessment checklists. (ISBN: 978-1-3055-7495-3).

Online Resources

Online resources are available to enhance the learning experience. Additional resources include:

- PowerPoint® presentations
- Anatomy and pathology animations
- Health care–related videos
- Mathematics tutorials

Redeeming an Access Code:

1. Go to: http://www.CengageBrain.com
2. Register as a new user or log in as an existing user if you already have an account with Cengage Learning or CengageBrain.com
3. Select **Go to My Account**
4. Open the product from the My Account page

Animations and Videos included on the Online Resources

Chapter	Animation Topic
4	Word Parts Work Together
4	Combining Word Roots
6	Anatomy of a Typical Cell
6	Body Planes
7	Shoulder Injuries
7	Skin
7	The Heart
7	The Blood
7	Lymphatic System
7	Respiration
7	Digestion
7	Urine Formation
7	Vision
7	Hearing
7	Endocrine System
7	Female Reproductive System
7	Male Reproductive System
10	Infection Control

Chapter	Video Topic
9	Body Mechanics
10	Pathogens
10	Sterile Gloves and the Sterile Field
11	Fire Safety
20	Thermometers (Chemical-dot)
20	Digital/Electronic Thermometers
20	Tympanic Thermometers
20	TPR and BP
20	Radial Pulse
20	Apical Pulse
20	Respiration
20	Blood Pressure
20	Taking a Patient's Blood Pressure

Math Tutorials for Chapter 5
Convert between Traditional and International Time
Convert between Celsius and Fahrenheit Temperature
Approximate Equivalents
The Metric System
The Apothecary System
The Household System
Ratios
Converting among Fractions, Decimals, Ratios, and Percents
Comparing the Size of Fractions, Decimals, Ratios and Percents
Calculate the Percentage of a Quantity
Reading and Writing Decimals
Fractions and Decimals
Converting between Fraction Types
Calculations with Fractions
Comparing the Values of Fractions and Decimals
Calculations with Decimals
Rounding of Decimals

Instructor Resources

Resources for instructors include:

- Cognero® Testbank makes generating tests and quizzes a snap. You can create customized assessments for your students with the click of a button. Add your own unique questions and print tests for easy class preparation.
- Customizable instructor slide presentations created in PowerPoint® focus on key concepts from each chapter.
- Electronic Instructor's Manual includes the following items to help instructors most effectively use the text in planning and teaching an introductory course:
  - Suggested answers to "Thinking It Through" and "Application Exercises" found in the text
  - Procedure check-off forms for evaluating skills
  - Suggestions for class activities
  - Teaching thinking skills
  - Answers to review questions found at the end of each chapter in the text
  - Answers to workbook exercises

MindTap

MindTap is a fully online, interactive learning experience built upon authoritative Cengage Learning content. By combining readings, multimedia, activities, and assessments into a singular learning path, MindTap elevates learning by providing real-world application to better engage students. Instructors customize the learning path by selecting Cengage Learning resources and adding their own content via apps that integrate into the MindTap framework seamlessly with many learning management systems.

The guided learning path demonstrates the relevance of fundamental topics common to all health care professions through engagement activities and interactive exercises. Learners apply an understanding of these fundamental topics through scenarios. These simulations elevate the study of fundamentals by challenging students to apply concepts to practice.

To learn more, visit www.cengage.com/mindtap

Infection Control Content at a Glance

Topic	Content Summary	Page Number(s)
Microbiology	General theory and terminology of microbiology, types of microbes, chain of infection, scope of the problem, and regulatory agencies.	219–225
Prevention through Asepsis	Discusses how to break the chain of infection by using standard, transmission, and neutropenic precautions. Methods of inhibiting or destroying microorganisms and surgical asepsis are introduced.	225–241
Procedures:		
10–1 Handwashing	These procedures show step-out directions and rationales with accompanying figures to illustrate the steps.	228–229
10–2 Nonsterile Gloves		231
10–3 Applying and Removing PPE		232–233
10–4 Sterile Gloves		241–242
The Risks	The most common contagions that health care professionals may encounter.	244–256
Reporting Accidental Exposure	OSHA regulations that apply to all health care facilities.	256

List of Vital Signs Procedures

Procedure Number	Procedure	Purpose	Page Number(s)
20–1	Temperature	Measures how much heat is in the body. An elevation may indicate that an infection or other disease process is present	420
20–2	Radial Pulse	Measures how fast the heart is beating when felt at the wrist	426–427
20–3	Apical Pulse	Measures how fast the heart is beating by listening over the heart with a stethoscope	428
20–4	Respirations	Measures how fast the patient is breathing	430
20–5	Blood Pressure	Indicates how hard the heart is working to distribute blood to all parts of the body	433–434

List of First Aid Procedures

Procedure Number	First Aid Procedure	Page Number(s)
21–1	Allergic Reactions	447–448
21–2	Bleeding and Wounds	449–452
21–3	Bone, Joint, and Muscle Injuries	454–455
21–4	Facial Injuries	456–458
21–5	Burns	460–461

(continued)

Procedure Number	First Aid Procedure	Page Number(s)
21–6	Drug-Related Problems	462–463
21–7	Poisonings	464
21–8	Temperature-Related Illnesses	465–466
21–9	Other Common Conditions	467–473
21–10	Applying a Triangular Sling	474
21–11	Applying a Spiral Wrap	475
21–12	Applying a Figure-Eight Wrap	476–477
21–13	Applying Bandage to a Finger	478

DEDICATION

To the future health care professionals who will dedicate their time and energy to taking care of those in need of their services. May your career be as rewarding to you as mine is to me.

—Dakota Mitchell

To David, for providing daily inspiration and continual encouragement.

—Lee Haroun

ABOUT THE AUTHORS

Dakota Mitchell has a Master's of Science degree in Nursing from the University of California, San Francisco, and a Master's in Business Administration degree from the University of Santa Clara. The combination of the two degrees provides a framework for understanding and functioning within the current and rapidly evolving world of health care today.

Dakota has 30-plus years of experience in health care, including education, management, and curriculum consultation. Besides many years in classroom and clinical teaching, she has developed and implemented unique and innovative health care programs at both the vocational and associate's degree levels.

Lee Haroun has a Master's of Art in Education from Portland State University (Oregon), a Master's in Business Administration from National University in San Diego, and a Doctorate of Education from the University of San Diego.

She has more than 35 years' experience in teaching and educational administration and has developed curricula for a variety of postsecondary programs, including occupational therapy assistant, health information professional, insurance coder, and patient care technician.

Lee is the author of *Career Development for Health Professionals* (Elsevier Science); co-author of *Teaching Ideas and Classroom Activities for Health Care* with Susan Royce (Cengage Learning); co-author of *Occupational Therapy Fieldwork Survival Guide* with Bonnie Napier-Tibere (F. A. Davis; out of print); and technical writer for *Essentials of Health and Wellness* by James Robinson and Deborah McCormick (Cengage Learning).

ACKNOWLEDGMENTS

The authors wish to acknowledge the help, support, and continual good humor of Laura Stewart, Managing Editor, and Deb Myette-Flis, Senior Product Manager, at Cengage Learning who patiently shepherded us through the process of producing a fourth edition. A special thank you to all the reviewers who offered many wonderful suggestions.

Patricia Fennessy, RN, MSN
Education Consultant
Connecticut Technical High Schools

Patricia F. Lassiter, PhD
Professor, Health Sciences and Related Studies

Daniel Lovasz, RN, MSN, DHA
Assistant Professor, Nursing
Charleston Southern University

Alice Macomber, RN, RMA, RPT, AHI, LXMO, CPI
Medical Assisting Instructor
Keiser University

Mark Schubert, RT(R), CI
Adjunct Faculty of Health Professions
Tidewater Community College

Alana Waters, MSN, RN
Health Sciences Faculty

ABOUT THIS BOOK

Objectives: Overview of chapter content and goals for learning. Review these before beginning to read the chapter and use the objectives to check your progress after completing the chapter.

Key Terms: List of important vocabulary and key concepts. Understanding vocabulary is critical to understanding the concepts presented in the chapter. Key terms are bolded and defined the first time they appear in the chapter. There is also a comprehensive glossary in the back of the book.

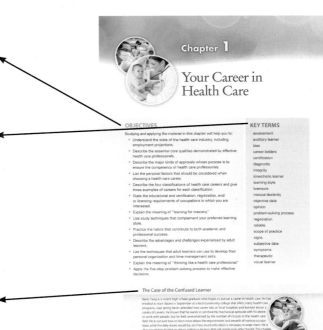

Chapter 1

Your Career in Health Care

OBJECTIVES

Studying and applying the material in this chapter will help you to:

- Understand the state of the health care industry, including employment projections.
- Describe the essential core qualities demonstrated by effective health care professionals.
- Describe the major kinds of approvals whose purpose is to ensure the competency of health care professionals.
- List the personal factors that should be considered when choosing a health care career.
- Describe the four classifications of health care careers and give three examples of careers for each classification.
- State the educational and certification, registration, and/or licensing requirements of occupations in which you are interested.
- Explain the meaning of "learning for mastery."
- Use study techniques that complement your preferred learning style.
- Practice the habits that contribute to both academic and professional success.
- Describe the advantages and challenges experienced by adult learners.
- List the techniques that adult learners can use to develop their personal organization and time management skills.
- Explain the meaning of "thinking like a health care professional."
- Apply the five-step problem-solving process to make effective decisions.

KEY TERMS

assessment
auditory learner
bias
career ladders
certification
diagnostic
integrity
kinesthetic learner
learning style
licensure
manual dexterity
objective data
opinion
problem-solving process
registration
reliable
scope of practice
signs
subjective data
symptoms
therapeutic
visual learner

The Case of...: These health care scenarios introduce chapter content and show why the material in the chapter is important for the competent health care professional. An application exercise at the end of the chapter refers back to the case.

The Case of the Confused Learner

Kevin Yang is a recent high school graduate who hopes to pursue a career in health care. He has enrolled to start classes in September at a local community college that offers many health care programs. Last spring Kevin attended two career fairs at local hospitals and learned about a variety of careers. He knows that he wants to combine his mechanical aptitude with his desire to work with people, but he feels overwhelmed by the number of choices in the health care field. He is not sure how to learn more about the requirements and rewards of various occupations, what the daily duties would be, and how much education is necessary to enter them. He is also unsure how to best go about making a decision that will significantly affect his life. This chapter includes basic information about a variety of health career areas and occupations, a problem-solving process that can be used to make effective personal and professional decisions, and tips on succeeding in a health career program.

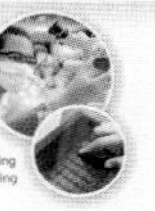

Fascinating Facts: Interesting information that is related to the chapter topics.

Fascinating Facts

In 2009, there were 39.6 million persons aged 65 and over, representing 12.9% of the total population. By 2030, this number will have grown to 72.1 million persons, who will make up 19% of the population.

Source: U.S. Department of Health & Human Services, Administration on Community Living, www.aoa.gov/AoARoot/Aging_Statistics/index.aspx

Tables: These provide summaries of related facts. Use them as study aids and for quick reference.

Table 1-17 Medical Laboratory Occupations

Career	Education	Testing and Licensure
Pathologist (MD)	4 years college preprofessional education 4 years medical school 4 years of graduate medical education (residency); 1 or 2 more years required for specialties	Licensed by states: 1. Graduate from accredited medical school 2. Complete specialized studies, internship, and residency 3. Pass written exam
Medical Laboratory Technologist (MT)	Bachelor's or master's degree	Licensed or registered in some states Certification available from: 1. American Medical Technologists 2. Board of Registry of the American Society for Clinical Pathology 3. Board of Registry of the American Association of Bioanalysts
Medical Laboratory Technician	Completion of certificate program or associate degree	Licensing or registration required in some states Certification available from: 1. American Medical Technologists 2. Board of Certification of the American Society for Clinical Pathology
Medical Laboratory Assistant	1- to 2-year training program or specific work experience	Voluntary certification from American Medical Technologists Association
Phlebotomist	On-the-job training or formal training program	Licensure required in California and Louisiana Certification is required by most employers and is available from: 1. National Phlebotomy Association 2. American Society for Clinical Pathology 3. Association of Phlebotomy Technicians 4. Several other organizations also test and certify phlebotomists

Boxes: These include special features and additional information that expand on and support the material presented in the chapter.

BOX 3–2

Code of Ethics

The Code of Ethics of the American Association of Medical Assistants (AAMA) shall set forth principles of ethical and moral conduct as they relate to the medical profession and the particular practice of medical assisting.

Members of AAMA dedicated to the conscientious pursuit of their profession, and thus desiring to merit the high regard of the entire medical profession and the respect of the general public which they serve, do pledge themselves to strive always to:

A. render service with full respect for the dignity of humanity;
B. respect confidential information obtained through employment unless legally authorized or required by responsible performance of duty to divulge such information;
C. uphold the honor and high principles of the profession and accept its disciplines;
D. seek to continually improve the knowledge and skills of medical assistants for the benefit of patients and professional colleagues;
E. participate in additional service activities aimed toward improving the health and well-being of the community.

Source: Reprinted with permission of the American Association of Medical Assistants, Inc.

Colored photos and illustrations: These reinforce important concepts and topics. Use them to increase your understanding of the material.

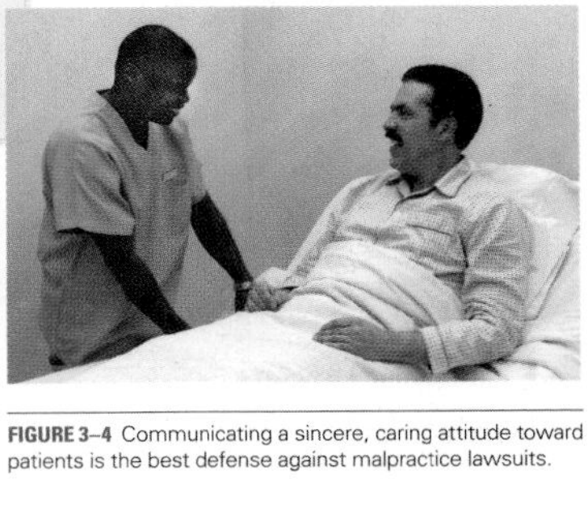

FIGURE 3–4 Communicating a sincere, caring attitude toward patients is the best defense against malpractice lawsuits.

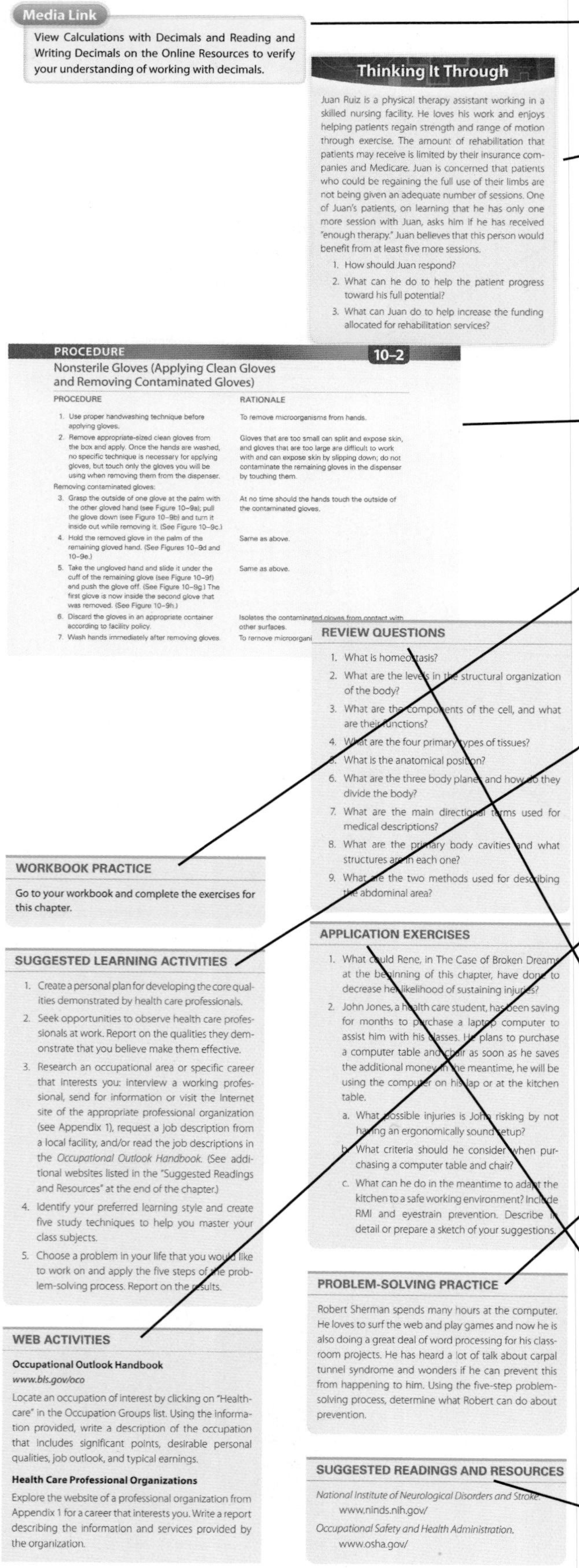
Media Link
View Calculations with Decimals and Reading and Writing Decimals on the Online Resources to verify your understanding of working with decimals.
Thinking It Through
Juan Ruiz is a physical therapy assistant working in a skilled nursing facility. He loves his work and enjoys helping patients regain strength and range of motion through exercise. The amount of rehabilitation that patients may receive is limited by their insurance companies and Medicare. Juan is concerned that patients who could be regaining the full use of their limbs are not being given an adequate number of sessions. One of Juan's patients, on learning that he has only one more session with Juan, asks him if he has received "enough therapy." Juan believes that this person would benefit from at least five more sessions.
1. How should Juan respond?
2. What can he do to help the patient progress toward his full potential?
3. What can Juan do to help increase the funding allocated for rehabilitation services?
PROCEDURE 10–2
Nonsterile Gloves (Applying Clean Gloves and Removing Contaminated Gloves)
PROCEDURE
RATIONALE
1. Use proper handwashing technique before applying gloves.
To remove microorganisms from hands.
2. Remove appropriate-sized clean gloves from the box and apply. Once the hands are washed, no specific technique is necessary for applying gloves, but touch only the gloves you will be using when removing them from the dispenser.
Gloves that are too small can split and expose skin, and gloves that are too large are difficult to work with and can expose skin by slipping down; do not contaminate the remaining gloves in the dispenser by touching them.
Removing contaminated gloves:
3. Grasp the outside of one glove at the palm with the other gloved hand (see Figure 10–9a); pull the glove down (see Figure 10–9b) and turn it inside out while removing it. (See Figure 10–9c.)
At no time should the hands touch the outside of the contaminated gloves.
4. Hold the removed glove in the palm of the remaining gloved hand. (See Figures 10–9d and 10–9e.)
Same as above.
5. Take the ungloved hand and slide it under the cuff of the remaining glove (see Figure 10–9f) and push the glove off. (See Figure 10–9g.) The first glove is now inside the second glove that was removed. (See Figure 10–9h.)
Same as above.
6. Discard the gloves in an appropriate container according to facility policy.
Isolates the contaminated gloves from contact with other surfaces.
7. Wash hands immediately after removing gloves.
To remove microorgani
REVIEW QUESTIONS
1. What is homeostasis?
2. What are the levels in the structural organization of the body?
3. What are the components of the cell, and what are their functions?
4. What are the four primary types of tissues?
5. What is the anatomical position?
6. What are the three body planes and how do they divide the body?
7. What are the main directional terms used for medical descriptions?
8. What are the primary body cavities and what structures are in each one?
9. What are the two methods used for describing the abdominal area?
WORKBOOK PRACTICE
Go to your workbook and complete the exercises for this chapter.
APPLICATION EXERCISES
1. What could Rene, in The Case of Broken Dreams at the beginning of this chapter, have done to decrease her likelihood of sustaining injuries?
2. John Jones, a health care student, has been saving for months to purchase a laptop computer to assist him with his classes. He plans to purchase a computer table and chair as soon as he saves the additional money. In the meantime, he will be using the computer on his lap or at the kitchen table.
a. What possible injuries is John risking by not having an ergonomically sound setup?
b. What criteria should he consider when purchasing a computer table and chair?
c. What can he do in the meantime to adapt the kitchen to a safe working environment? Include RMI and eyestrain prevention. Describe in detail or prepare a sketch of your suggestions.
SUGGESTED LEARNING ACTIVITIES
1. Create a personal plan for developing the core qualities demonstrated by health care professionals.
2. Seek opportunities to observe health care professionals at work. Report on the qualities they demonstrate that you believe make them effective.
3. Research an occupational area or specific career that interests you: interview a working professional, send for information or visit the Internet site of the appropriate professional organization (see Appendix 1), request a job description from a local facility, and/or read the job descriptions in the Occupational Outlook Handbook. (See additional websites listed in the "Suggested Readings and Resources" at the end of the chapter.)
4. Identify your preferred learning style and create five study techniques to help you master your class subjects.
5. Choose a problem in your life that you would like to work on and apply the five steps of the problem-solving process. Report on the results.
PROBLEM-SOLVING PRACTICE
Robert Sherman spends many hours at the computer. He loves to surf the web and play games and now he is also doing a great deal of word processing for his classroom projects. He has heard a lot of talk about carpal tunnel syndrome and wonders if he can prevent this from happening to him. Using the five-step problem-solving process, determine what Robert can do about prevention.
WEB ACTIVITIES
Occupational Outlook Handbook
www.bls.gov/oco
Locate an occupation of interest by clicking on "Healthcare" in the Occupation Groups list. Using the information provided, write a description of the occupation that includes significant points, desirable personal qualities, job outlook, and typical earnings.
Health Care Professional Organizations
Explore the website of a professional organization from Appendix 1 for a career that interests you. Write a report describing the information and services provided by the organization.
SUGGESTED READINGS AND RESOURCES
National Institute of Neurological Disorders and Stroke.
www.ninds.nih.gov/
Occupational Safety and Health Administration.
www.osha.gov/

Media Link: This feature directs the learner to numerous anatomy and pathology animations, and health-related videos on the Online Resources.

Thinking It Through: Located throughout the chapter, these exercises are a very important part of this text. The health care scenarios require you to think about the concepts presented in the chapter and use them to resolve typical problems encountered by health care professionals. Use the exercises to develop the thinking skills necessary to be a successful health care professional.

Procedures: A step-by-step format that helps you master basic hands-on skills. Pay special attention to the rationales that explain the reasons for the actions.

Workbook Practice: This feature directs the learner to even more learning tools in the workbook, including practice questions, image labeling, critical thinking scenarios, and skill assessment checklists.

Suggested Learning Activities: Try these interesting projects that include doing research on the Internet, reporting on observations from daily life, and visiting health care facilities.

Web Activities: Use these guided assignments to increase your research skills and learn more about the chapter content. Many of the activities refer you to specific websites.

Review Questions: The questions are keyed to the chapter objectives to ensure your mastery of the chapter content. Use them to check your learning and identify areas that need more study.

Problem-Solving Practice: Practice your skills with these typical, real-world problems encountered by learners and health care professionals.

Application Exercises: Opportunities to apply the chapter's major concepts to typical health care situations. Use these exercises to practice using your knowledge in ways similar to those you may encounter on the job.

Suggested Readings and Resources: Learn more about topics of interest from the books, articles, and websites listed in this section.

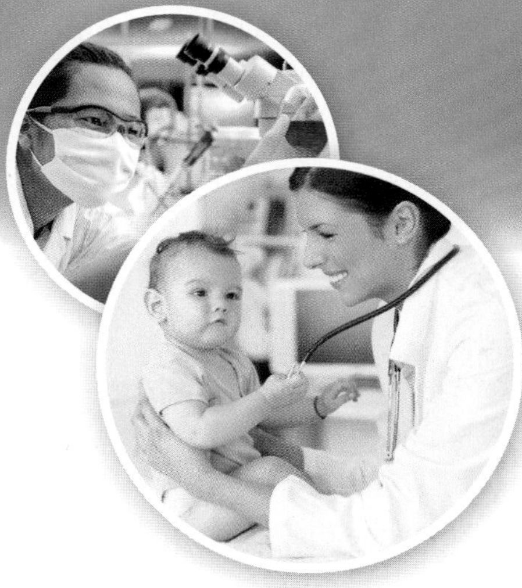

Unit 1

Health Care Today

This page intentionally left blank

Chapter 1

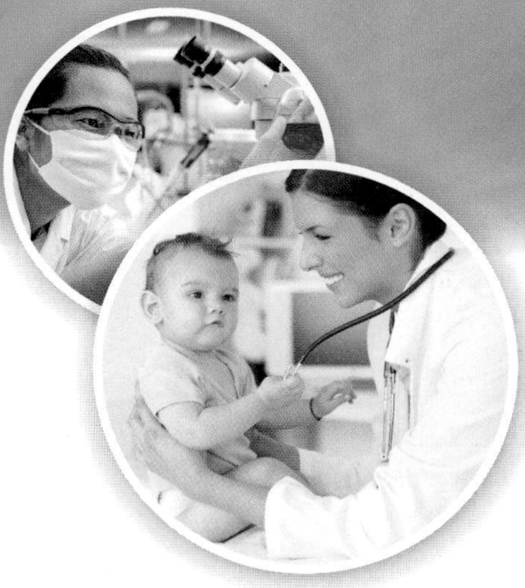

Your Career in Health Care

OBJECTIVES

Studying and applying the material in this chapter will help you to:

- Understand the state of the health care industry, including employment projections.
- Describe the essential core qualities demonstrated by effective health care professionals.
- Describe the major kinds of approvals whose purpose is to ensure the competency of health care professionals.
- List the personal factors that should be considered when choosing a health care career.
- Describe the four classifications of health care careers and give three examples of careers for each classification.
- State the educational and certification, registration, and/or licensing requirements of occupations in which you are interested.
- Explain the meaning of "learning for mastery."
- Use study techniques that complement your preferred learning style.
- Practice the habits that contribute to both academic and professional success.
- Describe the advantages and challenges experienced by adult learners.
- List the techniques that adult learners can use to develop their personal organization and time management skills.
- Explain the meaning of "thinking like a health care professional."
- Apply the five-step problem-solving process to make effective decisions.

KEY TERMS

assessment
auditory learner
bias
career ladders
certification
diagnostic
integrity
kinesthetic learner
learning style
licensure
manual dexterity
objective data
opinion
problem-solving process
registration
reliable
scope of practice
signs
subjective data
symptoms
therapeutic
visual learner

The Case of the Confused Learner

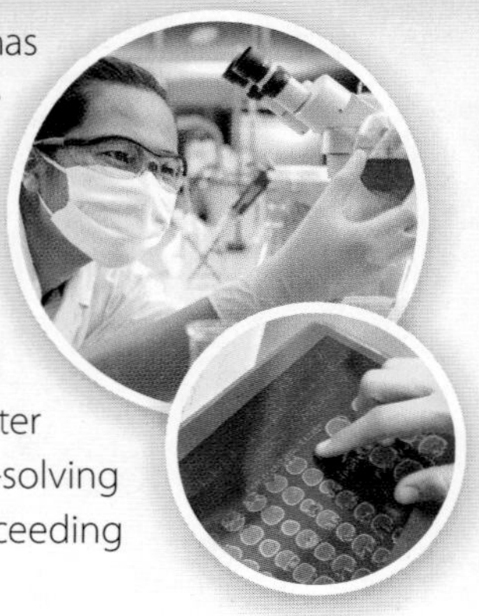

Kevin Yang is a recent high school graduate who hopes to pursue a career in health care. He has enrolled to start classes in September at a local community college that offers many health care programs. Last spring Kevin attended two career fairs at local hospitals and learned about a variety of careers. He knows that he wants to combine his mechanical aptitude with his desire to work with people, but he feels overwhelmed by the number of choices in the health care field. He is not sure how to learn more about the requirements and rewards of various occupations, what the daily duties would be, and how much education is necessary to enter them. He is also unsure how to best go about making a decision that will significantly affect his life. This chapter includes basic information about a variety of health career areas and occupations, a problem-solving process that can be used to make effective personal and professional decisions, and tips on succeeding in a health career program.

YOUR FUTURE IN HEALTH CARE

Health care services make up one of the largest industries in the United States, providing 14.3 million jobs in 2010 (Center for Health Workforce Studies, 2012). The need for health care professionals continues to grow. According to the Bureau of Labor Statistics, health care will generate 4.2 million new jobs in the 10-year period between 2010 and 2020. In fact, between 2010 and 2020, it is projected that employment in the health care industry will grow by more than 30%, more than two times that of the general economy. Currently, more than 13% of the U.S. labor force works in health care.

Many health care occupations are projected to have increases of over 30 percent. (See Table 1–1.) Ten of the 20 fastest growing jobs in all industries are health care–related. At the same time, four of the 20 occupations with the largest numerical increases are in health care: registered nurse; personal and home care aides; home health aides; nursing aides, orderlies, and attendants. (See Table 1–2.)

Careers in health care can be sources of great satisfaction. Health care professionals perform valuable services that make a significant contribution to the community. Each day their work makes a difference in the quality of life of those they serve. Whether you choose to work directly with patients or provide support services, be assured that what you do is important and of benefit to others.

As well as providing satisfaction, health care work makes many demands on those who pursue it. The work must be taken seriously because it affects the well-being of others. All tasks must be performed thoughtfully and conscientiously. Nothing can be taken for granted or done automatically, not even routine assignments. Health care professionals must be willing to devote their full attention to everything they say and do. Potential problems must be noted and addressed before they become critical. The consequences of mistakes can be devastating if, for

Table 1–1 Examples of Growing Health Care Jobs

Job	Projected Percentage Increase in Employment, 2010–2020
Home Health Aide	69%
Veterinary Technologists and Technicians	52%
Physical Therapist Assistant	46%
Physical Therapist Aide	43%
Occupational Therapy Assistant	43%
Dental Hygienist	38%
Dental Assistant	31%
Physician Assistant	27%
Surgical Technologist	24%

Source: Center for Health Workforce Studies. (2012). Health care employment projections: An analysis of Bureau of Labor statistics occupational projection, 2010–2020. *Available: www.healthit.gov/sites/default/files/chws_bls_report_2012.pdf*

Table 1–2 Occupations with the Largest Numerical Increases

Job	Numerical Increase in Positions, 2010–2020
Registered Nurses	712,000
Home Health Aides	706,000
Personal Care Aides	607,000
Nursing Aides, Orderlies, and Attendants	302,000
Medical Secretaries	210,000
Licensed Practical and Vocational Nurses	169,000
Physicians and Surgeons	168,000
Medical Assistants	163,000

Source: Center for Health Workforce Studies. (2012). Health care employment projections: An analysis of Bureau of Labor statistics occupational projection, 2010–2020. *Available: www.healthit.gov/sites/default/files/chws_bls_report_2012.pdf*

example, a prescription for medication is incorrect or the wrong procedure is performed.

Fascinating Facts

In 2009, there were 39.6 million persons aged 65 and over, representing 12.9% of the total population. By 2030, this number will have grown to 72.1 million persons, who will make up 19% of the population.

Source: U.S. Department of Health & Human Services, Administration on Community Living, www.aoa.gov/AoARoot/Aging_Statistics/index.aspx

Essential Qualities of Health Care Professionals

Although the specific duties performed in the many health care occupations vary, there are common core qualities required of everyone who works in health care. A learner whose goal is to become an effective health care professional must:

- Care about others: Have compassion. Apply knowledge and skills to decrease suffering and increase the well-being of others. When necessary, be willing to put the needs of patients ahead of one's own. Have respect for all people and help them regardless of their race, nationality, economic status, religion, age, or lifestyle preferences.
- Have **integrity**: Be honest at all times. Respect the privacy of others. Be loyal to the employer. Accept responsibility for one's actions.
- Be dependable: Be at work on time and as scheduled. Follow through and finish all assigned tasks. Perform work accurately and completely. Work without constant supervision and reminders.
- Work well with others: Strive to understand the feelings and needs of others. Be courteous and considerate. Practice good communication skills. Be a good team member by cooperating and contributing to the achievement of group goals. Take directions willingly from the supervisor.
- Be flexible: Be willing to adapt to changing conditions and emergencies. Do what is needed to carry out tasks. Acquire knowledge and skills necessary to keep up with advances in technology and changes in the way health care is delivered.
- Be willing to learn: Keep skills up to date. Ask questions, attend workshops, read professional publications, use the Internet, and continue to acquire new skills.
- Strive to be cost conscious: Look for ways to improve patient care while maintaining or lowering expenses. Work efficiently and take care not to waste supplies. (See Figure 1–1.)

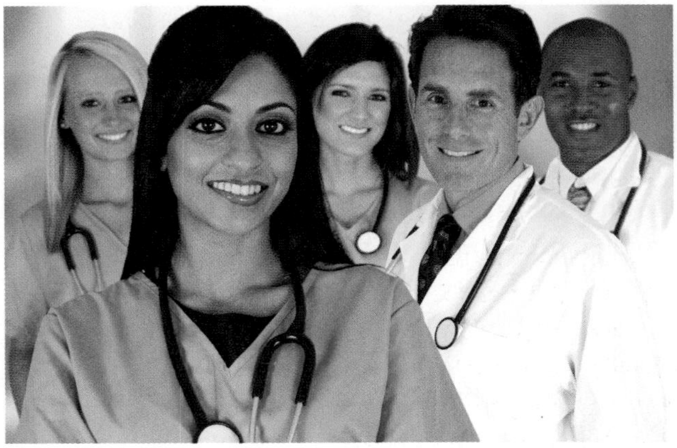

© Rob Marmion/Shutterstock.com.

FIGURE 1–1 Successful health care professionals work hard and exhibit the core qualities discussed in this chapter. At the same time, they enjoy the satisfaction of helping others.

STANDARDS FOR HEALTH CARE PROFESSIONALS

Standards for health care professionals have been established to protect the public from potential harm caused by incompetence. Testing, along with various approval and monitoring mechanisms, has been developed to determine whether professionals have met specific standards. The purpose of standards is to ensure that professionals master at least the minimum knowledge and skills necessary to safely and competently practice their professions. Learners should be aware that in addition to knowledge and skill standards, some occupations require background checks and drug testing. Individuals who have been convicted of certain crimes are prohibited from taking certification exams or practicing certain occupations.

Standards may be set by state boards or national professional organizations. There are several terms that designate various types of approvals. **Certification** is a general term that means a person has met predetermined standards. The process of becoming certified usually involves completing certain educational requirements and passing a professional examination. Most individuals who work in health care go through a certification process, although their title might not include the term *certified*. Examples of occupations that do include this term in their title are certified occupational therapy assistant, certified medical assistant, and certified nursing assistant.

Some occupations require **registration**, which means being placed on an official list (registry) after meeting the educational and testing requirements for the profession. Professionals who use this term in their title include registered nurse, registered respiratory therapist, and registered medical assistant.

Licensure is a designation that means the person has been granted permission to legally perform certain acts. Licenses are granted by government agencies, often the state. The specific occupations that require licensure vary from state to state. Some occupations are licensed in most, but not all, states. The word *licensed* does not usually appear with the title of licensed professions. For example, in the following list of licensed professions, only one includes the term: dentist, dental hygienist, physician, registered nurse, and licensed practical/vocational nurse.

The various types of approvals can be confusing. Certification and registration are often, but not always, required to work legally. Even when not required by law, they provide credibility and are preferred by many employers when hiring. Medical assisting is an example of an occupation in which voluntary certification or registration enhances the graduate's chances of being hired. Licensure, if required for a profession, is never voluntary.

Some professions have more than one form of approval. Medical assistants, for example, can be either certified or registered. Both approvals require meeting specific educational requirements and passing a national exam. The American Association of Medical Assistants grants the title "certified." The American Medical Technologists grants the title "registered."

Certification and licensing exams vary by occupation. Some consist of multiple-choice questions that are presented in a computerized format. Others contain case studies and ask questions to test the candidates' knowledge about handling situations that may be encountered on the job. Still others have a practical component that requires candidates to demonstrate their ability to perform certain tasks. In addition to occupational questions, some states test the knowledge of the laws that apply to health care occupations.

Another point that can be confusing is that some professions are licensed but use the title "registered." Nurses take a national exam that, when passed, entitles them to apply for a license in the state where they want to work. They can become licensed in any state as long as they follow the proper application process. In addition, they are listed in a registry. Although "registered nurse" is the title for the occupation, it is also a licensed profession.

Study the contents of Tables 1–8 and 1–9. Note the variety of titles and educational levels within the nursing and occupational therapy careers. As you can see, professional titles and the types of approval granted do not necessarily indicate the level of education achieved. For example, the educational requirements for a certified nursing assistant can be less than 200 hours of instruction; a certified occupational therapy assistant, however, must earn an associate degree. The titles given refer to the specific methods chosen by various organizations to ensure that their standards are met, rather than to the educational requirements. Furthermore, some titles may be acquired with varying amounts of education. Using the example of the registered nurse once again, we see that qualifying education can be either an associate or bachelor's degree.

It is essential that students understand what is necessary for them to work in their chosen occupation. Most examining and licensing boards require attendance at an accredited school and/or program. This means that the school and/or program meets the standards set by a specific professional organization. To become accredited, a school or program must formally apply for approval. Once the application is accepted, a team from the organization visits the campus to ensure that all standards are being met.

In addition to attending an accredited program, students must meet the following requirements before most professional exams can be taken:

- High school diploma or the equivalent
- Completion of specific courses
- Successful completion of the clinical portion of the training
- Not having been convicted of certain crimes

Once obtained, most certifications require specific amounts of continuing education. This is discussed further in Chapter 14. Individuals who fail to maintain the competency and conduct standards for their profession can lose their certification or license. The purpose of health care regulation is not to provide one-time approval. It is an ongoing effort to ensure that only qualified professionals are serving the public.

OCCUPATIONAL PROFILES

There are hundreds of job titles in health care and the number continues to grow. They require a wide range of skills and abilities. Each occupational area, such as radiology and physical therapy, has positions that require different amounts of education and training. Collectively, these levels are known as **career ladders**.

Learners who are pursuing occupations in health care should discover as much as possible about the requirements, responsibilities, and conditions of their areas of interest. This knowledge will enable them to make good career choices that match their preferences and abilities. For example, some individuals interested in health care would find the emergency medical technician's (EMT) job to be interesting and exciting. EMTs have opportunities to apply their skills to help others in significant ways, sometimes even saving lives. At the same time, the work is physically and emotionally demanding. It is often performed under difficult circumstances. Emergencies do not happen at convenient times and places. The schedules for EMTs include nights, weekends, and holidays, and they are called out to work in all types of weather conditions. All aspects of an occupation must be considered to increase the chances of choosing a career that will provide long-term satisfaction.

Learners who thoroughly explore the career areas that interest them will have a better chance of finding an occupation that matches their abilities and preferences. When choosing an occupation, learners should carefully consider the following factors about themselves:

- Educational background
- The amount of additional time they are willing to dedicate to their education
- Natural abilities
- The type of activities they most enjoy
- Preferences for workplace environment and conditions

The occupations described in this section are organized into four categories:

1. **Therapeutic** and Treatment
2. **Diagnostic**
3. Health Information Management
4. Environmental

Note that there is overlap among the categories. For example, although listed in the therapeutic and treatment section, a major responsibility of dentists and physicians is to diagnose their patients' conditions. And although dietetics is listed in the environmental category, nutrition experts prescribe diets as part of the treatment of health conditions such as diabetes and heart disease.

Occupational titles are further divided into specific career areas, such as dental and mental health. The educational and certification, registration, and/or licensing requirements for various occupational levels are presented in Tables 1–3 through 1–20. (Note that the abbreviations given in the tables for job titles assume that the individual has achieved the required approval, such as certification. For example, RN stands for *registered nurse*.) Following each table, occupations that generally require associate degrees or vocational training are described in more detail.

It is important for learners to keep in mind that the information in this chapter consists of brief overviews and contains only some of the hundreds

BOX 1–1

Examples of Health Care–Related Occupations

Art Therapist

Athletic Trainer

Audiologist

Health Educator

Medical Illustrator

Medical Librarian

Medical Photographer

Medical Writer

Music Therapist

Speech and Language Pathologist

of health care jobs available today. (See Box 1–1 for examples of additional occupations.) The growth projections cited are taken from the Bureau of Labor Statistics (2014). It is also important to note that there are more rungs on each career ladder than appear in the tables. For example, there are many nurse specialties, such as nurse anesthetist, clinical nurse specialist, and nurse practitioner, as well as doctoral degrees in nursing. Many health care providers earn advanced degrees beyond the basic requirements for their professions.

Learners should use the tables as a starting point and then thoroughly investigate all the career options in their areas of interest. Good starting points for career information include the following:

- The professional organizations for the various occupations. Contact information for these organizations is listed in Appendix 1.
- Occupational Outlook Handbook from the Bureau of Labor Statistics. Available at: www.bls.gov/ooh
- O*Net, sponsored by the U.S. Department of Labor. Available at: www.onetonline.org
- Education Portal. Available at: education-portal.com (It is not necessary to register and log in.)

Salaries have not been included for the various occupations. It is difficult to provide accurate, up-to-date information that applies to all geographic areas, individual facilities, and current economic conditions. Learners are encouraged to check the latest statistics provided by the Bureau of Labor to see current median salaries for occupations of interest.

On-the-job training, in which individuals learn necessary job skills after being employed, is being replaced in many occupations by formal training. For example, aide-level positions are being assigned more responsibilities, and classroom training is becoming necessary. Today's health care facilities need individuals who have current skills, are able to think for themselves, and can start immediately as contributing members of the health care team.

Therapeutic and Treatment Occupations

Therapeutic and treatment occupations provide services that assist patients to regain or attain maximum wellness. They may involve direct patient care, such as nursing, or provide services that contribute to the patient's recovery, such as the pharmacy professions. The majority of health care occupations fall into this category.

Dental Occupations

Dental professionals treat diseases and conditions of the teeth and soft tissues of the mouth. They perform preventive measures, restore missing and defective teeth, diagnose and treat diseases of the gums, perform cosmetic dentistry, and provide patient education. (See Table 1–3.)

Dental Hygienist

The primary responsibility of a dental hygienist is to provide preventive dental care. This is accomplished by cleaning the teeth with special instruments and equipment, examining the mouth and taking X-rays, and providing patient education about dental care. Although hygienists perform their work independently, they are under the supervision of a dentist. Work schedules are often flexible, and many hygienists work part-time and/or for more than one dentist. The work involves prolonged patient contact, standing and reaching, and requires the ability to get along well with others. Good **manual dexterity** (skill working with the hands) and hand–eye coordination are essential. This is one of the 20 fastest growing health care occupations, with some parts of the country reporting a significant shortage of hygienists.

Dental Assistant

Dental assistants are trained to perform a variety of duties in the dental office. They may work closely with

Table 1–3 Dental Occupations

Career	Education	Testing and Approval
Dentist (DDS or DMD)	2–4 years college preprofessional education 4 years dental school 2–4 years additional education if seeking specialty	Licensed by states: 1. Graduate from accredited dental school 2. Pass written and practical exams
Dental Hygienist (RDH)	Associate or bachelor's degree 2–4 years depending on program requirements	Licensed by states: 1. Graduate from accredited dental hygiene school 2. Pass national board exams administered by American Dental Association Joint Commission on National Dental Examinations 3. Pass state and/or locally administered clinical exams 4. Pass state exam covering dental hygiene law
Dental Assistant (CDA or RDA)	1–2 year educational program (recommended) or on-the-job training	Requirements vary by state; voluntary certifications available through Dental Assisting National Board
Dental Laboratory Technician	On-the-job training or 2-year associate degree program	Voluntary certification available from National Association of Dental Laboratories and/or National Board for Certification in Dental Laboratory Technology

the dentist by preparing patients for treatment, passing instruments, and suctioning the mouth during procedures performed by the dentist. Laboratory duties may include sterilizing and preparing instruments, creating casts of the teeth, and making temporary crowns. Administrative dental assistants greet patients, schedule appointments, keep patient records, send bills, and perform other clerical duties as needed. Dental assistants must have good manual dexterity, the ability and willingness to follow directions, and good interpersonal skills. This occupation is experiencing positive growth and provides excellent job opportunities.

Dental Laboratory Technician

Dental laboratory technicians make the items used by dentists to replace and restore teeth, such as crowns, bridges, and dentures. These are fabricated using models of the patient's mouth and involve working with plaster, wax, metal, and porcelain. Small hand-held tools, grinding and polishing equipment, and heat sources for melting and baking are used. The work is precise and very delicate. Successful technicians are patient and steady-handed and have good vision, especially the ability to discriminate colors, needed for matching replacements to remaining teeth. Growth in the number of jobs is expected to be lower than average because improved dental care has decreased the need for dentures.

Emergency Medical Occupations

Emergency medical technicians provide quick response service to victims of medical emergencies. All EMTs are qualified to give life support and immediate care such as restoring breathing, controlling bleeding, administering oxygen, bandaging wounds, and treating a person for shock. EMTs transport victims to health care facilities and provide necessary care en route. Intermediate EMTs have additional skills that include administering fluids intravenously and using a defibrillator to administer an electrical shock to a person whose heart has stopped. Paramedics are qualified to administer drugs, interpret electrocardiograms (measurements of the heart's electrical activity), and perform various invasive procedures (involving puncture or insertion of an instrument or material into the body). EMTs must be emotionally stable, able to deal with stressful situations, physically coordinated, able to move quickly and easily, and able to lift and carry heavy loads. EMTs are employed by rescue squads, police departments, and fire departments, and employment is expected to grow rapidly. (See Table 1–4.)

Massage Therapy Occupations

Massage therapists use different types of massage, such as Swedish, deep tissue, and reflexology, to treat ailments and injuries; decompress tired muscles; reduce stress; and promote wellness. There are dozens of specialties, or types of massage, each designed to achieve specific results.

A large percentage of massage therapists are self-employed, with the remainder working in settings ranging from physician and chiropractors' offices to fitness centers to spas. Massage therapy is physically demanding, as it requires standing and repetitive movements. Working with clients requires good communication, empathy, and the ability to make clients feel comfortable with the personal nature of massage treatment. (See Table 1–5.)

Medical Office Occupations

Medical office personnel treat patients who are seeking to maintain or improve their health or who need treatment for illnesses and injuries. Medical offices are staffed by a physician who may be either a medical doctor (MD) or a doctor of osteopathic medicine (DO). MDs and DOs receive similar training and perform similar functions. The major difference is that osteopathic physicians place more emphasis on the musculoskeletal system. Doctors of osteopathy also tend to approach medicine more holistically, meaning that they consider mental and emotional as well as physical health.

Physicians may provide general care or they may specialize in what and who they treat. (For a list of medical specialties see Box 1–2.)

In addition to the physician, medical offices need support staff to assist with patient care and to perform clinical, laboratory, and administrative duties. (See Table 1–6.) (Note: Physicians and occupations designated as "medical office support staff" also work in other settings, such as large clinics, hospitals, rehabilitation centers, etc.)

Medical Assistant

Medical assistants must be prepared to carry out a wide variety of duties. They may work closely with the physician and perform clinical tasks. Known as clinical or "back office assistants," their duties include preparing patients, taking vital signs, helping the physician with exams and procedures, and performing a variety of tests and procedures on patients. Medical assistants may also choose to concentrate on administrative or "front office tasks," which include receiving patients, answering the telephone, maintaining patient records, and handling insurance and billing duties. In small offices, the medical assistant may have both front and back office assignments. Medical assistants must be able to follow directions, work accurately, get along well with others, and have good manual dexterity. The occupation is expected to grow much faster than average for all occupations through the year 2022.

Mental Health Occupations

Mental health professionals provide care, treatment, counseling, and activities for patients with mental, emotional, and/or psychosocial (combination of mental and social) problems. These services are provided for patients in a wide variety of settings, including medical offices dedicated to the practice of psychiatry, psychiatric hospitals, halfway houses, general hospitals, clinics dedicated to treating substance abuse problems, group homes, and prisons. Diagnoses encountered range from mild anxiety disorders, in which patients experience temporary feelings of distress, to serious conditions, such as schizophrenia, that result in behaviors that are unsafe for both the patient and the public. (See Table 1–7.)

Mental Health Technician

Mental health technicians work with patients under the direction of a psychiatrist, psychologist, or registered nurse. They carry out care plans, assist with group activities, listen to patients and provide encouragement, and note behavior. The work requires a strong desire to help others, patience, understanding, excellent oral communication skills, and emotional stability. Employment growth is expected to be slower than average for all occupations.

Table 1–4 Emergency Medical Occupations

Career	Education	Testing and Certification
Paramedic	Typically 1–2 years; may result in a certificate or associate degree	Licensed by states: Most states require certification from the National Registry of Emergency Medical Technicians, which includes the following: 1. Complete a state-approved paramedic course that meets or exceeds the U.S. Department of Transportation National Standard Curriculum 2. Pass written and practical exams 3. Pass a state-approved psychomotor exam
EMT-Intermediate/99 EMT-Intermediate/85	Training requirements vary by state. Typically consist of 30–350 hours of training, depending on the scope of practice	Licensed by states: Most states require certification from the National Registry of Emergency Medical Technicians, which includes the following: 1. Complete a state-approved EMT-Intermediate/99 or EMT-Intermediate/85 course that meets or exceeds the U.S. Department of Transportation National Standard Curriculum 2. Pass written and practical exams 3. Pass a state-approved psychomotor exam
EMT-Basic	Training requirements vary by state, typically at least 100 hours	Licensed by states: Most states require certification from the National Registry of Emergency Medical Technicians, which includes the following: 1. Complete a state-approved EMT-Basic course that meets or exceeds the U.S. Department of Transportation National Standard Curriculum 2. Pass written and practical exams 3. Pass a state-approved psychomotor exam
First Responder/ Emergency Medical Responder	Training requirements vary by state	Licensed by states: Most states require certification from the National Registry of Emergency Medical Technicians, which includes the following: 1. Complete a state-approved paramedic course that meets or exceeds the U.S. Department of Transportation National Standard Curriculum 2. Pass written and practical exams 3. Pass a state-approved psychomotor exam

Note: Some states have their own certification programs and different names and titles for emergency service personnel.

Table 1–5 Massage Therapy Occupations

Career	Education	Testing and Certification
Massage Therapist	Requirements vary by state and locality; ranges from 3 to 24 months	Most states regulate and require formal education and national or state licensure or certification. In addition, some cities, towns, and counties have their own regulations and licensing requirements. Certification required for licensure in many states is offered by the National Certification Board for Therapeutic Massage and Bodywork (NCBTMB). Some states also require practical exams.

BOX 1–2

Medical Specialists

Physicians who specialize in treating specific parts of the body:

Cardiologist	Heart and blood vessels
Dermatologist	Skin
Endocrinologist	Endocrine system (glands)
Gastroenterologist	Stomach and intestines
Gynecologist	Female reproductive organs
Internist	Internal organs, including the lungs, heart, glands, intestines, and kidneys
Nephrologist	Kidneys
Neurologist	Brain and nervous system
Ophthalmologist	Eyes
Orthopedist	Muscles and bones
Otolaryngologist or Otorhinolaryngologist	Ear, nose, and throat
Proctologist	Lower part of the large intestine
Psychiatrist	Mind
Urologist	Kidneys, bladder, and urinary system

Physicians who perform specific kinds of work:

Anesthesiologist	Administers medication to cause loss of sensation or feeling during surgery
Emergency Physician	Treats acute illnesses and injuries
Oncologist	Diagnoses and treats tumors (cancer)

(continued)

Pathologist	Diagnoses disease by studying changes in organs, tissues, and cells
Physiatrist	Treats conditions associated with physical medicine and patients in need of rehabilitation
Plastic Surgeon	Performs corrective surgery to repair injured or malformed body parts
Radiologist	Uses X-rays and radiation to diagnose and treat diseases
Sports Medicine Physician	Prevents and treats injuries sustained in athletic events and physical activities
Surgeon	Performs surgery to correct deformities and treat injuries and diseases
Thoracic Surgeon	Performs surgery on the lungs, heart, and chest cavity
Physicians who work with specific populations:	
Family Practice Physician	Promotes wellness and treats individuals in all age groups
Gerontologist	Promotes wellness and treats older persons
Obstetrician	Assists women with pregnancy and childbirth
Pediatrician	Promotes wellness and treats children

Table 1–6 Medical Office Occupations

Career	Education	Testing and Certification
Physician (MD, DO)	4 years college preprofessional education 4 years medical school MD: 3–8 years of graduate medical education (residency) DO: 1-year internship and a 2- to 6-year residency	Licensed by states: 1. Graduate from accredited medical school 2. Complete graduate medical education 3. Pass written examination
Physician's Assistant (PA)	Varies. 2–4 years college + 24-month (minimum) PA program	Requirements vary by state; most require passing the exam administered by National Commission on Certification of Physician's Assistants
Medical Assistant Administrative and/or Clinical (MA, CMA, RMA) Certified Medical Assistant (CMA) Registered Medical Assistant (RMA)	Certificate program or associate degree	Specific tasks, such as giving injections, regulated by some states. Optional certification through exam administered by American Association of Medical Assistants. Optional registration through exam administered by American Medical Technologists

Table 1–7 Mental Health Occupations

Career	Education	Testing and Certification
Psychiatrist (MD)	4 years college preprofessional education 4 years medical school 4–7 years of medical graduate education (residency)	Licensed by states: 1. Graduate from accredited medical school 2. Complete specialized studies, internship, and residency 3. Pass written exam
Clinical Psychologist (PhD, PsyD)	4 years college 2–3 years graduate school (master's degree) 2–4 years (doctorate)	Licensed by states: Pass written exam
Clinical Social Worker	4 years college 2–3 years graduate school, including supervised experience (master's degree)	Licensed by states: Pass written exam
Psychiatric Clinical Nurse Specialist	Licensure as RN 2–3 years graduate school (master's or doctoral degree)	Licensed by states: 1. Requirements vary by state but include passing a written exam
Mental Health Technician	Certificate or associate degree in human services or mental health	Licensed by some states
Psychiatric Aide	Some states require formal training program	Varies by state

Psychiatric Aide

Psychiatric aides assist other health care professionals and provide help with the physical needs of patients, such as hygiene and feeding. They provide companionship for patients and may help escort patients within or outside the care facility. Aides must be patient, caring, and responsible. Average growth in job opportunities is expected for this occupation. (Note: Psychiatric aides generally have less formal education than mental health technicians. In some states, however, the two job titles refer to the same level of education and work duties.)

Nursing Occupations

Nurses promote health and provide care and treatment for patients with all types of health problems. Nursing care is carried out through the application of a structured process to determine each patient's needs, develop individual care plans, implement the plans, and then evaluate their effectiveness. An important responsibility of the nurse is to provide education to patients and their families regarding self-care and health maintenance. (See Table 1–8.)

Registered Nurse

Registered nurses provide a wide variety of patient care services. They give direct patient care or supervise other personnel who do so, serve as patient advocates (support the interests of patients), and provide patient education. They are often the professionals who coordinate the overall care of patients by interacting with all other health care professionals involved. Registered nurses can achieve many educational levels and pursue a great number of specialties. Opportunities range from direct patient care to management of a hospital department. Specific day-to-day activities are determined by the work setting, which may be a hospital, clinic, long-term care facility, school, prison, or patients' homes. Registered nurses must be caring and responsible, have excellent assessment and communication skills, and be emotionally stable and able to both follow

Table 1–8 Nursing Occupations

Career	Education	Testing and Certification
Certified Registered Nurse Anesthetist (CRNA)	Be a registered nurse Complete specialized education leading to a master's degree	Licensed by states: Pass a national certification exam
Nurse Practitioner (CRNP)	Be a registered nurse Complete additional educational and clinical practice requirements (most are master's or doctoral degree programs)	Licensed by states: Pass a national certification exam
Registered Nurse (RN)	4-year (bachelor's) college degree (preferred by most and required by many hospitals) or 2-year (associate) degree	Licensed by states: 1. Graduate from approved program 2. Pass the National Council Licensing Examination for Nurses (N-CLEX)
Licensed Practical/Licensed Vocational Nurse (LPN/LVN)	1- or 2-year state-approved associate degree or diploma program	Licensed by states: 1. Graduate from approved program 2. Pass national licensing exam
Certified Nursing Assistant (CNA)	States have various training requirements for classroom and clinical experience Programs must meet specific federal minimum standards Typical program is at least 8 weeks	All states require certification for work in long-term care facilities Requirements guided by federal regulations established by the Omnibus Budget Reconciliation Act of 1987 (OBRA) Certification requirements vary for other work environments
Patient Care Technician/Patient Care Assistant	Vocational training program	Certification required if nursing assistant duties are included. Voluntary certifications available: 1. National Health Association 2. National Center for Competency Testing
Home Health Aide	States have various training requirements for classroom and clinical experience. Some types of employers require formal training.	Approval requirements vary by state under guidance of OBRA Voluntary certification available from the National Association for Home Care and Hospice

orders and supervise others. Registered nursing is one of the most versatile careers in any field. It is one of the occupations projected to have the largest number of job openings during the period 2012 to 2022. In fact, many areas of the United States are reporting severe shortages of qualified registered nurses. It is estimated that by 2020, 1.2 million registered nurses will be needed nationwide. (Center for Health Workforce Studies, 2012). (See Figure 1–2.)

Licensed Practical/Vocational Nurse

Licensed practical nurses (known as licensed vocational nurses in California and Texas) provide basic patient care under the direction of physicians and

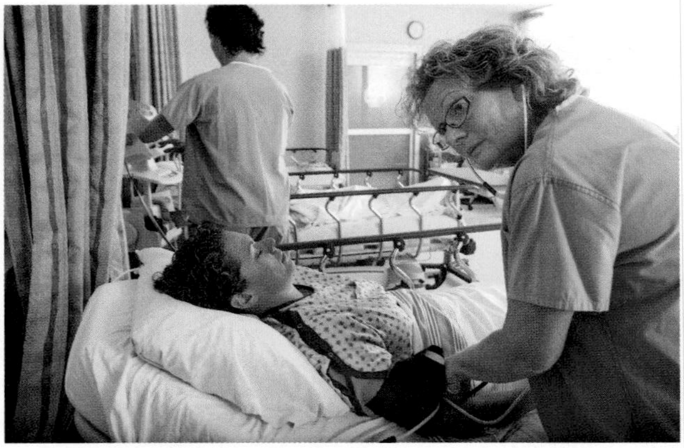

FIGURE 1–2 As older nurses retire, there will be a great need for newly trained registered nurses.

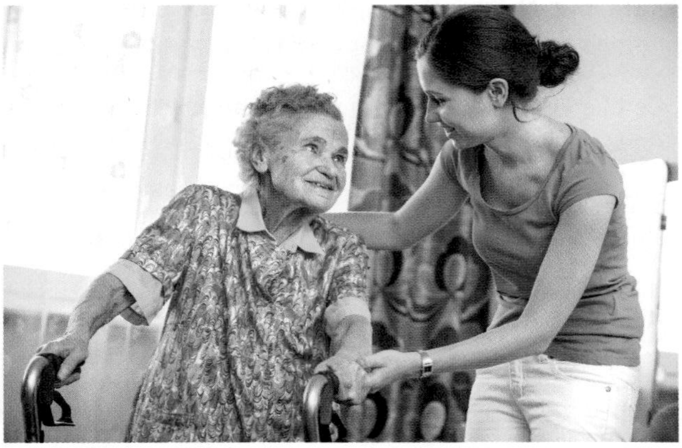

FIGURE 1–3 Home health aide is a fast growing occupation. Aides must be compassionate, patient, and interested in helping the elderly and disabled.

registered nurses. Most practical nurses carry out bedside tasks that include taking vital signs, administering medications, applying dressings and hot and cold packs, treating bedsores, and giving various comfort measures. They are also responsible for recording patient information. Practical nurses must be caring, responsible, emotionally stable, and able to follow directions and work under supervision. Job opportunities vary by region. Most new jobs are in residential care facilities and home health environments. Employment growth is expected to be much faster than average for all occupations.

Certified Nursing Assistant

Nursing assistants work under the supervision of nursing staff to help care for patients' basic needs. They may take vital signs, assist patients with hygiene and feeding, give comfort measures, change bedding, and help transport patients. The variety and level of duties depend on state laws, the amount of training, and the needs of the facility. Assistants must be patient, caring, dependable, and able to follow directions. This is a fast-growing occupation, especially for individuals who are also qualified to work as home health aides.

Patient Care Technician

The work of patient care technicians is similar to that of nursing assistants. They work under the supervision of physicians or nurses, taking vital signs; collecting specimens; and assisting patients with eating, hygiene, and grooming. Patient care technicians work in hospitals, clinics, and rehabilitation facilities.

Home Health Aide

Home health aides help the disabled, elderly, and chronically ill. Their work is similar to that of certified nursing assistants. In fact, many patient care technicians have nursing assistant certification. In some states they are allowed to give mediations to clients and take vital signs. They may work in patients' homes or in a care facility, assisting with moving patients, providing personal care, and dressing. In the client's home, duties may include preparing meals, providing companionship, doing light housekeeping, and providing transportation. This is one of the fastest growing of all occupations, including health care. (See Figure 1–3.)

Occupational Therapy Occupations

The purpose of occupational therapy is to help individuals attain the highest level of self-sufficiency possible. Difficulties in performing the activities of daily living can be the result of physical, mental, or emotional problems caused by disease, injury, or congenital (present at birth) conditions. Occupational therapists evaluate patients, set goals to increase their function and lessen their limitations, and create treatment plans to achieve these goals. Treatment may involve individual or group activities, exercise, providing adaptive equipment such as splints and special tools, and teaching patients new ways to perform daily tasks. (See Table 1–9.)

Occupational Therapy Assistant

Occupational therapy assistants work under the supervision of occupational therapists. They carry out

Table 1–9 Occupational Therapy Occupations

Career	Education	Testing and Licensure
Occupational Therapist (OTR)	Master's degree (minimum) or doctorate	Licensed in all states National registration: 1. Graduate from program accredited by American Occupational Therapy Association (AOTA) 2. Pass national exam administered by National Board for Certification in Occupational Therapy (NBCOT)
Occupational Therapy Assistant (COTA)	2-year (associate) college degree	Licensure or certification required in most states National certification: 1. Graduate from program accredited by AOTA 2. Pass national exam administered by NBCOT
Occupational Therapy Aide	Certificate program or on-the-job training	None

rehabilitative activities and exercises prescribed in treatment plans prepared by occupational therapists. Other important duties include patient education, monitoring patient progress, and preparing reports for the therapist. Typical tasks include teaching a patient to use special devices that enable the performance of everyday tasks, such as reaching, dressing, and cooking; assisting with a stretching exercise; and making a hand splint. Occupational therapy assistants must have good communication skills, be patient and caring, and be sensitive to the needs of people who suffer from a variety of disabilities. The number of new positions is expected to grow rapidly.

Occupational Therapy Aide

Aides help therapists and assistants by performing supportive duties such as preparing supplies for activities, assisting with patient transfers, helping with patient treatments and activities, and cleaning activity areas. Some aides are cross-trained to assist other rehabilitation professionals such as physical therapists. Rehabilitation skills may be combined with nursing assistance training and certification. Aides must be responsible and able to follow directions. For aides who are also certified nursing assistants, the number of positions is expected to grow rapidly.

Pharmacy Occupations

Pharmacy professionals prepare and dispense medications to promote patient wellness and recovery, as well as pharmaceutical products used to diagnose health conditions. Important duties also include educating patients about the proper use of medications and ensuring that patients are not given drugs that will cause harm because of allergic reactions or negative interactions with other drugs. (See Table 1–10.)

Pharmacy Technician

Pharmacy technicians work under the supervision of a licensed pharmacist. They fill orders for drugs, stock medication carts, record and store incoming drug supplies, and reorder inventory as needed. They also assist in maintaining paperwork and records required for controlled drugs (have potential for abuse). Pharmacy technicians must be responsible, detail oriented, and able to follow directions exactly. Job opportunities are expected to grow faster than average for all occupations, especially for technicians who are certified.

Physical Therapy Occupations

The purpose of physical therapy is to help patients improve their physical functions by increasing muscle strength, range of motion, movement, and by decreasing pain. This is accomplished through assessment and the creation and implementation of treatment programs that may include exercise, massage, and the use of modalities such as heat, cold, and electrical stimulation. Physical therapists teach patients to perform exercises and use equipment, such as canes and crutches. (See Table 1–11 and Figure 1–4.)

Table 1–10 Pharmacy Occupations

Career	Education	Testing and Licensure
Pharmacist (PharmD)	2–3 years college 3–4 years pharmacy school (doctoral degree)	Licensed by states: 1. Graduate from college of pharmacy accredited by the American Council on Pharmaceutical Education 2. Pass the North American Pharmacist Licensure Exam (NAPLEX) 3. Most states also require passing the Multistate Pharmacy Jurisprudence Exam (MPJE)
Pharmacy Technician	Up to 1 year on-the-job-training or 1- or 2-year college certificate program or associate degree	A few states require licensure, certification, or registration Voluntary national certification available through examination administered by Pharmacy Technician Certification Board and the Institute for Certification of Pharmacy Technicians
Pharmacy Aide/ Helper/Clerk	High school diploma and on-the-job-training or vocational training program	None

Table 1–11 Physical Therapy Occupations

Career	Education	Testing and Licensure
Physical Therapist (PT)	Doctorate	Licensed by states: 1. Graduate from program accredited by the Commission on Accreditation in Physical Therapy Education (APTE) 2. Pass exam administered by the Federation of State Boards of Physical Therapy
Physical Therapist Assistant (PTA)	2-year (associate) college degree	Many states require licensure, certification, and/or registration: 1. Graduate from program accredited by APTE 2. Pass exam administered by the Federation of State Boards of Physical Therapy
Physical Therapist Aide	On-the-job-training or vocational training program	None

Physical Therapist Assistant

Assistants work with patients under the supervision of a physical therapist to carry out treatment plans. They teach and supervise exercises, apply modalities, perform massages, assist patients with ambulatory devices such as walkers and canes, and document progress. Physical therapist assistants must be patient and encouraging and have the physical strength to assist patients with exercises. This occupation is projected to be among the fastest growing in the next several years.

Physical Therapist Aide

Aides support the work of therapists and assistants by preparing and cleaning equipment and therapy areas, assisting with treatments, transporting patients, and ordering and maintaining supplies. Aides must be responsible and able to follow directions.

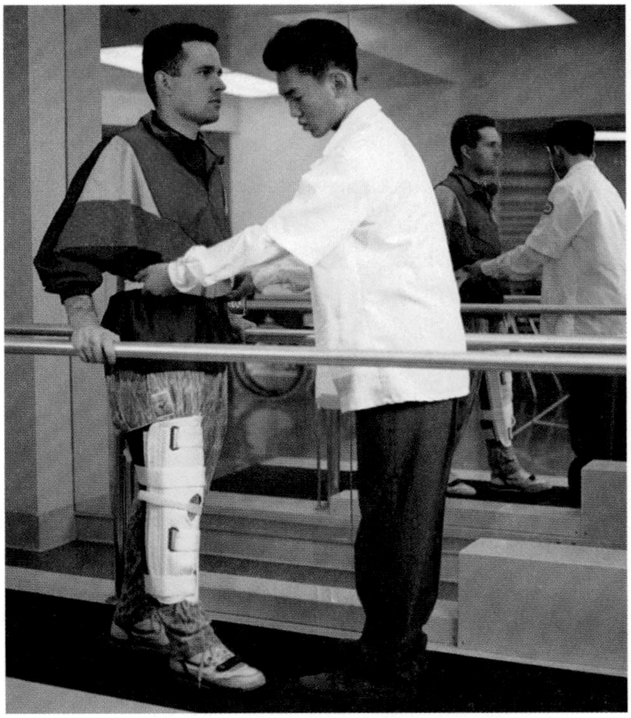

FIGURE 1–4 Physical therapist assistants help patients improve their physical function after accidents, surgery, and illness.

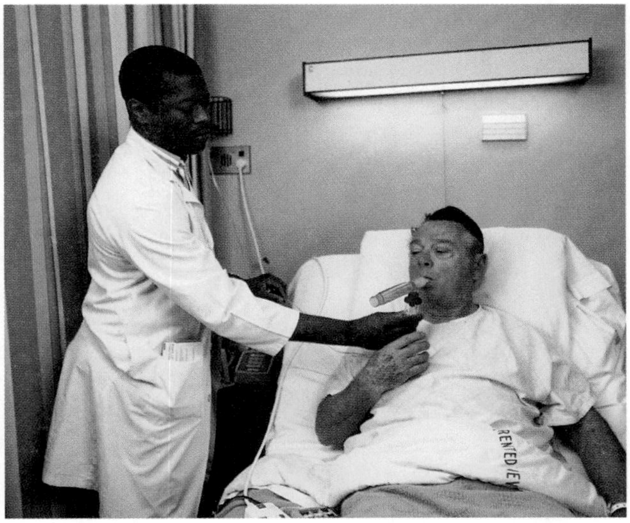

FIGURE 1–5 Respiratory therapists administer medications and treatments to patients who have lung and heart disorders.

Respiratory Therapy Occupations

Respiratory therapy involves evaluating, treating, and caring for patients with breathing disorders. Respiratory therapists assist patients who cannot breathe on their own because of conditions such as heart disease, acute diseases (lasting a short time but relatively severe) such as pneumonia, or chronic diseases (lasting a long time) such as emphysema. (See Table 1–12 and Figure 1–5.)

Respiratory Therapist

Respiratory therapists perform a variety of tasks to assist patients with breathing. These include using special instruments to measure lung capacity and drawing blood samples to test for levels of oxygen and other components. Therapists provide patients with oxygen and connect those who cannot breathe on their own to ventilators. The monitoring and maintenance of equipment are critical to a patient's well-being. Therapists also administer aerosol medications and perform chest physiotherapy, which involves thumping and vibrating the patient's chest cavity to remove mucus from the lungs. Respiratory therapists must have good technical aptitude and be attentive to detail and able to work under stress. Jobs are expected to grow faster than average for all occupations.

Surgical Occupations

Surgical procedures vary from minor to extremely complex and from emergency to elective. The types of surgery available, and their complexity, are growing at a fast rate. Many people are alive today as a result of modern surgery. Surgical occupations involve the care of the patient before, during, and after surgery. (See Table 1–13 and Figure 1–6.)

Table 1–12 Respiratory Therapy Occupations

Career	Education	Testing and Licensure
Respiratory Therapist (RRT, CRT)	Associate or bachelor's degree	Licensed in all states except Alaska: 1. Graduate an accredited program (accepted approval agencies vary by state) 2. Pass exam administered by the National Board for Respiratory Care

Table 1–13 Surgical Occupations

Career	Education	Testing and Licensure
Surgeon (MD or DO)	4 years college preprofessional education 4 years medical school MD: Up to 6 years of graduate medical education (residency) DO: 1-year internship and 3- to 5-year residency	Licensed by states: 1. Graduate from accredited medical school 2. Complete specialized studies, internship, and residency 3. Pass written exam
Surgical Physician Assistant	Varies; 2–4 years college + 2-year PA program + 2-year surgical assistant master's degree program	Licensed by states. Must pass exams administered by the National Commission on Certification of Physician's Assistants
Certified Surgical Technician (CST), Operating Room Technician (ORT), Surgical Technologist	9-month to 2-year program leading to certificate or associate degree Clinical experience	Some states require certification or registration by passing exam administered by National Board of Surgical Technology and Surgical Assisting

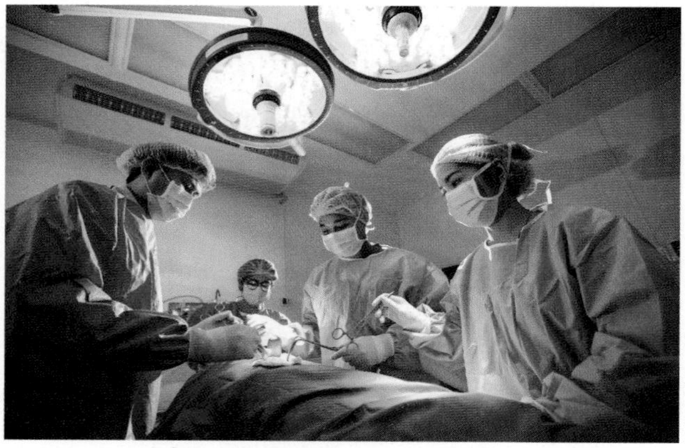

FIGURE 1–6 Surgical technologists prepare patients for surgery, set up instruments and supplies, and assist during surgery by passing instruments and supplies.

Surgical Technologist/Surgical Technician/Operating Room Technician

The health care professionals who are trained to perform important functions in the operating room may work under a variety of job titles. Duties include sterilizing and setting up instruments, preparing equipment and linens in the operating room, and preparing patients for surgery and transporting them to the operating room. During surgery, technicians may perform a variety of tasks: pass instruments to the surgeon, hold retractors (instruments that open or draw back tissue, bone, etc.), cut sutures, operate lights and equipment, and assist with the preparation of specimens. Work in surgery requires excellent manual dexterity, attention to detail, the stamina to stand for long hours, and the ability to respond quickly. Employment is expected to grow much faster than average for all occupations.

Veterinary Occupations

Veterinary professionals provide medical treatment and preventive care for many types of animals who fill a variety of roles: pets; food sources for humans; entertainment, such as zoo animals and racehorses; and animals used in laboratory experiments. Pet care has become a multibillion industry in the United States as more people acquire pets as companions and consider them to be members of the family. Although most veterinary practices work with small animals, some work with livestock and other large animals. Others specialize in more exotic animals such as alpacas and ostriches. Keeping livestock healthy contributes to human health by ensuring the health and safety of our meat, egg, and milk supply. (See Table 1–14 and Figure 1–7.)

Veterinary Technologists and Technicians

Veterinary technologists and technicians work under the supervision of a veterinarian in diagnosing and

Table 1–14 Veterinary Occupations

Career	Education	Testing and Licensure
Veterinarian (DVM or VMD)	3–4 years college preprofessional education 4 years veterinary college 2- to 5-year internship/residency required for specialties	Licensed by states: 1. Graduate from accredited veterinary school 2. Pass the North American Veterinary Licensing Exam (NAVLE) 3. Many states administer exam covering state laws and regulations
Veterinary Technologist	Bachelor's degree	Regulation varies by state. All states require credentialing exam. Most use National Veterinary Technician (NVT) exam Voluntary certification for work in research facility is administered by the American Association for Laboratory Animal Science
Veterinary Technician	2-year associate degree	Regulation differs by state Almost all states require credentialing exam Most use NVT exam Voluntary certification for work in research facility is administered by the American Association for Laboratory Animal Science
Veterinary Assistant	On-the-job training or college certificate program	No licensing required

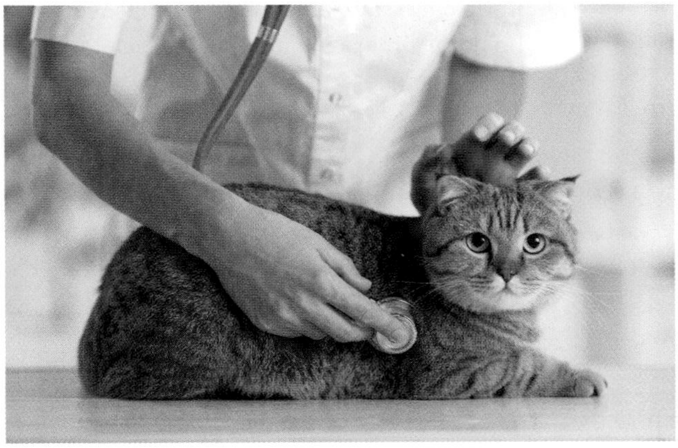

FIGURE 1–7 Veterinary technologists and technicians assist veterinarians as they diagnose and treat various types of animals.

treating animals. Their duties are similar and include conducting laboratory tests, taking blood samples and X-rays, cleaning an animal's teeth, assisting in surgery, and educating animal owners. Individuals who work in veterinary careers must like animals and enjoy working with them. The work can be physically and emotionally demanding, as when large animals must be restrained or beloved pets are euthanized. Technologists and technicians must be able to work responsibly under supervision, communicate well, and demonstrate empathy for the owners of the animals they treat. The most common employment settings include private veterinary clinics, animal hospitals, and research facilities. These are expected to be very fast growing occupations.

Vision Care Occupations

Vision care professionals perform the important work of assisting up to 75% of Americans who use some form of corrective lens. In addition to working to correct vision problems, they identify and treat diseases of the eye, provide education and care to maintain good vision and eye health, and make eyeglasses. (See Table 1–15.)

Ophthalmic Technician

Ophthalmic technicians assist ophthalmologists in their work with patients. They take care of equipment,

Table 1–15 Vision Care Occupations

Career	Education	Testing and Licensure
Ophthalmologist (MD)	4 years college preprofessional education 4 years medical school 4–7 years graduate medical education (internship and residency)	Licensed by states: 1. Graduate from accredited medical school 2. Complete specialized studies, internship, and residency 3. Pass written exam
Optometrist (OD)	3–4 years college 4 years college of optometry 2+ years residency required to specialize in specific types of optometry	Licensed by states: 1. Graduate from accredited optometry school 2. Pass written and clinical state board exams or exam administered by National Board of Examiners in Optometry 3. Many states require exam on state law
Ophthalmic Medical Technologist	Associate or bachelor's degree	Requirements vary among states Voluntary certification from the Joint Commission on Allied Health Personnel in Ophthalmology (JCAHPO)
Ophthalmic Technician	1-year certificate or diploma program	Requirements vary among states Voluntary certification from the JCAHPO
Optician	On-the-job training or 2- to 4-year apprenticeship or vocational or associate degree program (apprenticeship means formal on-the-job training with specific conditions and goals). Some states require formal training to qualify to take certification exams.	Licensed or certified in 23 states Requirements vary Certification available through American Board of Opticianry and National Contact Lens Examiners
Ophthalmic Assistant	On-the-job training or formal education ranging from 2 weeks to 2-year associate degree	Optional certification: 1. Complete educational program 2. Clinical experience 3. Pass national exam administered by JCAHPO
Ophthalmic Laboratory Technician	On-the-job training or 6- to 12-month vocational training program	Voluntary certification available from American Board of Opticianry and National Contact Lens Examiners: 1. Possess high school diploma 2. Pass examination
Optometric Assistant/Technician	On-the-job training or vocational program	Voluntary certification available from American Optometric Association, Commission on Paraoptometric Certification

record patient histories, perform eye tests, assist with surgery, and carry out office maintenance duties. Good manual dexterity, observation skills, and attention to detail are important characteristics for success in this occupation. Job growth is expected to be at least average.

Ophthalmic Laboratory Technician

Ophthalmic laboratory technicians make eyeglass lenses following prescriptions prepared by ophthalmologists and optometrists. They use special equipment to cut, grind, edge, and finish eyeglass lenses. Lenses must then be checked for accuracy. The job sometimes includes inserting lenses into frames. Technicians must have good manual dexterity, attention to detail, and the ability to follow directions. Job growth is expected to be low because the occupation is small.

Diagnostic Occupations

Professionals in diagnostic occupations help identify and/or determine the causes and extent of diseases and injuries so that proper treatment can be planned. They also monitor patient progress over time to determine if treatment is effective. Occupations may involve working directly with patients to perform tests and collect specimens, operating complex equipment, and carrying out tests in a laboratory setting.

Diagnostic Imaging Occupations

Diagnostic imaging uses a variety of techniques and machines to view structures and functions inside the body. Many diseases and injuries can be diagnosed without carrying out invasive procedures. Equipment is used that employs X-rays, sound waves, magnetic fields, and radioactive substances. (See Chapter 18 for more information on computerized imaging techniques.) The ongoing development of noninvasive diagnostic methods has resulted in new specialties and occupational areas, such as magnetic resonance imaging (MRI) technologist. (See Table 1–16.)

Radiologic Technologist/Radiographer

Radiographers perform X-ray procedures. They explain procedures to patients, position them properly, provide shielding against excessive exposure to X-rays, operate equipment, and develop film. This work requires great attention to safety factors, a high degree of technical aptitude, the ability to communicate well with patients, the stamina to stand for long periods, and the ability to work under emergency conditions. Faster than average employment growth is expected. Radiographers who learn a variety of specialties, such as skull X-rays and mammography, will have the best chances for employment.

Diagnostic Medical Sonographer

Sonographers operate equipment that uses sound waves (ultrasound) to produce images of soft tissue. The technology allows the movement of internal structures to be viewed on a screen, as well as the creation of images on film. Sonographers can specialize in cardiac, vascular, or abdominal areas. A common use of ultrasound, because of its safety, is to observe the developing fetus. Sonographers must have good math and technical aptitude, the ability to communicate with patients, and accurate work habits. Employment growth is expected to be much faster than for all occupations.

Limited X-ray Machine Operator

Limited X-ray machine operators are licensed personnel whose duties are similar to those of a radiologic technologist, but are more limited in scope. This position does not exist in all states and may have another title, such as radiologic technician or radiographic assistant.

Cardiovascular Technologist and Diagnostic Vascular Technologist

Cardiovascular and diagnostic vascular technologists assist physicians in the diagnosis and treatment of heart, vein, and artery disorders. They are qualified to perform noninvasive tests using ultrasound as well as to assist with invasive procedures, such as cardiac catheterization, which is the insertion of a small tube through the blood vessels to the heart. Technologists prepare patients for procedures and monitor them throughout. They must work accurately, handle stress well, and have high technical aptitude. Employment growth is expected to be faster than average, but the number of positions is not high because the occupation is small.

Electrocardiography Technician

Electrocardiography records the electrical action of the heart. The electrocardiograph (ECG) technician attaches electrodes to the specific points on the patient and manipulates switches on a machine to trace the

Table 1–16 Diagnostic Imaging Occupations

Career	Education	Testing and Licensure
Radiologist (MD or OD)	4 years college preprofessional education 4 years medical school 5–7 years of graduate medical education (residency)	Licensed by states: 1. Graduate from accredited medical school 2. Complete specialized studies, internship, and residency 3. Pass written exam administered by American Board of Radiology
Registered Radiologic Assistant	Bachelor's degree	Licensed in most states Voluntary registration from the American Registry of Radiologic Technologists (ARRT): 1. Graduate from accredited program or meet other specified requirements 2. Pass certification exam
Radiologic Technologist (RT)/Radiographer	Associate or bachelor's degree	Licensed in most states Voluntary registration from ARRT: 1. Graduate from accredited program or meet other specified requirements 2. Pass certification exam
Computed Tomography Technologist	Associate or bachelor's degree plus on-the-job training or training from manufacturer	Same as radiographer plus additional specialty exam
Magnetic Resonance Technologist	Be a registered radiographer Associate or bachelor's degree plus on-the-job training or training from manufacturer	Same as radiographer plus additional specialty exam
Positron Emission Tomography Technologist	Be a registered radiographer Associate or bachelor's degree plus on-the-job training or training from manufacturer	Same as radiographer plus additional specialty exam
Diagnostic Medical Sonographer	Certificate program or associate or bachelor's degree (associate degree most common)	Some states require licensure Voluntary certification available from American Registry of Diagnostic Medical Sonographers (ARDMS): 1. Graduate from accredited program or meet other requirements 2. Pass national exam
Limited X-ray Machine Operator	Diploma or certificate program	Certification and title of position vary by state. Most states (32 currently) require licensure. Some require specific education from an accredited program and passing a certification exam

(continues)

Table 1–16 Diagnostic Imaging Occupations (continued)

Career	Education	Testing and Licensure
Cardiovascular Technologist/ Diagnostic Vascular Technologist	Associate or bachelor's degree	Some states require licensure Registration available with ARDMS Certification available from Cardiovascular Credentialing International
Electrocardiography Technician	On-the-job training or 6- to 12-month vocational education program	Certification available from the National Center for Competency Testing and the National Healthcareer Association
Neurodiagnostic Technologist/ Electroneurodiagnostic Technologist/ Electroencephalographic Technologist	Associate degree (preferred) or formal training program of 1–2 years leading to a diploma or on-the-job training	Some states require certification Certification available from American Board of Registration of Electroencephalographic and Evoked Potential Technologists

electrical activity on graph paper. This skill is often included in the training of other patient care occupations, such as medical assisting. The number of jobs for ECG technicians who are not trained to perform other tasks in addition to this specialty is expected to grow at a slower-than-average rate.

Neurodiagnostic Technologist/Electroneurodiagnostic Technologist/Electroencephalographic Technologist

Electroneurodiagnostics is the monitoring, recording, interpreting, and study of the entire nervous system using various tests and instruments. Electroencephalic technology refers specifically to the recording and study of the brain's electrical activity. Technologists take patient histories, apply electrodes to the scalp, operate recording and monitoring instruments, and monitor patients during procedures. They should have good manual dexterity and vision, technical aptitude, and excellent communication skills.

Medical Laboratory Occupations

Work in medical laboratory occupations involves collecting and studying specimens from the human body. These include blood and other body fluids, tissues, and cells. Many kinds of tests are available to detect the presence of disease and determine its cause. The work requires the use of specialized equipment, such as microscopes and cell counters, and various chemicals. (See Table 1–17 and Figure 1–8.)

Medical Laboratory Technician

Laboratory technicians perform routine tests, which can require preparing slides, counting cells, and using sophisticated equipment. The work can also involve caring for and cleaning the equipment, maintaining supplies, and keeping records. Laboratory technicians must have good manual dexterity, great attention to detail and accuracy, and good observation skills. Employment projection is expected to be much faster than for all occupations.

Medical Laboratory Assistant

Laboratory assistants perform routine tests and tasks that are less complex than those for which the technician is qualified. The necessary qualities and job outlook are similar to those of the technician.

Phlebotomist

Phlebotomists draw blood from patients for medical testing and from blood donors. In addition to good manual dexterity, they must be calm and reassuring and able to work with individuals who fear blood and needles. Employment growth is expected to be much faster than for all occupations.

Health Information Management Occupations

Individuals who work in health information management occupations gather, analyze, organize, store,

Table 1–17 Medical Laboratory Occupations

Career	Education	Testing and Licensure
Pathologist (MD)	4 years college preprofessional education 4 years medical school 4 years of graduate medical education (residency); 1 or 2 more years required for specialties	Licensed by states: 1. Graduate from accredited medical school 2. Complete specialized studies, internship, and residency 3. Pass written exam
Medical Laboratory Technologist (MT)	Bachelor's or master's degree	Licensed or registered in some states Certification available from: 1. American Medical Technologists 2. Board of Registry of the American Society for Clinical Pathology 3. Board of Registry of the American Association of Bioanalysts
Medical Laboratory Technician	Completion of certificate program or associate degree	Licensing or registration required in some states Certification available from: 1. American Medical Technologists 2. Board of Certification of the American Society for Clinical Pathology
Medical Laboratory Assistant	1- to 2-year training program or specific work experience	Voluntary certification from American Medical Technologists Association
Phlebotomist	On-the-job training or formal training program	Licensure required in California and Louisiana Certification is required by most employers and is available from: 1. National Phlebotomy Association 2. American Society for Clinical Pathology 3. Association of Phlebotomy Technicians 4. Several other organizations also test and certify phlebotomists

Note: All of the above careers require completion of various amounts of training in order to take professional exams.

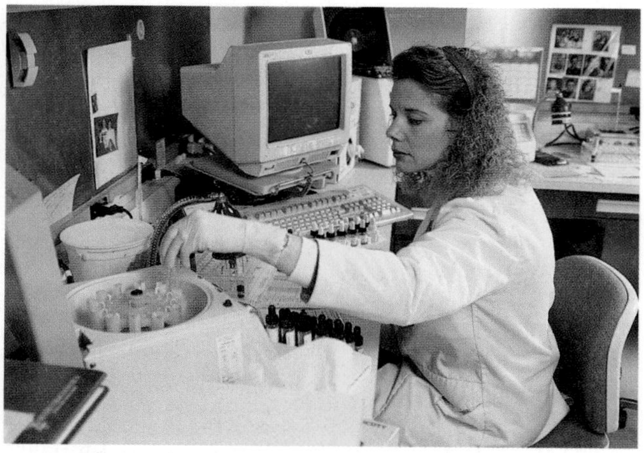

FIGURE 1–8 Medical laboratory workers perform manual and computerized tests to detect the presence of disease.

and document patient information. Consistent patient care, as well as regulatory compliance, depends on complete and accurate records. The increasing emphasis on monitoring the cost of health care delivery and the outcomes of patients who undergo treatment has increased the need for high-quality medical recordkeeping, with employment projections much faster than average for all occupations. (See Table 1–18.)

Registered Health Information Technician

Health information technicians perform a variety of tasks related to the collection and organization of patient data. They organize patient records, perform coding (the assignment of predetermined numbers that designate specific diagnoses and procedures),

Table 1–18 Health Information Management Occupations

Career	Education	Testing and Licensure
Registered Health Information Administrator (RHIA)	Bachelor's or master's degree	Voluntary registration available from American Health Information Management Association (AHIMA): 1. Complete educational program approved by the Commission on Accreditation for Health Informatics and Information Management Education (CAHIIM) 2. Pass national exam administered by AHIMA
Registered Health Information Technician (RHIT)	Associate degree	Voluntary registration available from AHIMA: 1. Complete educational program accredited by CAHIIM 2. Pass national exam administered by AHIMA
Medical Transcriptionist (MT)	Certificate program or associate degree	Voluntary certification available from Association for Healthcare Documentation Integrity
Certified Coding Specialist (CCS)	Associate degree (preferred) or on-the-job training or coding seminars	Voluntary certification (Certified Coding Specialist [CCS]) available from AHIMA: 1. High-school diploma 2. Complete educational program accredited by CAHIIM 3. Written exam
Medical Records Clerk	On-the-job training	None

enter data from paper records into computerized recordkeeping systems, and compile data for reports. Good organizational skills, a high degree of accuracy with details, and good computer aptitude are necessary for success in this field. Job prospects are expected to be very good.

Medical Transcriptionist

Transcriptionists prepare written medical reports. A variety of reports are used in health care to describe all types of findings and procedures. They include topics ranging from descriptions of surgeries to reports documenting autopsies (examination of organs and tissues performed after death to determine cause of death). Transcriptionists must sit and concentrate for long periods; be able to hear and interpret spoken language that includes medical terms; have excellent grammar, spelling, and computer software skills; and produce consistently accurate work. Employment prospects are expected to be about average as compared to all occupations.

Certified Coding Specialist

Medical coders classify medical data contained in patient records. Codes are assigned from the two major coding systems, the ICD-10-CM (diagnoses) and CPT (procedures). With experience and additional training, coders can achieve positions such as coding supervisor and compliance officer. A high level of accuracy and attention to detail is necessary for success as a coder. Job prospects are expected to be good.

Environmental Occupations

Individuals who work in environmental occupations develop and maintain therapeutic environments necessary to support patient care. Responsibilities include providing food services, cleaning and maintaining facilities and equipment, managing resources, and creating pleasant surroundings.

Nutrition and Dietary Service Occupations

Dietary service professionals support patients by planning and providing nutritious foods that are essential to the healing process. Therapeutic diets are sometimes prescribed by physicians for patients with specific health problems and conditions, such as high blood pressure and diabetes, and following abdominal surgery. (See Table 1–19.)

Table 1–19 Dietary Service Occupations

Career	Education	Testing and Licensure
Dietitian (RD)	Bachelor's degree (minimum)	Licensure, certification, or registration required in most states. Registration available from American Dietetic Association (ADA): 1. Complete educational program approved by ADA 2. Complete supervised experience 3. Pass national exam administered by Commission on Dietetic Registration
Dietetic Technician (DTR)/ Dietetic Assistant	Associate degree	Completed educational program approved by ADA Voluntary registration available from Commission on Dietetic Registration
Dietetic Aide	Certificate program in food services or on-the-job training	None

Dietetic Technician

Dietetic technicians work under the supervision of dietitians and perform tasks related to all aspects of food planning and preparation. They assist with creating menus, testing recipes, ordering food and supplies, and preparing meals. Some technicians work with patients to learn their food preferences and design special diets as ordered by a physician. Dietetic technicians must have good communication skills and be attentive to detail and able to follow specific directions. The projected employment rate is expected to be good.

Biomedical Engineering

The application of engineering to health care has resulted in the creation of sophisticated medical equipment that helps in diagnosing, treating, and monitoring patient conditions. Life-enhancing and lifesaving inventions resulting from biomedical engineering include the heart–lung machine, cardiac pacemakers, surgical lasers, and ultrasound technology. All engineering specialties, including electrical, mechanical, computer, and chemical, have been applied to seeking improvements in health care. (See Table 1–20.)

Biomedical Equipment Technician

Biomedical equipment technicians are specially trained to work on medical equipment that requires continual and competent maintenance to provide accurate diagnoses and reliable service to treat and monitor patients. Duties of the technician include installing, testing, servicing, and repairing all types of equipment. Technicians may specialize in one area, such as radiology or clinical laboratory equipment. Work in this area requires excellent manual dexterity, hand–eye coordination, mechanical aptitude, and interest in technology. Projected employment is expected to be much faster than average.

GETTING OFF TO A GOOD START

Health care educational programs are designed to prepare learners to succeed in the workplace. Instructors dedicate themselves to helping learners who put forth the necessary effort to graduate and become employed. Take advantage of the learning opportunities available in your school and commit yourself to doing your best toward becoming a competent, qualified health care professional.

Learning for Mastery

Health care professionals must know what they are doing. Mistakes on the job can result in serious consequences. Therefore, it is essential that learners commit to learning the material presented in their courses. Learning means more than just memorizing facts. It means striving to understand and remember

Table 1–20 Biomedical Engineering Occupations

Career	Education	Testing and Licensure
Biomedical Engineer	Bachelor's degree or higher	Licensed for some employment positions in some states Many states require passing exams administered by National Council of Examiners for Engineering and Surveying Certification also available from International Certification Commission for Clinical Engineering and Biomedical Technology (ICC): 1. Complete degree in engineering 2. Have at least 3 years experience as hospital clinical engineer 3. Pass both written and oral exams
Biomedical Equipment Technician	Associate degree	Certifications available from ICC: 1. Associate degree in biomedical engineering or specific combinations of training and experience 2. Pass written exam

information so that it can be applied to new situations. This understanding provides a basis for thinking like a health care professional, which was discussed earlier.

Learners who do only the minimum necessary to pass tests may think they are learning, but in reality, they are not likely to have acquired the long-term knowledge necessary to perform on the job. Learners who study to understand *and always search out the why of the subject* increase their chances of becoming highly competent health care professionals who can think on their feet and meet new challenges as they arise. If necessary, spend some time now working to improve your study skills: taking notes, reading, writing, and preparing for tests. See the suggested websites at the end of the chapter.

Getting the Most from Your Studies

People learn in different ways. One often-used method categorizes these differences by the senses used to receive and process new information. These categories are known as **learning styles**, and they are:

1. **Visual learner**: Learns best from seeing printed materials, images, colors, drawings, diagrams, maps, and films. Visual learners may find it difficult to follow lectures unless the instructor writes on the board, shows overheads, or demonstrates with models. They learn most easily from reading and studying drawings and charts.
2. **Auditory learner**: Learns best from hearing lectures, music, tapes, or rhymes. Auditory learners often find it difficult to follow printed material. They learn most easily when new material is explained orally.
3. **Kinesthetic learner**: Learns best from hands-on activities such as labs, practice, experiments, projects, games, and movement. Kinesthetic learners often do not really understand how to perform a procedure until they have performed it themselves. They even learn theoretical material best when activity is involved.

Although no one learns in only one way, each person has a dominant learning style or preference. Students who pay attention to their style can develop study techniques to get the most from their study time. For example, there are a variety of ways to learn the first aid techniques presented in Chapter 21:

- Visual: Study the illustrations in the text; watch a first aid video; make colored illustrations describing the procedures; read the chapter silently.

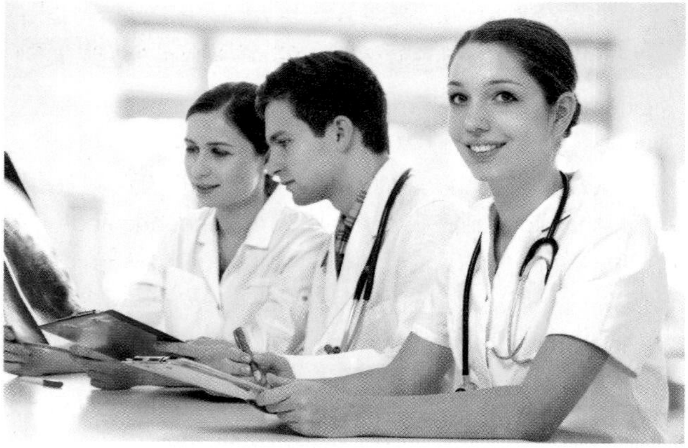

FIGURE 1–9 Individuals learn in different ways: by seeing, listening, and doing.

- Auditory: Listen to taped explanations of the techniques; read the chapter aloud; create rhymes to help remember information.
- Kinesthetic: Practice performing the techniques; read the chapter while pointing and moving finger down page; write in the book; study while standing up or moving about.

The more senses used in learning, the greater the chance that the information will be understood and remembered. This is why it is important for learners to read assignments before class (visual), attend all lectures (auditory), and participate fully in lab sessions (kinesthetic). (See Figure 1–9.)

Returning Adult Learners

Many learners who enroll in health care programs are adults returning to school after working in other fields, raising families, and/or handling other adult responsibilities. Some adults find the experience of attending classes stressful and wonder if they have what it takes to study and learn new information and skills.

These fears are natural, but the fact is that most adults have acquired life experiences and skills they can apply to their learning which, in many cases, will help them become excellent students. For example, holding down a job contributes to the ability to set priorities, communicate, demonstrate dependability, and apply practical skills such as math. The self-confidence developed as a result of handling adult responsibilities can be applied to reviewing one's study skills, including those that may not have been used for many years.

Perhaps the most pressing problem for adult students is finding the time to fulfill all their responsibilities: attending classes, studying, caring for the family, and perhaps holding down a full- or part-time job. Practicing good time management and personal organization skills, such as the following, can be helpful in handling the additional work of attending school:

- Start each day with a list of what needs to be accomplished, ranked from most to least important.
- Advise others of your study schedule. Plan care or activities for your children to allow you the time needed.
- Schedule time, even if for short periods, with family members. Some children enjoy doing homework with mom or dad.
- Create personal organization techniques, such as clustering errands, keeping things in repair, and planning backups to prevent wasting time and energy.
- Ask for help when you need it. Delegate tasks at home. Let the children fix dinner once or twice a week.

Establishing Good Work Habits

As a learner, you have many opportunities in school to begin to practice good workplace habits. Work hard now to develop the skills that will make you a valuable employee. At the same time, you can be acquiring habits that also contribute to academic success. The qualities essential for health care professionals that were listed at the beginning of the chapter can be applied in the classroom, in the lab, and at the clinical (externship/internship/fieldwork) site:

- Care about others: Show respect and consideration for instructors and classmates. Be kind to everyone, regardless of his or her background. Refrain from talking during lectures. Prepare for classes so the instructor does not need to take time to answer questions about material covered in the reading or study assignments. Practice courtesy in the classroom and throughout the school. Volunteer to help others, as needed or as possible.
- Have integrity: Do your own work. Never copy the homework assignments of others or cheat on exams. Always tell the truth. Never share anything told to you in confidence.

- Be dependable: Be at school on time and attend all classes. Complete assignments on time. Strive for accuracy in all written and practical assignments. Follow through on all obligations and anything you have volunteered to do.
- Work well with others: Be understanding of the needs of instructors and classmates. Participate in class. Do your share when working on group assignments.
- Be flexible: Accept instructional differences, changes in class schedules, and other unexpected occurrences. Be willing to cooperate as needed.
- Be willing to learn: Take your studies seriously. Make school a high priority. Dedicate sufficient time to studying throughout the length of each course to ensure maximum learning.

Learning to Think Like a Health Care Professional

A common problem in health care today is that many graduates spend months, or even years, accumulating information, but are unable to apply it when it is needed on the job. The lack of effective thinking skills is a primary reason for this unfortunate situation. Regardless of the health care area or occupational level chosen by learners, it is essential that they learn to *think* like health care professionals. This type of thinking actually involves many skills and, in this text, has the following meanings:

- Learning for understanding, not simply to memorize facts
- Applying learned material to new situations
- Having an organized approach to problem solving
- Basing decisions on facts, rather than on emotional reactions or **biases** (opinions made before facts are known)
- Drawing on many facts and creating relationships among them
- Locating reliable sources of information with which to make decisions
- Basing decisions on ethical principles (see Chapter 3)
- Practicing good communication skills when gathering and distributing information (see Chapters 16 and 17)
- Understanding exactly what one is legally allowed to do in one's profession, known as **scope of practice**

One of the major goals of this text is to provide learners with opportunities to practice thinking like a health care professional. The discussion on thinking is being presented at the beginning of the text so that learners will have maximum time to apply and practice thinking skills. The "Thinking It Through," "Application Exercises," and "Problem-Solving Practice" features, which appear in every chapter, encourage learners to apply thinking skills to the topics presented.

Thinking proficiently is much more than an academic skill. Although it is true that it is achieved through training and practice, its use is not restricted to school and certainly not to textbook exercises. It should be applied to the personal, as well as professional, areas of life. For example, buying a certain puppy simply because it is cute and seems the friendliest is an emotional decision. An informed, thinking decision involves some research to learn about available breeds, physical and personality characteristics, common health problems, and methods of training. Knowing these facts will help ensure that the puppy selected best fits the new owner's lifestyle and will be a suitable companion. Knowing ahead of time helps prevent future regrets.

Thinking like a health care professional can be described as an "examined process." This means not simply accepting situations without observing and thinking about the meaning of what is observed. Effective thinkers are aware of their thoughts and of why and how they are acting or making decisions.

As stated earlier, nothing in health care work can be done routinely and without thinking. Mindless actions occur as the result of not paying attention or basing decisions on ideas that have been accepted "just because." These ideas may come from family members, friends, personal experiences, television, movies, and magazines. Health care professionals must learn to think for themselves, gather facts, and use their own observations for making decisions. (See Figure 1–10.)

Using Questions in Thinking

An effective way for learners to start improving thinking skills is to ask themselves questions about what they are learning or doing. Questions serve to gather information, expand one's view of a subject,

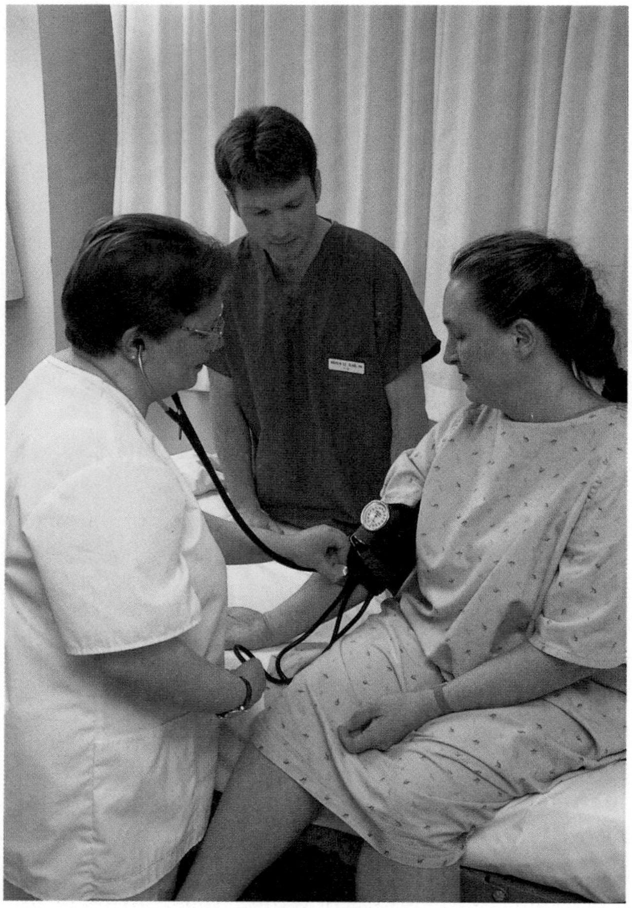

FIGURE 1–10 Observing carefully, asking questions, and thinking about what you are doing are essential in health care work.

and stimulate the mind. They help ensure that actions are not based on false assumptions or insufficient information.

Questions may be asked mentally (to oneself) or of others. Think of the five *W*s plus the one *H*: What, When, Where, Why, Who, and How. The following examples show how questions can be used to promote thinking:

- When learning new information, ask *why* it is important and to *whom? How* does it relate to what is already known?
- When working with patients, ask *what* might work best for them and *when* it should be done.
- When sharing important information with a coworker, ask yourself *what* you know about this person that will help you communicate most effectively.
- When working in a health care facility, consider *how* your work habits might be changed to improve overall efficiency.

Learners commonly believe that the role of their instructors is to *tell* them rather than *ask* them. In reality, instructors who continually ask questions that require learners to explain their answers and actions are encouraging them to think like health care professionals. Some instructors even respond to a learner's question with another question. Their intention is to teach learners to begin to think for themselves and trust that they are capable of finding the answer. Instructors also use questioning to guide learners in pulling known facts together, making connections, and applying what they know to new situations. For example, a respiratory therapy learner is working with a hospitalized patient. He has studied the illness presented by the patient and knows how to perform the prescribed breathing treatments. Through questioning, the instructor guides this learner to explain why these particular treatments have been prescribed. The learner is encouraged to consider the nature of the illness and the properties of the treatments and medications, and draw conclusions about the relationships among these factors.

Problem-Solving Process

Important applications of thinking skills are problem solving and decision making, two very important competencies for health care professionals. There are a variety of problem-solving and decision-making models. This book presents a five-step **problem-solving process** to help learners and health care professionals approach problem solving in an organized manner.

Step One—Identify the Problem

Identifying problems is not always as simple as it sounds. Factors that are described as *the problem* are often only *symptoms* of the problem. For example, Jamie, a radiologic technologist, does not receive the high scores she had hoped for on her performance review at work. When she receives the rating "poor" in the dependability category, she feels upset and believes that her problem is "receiving a poor evaluation because her supervisor dislikes her."

Identifying the real nature of problems requires a willingness to observe, pay attention, and confront difficult issues. Problem solvers must look beyond what seems obvious and use questions effectively to identify the real situation. Denying problems does not make them go away. Problems that are not addressed tend to get worse, because no action is being taken to resolve them. In Jamie's case, she must be willing to speak frankly with her supervisor about her low rating. It turns out that the real problem is actually what *caused* the poor evaluation, not the evaluation itself. In Jamie's case, it is her frequent tardiness.

Jamie's first reaction is, "I can't help it. My car is old and breaks down a lot." When her car won't start, she must rely on family and friends to drop her off at work. Their schedules are not the same as Jamie's, so she often arrives late.

Taking the time to think about what she has said ("I can't help it"), Jamie realizes that being at work on time is her responsibility. She is now able to identify the real problem: lack of reliable transportation. This enables her to start seeking effective solutions. Accepting responsibility for a problem makes it possible to start doing something about it.

Step Two—Gather Information

Good problem solving is based on having accurate and reliable information. Acting on assumptions (untested ideas), **opinions** (beliefs not based on facts or knowledge), and emotions is likely to result in poor decisions. In health care, gathering information is also known as **assessment**. There are many methods for gathering information:

- Review what is already known: What knowledge do I have about the problems or situation? About the causes? About possible solutions?
- Collect **objective data**: What can be observed? Measured? Tested? What are the facts? When working with patients, objective data are called **signs**.
- Collect **subjective data**: How do I feel about a situation? What do I want? What do others want? When working with patients, subjective data refer to what is reported by the patient, such as pain and feeling nauseated. Also known as **symptoms**, they cannot be directly observed or measured by the health care professional, but nevertheless must be taken into account.
- Conduct research: What are the facts? Are they from a **reliable** (trustworthy) source? How do I know? Are they scientifically based? (Can they be tested?)
- Ask for help: Who has useful knowledge? Are there experts available who can give me reliable information and help me find a solution?

When she starts out, Jamie finds the idea of solving her transportation problem overwhelming. The only solution that makes sense to her is buying a new car, but she knows that she probably cannot afford one at this time. When she puts her fear aside and commits herself to gathering information, she discovers the following:

- Carpools have been organized at the facility where she works.
- The most economical new car for sale in her area costs $15,595.
- *Consumer Reports* magazine has a recent article about purchasing used cars and publishes annual reports on the performance of most auto models manufactured over the past 10 years.
- Her credit union sponsors car sales to help buyers who have limited funds to spend. They also offer low-interest loans to buyers who qualify.
- A cousin has an older car that he wants to sell.
- There is a bus route within half a mile of her apartment.
- A local college offers a workshop that teaches people how to buy a car.
- The local high school has an auto-mechanic training program. For a small fee, students will check over used cars before they are purchased.

Step Three—Create Alternatives

The third step in problem solving is to create a list of alternatives. Ideas for solutions and actions are generated based on the information collected. All possibilities should be considered before one is selected. Some alternatives may prove, on further investigation, to be impractical or unworkable. It is essential to think through each one and consider the likely consequences, both positive and negative.

Based on her research, Jamie creates the following list:

1. Take the bus to work. When the weather is nice, walking to the bus stop will be a good form of exercise. In rainy weather, common about five months of the year where she lives, getting to the bus stop without getting soaked is not likely.

Thinking It Through

Linda Stevens, LPN, works on a medical floor at the local hospital. One of the patients she has been assigned to take care of is Frank Gibbons, a 72-year-old newly diagnosed with diabetes (a condition in which the body does not produce enough insulin to control blood sugar levels). Part of Linda's process of preparing to care for her patients is to review the patients' charts for any new physician orders. She notes that Dr. Romero was in the previous evening and ordered the patient's blood sugar to be checked at 8 a.m. According to the results, insulin is to be given. (The higher the level of blood sugar, the greater the amount of insulin that is given, based on a formula defined by the physician.) Linda is a "thinking nurse" and starts to question if this is an appropriate order. She realizes that breakfast trays arrive at 7:30 a.m. on her floor and that Mr. Gibbons will already have eaten when she checks his insulin level at 8 a.m. She knows that after eating, a person's blood sugar normally increases for a few hours. This is why blood sugar tests are usually ordered when the patient has not eaten for a number of hours. Linda reasons that if she calculates the amount of insulin based on the temporarily elevated blood sugar levels, Mr. Gibbons will receive too much insulin and may have a negative reaction. Linda calls Dr. Romero to clarify the order. Dr. Romero states that he believed the breakfast trays did not arrive until 8:30 a.m. He thanks Linda for catching the error and changes the order.

- What might have happened if Linda had simply performed the blood sugar test exactly as ordered?
- Do you think Linda should have been considered responsible for the error if she had followed the orders exactly?
- Review the five *Ws* and *How* question in relation to this situation. Give examples of questions that Linda may have asked herself.

Also, the bus ride takes about 30 minutes longer, each way, than driving to work.

2. Take the workshop on how to buy a car, then purchase a used one through the credit union. The monthly car payments and higher insurance rates will mean having to budget carefully to meet all expenses. Chances of buying a "lemon" can be reduced by using the service offered at the high school.
3. Continue to rely on others for rides to work. (Nonaction is also an alternative.)
4. Ask her father for a loan to buy a new car. While Jamie would like to have a shiny new car, she has been financially independent for several years and prefers to remain that way.

Some potential alternatives do not appear on the above list because of information acquired during step two:

1. Carpool participants must have a reliable vehicle of their own. This might be an alternative later, if she purchases a dependable car.
2. Her cousin's car has more than 175,000 miles and is not one of the more reliable models, according to the reports she studied.

Step Four—Choose an Alternative and Take Action

Step four is critical. A common difficulty in problem solving and decision making is failure to act. Opportunities are missed and accomplishments not realized when there is no follow-through.

Jamie decides to combine two alternatives. There are five months of dry weather ahead, so she decides to take the bus to work. She will use the extra riding time to read and keep up with advances in radiology. In October, she plans to buy a used car. In the meantime, she will create a personal budget to control expenses, save money, and learn more about how to buy a car and which model is likely to give her the best value.

Step Five—Evaluate and Revise as Needed

Evaluation means reviewing the results of the actions taken. Even well-thought-out plans can prove to be ineffective or have unexpected, negative consequences. And circumstances can change. It is sometimes necessary to make adjustments or choose another alternative. It may even require going back to step two to gather additional information and go through the process again.

When applying the process to health care work, it is important to remember that the needs of patients and facilities may change and/or additional information may become available. This can affect the process and force revisions to be made before the entire process has been completed. Problem solving is a continual process.

WORKBOOK PRACTICE

Go to your workbook and complete the exercises for this chapter.

SUGGESTED LEARNING ACTIVITIES

1. Create a personal plan for developing the core qualities demonstrated by health care professionals.
2. Seek opportunities to observe health care professionals at work. Report on the qualities they demonstrate that you believe make them effective.
3. Research an occupational area or specific career that interests you: interview a working professional, send for information or visit the Internet site of the appropriate professional organization (see Appendix 1), request a job description from a local facility, and/or read the job descriptions in the *Occupational Outlook Handbook*. (See additional websites listed in the "Suggested Readings and Resources" at the end of the chapter.)
4. Identify your preferred learning style and create five study techniques to help you master your class subjects.
5. Choose a problem in your life that you would like to work on and apply the five steps of the problem-solving process. Report on the results.

WEB ACTIVITIES

Occupational Outlook Handbook

www.bls.gov/oco

Locate an occupation of interest by clicking on "Healthcare" in the Occupation Groups list. Using the information provided, write a description of the occupation that includes significant points, desirable personal qualities, job outlook, and typical earnings.

Health Care Professional Organizations

Explore the website of a professional organization from Appendix 1 for a career that interests you. Write a report describing the information and services provided by the organization.

Study Guides and Strategies

www.studygs.net

Click on "Problem solving/decision making." Read the information and list five strategies you believe might help you with problem solving.

REVIEW QUESTIONS

1. List the seven core qualities that every health care professional should demonstrate.
2. Give examples of behavior that demonstrate each core quality.
3. List and describe the three major types of approvals that certify the competency of health care professionals.
4. What are the four major categories of health care occupations? Describe the type of work performed in each.
5. What are the educational and licensing requirements of the health care occupation in which you are most interested?
6. What is the meaning of "learning for mastery"?
7. Describe the three learning styles and provide two examples of appropriate learning activities for each.
8. What are some skills that adult learners bring from their life experience when they return to school to study a health career?
9. What are five techniques that adult learners can use to stay organized and manage their time efficiently?
10. How can the core health care professional qualities be applied at school?
11. What does it mean to "think like a health care professional"? Give two examples.
12. What are the five steps in the problem-solving process?

APPLICATION EXERCISES

1. Refer back to The Case of the Confused Learner at the beginning of the chapter. Using the information in this chapter, list your recommendations for occupations that Kevin should investigate.
2. Juan has always been interested in helping people. He also likes science and has maintained good grades throughout high school in chemistry, biology, and physics. He has enrolled in the local community college and is taking "Introduction to Health Care." Juan thinks that a career in health care might be for him, but he doesn't feel that he knows enough to make a career decision at this time. He's not sure what's out there or what jobs would be appropriate for him.
   a. What does Juan need to know in order to conduct an effective career search?
   b. Describe how he can use the problem-solving process to help him make a tentative career decision.
   c. Explain methods that Juan can use to research and learn more about different career options.

PROBLEM-SOLVING PRACTICE

Brenda has thought about being a dental assistant for a long time and has just enrolled in a one-year educational program. She wants to do well in school, but she is having trouble finding reliable day care for her two young children. Describe how she might use the five-step problem-solving process to ensure that she attends all her classes and that her children receive proper care.

SUGGESTED READINGS AND RESOURCES

Adult Student.com. www.adultstudent.com

Education-Portal. Articles and videos for researching careers. http://education-portal.com

Explore Health Careers. www.explorehealthcareers.org

Mind Tools. Information on essential career skills such as problem solving, decision making, and memory improvement. www.mindtools.com

Occupational outlook handbook. 2014 edition. Online version. www.bls.gov/oco/home.htm

*O*Net*. Detailed information about occupations, including skills and aptitude needed, and tasks performed. Sponsored by the U.S. Department of Labor. www.onetonline.org

Study Guides and Strategies. Information on time management, learning, thinking, studying, problem solving, decision making, and specific study skills. www.studygs.net

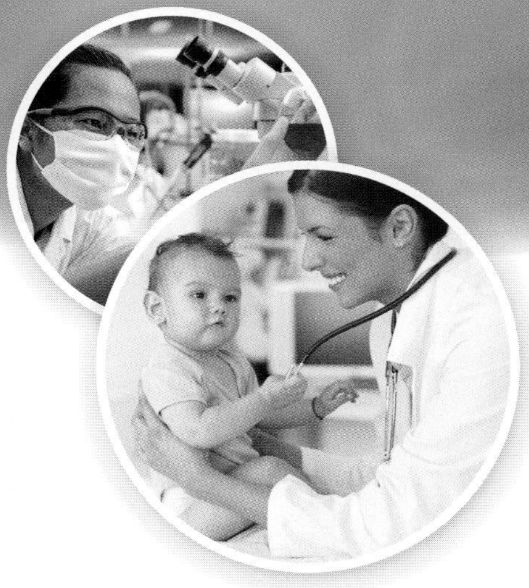

Chapter 2

Current Health Care Systems and Trends

OBJECTIVES

Studying and applying the material in this chapter will help you to:

- Describe 10 significant events in the history of health care that changed the way care was delivered.
- Describe the major forces in the health care industry today.
- Describe the levels of care offered by the modern hospital.
- List 10 ambulatory health care facilities and give examples of the type of services offered by each one.
- Describe the major types of long-term care facilities.
- Provide examples of health care services and care that can be provided in the patient's home.
- Explain the purpose of hospice.
- List typical services offered by federal, state, and local health agencies.
- Explain the concept of wellness.
- Describe the types of complementary and alternative medicine being practiced in the United States today.
- List five challenges facing health care today and explain how the health care professional can contribute to their resolution.

KEY TERMS

acupuncture

adult foster home (also called adult foster care)

alternative medicine

Alzheimer's disease

assisted living residence

chiropractic

complementary medicine

continuing care community

dementia

expanding consciousness

gene therapy

guided imagery

holistic medicine

homeopathy

hospice

inpatient

integrative medicine

intermediate nursing care facility (INCF)

massage therapy

Medicaid

(continues)

KEY TERMS (continued)

- medical mall
- medication adherence
- nursing homes
- opioids
- osteopathy
- outpatient services
- palliative
- pandemic
- psychiatric hospital
- psychosomatic
- skilled nursing facility (SNF)
- targeted drug therapy
- vital statistics
- wellness

The Case of the Confused Daughter

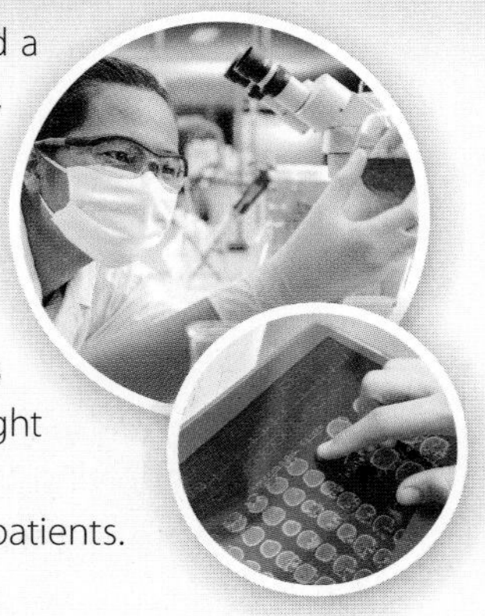

Until recently, Dora Freemont, age 87, lived alone in a small apartment. Last week she suffered a slight stroke. After several days in the hospital, she is ready to be discharged. Her daughter, Sally, is very concerned that her widowed mother is no longer capable of living alone and handling all her housekeeping and personal needs. She shares her concern with Angela Cisneros, one of the nurses who cared for her mother during her hospital stay. Sally is very worried and fears she will have to quit work in order to help take care of her mother. Angela knows that there are a variety of long-term care facilities and a number of options available for Mrs. Freemont. She refers Sally to the hospital social worker, who explains these options and discusses with her which might be most appropriate for her mother.

This chapter provides learners with important information they can use to assist their future patients. It also helps learners understand the many settings in which they can seek employment.

THE HEALTH CARE INDUSTRY TODAY

The health care industry is the largest service employer in the United States. Federal economists report that in 2013, the amount spent on health care was $2.9 trillion or an average of $9255 per person. Further, it is projected that between 2013 and 2023, the cost of health care will grow an average of 5.7% annually (Centers for Medicare and Medicaid Services, 2013). Many factors are shaping the delivery of health care today. It is important for health care professionals to understand the characteristics of and forces behind this enormous industry. These will surely influence their working conditions, as well as determine what it takes for them to be successful on the job.

Technological Advancements

The long history of health care was marked by gradual change until the beginning of the 20th century. Table 2–1 contains a summary of significant events in the history of medicine. Starting about 100 years ago, the rate of discovery and change increased rapidly so that in the last few decades, medical technology and diagnostic and treatment methods advanced more than in the previous 100 years. At the beginning of the 1900s, the major killers were infectious diseases, the leading causes being influenza and pneumonia. Between 1918 and 1919, an influenza **pandemic** killed between 20 and 40 million people across the globe. Physicians at that time had a limited number of treatment techniques available. Because of the discovery of penicillin and antibiotics, along with the widespread use of immunizations, many infectious diseases are almost unheard of today.

Modern discoveries and inventions build upon one another, increasing the rate of growth of new developments. There are now an amazing number of treatments, including organ transplantation, microscopic and robotic surgery, **gene therapy**, and **targeted drug therapy**. Pharmaceuticals are the leading prevention and treatment option today, and new drugs are being developed rapidly. Keeping informed about these changes and learning to use and apply new equipment and techniques will be a continual and interesting challenge for the health care professional of the 21st century. (See Chapter 14 to learn more about continuing education in health care and Chapter 18 for more information about technology in health care.)

Table 2–1 History of Health Care

Time Frame	Event	Impact
Ancient Times (???–A.D. 400)	Study of fossilized bones and Egyptian mummies indicates many modern health conditions, such as arthritis, infectious bone diseases, appendicitis, arteriosclerosis, and urinary and intestinal diseases.	Health care problems and diseases have been with us from the beginning of human life.
	Belief system based on supernatural rather than natural laws. Causes of disease were expected to be supernatural (caused by spirits, ghosts, or gods).	Home remedies were used and rituals performed to drive away the evil spirits. Examples of rituals are creating loud noises, beating the ill person, or bloodletting.
		Preventive medicine consisted of wearing amulets and mutilating or painting the body to ward off evil spirits.
	Life span was only 20–35 years.	Chronic illnesses were rare.
	Hippocrates of Cos (460–379 B.C.) was the most famous Greek physician of ancient times. He stressed observation and conservative treatment. Believed that health was the balance of four humors.	Called the "Father of Medicine," he used dietetics as a means of balancing the humors. Only if diet failed would he resort to drugs or surgery.
Medieval Times (A.D. 400–1350)	Two plagues (in A.D. 543 and 568) killed majority of the people and led to breakdown in civilization.	Monks preserved written medical texts and monasteries served as centers of learning to maintain knowledge.
	Christianity became an increasing center of power. Believed that disease was punishment for sins, possession by devil, or result of witchcraft.	Christians emphasized saving the soul, not the body. Treatment methods were prayer, penitence, and the assistance of saints. Any cure was considered a miracle.
	At the Council of Tours in 1163, the Catholic church proclaimed that "blood is not to be shed" by physicians.	Because most physicians were clergymen in the Catholic church, these practitioners were no longer able to perform surgery.
	The title of Doctor became known and major medical legislation was written in 1140 and 1224 that specified a 9-year curriculum with state examinations and licenses.	Medicine became an official profession, although there were not enough physicians for the population. As a result, lower-class citizens still relied on barbers and lay healers.
	Black Plague of 1348 killed a large percentage of European population.	Concept of quarantine as preventive measure was recognized.
	Network of hospitals were built.	Marked a new and more humane approach toward the ill. Hospitals were primarily a refuge for the sick, old, disabled, or homeless.
Renaissance (1350–1650)	Revival of learning and science. Tremendous growth in inquiry of how the body was structured and how it worked. Numerous autopsies were performed.	First attempts to connect autopsy results with clinical observations made during life. Accurate anatomical drawings were now available for study.

(continues)

Table 2–1 History of Health Care (continued)

Time Frame	Event	Impact
	Despite the new advances, it was still a time of tremendous filth in the cities and among their people, characterized by the spread of disease and extreme superstitions.	Criticisms of the old ways were frequently met with hatred.
	Study of botany (plants) greatly expanded as travel between countries increased.	Plants were the main source of drugs; 500 new plant species were categorized and the first modern pharmacopoeia written.
	Girolamo Fracastoro wrote a book in 1546 in which he presented the first theory of contagious diseases.	Theory was not taken seriously and would not be proven for several centuries. High incidence of infections continued as handwashing and hygiene were not considered important (e.g., a physician would perform autopsy and then go do surgery without washing his hands).
	Printing press invented.	Allowed for widespread distribution of new information and books.
	Invention of gunpowder resulted in numerous gunshot wounds during frequent wars.	Need for surgical treatment of wounds elevated barber-surgeons to a higher status.
17th Century	Increasing interest in experimentation and observation.	Studies in anatomy continued, but the study of physiology (how the body functions) was also now investigated.
	William Harvey, an Englishman, stated that blood circulates throughout the body within a continuous network of vessels. Only the mechanical aspects of the system were addressed.	Vehemently opposed at first, this discovery led to the realization that medications could be injected into the circulatory system, and blood could be transfused. After many failed attempts, it fell out of favor for several centuries.
	In 1666, Anton van Leeuwenhoek invented the microscope.	Study of microscopic anatomy and visualization of organisms were now possible. Germs were only viewed under the microscope; the connection with disease came several centuries later.
	Quinine imported from Peru as a cure for malaria.	Separated malaria from other types of fevers. Confirmed the idea that specific diseases have specific cures.
	The study of the brain and psychology was of interest. (Prior to this time, a common belief was that the soul resided in the pineal gland and the rest of the body was purely mechanical in nature.)	Nervous system and stimulation of muscles discovered. The long-believed theory that mucus from a head cold was produced by the brain was disproved.

(continues)

Table 2–1 History of Health Care (continued)

Time Frame	Event	Impact
18th Century	Researchers and theorists still struggled with an explanation of how the body functioned.	Three theories were proposed. First, that the body functioned like a hydraulic pump that was run by an undefined fluid flowing through the nervous system. Second, that every disease was the result of overstimulation or inability to respond to stimulation. Treatment was then either a depressant or a stimulant (e.g., opium and alcohol). Third, that direct clinical observation should be used to define and categorize diseases. (This led to the absurd description of 2400 different diseases; the same diseases were listed many times, just because the symptoms varied slightly between cases.)
	Surgery became a respected form of treatment in France after the court physician successfully repaired an anal fistula for King Louis XIV.	Surgery was upgraded from a craft to an experimental science. Procedures were developed that could cure problems that were treatable only through surgery.
	In 1761, Giovanni Battista Morgagni of Padua published a comprehensive book titled *On the Sites and Causes of Disease.*	Emphasis changed from concentration on general conditions and humors to specific changes in organs.
	Techniques for measuring blood pressure and temperature were developed.	Measurements of vital signs were used to monitor patient status.
	Science of chemistry came of age.	Digestion was now seen as a chemical process, rather than a purely mechanical process or one of putrefaction.
	The philosophy of "enlightenment" was developed, which stressed the rational approach to problems and dissemination of knowledge for others to study.	Numerous studies and experiments added rapidly to the expanding base of knowledge. Sharing of knowledge with others added to the increasing pace of progress.
	Focus went from belief in the devil and "possession" to recognition of mental illness as a disease. Previously, patients were locked up in filthy conditions, as mental illness was thought to be due to possession, sin, crime, or vice.	Mentally ill patients were released from their chains and treated in a more humane way.
	Preventive health came to the forefront in the form of public health.	Sanitary reform was initiated in hospitals, prisons, and military. Personal hygiene also improved dramatically.
	Interest in child health increased.	Decreased the appalling rate of deaths in infants and children.
	Edward Jenner (1749–1823) demonstrated that vaccination with cowpox provides immunity for smallpox.	Countless lives were saved. It opened the door into investigation for other vaccines to be developed.

(continues)

Table 2–1 History of Health Care (continued)

Time Frame	Event	Impact
19th Century	Industrial Revolution created growth of city population as peasants flooded into the city. Hospitals were built that could hold many patients.	Large hospital populations allowed for the clinical observation of many cases, followed by autopsy when a patient died.
	Advances in physiology continued.	Emphasis moved from individual organs to the identification of more specific tissues. For example, inflammation of the heart was now stated as endocarditis, pericarditis, or myocarditis (inflammation of one of the three layers of the heart).
	Tremendous increase in medical knowledge was acquired and documented. Physicians and surgeons were united into one profession.	Many first-time surgical operations were performed, such as tracheostomy and removal of thyroid and uterus. Medical profession started to develop specialty areas, such as pediatrics, psychiatry, dermatology (skin), public health, and preventive medicine.
	Medicine based on observation and autopsies had offered all it could to the field. Further advances would need the study and application of the sciences.	Study shifted from practicing physicians to full-time scientific researchers.
	More powerful microscopes were developed.	Human tissue could now be seen at the cellular level.
	Advances were made in chemistry.	Laboratory tests for diagnostic purposes became common. Metabolism and dietetics came under scientific study. Pharmacology was established as a new science.
	Dentists introduced anesthesia, and this practice expanded to major surgical procedures.	Large-scale surgery could now be done. Death rate fell as anesthesia decreased shock and the need for speed in surgery.
	Elizabeth Blackwell (1821–1910) was the first woman MD in the United States. She opened the first nursing school in the United States in 1860.	Medical education opened for the first time to a female. Nursing was established as a profession in the United States.
	Louis Pasteur (1822–1895), a chemist, proved that specific microorganisms called bacteria are the cause of specific diseases in both humans and animals.	The results of his work led to the development of the germ theory.
	It was discovered that infectious microorganisms are carried by various means (e.g., humans, animals, mosquitoes, food). Specific identification of microorganisms led to the development of vaccines for prevention.	Revolutionized the ability to prevent, diagnose, and treat infectious diseases. Then in 1864, Lord Joseph Lister, MD, applied the germ theory to his surgical practice by reasoning that microorganisms could also fall into open surgical wounds.

(continues)

Table 2–1 History of Health Care (continued)

Time Frame	Event	Impact
	Anesthesia, asepsis, and invention of a variety of surgical instruments changed the face of medicine forever.	Previously the public viewed hospitals as a place one went to die. Now there was hope of recovery for the first time. Many more advanced surgeries could be performed (e.g., on joints, abdomen, head, spinal column).
	Psychiatry had come to a dead end as it eluded the scientific advances of the day. No satisfactory explanation of mental illness could be given.	Sigmund Freud (1856–1939), an Austrian neurologist, and Joseph Breuer developed the theory of psychoanalysis and presented it to the public in their book on hysteria in 1893. The theory was based on using hypnosis to allow patients to recall prior traumatic and repressed events. Freud later discarded hypnosis and based his new theory on repression of sexual urges as the central theme of psychological illnesses.
	Preventive medicine made great strides as pasteurization, vaccination, asepsis, and sanitation were implemented.	Life span increased from 40 years in 1850 to 70 years in 1950 due primarily to preventive, not curative, measures.
20th Century	In 1921, Karl Landsteiner of Vienna discovered blood groups.	Made transfusion of blood products safe for the first time in history.
	Insulin was extracted and tested for treatment of diabetes.	Diabetes was no longer considered a fatal disease, but could be managed with injections of insulin.
	Large-scale vaccination programs were conducted.	Many commonly feared infectious diseases were eradicated. But the influenza epidemic of 1918 that killed 20 million brought reality back after the euphoria of success.
	New diagnostic and therapeutic techniques were developed. The field of biomedical engineering was advanced with the invention of the computer.	X-rays, electrocardiograph (ECG), electroencephalograph (EEG), ultrasound, pacemakers, dialysis, and tomography provided physicians with more diagnostic and therapeutic tools.
	Vitamins were discovered; the United States took the leadership role in this research.	The belief that all diseases were caused by microbes was disproved when lack of certain vitamins was linked to various diseases (e.g., scurvy, beriberi).
	New synthetic drugs were developed to treat specific problems.	Chemotherapy was used to fight cancer. Antibiotics were developed to fight various infections caused by bacteria. Medications for treating allergies were developed.
	Life span increased 70–80 years.	Geriatrics became a specialty. Chronic illnesses were very common.

(continues)

Table 2–1 History of Health Care (continued)

Time Frame	Event	Impact
	Mental illness became an increasing problem in modern society.	Shock treatment and psychosurgery were replaced with new drugs and psychotherapy. Tranquilizers, used to calm patients, changed the approach to and assessment of mental patients.
	The end of the 19th and beginning of the 20th centuries were so laboratory and science based, with increasing specialization, that the patient focus was lost. It has always been known that mental processes can profoundly affect bodily illnesses and symptoms or even cause them, but this was lost in the science of medicine.	The increasing specialization continued to cloud this issue as specialization broke the individual into various parts rather than treating the patient as a holistic being (i.e., different physicians are seen for cardiac, intestinal, and neurological conditions; one physician may diagnose the problem and another do the surgery).
	Other health care specialties developed as the knowledge base increased (e.g., physical therapy, occupational therapy, speech therapy).	Increased number of practitioners came in contact with the patient and viewed the concerns from a specialty focus versus holistic perspective.
	Health care costs increased due to increased specialization of knowledge and cost of technological advancements, which put health care services beyond the reach of many.	This social issue had been present for many centuries, but increased literacy, availability of information, and global awareness increased the dissatisfaction of those unable to access health care. The question was raised, "Does everyone have an equal right to health care?"
	Surgical techniques and anesthesia methods made great advancements. Transplantation of organs was now possible.	Heart, brain, and prosthetic joint replacements were performed. Definition of death was changed from cessation of heart and lung function to demonstration of brain death by EEG.
	People could be kept alive by mechanical means beyond the point of having any quality of life.	Emphasis was placed on people having written living wills to specify what they do and do not want done to prolong their lives. In 1975, the New Jersey Supreme Court ruled that the parents of a comatose woman could authorize the removal of life support systems.
	Patients with terminal illnesses publicly expressed the wish to die with dignity.	England opened the first hospice in 1967. Dr. Jack Kevorkian argued that patients should be allowed to request assistance to end their lives. Between 1990 and 1998, he participated in a number of physician-assisted suicides.
	Development of new and faster machines (e.g., automobiles, airplanes, various recreational vehicles) caused many accidental injuries.	Trauma medicine became a specialty.

(continues)

Table 2–1 History of Health Care (continued)

Time Frame	Event	Impact
	Mass media became available to public (e.g., television, radio, newspapers, Internet). Medical physicians were often seen as cold and uncaring as a result of their focus on trying to find a diagnosis.	Quackery medicine had greater access to the public, generating huge sales of products. Outrageous claims of quick-acting results and complete cures requiring very little effort were a strong draw compared with other forms of health care.
	Scientific approach was used almost exclusively. Traditional medicine primarily based on diagnosis and then treatment with synthetic medications and surgical procedures. Rejection of herbal and alternative therapies by many traditional medical practitioners.	Practitioners of traditional medicine rejected the "old methods" that had been useful in the past but had not been scientifically proven. People flocked to herbalists and alternative therapists in search for more natural therapies, but lack of regulation in these areas resulted in many abuses.
	Genetic research into cause of certain diseases and conditions.	Identification of specific genes related to certain conditions, but how to alter to prevent condition was yet to be discovered.
	In 1978, the first "test tube" baby was born in England.	Opened up opportunity for couples previously unable to have children.
	In 1981, acquired immunodeficiency syndrome (AIDS) was identified as a disease.	Huge challenge to medical research that resulted in medications that prolonged life but did not cure the disease.
	First successful cloning of sheep in 1997.	Opened door for human cloning and growth of organs for transplantation.
21st Century and Beyond—What Is Possible?	Some of the hopes for the new millennium: • Vaccine to prevent human immunodeficiency virus (HIV) • Cure for AIDS • Cure for obesity • Cloning of organs for transplantation to overcome extreme difficulty in finding suitable organ donors • Development of medication specific to a person's genotype to optimize treatment • Cures for heart disease, hypertension, and cancer • More effective treatment and cure for mental illnesses • Preventive health and alternative therapies used in a complementary way with practice of traditional medicine • Life span of healthy living expanded to 100+ years • Less invasive diagnostic and therapeutic treatments and medications with less harmful side effects	When health care professionals several centuries into the future look back at the 21st century, they will be astounded. This reaction would be similar to ours when we look back to previous centuries and are mystified by the ignorance and resulting unnecessary human suffering.

Specialization

Another significant trend in health care over the last 30 years has been the specialization of medicine (Williams, 2005). (Recall the large number of physician specialties listed in Box 1–2.) This has had several important effects on health care delivery:

- Diagnosis and treatment are improving as physicians and other practitioners concentrate on specific areas of expertise, such as endocrinology and cardiology.
- Medical practice is more technical and fragmented, because specialists treat one aspect, rather than the patient as a whole.
- The cost of providing health care has increased.
- Long-term relationships between physicians and their patients are breaking down because one physician no longer provides all or most of the needed care.

Specialization has created many employment opportunities for health care professionals. At the same time, it has increased the need for caring attitudes and effective communication with patients. Lifelong relationships developed between physicians and their patients are rare today. Much of the care is provided to patients by professionals they do not know. Therefore, you may play an important part in helping patients understand and have confidence in the care they are receiving.

Aging Population

Improvements in medical care, especially the development of new drugs and surgical techniques, have lengthened the average life span. Life expectancy for a male born in 1900 was 46 years, and 48 years for a female. This increased dramatically; for the total population in 2010, life expectancy was 78.7 years for a male and 81 years for a female (Centers for Disease Control and Prevention [CDC], May 2014).

A second reason for the growing number of seniors is the continuing aging of the group known as the "baby boomers." An unusually large number of births occurred during the years following the end of World War II, starting in 1946 and lasting until 1964. These individuals have started and will continue entering their period of heaviest use of the health care system over the next 20 years. (See Figure 2–1.)

Older persons are the heaviest users of health care services. The tremendous growth of this segment of the population is putting increased demands on all types of services, including the following:

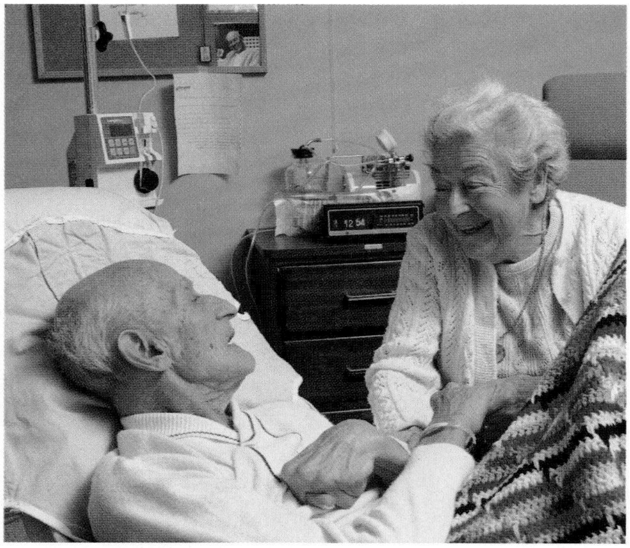

FIGURE 2–1 Today's growing population of older patients is putting increasing demands on the modern health care system.

- Facilities that provide long-term care for older persons unable to live in their own homes
- Treatment and care devoted to chronic (persisting for a long time, not cured quickly) problems that develop in people who live longer
- Home care services ranging from housekeeping duties to high-level nursing care
- Increasing incidence of Alzheimer's disease (discussed later in this chapter)

Fascinating Facts

It seems incredible that the importance of handwashing to prevent the spread of infection, a basic health care practice now taken for granted, was discovered less than 200 years ago. Ignaz Semmelweis, working in a hospital maternity ward in Vienna, became concerned about the high death rate of new mothers. He observed that it occurred most often among women who were assisted in childbirth by physicians who came directly from performing autopsies. Amazingly, his beliefs were rejected by colleagues. This is an example of how new ideas are often met with resistance and how being open to change can improve—and even save—the lives of many.

Increasing Costs

The cost of providing health care has increased dramatically over the past few decades. While every product and service has steadily increased in price over the years, health care costs have grown at a faster rate than almost anything else. This is due to several factors:

- Technological advances, resulting in the use of very expensive equipment and supplies
- Increasing number of elderly citizens, resulting in higher numbers of patients seeking services
- Rising prices of pharmaceutical products, which make up the most widely used methods of treatment
- Increasing number of diagnostic tests and treatment options available
- Extensive use of diagnostic tests to both help patients and protect physicians against malpractice lawsuits
- Lack of competition in some areas that decreases efficiency and does not provide incentives to lower costs
- Rising expectations of patients that health care should provide more effective solutions
- More effective treatments that encourage increasing numbers of patients to seek medical care
- Poor distribution of physicians and other health care providers

  (Source: Adapted from *Introduction to Health Services* [7th ed.], by S. J. Williams and P. R. Torrens, 2008, Clifton Park, NY: Delmar Cengage Learning.)

Two other factors that contribute to high health care costs are waste and fraud. In 2012, the Institute of Medicine reported that about 30 cents of every dollar, or $750 billion, spent annually on health care is wasted on unneeded care, huge amounts of paperwork, and fraud. (Alonso-Zaldivar, 2012). The report broke this amount into six categories of waste:

$210 billion	Unnecessary services
$190 billion	Excess administrative costs
$130 billion	Inefficient delivery of care
$105 billion	Inflated prices
$55 billion	Prevention failures
$75 billion	Fraud

The report suggested that health care costs could be better controlled without decreasing the quality of care. Reforms suggested include demanding greater accountability from hospitals and major medical groups and encouraging more collaboration among medical professionals (Alonso-Zaldivar, 2012).

In response to skyrocketing health care costs, new methods have been and continue to be developed to deliver and pay for health care. At the same time, efforts are being made to control costs. (See Chapter 22.) Figure 2–2 shows where U.S. health care dollars originated and were spent in 2013.

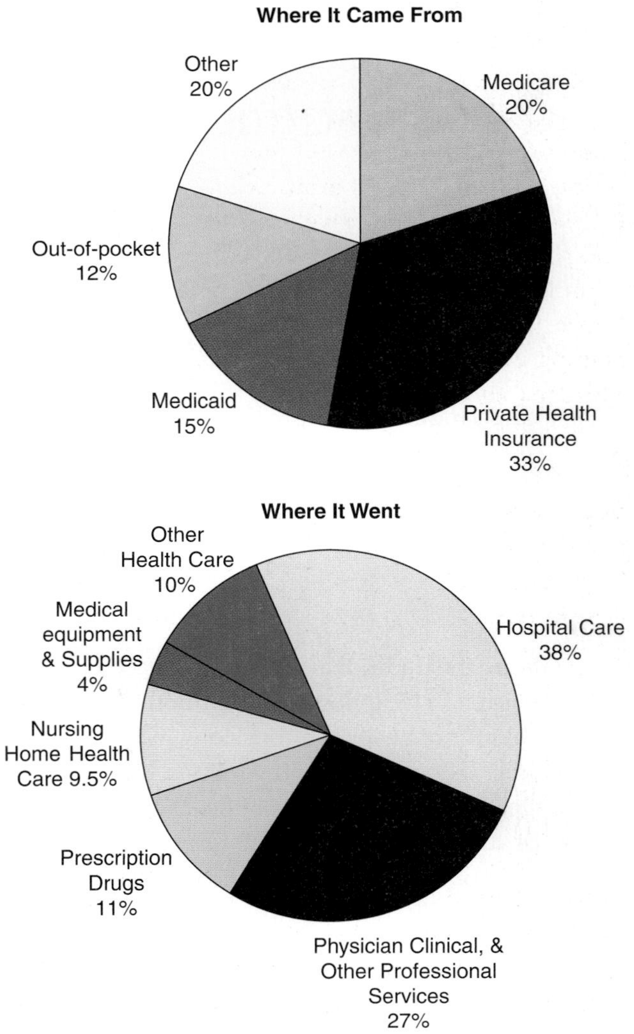

FIGURE 2–2 Health care spending in the United States—2013.

Thinking It Through

Joseph Appleton's primary care physician has referred him to Dr. Nester, an oncologist (physician who specializes in diagnosis and treatment of cancer). Preliminary tests show that Mr. Appleton may have colon cancer. Mr. Appleton, age 77, is uncomfortable about visiting a specialist he has never met. He is especially distraught about the possibility of having a life-threatening illness and does not understand why the physician he has seen for many years cannot take care of the problem. Carmen Rodriguez, Dr. Nester's medical assistant, greets Mr. Appleton on his first visit to the office.

1. Discuss the changes in health care delivery that have led to the referral of patients to specialists.
2. What can Carmen do to help Mr. Appleton feel more comfortable?

HEALTH CARE FACILITIES AND SERVICES

A wide variety of health care facilities are available that offer many services for patients with all types of needs. They range in size from a private physician's office to nationwide health care systems that include hospitals, clinics, and long-term care facilities. (See Figure 2–3.) Health care facilities offer many kinds of services, ranging from preventive care to emergency treatment; from routine physical exams to in-home assistance for dying patients. There are many kinds of employment settings for today's health care professional.

Hospitals

Hospitals are the traditional facilities for the care of the ill and injured. The following conditions accounted for the majority of hospital admissions in 2012: births, pneumonia, osteoarthritis (fractures), heart attack and congestive heart failure, septicemia, mood disorders, cardiac dysrhythmias (abnormal heart beat), and chronic obstructive pulmonary disease (COPD) (Pfuntner, Wier, & Stocks, 2013). In the past, most patients remained in the hospital for all care needed until they were able to return home. The cost of hospital care has increased so dramatically that other means of patient care have been developed to limit the number and length of patient stays. Hospitals are now just one of many facilities that provide patient care.

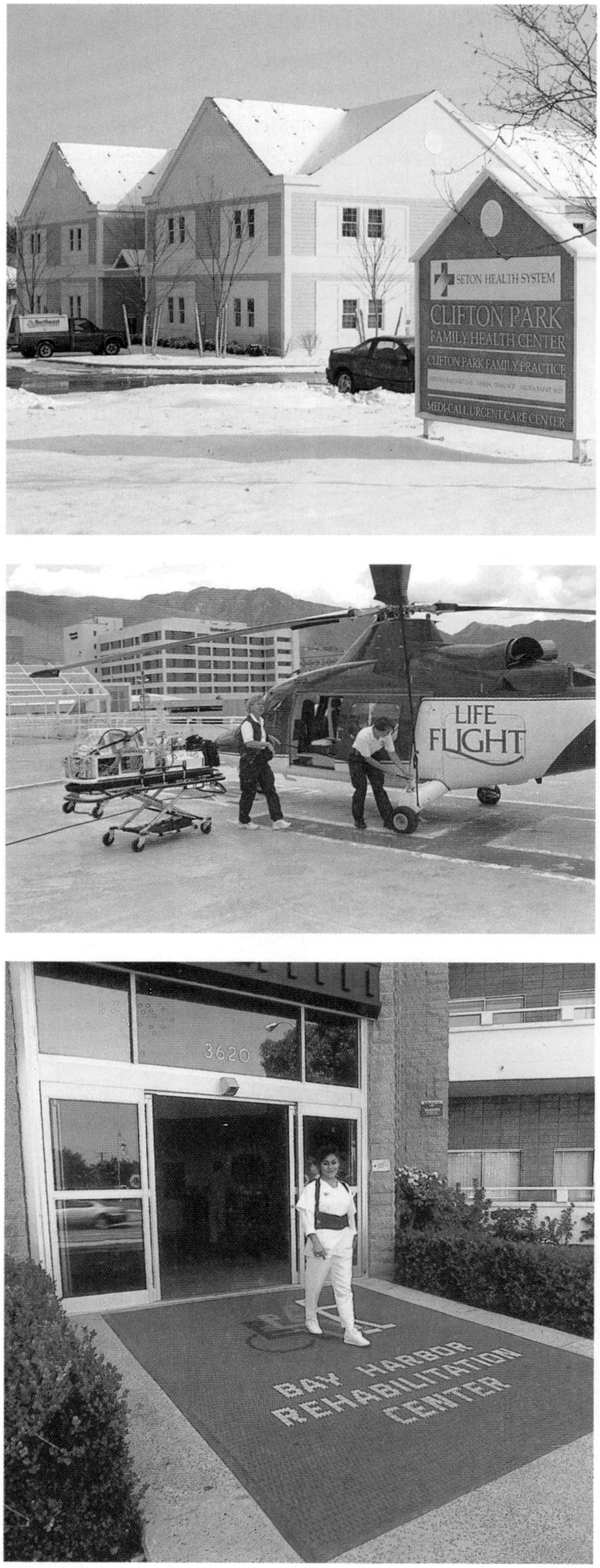

FIGURE 2–3 Health care professionals are employed in a wide variety of settings.

The trend is for hospitals to be high-tech facilities that specialize in serving patients who need sophisticated treatment and 24-hour nursing care. The various levels of care offered by hospitals include the following:

- Trauma center: Offers comprehensive services for life-threatening injuries. Specific criteria must be met to quality as a trauma center, such as having certain sophisticated diagnostic equipment and trauma surgeons available.
- Emergency department: Treats conditions that occur suddenly and require immediate attention. Examples include serious injuries from accidents and heart attacks.
- Intensive care unit (ICU): Provides specialized equipment and continuous care and monitoring for patients with serious illnesses or injuries. Offers continuous nursing care with one or two patients per nurse.
- Cardiac care unit (CCU): Provides specialized equipment and continuous care and monitoring for patients with serious heart conditions. Offers continuous nursing care with one or two patients per nurse.
- Definitive observation unit or step-down unit: Offers continuous nursing care, although less frequent than in an ICU or CCU.
- General unit: Provides care for patients who are seriously ill but do not need a high level of specialized equipment and continuous nursing care. There may be 10 or more patients per nurse.
    - Surgical floor: Provides care for patients recovering from surgery.
    - Medical floor: Provides care for patients with conditions such as infections and diabetes.
- Transitional care unit (TCU): Provides lower-level care while patients' needs are assessed and arrangements made to release patients to return home or enter another care facility.

Some hospitals also have rehabilitation units, which provide treatment for musculoskeletal, neurological, and orthopedic conditions. Rehabilitation focuses on helping patients regain as high a level of normal function as possible.

Other hospitals offer specialized care for certain populations, such as children, or specific conditions, such as burns or psychiatric conditions. **Psychiatric hospitals** offer treatment to individuals with psychiatric and behavioral disorders, including assistance with crises, medication management, counseling, and monitoring of activities of daily living. Patients may be treated on an outpatient or **inpatient** (hospitalized) basis, depending on their needs.

The modern hospital faces the challenge of controlling expenses and at the same time maintaining a certain occupancy rate (number of patients) in order to meet its operating costs. A variety of approaches have been developed to resolve this conflict:

- Diversification of services. Examples include offering rehabilitation, outpatient surgery, and long-term care in lower-tech wings or separate buildings.
- Elimination of services that duplicate those offered at nearby hospitals.
- Merging with other hospitals to share expenses and avoid duplication of services.
- Joining a large health care system that also operates clinics, nursing homes, diagnostic centers, home health agencies, and so on.
- Being purchased by a national corporation that owns and manages many hospitals.

A serious problem faced by many hospitals is the number of uninsured individuals who use emergency departments to receive care that could be provided by a clinic, physician, or other less costly provider. By law, emergency departments must give basic needed care. In many cases, patients who cannot afford routine care wait until their condition is critical before seeking help. What might be a $150 visit to a physician becomes a $1500 emergency-department expense for which the hospital is not reimbursed. Some hospitals, unable to afford the burden of providing free care, have closed their emergency departments. Others have set up hospital clinics that offer basic care to walk-in patients. This problem is being relieved by the Patient Protection and Affordable Care Act (discussed in Chapter 22) that has helped millions of Americans obtain health insurance. A remaining problem, however, is educating patients who have never had health insurance to seek primary care physicians and not rely on emergency departments for routine and nonemergency care.

Changes will continue to be made as hospitals seek ways to control costs and at the same time provide adequate services for the communities they serve. Maintaining quality of care is another concern, and many hospitals seek voluntary accreditation from the Joint Commission, a private, nonprofit organization whose purpose is to encourage the attainment of high standards of institutional medical care. It establishes guidelines for the operation of hospitals and other facilities, such as ambulatory surgery centers, long-term care facilities, and laboratories, and conducts inspections to ensure that standards are being met.

Health care professionals who are employed at approved facilities by the Joint Commission should become familiar with the standards that regulate the duties and areas for which they are responsible. Being accredited is very important because Medicare and many insurance companies will not pay for services provided at nonaccredited facilities.

Ambulatory Services

Ambulatory services are those that do not require hospitalization. Also known as **outpatient services**, they are provided by the many diagnostic, treatment, and rehabilitation facilities that account for most patient care activities. Many procedures that were previously performed in hospitals are now done on an outpatient basis. For example, a growing number of surgeries are now performed in ambulatory surgery centers with some patients being discharged one to three hours after surgery.

The physician's office is the location of the majority of ambulatory services. Ambulatory care is also provided by comprehensive facilities that offer a variety of services. A large clinic, for example, may have on-site radiographic and laboratory services. Other facilities are freestanding and offer one type of specialized service, such as an imaging center that only performs X-rays and ultrasound procedures. These facilities accept patients on a referral basis from professionals throughout the area. Table 2–2 lists common ambulatory settings and their services.

Long-Term Care Facilities

Various forms of long-term care are available for people who do not need to be hospitalized but are unable to live at home. This is one of the fastest growing areas in health care and offers an increasing number of services for patients and employment opportunities for health care professionals. There are many types of long-term care:

- **Nursing homes**: There are two types of facilities commonly referred to as nursing homes:
  - **Skilled nursing facility (SNF)**: Provides nursing and rehabilitation services on a 24-hour basis. Includes regular medical care for patients with long-term illnesses and those recovering from illness, injury, or surgery.
  - **Intermediate nursing care facility (INCF)**: Provides personal care, social services, and regular nursing care for individuals who do not require 24-hour nursing but are unable to care for themselves.
- **Adult foster home**: Provides 24-hour personal care and supervision for a small number of residents (five is typically allowed by state regulations) in a family-type home or similar setting.
- **Assisted living residence**: Provides housing, meals, and personal care to individuals who need help with daily living activities but do not need daily nursing care. The level of assistance provided depends on individual needs. This type of residence is also known by other names, such as supportive housing, residential long-term care facilities, adult residential care facilities, board-and-care, and rest homes.
- **Continuing care community**: Provides a variety of living arrangements that support lifestyles as they change from independent living to the need for regular medical and nursing care. Additional services, such as meals and daily nurse visits, can be contracted for as required.

Providing quality care for an aging population will be one of society's biggest challenges in the coming decades. The expense of such care is not covered by Medicare, except for short periods of time in a nursing home under certain conditions. The burden on individuals can be heavy, as the average cost of a skilled nursing home ranges from $4000 to $9000 per month. Long-term care insurance policies are available, but many people do not purchase these because of the relatively high cost or their inability to qualify for a policy. Other challenges include improving and maintaining the quality of care in long-term care facilities so that older Americans can live out their lives in a supportive, non-warehousing environment.

Home Health Care Providers

The provision of home health services is growing rapidly with various levels of services and care being

Table 2–2 Ambulatory Facilities

Facility	Services Offered
Adult Day Care	Activities, meals, and supervision for adults who need assistance, such as older persons and developmentally disabled persons
Dental Offices	Prevention, diagnosis, and treatment of problems with the teeth
Diagnostic Centers	Procedures, such as radiography, to determine the cause and nature of diseases and injuries
Emergency and Urgent Care Centers	Care for conditions that need immediate attention
Health Care Services in Companies, Schools, and Prisons	Basic and preventive care for employees, students, and prisoners
Laboratories	Clinical labs draw blood and collect urine and other samples, and perform tests that provide information needed to diagnose, treat, or prevent disease. Dental labs make false teeth, crowns, and corrective devices for the mouth
Medical Offices	Prevention, diagnosis, and treatment of all types of health conditions
Rehabilitation Centers	Therapies to help patients regain maximum physical and mental function; types include physical, occupational, speech, and hearing. Specialized centers help patients overcome problems with substance abuse
Specialty Clinics and Offices	Treatment for specific conditions such as cancer and venereal disease; rehabilitative services such as hand therapy, psychological counseling, and many others
Surgical Centers	Outpatient surgeries that do not require hospitalization
Wellness Centers	Routine physicals; preventive measures such as immunizations; educational programs about nutrition, exercise, and so on

provided to patients in their homes. Several factors have caused this trend:

- Shorter hospital stays
- Increase in the older population
- Advances in equipment that allow more technical procedures to be carried out in the home
- Desire of individuals to remain in their homes as they age

A wide range of professionals deliver care to patients in their homes:

- Registered and practical/licensed vocational nurses: Educate patients about self-care; administer medications, including intravenous (IV) therapy (administered through the veins); check progress; and change dressings, check the healing of wounds, and remove sutures following surgery.
- Physical therapists and physical therapist assistants: Recommend and teach physical exercises, work with patients to increase physical stamina and movement, monitor progress following injury or surgery.
- Occupational therapists and occupational therapy assistants: Assist patients in attaining maximum function and performing activities of daily living (ADLs), such as eating, bathing, and toileting, as independently as possible.
- Speech therapists: Help patients recover speech and ability to swallow.
- Medical social workers: Provide supportive counseling, assist with financial planning and arranging for in-home help or placement in the appropriate facility.
- Certified nursing assistants/home health aides: Provide personal care such as bathing and grooming, and follow care plans developed and monitored by a registered nurse or other designated professional.

Medicare pays for medically related home health services only when it is expected that the person who is homebound will improve and recover. Although nonmedical services are also available to help individuals with shopping, cooking, cleaning, and other housekeeping tasks, these are not considered medical in nature and are not usually covered by health insurance plans.

Some of the occupations showing the largest numerical increase in employment involve home health care (Bureau of Labor Statistics, 2014). At the same time, quality of care becomes a concern when health care providers work in off-site locations without direct supervision. In response to these concerns, states require the licensing of home health agencies. The types of care that may be performed in the home by various health care personnel are strictly regulated by both state law and insurance reimbursement guidelines. Medicare and most insurance companies will cover only those services provided by specific personnel.

Hospice

Hospice provides **palliative** (relieves but does not cure) care and support to dying patients and their families. It involves a team of professionals and volunteers who provide medical, emotional, and spiritual assistance. The emphasis of hospice is to make the patient's last days as pain-free and meaningful as possible. Care may be provided in a special facility, known as a hospice, in a care facility, or in the patient's home. After the patient dies, continuing support is available for the family.

Consolidation of Health Care Services

Mainly due to efforts to control costs, many health care facilities are combining under the same ownership. In this way they enjoy a number of advantages:

- Buy supplies in large quantities, thus negotiating for better prices
- Share expensive equipment
- Avoid duplication of laboratory and diagnostic services
- Share knowledge and management expertise
- Consolidate services and prevent duplication

Multiservice systems offer patients more coordinated health care, a sort of "one-stop shopping." For example, following a hospital stay, a patient can be transferred to the system's skilled nursing facility and at the same time be referred to its rehabilitation services. Some systems include a home health division.

An advantage of consolidation for patients is that they may experience more consistent care and better follow-through when dealing with one system. A disadvantage to consolidation is that there are fewer choices for health care consumers. There is the danger, too, that the lack of competition will result in higher prices and lower quality. Government regulation and patient demands help prevent these problems and ensure that large health care systems are accountable and maintain good patient care as their first priority.

New Types of Health Care Facilities

The high cost of health care, in terms of both facilities' and physicians' fees, has encouraged the development of alternative sites to provide medical care. Pharmacies, for example, now offer immunizations. Going a step further, the CVS chain of drugstores opened MinuteClinics in which nurse practitioners diagnose patients, decide on treatments, and then prescribe the needed medication. The typical cost for the patient runs from $79 to $99. When necessary, patients are referred to a physician or the local emergency department. CVS predicts that this service not only can save the lives of patients who do not have a primary care physician or are unable to pay for medical care, but can save hundreds of billions of dollars in annual health care costs (Gray, 2015).

Some areas of the country have more hospitals than necessary to service their communities, leading in some cases to overutilization and higher health care costs. At the same time, many shopping malls are becoming vacant as Americans change their shopping habits. To take advantage of the vacated buildings and provide truly needed services, health care providers and investors are developing **medical malls**, facilities that provide a variety of outpatient services, some of which were previously provided by the hospitals. Box 2–1 lists examples of typical services.

This grouping of services, especially those previously provided by high-cost hospitals, in one location is believed to reduce costs in addition to making needed health care more convenient for patients, especially the elderly. Several medical malls in New Jersey have adult day care centers whose employees can take seniors out for services located nearby, such

BOX 2–1

What Might You Find in a Medical Mall?

- Physicians' offices
- Same-day surgery
- Adult day care
- Urgent care
- Substance abuse treatment
- Medical lab
- Home health care agency

as physician visits and eye exams. This type of all-inclusive care may be a less expensive alternative to nursing home stays for some patients.

Government Health Services

Federal, state, and local governments provide a variety of important services to protect and promote the health of the American public. Supported by taxpayers, agencies have been created that concentrate on conducting research, creating and enforcing regulations, and providing educational materials and activities. Four of the major federal health-related agencies are shown in Table 2–3. Other U.S. Department of Health and Human Services agencies include the Administration on Aging, the Agency for Toxic Substances and Disease, the Indian Health Service, and the Substance Abuse and Mental Health Services Administration.

State and local health departments receive monetary and administrative support from the federal government. The following lists include examples of typical services offered.

State Health Departments

- License health care personnel, hospitals, and nursing homes
- Monitor chronic and communicable (contagious) diseases
- Provide laboratory services
- Provide emergency medical services
- Establish health data systems
- Conduct public health planning
- Provide mental health services

Local Health Departments

- Collect **vital statistics** (births and deaths)
- Conduct sanitation inspections
- Provide health education
- Screen for diseases such as cancer and diabetes
- Carry out insect control measures
- Supervise water and sewage systems
- Provide immunizations
- Operate venereal disease clinics
- Provide mental health and substance abuse counseling

(Adapted from Williams, 2005)

Government services provide a variety of employment opportunities for health care professionals. Everyone who works in health care, whether public or private, must understand the regulations of these agencies and how they affect their occupation. For example, the Centers for Disease Control and Prevention (CDC) has developed standard precautions for the safe handling of body fluids. These are essential for health care professionals who have contact with patients and are explained in Chapter 10.

Table 2–3 Health-Related Agencies of the Federal Government

National Institutes of Health (NIH)	Centers for Disease Control and Prevention (CDC)
Twenty-seven institutes and centers that conduct and support all types of medical research	Research ways to control the spread of diseases that are contagious, caused by environmental conditions, or spread by animals and insects
U.S. Department of Labor Occupational Safety and Health Administration (OSHA)	**Food and Drug Administration (FDA)**
Develops and enforces minimum health and safety standards (which employers must follow) for all of America's workers	Ensures that foods are safe, pure, and wholesome; that therapeutic drugs are safe and effective; and that cosmetics are harmless

TRENDS IN HEALTH CARE

New approaches to health care are constantly being developed due to several factors:

- Discoveries about the causes of disease and methods of treatment
- Access to information about the health care practices of other cultures
- Search for less invasive and less costly alternatives to surgery and drugs
- Growing interest in the use of natural products
- Belief that the mind and body are more closely connected than previously thought
- Emphasis on preventing rather than simply curing disease
- Increasing number of patients who want to assume more responsibility for their health by participating in preventive and self-care practices
- More patients conducting their own research and taking an active role in making decisions about their treatment and care through access to websites such as http://medlineplus.gov and www.mayoclinic.com
- Desire for increased humanization of medicine through touch, massage, and other hands-on methods
- Increased direct-to-consumer advertising of drugs and medical supplies and services

Wellness

Wellness is the promotion of health through preventive measures and the practice of good health habits. There are a growing number of people who believe that more emphasis should be placed in health care on the maximization of good health. This goes beyond the traditional view of health as the absence of disease. Wellness centers have been established to offer services such as routine physicals, immunizations, nutrition and exercise classes, and educational programs on disease prevention.

An important part of the wellness concept is the emphasis on the need for patients to take responsibility for their own health. Encouraging patients and teaching them about the basic principles of health promotion and self-care are increasingly important tasks of health care professionals. This is especially important today as we find ourselves in a contradictory situation: We understand the importance of personal habits on health but at the same time are experiencing increasing rates of health risks such as obesity and lack of physical exercise. (See Chapter 12 for more information about the relationship between lifestyle and health.) Stephen Williams, a professor of public health, states it very well: "We cannot expect to be rescued from every source of morbidity [being diseased] and mortality [death] by the nation's health care system if we do not individually and collectively emphasize prevention of disease and illness in the first place" (Williams, 2005).

Some traditional health care providers are becoming more interested in extending the definition of health to mean more than the absence of disease. Margaret Newman, RN, developed a theory she calls **expanding consciousness**. She realized that many of her patients would never be "well" in the traditional sense. They would be living with an incurable disease or the results of an injury for the rest of their lives. Newman developed a nursing approach to assist patients in making their lives as meaningful as possible by focusing on their possibilities rather than on their limitations (Newman, 2010).

Fascinating Facts

Public health agencies were established early in our country's history, at the time of the colonies. Plymouth Colony collected vital statistics such as births and deaths. And Paul Revere, famous for his midnight ride at the beginning of the Revolutionary War, was the head of Boston's board of health in the late 1700s (Williams, 2005).

Complementary, Alternative, and Integrative Health

Complementary and alternative medicine (CAM) refers to health care systems, practices, and products that have not traditionally been performed by conventional Western medical practitioners. This category covers a wide range and include practices such as using herbs and plants to treat symptoms, teaching patients meditation as a way to promote healing, and acknowledging the influence of the mind on physical symptoms. Although many health care providers do not accept the claims made for these techniques, a growing number of traditionally trained physicians, nurses, and others are conducting studies and adopting methods that were once considered to be unscientific and ineffective.

Complementary medicine is used *together with* conventional medicine. One example is using meditation, along with medication, to help patients lower their blood pressure. **Alternative medicine** refers to practices when used *instead of* conventional medicine. One example is when a patient chooses to use acupuncture rather than surgery to treat back pain. The National Center for Complementary and Integrative Health (NCCIH) reports that the use of true alternative medicine is not common; most people combine non-mainstream with conventional Western medical practices.

Integrative medicine is the term for this combination of conventional medicine with CAM. For example, a patient receiving chemotherapy for cancer may practice meditation and take nutritional supplements to manage symptoms and side effects (NCCIH, 2015). Table 2–4 lists the wide variety of nontraditional approaches to health care.

Complementary and alternative approaches are becoming increasingly popular among patients. Methods once considered to be alternative, such as massage, are increasingly being incorporated into treatment plans. Nearly 40% of Americans use some form of complementary medicine. Table 2–5 lists the 10 most common complementary methods used in 2005 (NCCIH, 2015).

Health care professionals are likely to come into contact with one or more forms of complementary or alternative medicine. Patients may ask opinions about something they have heard about; a friend or family member may seek these services; or their employer may be exploring the use of integrative medicine. Because the effectiveness and safety of many popular nontraditional therapies have not been proven, it is important for health care professionals to be aware of the various forms of complementary therapies so they can make intelligent decisions and direct patients to reliable sources of information where they can learn more for themselves. It is recommended that providers inform themselves through reading, attending workshops and seminars, and asking questions. The NCCIH, part of the National Institutes of Health, is a reliable source of information and can be accessed at https://nccih.nih.gov

CAM is susceptible to health fraud, the deceptive sale or advertising of services and products that claim to be effective against various health conditions. The U.S. Food and Drug Administration (FDA) considers the following to be signs that a product may be fraudulent:

- Claims that the product is a quick, effective cure for a wide variety of health problems
- Suggests that the product is based on a "scientific breakthrough," "miraculous cure," or "secret ingredient"
- Uses text with impressive-sounding terms that are not defined elsewhere
- Provides undocumented case histories of amazing results
- Has limited availability and requires payment in advance

Certain diseases and conditions are reportedly often the targets of false remedies. These include cancer, AIDS, arthritis, obesity and overweight, sexual dysfunction, and diabetes. Patients should be warned to check with their health care provider and to research the advice of government agencies, such as the FDA, before purchasing remedies online. Not only are many substances useless, some can be dangerous and cause serious health problems.

Holistic Medicine

Holistic medicine is a general term to designate the belief that the traditional view of medicine must be expanded. All aspects of the individual—physical, mental, emotional, spiritual, and environmental—contribute to states of health and disease. In other words, the entire person must be considered when making therapeutic decisions. The prevention of disease, rather than simply the relief of symptoms, is emphasized. Patient education and participation in the healing process are encouraged.

There is a growing interest in holistic medicine today as evidence mounts that the mind has a powerful effect on physical health. Disorders caused by mental or emotional factors are known as **psychosomatic**. Researchers now know that these illnesses are not "all in one's head" but that physical symptoms can be the result of what is happening in the mind. It is believed that a high percentage of visits to physicians' offices are due to psychosomatic disorders.

Holistic medicine providers tend to combine traditional and nontraditional treatments and emphasize that:

- Prevention is preferable to treatment.
- Patients must accept responsibility for their own health.

Table 2–4 Complementary and Alternative Approaches to Health

Category	Examples
Whole Medical Systems	• Homeopathic medicine: assist the body to heal itself of symptoms by giving very small quantities of a substance that produces the symptoms ("like cures like").
Complete systems of theory and practice	• Naturopathic medicine: assist the body to use its own healing power with methods such as exercise and medicinal plants. • Traditional Chinese medicine: ancient system based on balancing and maintaining the body's vital energy flow ("qi," pronounced "chee"); treatments include acupuncture and herbs. • Ayurveda: 5000-year-old system practiced in India; treatments include herbs, massage, and yoga.
Mind–Body Medicine	• Patient support groups
Enhance the mind's influence on the body	• Meditation • Prayer • **Guided imagery** • Creative outlets, such as art and music • Yoga
Natural Products	• Aromatherapy: scent of essential oils from plants is inhaled
Use substances found in nature	• Herbs • Dietary supplements • Use of natural products, such as shark cartilage
Manipulative and Body-Based Practices	• Chiropractic manipulation
Move parts of the body to regain health and function	• Osteopathic manipulation • Massage
(Manipulation: controlled force to a joint beyond its normal range of motion)	• Reflexology: application of pressure to parts of the feet that are believed to be connected to specific parts of the body • Relaxation exercises
Energy Therapies	• Biofield therapies: manipulate the fields of energy believed to surround and penetrate the body; practitioners use their hands to channel and balance this energy. Therapies include:
Involve the use of energy fields and pathways	○ Qi gong: combines movement, meditation, and controlled breathing ○ Reiki: practitioners attempt to transmit universal energy to a person to heal the spirit and thus the body ○ Therapeutic (healing) touch: patient's energy field is altered when energy is passed from the practitioner's hands to the patient • Bioelectromagnetic-based therapies: unconventional use of electromagnetic fields, such as using magnets to relieve pain

- Stress is an important factor in health and should be reduced.
- Proper nutrition and exercise are essential.
- Attitude has a powerful effect, both positive and negative, on the body and its functioning.

Osteopathy and Chiropractic

Osteopathy and chiropractic health care practices have become so widely accepted that they are no longer generally considered to be alternative. **Osteopathy** is based on the belief that the body can protect itself

Table 2–5 Ten Most Common Complementary Health Approaches Among Adults—2007

Approach	Percentage of U.S. Adults Who Used
Natural Products	17.7%
Deep Breathing	12.7%
Meditation	9.4%
Chiropractic and Osteopathic	8.6%
Massage	8.3%
Yoga	6.1%
Diet-based Therapies	3.6%
Progressive Relaxation	2.9%
Guided Imagery	2.2%
Homeopathic Treatment	1.8%

Source: Barnes, P.M., Bloom, B., & Nahin, R.L. (2008). Complementary and alternative medicine use among adults and children: United States, 2007. National Health Statistics Reports; *no 12. Hyattsville, MD: National Center for Health Statistics.*

against disease if the musculoskeletal system, especially the spine, is in good order. The importance of good nutrition and favorable environmental conditions is also emphasized. Osteopathic physicians receive training that is similar to that of traditional doctors of medicine (MDs). They can prescribe drugs, perform surgeries, and have staff privileges at most hospitals. Osteopaths take the same state licensing examinations as MDs.

Chiropractic is based on the belief that pressure on the nerves leaving the spinal column causes pain or dysfunction of the body part served by that nerve. Treatment involves manipulation of the spine to correct misalignments. Chiropractors are not allowed to prescribe drugs, but may recommend nutritional and herbal remedies. Every state has licensure requirements for chiropractors. (See Figure 2–4.)

Massage Therapy

Massage therapy is widely recognized, when administered by a trained practitioner, as a beneficial health practice. It involves using pressure or friction on the body. By enabling the muscles to relax, massage therapy promotes better blood circulation, faster healing of injuries, and pain relief. It is often recommended to supplement other forms of therapy and to provide an effective method of stress relief. Many types of formal training programs are available for people who wish

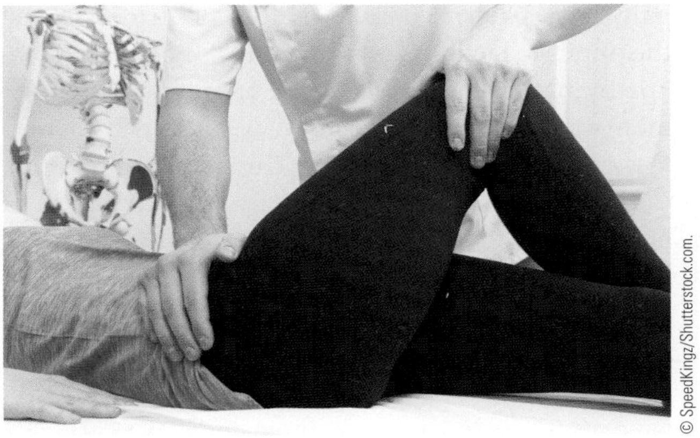

FIGURE 2–4 Osteopaths, chiropractors, and physical therapists may include manipulation of the joints as part of a treatment plan.

to practice massage therapy. Most states and localities require therapists to be licensed.

Naturopathy

Naturopathic medicine is based on the belief that the human body has its own natural healing ability. Naturopathic doctors (NDs) teach their patients to use diet, exercise, lifestyle changes and cutting-edge natural therapies to enhance their bodies' ability to ward off and combat disease. They combine traditional medicine and natural remedies when developing treatment plans for their patients (American Association of Naturopathic Physicians, 2014). Naturopathic physicians seek the causes of symptoms and believe the whole person, not just the symptoms, must be treated. Seventeen states, the District of Columbia, and the United States territories of Puerto Rico and the U.S. Virgin Islands have licensing laws for naturopathic doctors.

Homeopathy

Homeopathy is a method of treatment developed by a German physician in the early 1800s based on the idea of stimulating the body's own healing responses. Disorders are treated with very small amounts of the natural substances that cause the symptoms of the disorder in healthy people. For example, exposure to onions causes the same runny nose and eyes as are experienced with a head cold. Therefore, very diluted amounts of plants in the onion family are administered to treat cold symptoms. Belladonna, secured from a poisonous European plant, is widely used in homeopathy to treat a variety of symptoms, including pain. It has been used in traditional medicine to dilate the pupils to facilitate examination of the eyes. Homeopathy has been practiced in Europe and India for more than 200 years and is used by some medical professionals in the United States. Three states—Arizona, Connecticut, and Nevada—require practitioners of homeopathy to be licensed by the state homeopathic licensing board.

Energy Theories

Theories about the existence and importance of body energy originated in Asia thousands of years ago. There is growing interest today in therapies that claim to encourage the free flow of energy throughout the body. This flow, it is believed, is necessary to promote and maintain good health. Acupuncture may be the oldest application of this theory. Developed by the Chinese more than 5000 years ago, it involves the insertion of tiny needles into specific points in the body to relieve energy blocks. This treatment is becoming accepted in the United States as people who receive it find relief from various health problems.

CHALLENGES IN HEALTH CARE TODAY

The tremendous medical progress made during the last century continues into the new millennium. At the same time, our country faces many challenges in effectively delivering the results of this progress to all who need it. These challenges represent complex problems that affect millions of people. Problems of this size are not easy to solve. Finding solutions that satisfy the needs of everyone is very difficult. Some diseases, such as Alzheimer's, remain without a cure. Others, such as cancer, are sometimes curable and sometimes not, despite years of research and testing.

It is important for the health care professional to be aware of major health care issues. They will affect where and how you perform your job, as well as influence your relationships with patients and other members of the health care team.

Providing Affordable Health Care

In response to the fact that millions of Americans lacked health insurance, the Patient Protection and Affordable Care Act was signed into law in 2010. (The law is discussed in more detail in Chapter 22.) However, the insurance that Americans can now purchase can be expensive and may come with deductibles of several thousand dollars. This situation is especially challenging for the unemployed and the working poor (people who are employed but work part-time and do not qualify for employer-provided health insurance). It is even out of reach for many middle-class Americans, with reportedly one third unable to afford required deductibles (Altman, 2015). Although government subsidies are available for millions of Americans, the high cost of health care still presents a problem for many individuals. Another group that struggles with health care costs are low-income seniors. Medicare, a government-run insurance program for persons age 65 and older and the disabled, pays for only 80% of certain costs and many seniors cannot afford to purchase supplemental insurance to cover the remaining 20%, which can be substantial for a major health event.

A potential problem with government subsidies is that when not enough taxes can be collected to support the costs, services must be cut. This is an especially serious concern when the economy is weak and unemployment is high, which results in decreased tax revenues. Many economists have warned that Medicare is in danger of running out of funding (Social Security Administration, 2014). The problem is worsened by fraudulent claims paid out by Medicare. Although sources vary widely in estimates ranging from $17 billion to more than $100 billion in losses, it is known that many false claims are paid out each year. The Federal Bureau of Investigation is the primary agency for exposing and investigating health

Thinking It Through

Craig Oakley is a physical therapy assistant who does home visits for a rehabilitation service. One of his patients, Mr. Singh, suffers from rheumatoid arthritis and has asked Craig's opinion about taking Chinese herbal remedies that he has read help restore joint health.

1. How should Craig respond?
2. What are some of the resources he can consult in order to find out more about the treatment?
3. What precautions should Craig follow when speaking with Mr. Singh about complementary and alternative therapies?

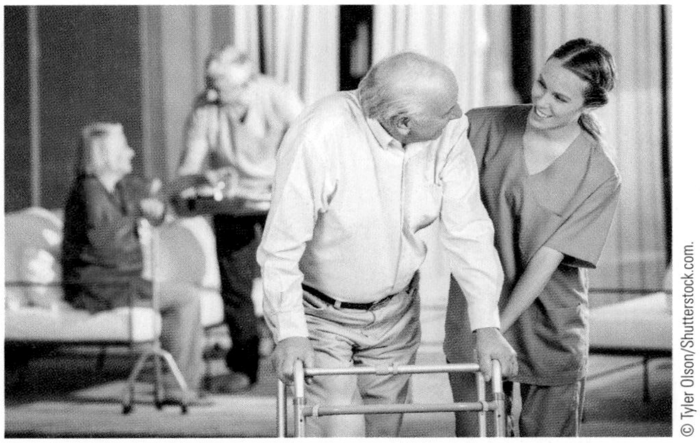

FIGURE 2–5 Health care professionals can help seniors live the highest quality of life possible as they age.

care fraud and penalties have been increased recently. It is hoped that the combination of cutting fraudulent claims for Medicare reimbursement, raising taxes, and promoting efficiencies in the delivery of health care will support the future costs of the health care system.

Providing Long-Term Care

The increasing population of older persons, discussed previously, means that an increasing number of people will need some sort of care as they age and experience health problems. As a result of medical advances many people are living beyond their ability to care for themselves. Some suffer from chronic conditions and require 24-hour nursing care. (See Figure 2–5.)

The costs of nursing facilities and other long-term care housing are increasing as much as 5% annually. The cost varies widely from state to state. Table 2–6 contrasts projected annual costs of various types of long-term care in Texas and New York.

Covering these costs will be a challenge. Medicare currently covers only short-term stays in a nursing home following a hospitalization and provides no coverage for assisted living. Long-term care insurance is available, but because of the increasingly high expense of paying for care, many insurance companies no longer sell this type of policy, and those that do, charge more for coverage than many Americans can afford. The states' **Medicaid** programs cover nursing home care, but it is not known if there will be adequate funding to cover the projected rise in expenses. (Medicaid is a federally funded program for low-income individuals.) (See Table 2–6.)

Improving Social Conditions

Many social problems affect the country's health care delivery systems, as well as the health of the nation as a whole. For example, the nearly 25% of Americans who do not graduate from high school have a higher rate of health problems than those who do finish high school. People living in poor neighborhoods that lack grocery stores, farmers' markets, and safe outdoor space for children to play and adults to walk experience higher rates of obesity, diabetes, and related health conditions. Table 2–7 lists a number of social conditions that can produce negative consequences for individual health, as well as for health care delivery systems.

The sad result of poverty and other social problems is that those who most need health care services are the least able to pay for them, even when

Table 2–6 Annual Costs of Long-Term Care Services

	Texas		New York	
Type of Service	2012	2017	2012	2017
Homemaker Services	$41,070	$62,596	$45,760	$77,503
Home Health Aide	$41,184	$54,812	$50,336	$83,600
Adult Day Care	$8,580	$13,803	$19,500	$148,175
Assisted Living—Private One Bedroom	$40,035	$153,394	$47,400	$135,796
Nursing Home: Semi-private Room Private Room	$47,538 $61,320	$88,563 $108,002	$120,998 $125,732	$135,371 $387,949

Sources: http://longtermcare.gov/cost-of-care-results/?state=US-TX and http://longtermcare.gov/cost-of-care-results/?state=US-NY

Table 2–7 Social Conditions That Affect Health and Health Care Systems

Condition	Impact on Health and Health Care System
Breakdown of Family Unit and Children Born to Single Women	Poverty among women and children. Lack of access to prenatal care, immunizations for children, and other preventive measures
Homelessness	Lack of access to medical care. Malnutrition and poor hygiene. Difficult to contact patient for follow-up care. An increasing number of families and children now number among the homeless
Violence	Use of emergency and other health care services. Inability of many victims to pay
Substance Abuse	Increased violence and susceptibility to disease. Inability to care for self and family
Spousal and Child Abuse	Need for health and protective services. Use of emergency department services for injuries
Poverty and Malnutrition	Poor health and inability to access health care. Lack of prenatal care
26% of Americans Live Alone	Need outside assistance when ill or injured. Lack of emotional support

Sources: Adapted from Essentials of Health Services, *by S. J. Williams, 2005, Clifton Park, NY: Delmar Cengage Learning. U.S. Census Bureau, www.census.gov/Press-Release/www/releases/archives/families_households/006840.html*

governmental and other services are available. People who do not seek preventive care and practice good health habits are more likely to develop serious conditions that result in more suffering as well as higher expenses for the health care system.

Maintaining the Quality of Care

The skyrocketing costs of health care have prompted all levels of government, as well as providers of health care, to initiate cost controls. This has caused widespread concern that quality of care is being sacrificed to cut expenses. A related area of concern is that for-profit insurance and health care organizations may emphasize profits more than providing high-quality patient care. Complaints reported by residents in nursing homes, discussed later in this section, may be related to the growth of for-profit facilities.

Some current methods of paying physicians and other providers for their services encourage them to provide less rather than more care. Reviewers who work on behalf of insurance companies make many decisions about patient care. The purpose is to determine whether the proposed procedures are medically necessary and whether lower cost alternatives are available. Permission is required in advance for certain procedures, a process called "preauthorization." For example, nonemergency hospital admissions and surgeries commonly require approval. Reviewers may or may not have extensive medical training. Their decisions are based on what is known about the "average patient" under the same or similar circumstances. Reviewers can make a variety of decisions. For example, they can:

- Approve the procedure as recommended by the physician
- Deny the procedure
- Require surgery to be performed as an outpatient service (patient does not occupy a bed in the facility, such as a hospital)
- Approve a different, usually less-costly method
- Approve a limited number of treatments

Under the Patient Protection and Affordable Care Act, patients have the right to appeal a health insurance company's decision to deny payment for a claim or to terminate their health coverage. However, the process required may discourage many patients or, if they proceed, may result in delays before they can receive the care their provider believes they need.

Many physicians feel they have lost control of the practice of medicine to business interests or government agencies, such as the Centers for Medicare and Medicaid. Accustomed to having the authority to make decisions about the best care for their patients, they are frustrated by what they see as interference from nonmedical personnel or those with financial interests.

Patients, in turn, believe the decisions of their physicians are being questioned and have concerns about the resulting quality of care. They worry that they are being denied needed procedures and treatments and that their health is being sacrificed for the sake of increasing profits.

At the same time, other health care experts point out that the number of unnecessary surgeries and other procedures, especially those used for diagnosis, have decreased. They believe that patient care has not suffered but has actually been improved by efforts to prevent the overuse of available techniques.

Another area of concern is the quality of the nation's nursing homes. Many for-profit facilities have been accused of providing inadequate care in order to raise profits. To address this issue, in 2015 the federal government raised its rating standards for the more than 15,000 facilities providing nursing care. Criteria for these ratings include adequate staffing at appropriate professional levels, health and fire safety measures, and quality of care (lack of pressure sores in patients, etc). The public has access to the ratings of nursing homes nationwide at www.medicare.gov/NursingHomeCompare. The health care professionals who fill the many future jobs in long-term care facilities need to be aware of the government oversight of these facilities and the importance of providing high-quality care to America's elderly and disabled patients. (See Figure 2–5.)

Restoring confidence in the system while at the same time controlling costs is a major challenge to ensuring continued quality of care. As a health care professional, you can help restore this confidence by providing the best care possible and supporting the decisions of the professional for whom you work.

Treating Alzheimer's and Other Forms of Dementia

Dementia is a condition marked by a decline in memory and/or other thinking skills. It is caused by damage to the nerve cells in the brain. **Alzheimer's disease** is the most common dementia, accounting for 60% to 80% of cases. Alzheimer's is a progressive disease that eventually affects basic body functions and results in death. It is now ranked as the sixth leading cause of death in the United States.

Alzheimer's is increasingly challenging the health care system's ability to handle the growing number of cases. As the population ages and people live longer because of advances in treating other diseases, more and more Americans are being diagnosed with this disease: one in nine individuals age 65 and over and one in three people age 85 and over. In 2014, 5.2 million Americans had Alzheimer's or another form of dementia and this number is expected to grow to 7.1 million in 2025 and 13.6 to 16 million in 2050 (Alzheimer's Association, 2014).

The need for care of dementia patients in terms of facilities and cost is of concern. Two thirds of patients with Alzheimer's live their last years or months in a nursing home. At the same time, few can afford the cost of this care so payment is made by government programs, such as Medicare and Medicaid. In 2014, Medicare and Medicaid were expected to pay $150 billion for all dementia care, including hospice. According to the Alzheimer's Association, it is "one of the costliest chronic diseases to society." Total costs of care is estimated to reach $1.2 trillion in 2050 (this doesn't account for inflation) (Alzheimer's Association, 2014).

There will be a growing need for trained caregivers to work with patients suffering from dementia. Patience, understanding, and the knowledge to safeguard individuals who have difficulty communicating and are experiencing changing patterns of behavior are required. These changes can include the inability to recognize themselves or others, fear and anxiety, and paranoia. While the work can be challenging, it can also be very satisfying to help provide the best possible quality of life for some of our society's most vulnerable members.

Addressing Public Health Concerns

The United States faces challenges in its efforts to safeguard the health of the public. Monitoring and researching health issues must be ongoing. For example, although most infectious diseases are under control in this country, there are increasing concerns about a pandemic occurring in the near future. The global outbreak in 2009 of influenza caused by the H1N1 virus demonstrated how difficult it can be to respond quickly as the United States encountered slow-downs in its efforts to develop an effective vaccine. More recently the entry into the United States of individuals with Ebola, a frequently fatal viral disease transmitted through contact with an infected person's bodily fluid, heightened concerns about the effectiveness of existing screening and infection control measures. (See Chapter 10 for information about infection control.) Fortunately, Ebola infected only a few Americans who were working in West Africa where the disease reached epidemic proportions. A nurse in Texas who treated an Ebola patient also contracted the disease. Her illness was the result of poor protocol in screening for the infection, which prompted the development and enforcement of more effective safety measures for health care professionals.

Encouraging Medication Adherence

Medication adherence means taking medications correctly: the right dosage at the right time and as often as prescribed. The failure of medication adherence in the United States accounts for $100 billion to $289 billion in annual preventable medical costs, 30% to 50% of treatment failures, and 125,000 deaths annually (CDC, 2013). The following statistics contain more facts about the lack of medication adherence:

- Between 20% and 30% of prescriptions are never filled.
- Medication is not continued for the time period prescribed in 50% of cases.
- Only 51% of patients treated for hypertension (high blood pressure) stay with their prescribed long-term therapy.
- Nonadherence to medications that protect the heart increases deaths from heart disease by 50% to 80% (CDC, 2013).

Many reasons account for this high rate of nonadherence, including the high cost of medications and their side effects. The main problem, however, is believed to be communication: Patients do not understand the purpose and importance of their medications and/or how to take them. As the CDC states, "Communication is the key!" (CDC, 2013). Chapters 15 and 16 contain information about how health care professionals can better communicate with patients.

Preventing Prescription Drug Overuse

A health care challenge that is the opposite of nonadherence is the overuse of painkillers. Since 1999 prescriptions for painkillers have nearly quadrupled and deaths from drug overdoses have tripled. Although prescriptions have leveled off since 2010, in 2013 almost two million Americans were abusing painkillers: taking too many or when not needed or when not prescribed for them. More than 15,500 people die annually from overdoses (CDC, April 2015).

Measures being taken to prevent overdoses and death include the following:

- Creating safe prescribing guidelines for providers
- Regulating pain clinics
- Identifying fraudulent prescriptions
- Teaching patients other methods for controlling pain
- Educating patients about the risks of **opioids**
- Improve access to naloxone, the antidote to opioid overdose

Preventing Antibiotic Resistance

Antibiotics are drugs that fight infections caused by bacteria. They are not effective against viruses, the microorganisms that cause colds and flu as well as other illnesses. Antibiotic resistance occurs when the bacteria the drugs target change in ways that reduce or eliminate the effectiveness of antibiotics to destroy them. According to the CDC, antibiotic resistance "is one of our most serious health threats," causing two million illnesses and 23,000 deaths each year (CDC, March, 2013). This is because as bacteria become resistant, they become increasingly difficult or even impossible to treat. Drug-resistant organisms are discussed in more detail in Chapter 10. (See Figure 2–6.)

Encouraging Personal Responsibility for Health

The four leading causes of death in the United States—heart disease, cancer, chronic lower respiratory disease, and stroke—are often influenced

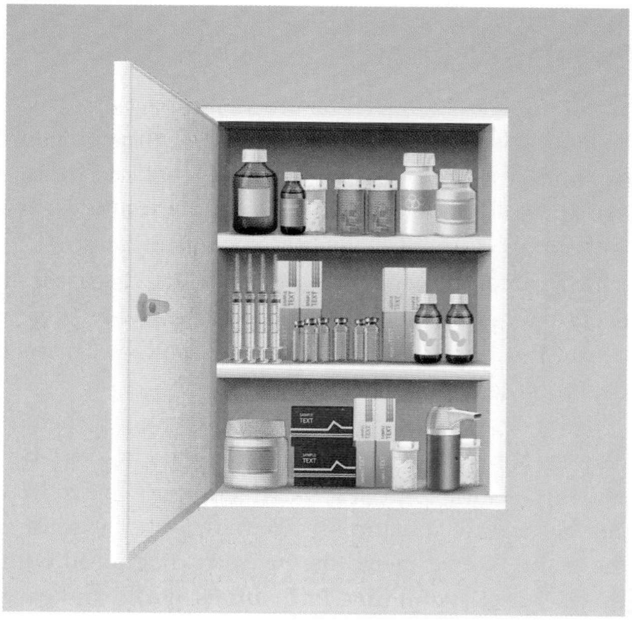

FIGURE 2–6 Prescription medications are the most commonly used treatment in the United States but must be used as directed—no more and no less.

by lifestyle choices. Many chronic diseases, such as diabetes, are also linked to personal behaviors. Individuals have control over the habits that contribute to the state of their health. The following behaviors have been identified as contributing to healthier and longer lives:

- Not smoking
- Getting enough sleep
- Eating moderately and maintaining a balanced diet and normal weight
- Exercising regularly
- Avoiding alcohol or drinking in moderation
- Practicing preventive measures such as getting immunizations and wearing seat belts
- Using stress reduction techniques
- Getting recommended screenings, such as mammograms and colonoscopies
- Taking needed medications correctly and on time

Individuals must also realize that modern medicine has limitations and that new technological advances do not guarantee that every disease can be cured and every injury repaired. On the other hand, nearly everyone can improve his or her own health and quality of life by making positive lifestyle choices.

IMPLICATIONS FOR HEALTH CARE PROFESSIONALS

Meeting the challenges that face our health care system is everyone's responsibility. Health care professionals are in the fortunate position of being able to positively influence this important area of life. Some steps they can take to help meet these challenges are:

- Keep informed of important issues by reviewing appropriate websites, attending workshops, reading professional journals, and participating in professional organizations.
- Contribute to the delivery of high-quality service by pledging to perform duties to the best of their ability. Chapter 23 discusses specific ways that health care professionals can improve the quality of their performance and give excellent customer service.
- Model good health habits and learn to provide effective patient education. (See Chapters 12 and 16.)

WORKBOOK PRACTICE

Go to your workbook and complete the exercises for this chapter.

SUGGESTED LEARNING ACTIVITIES

1. Look for articles about health care trends and challenges on the Internet, and in the newspaper and magazines. Which trends are mentioned most frequently? How do you think they will affect your future career as a health care professional?
2. Visit some of the health care facilities described in this chapter. What services do they offer? What types of employment opportunities are available?
3. Conduct a search of websites for major hospitals and health care systems in your area. What kind of information is available?
4. Investigate the services provided by your local public health department.
5. Explore complementary and alternative therapies practiced in your area. Interview a practitioner about the theory on which his or her therapy is based.
6. Learn more about the factors that contribute to cancer, heart disease, chronic lower respiratory disease, and stroke. Explore the websites of the American Cancer Society, the American Heart Association, the American Lung Association, and the National Stroke Association. Explore other sources on the Internet using the key words "cancer prevention," "heart disease prevention," "chronic lower respiratory disease prevention," and "stroke prevention."

WEB ACTIVITIES

Kaiser Family Foundation

www.kff.org

Choose a topic to explore. Based on what you learn, what changes do you think might take place in health care in the next 10 years? What might be done to control health care costs in the United States?

National Institutes of Health—National Center for Complementary and Integrative Health

https://nccih.nih.gov

Choose five therapies to explore and write a paragraph about each.

National Library of Medicine—Medline Plus
www.medlineplus.gov

Click on "Health Topics," and then choose a topic to explore under "Health and Wellness." Write a summary of what you learn, including how you might apply this information to your future work in health care.

REVIEW QUESTIONS

1. What are five events in the history of health care that improved the delivery of care for patients?
2. Briefly describe the major forces that are shaping the health care industry today.
3. What levels of care are typically provided in a modern general hospital?
4. What are 10 common ambulatory health care facilities? What type of services does each one offer?
5. What are the major types of long-term care facilities? What type of care is offered by each?
6. What are five typical services offered by federal health agencies? State agencies? Local agencies?
7. What services are provided by hospice professionals?
8. What are the factors influencing the increased interest in new approaches to health care?
9. What is meant by the term *wellness*?
10. Describe five types of complementary therapies being practiced in the United States today.
11. What are the major challenges facing health care today? How can the health care professional contribute to their resolution?

APPLICATION EXERCISES

1. Refer to The Case of the Confused Daughter at the beginning of the chapter. Put yourself in the place of the social worker. What information would you give Mrs. Freemont and her daughter?
2. Jim Parker has been working as a licensed practical nurse for seven years. Most of his career has been spent working in a community hospital providing direct patient care. Jim has been thinking about other settings in which he can apply his nursing skills.
   a. Describe at least five facilities that might offer employment opportunities for Jim.
   b. What type of patients should he expect to work with in each one?

PROBLEM-SOLVING PRACTICE

A growing number of children in Trueville, USA, are becoming overweight and obese. A group of concerned citizens has organized a committee to find ways to help children in the community attain normal weights and raise their levels of fitness. How might the committee use the five-step problem-solving process?

SUGGESTED READINGS AND RESOURCES

American Association of Naturopathic Physicians. www.naturopathic.org

American Cancer Society. www.cancer.org

American Heart Association. www.americanheart.org

American Hospital Association. www.aha.org

American Stroke Association. www.strokeassociation.org

Centers for Disease Control and Prevention. www.cdc.gov

Centers for Disease Control and Prevention. Antibiotic resistance threats in the United States, 2013. www.cdc.gov/drugresistance/threat-report-2013/

Centers for Medicare and Medicaid. www.medicare.gov

Expanding Consciousness. www.healthasexpanding-consciousness.org

Food and Drug Administration. www.fda.gov

The Joint Commission. www.jointcommission.org

Medline Plus. http://www.nlm.nih.gov

National Association for Home Care and Hospice. www.nahc.org

National Center for Complementary and Alternative Medicine. https://nccih.nih.gov

National Center for Health Statistics. www.cdc.gov/nchs

National Hospice and Palliative Care Organization. www.nho.org

National Institutes of Health. www.nih.gov

Occupational Safety and Health Administration. www.osha.gov

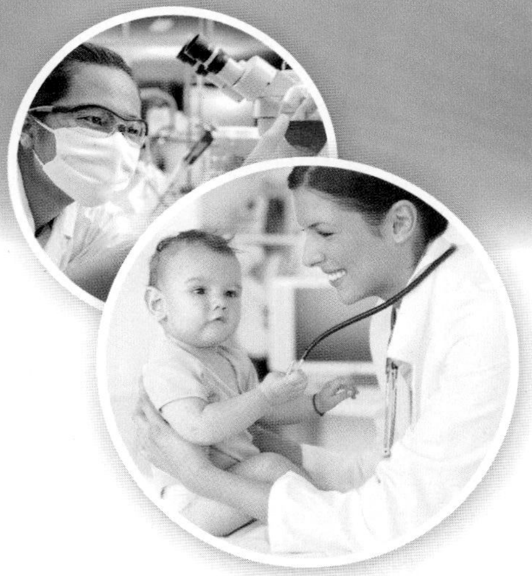

Chapter 3

Ethical and Legal Responsibilities

OBJECTIVES

Studying and applying the material in this chapter will help you to:

- Explain the meaning of ethics and its importance in the practice of health care.
- State the purpose of professional codes of ethics.
- Explain the meaning of values and how they influence personal and professional behavior.
- Describe the relationship between ethics and law.
- List the eight major ethical principles that apply to health care and give examples of the laws that support each.
- Explain how each of the following presents ethical challenges to the health care community: euthanasia, organ transplants, and rationing of care.
- Explain the importance of patient consent and the possible consequences when actions are taken without the patient's consent.
- Give the definitions of express and implied consent.
- Describe the two major components of advance directives.
- List the signs of child and elder abuse and state the actions that health care professionals should take in cases of suspected abuse.
- Explain the purpose of the federal schedule of controlled substances.
- Describe the importance of patient confidentiality and possible legal consequences when it is breached.
- Give examples of how the health care professional applies ethics on the job.

KEY TERMS

adult
advance directive
agent
assault
autonomy
battery
breach of contract
code of ethics
confidentiality
consent
contract
damages
defamation of character
designation of health care surrogate
discreet
emancipated minor
ethical dilemma
ethics
euthanasia
express consent
express contract
false imprisonment
fraud

(continues)

KEY TERMS (continued)

implied consent	justice	malpractice	protocols
implied contract	legislation	mercy killing	respondeat superior
informed consent	libel	negligence	slander
invasive procedures	living will	principles	values

The Case of the Missing Consent Form

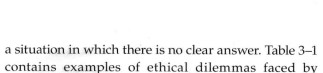

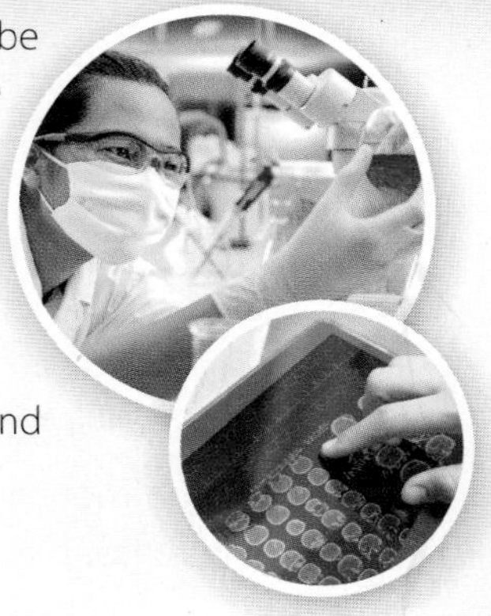

Mrs. McChesney is bringing her 3-year-old son, Sammy, to Dr. Michaels for a minor surgery to be performed in the physician's office. Medical assistant Gretchen Mills scheduled the surgery in the appointment book. Last night she checked to be sure that the necessary instruments and supplies were prepared and that an appropriate room was ready. When checking Sammy's file on the day of the surgery, she cannot find a consent form, signed by Mrs. McChesney, to authorize the surgery. Proceeding with the procedure without this having been completed could have serious legal implications.

Health care professionals must understand and help their facilities follow ethical principles and meet legal requirements.

THE PURPOSE OF ETHICS

Over the centuries human beings have struggled to answer questions about the meaning of life and how to properly conduct themselves. **Ethics** is a system of **principles** (fundamental truths) a society develops to guide decisions about what is right and wrong. Ethics helps people deal with difficult and complex problems that lack easy answers.

The ethical principles adopted by a society are influenced by religion, history, and the collective experiences of the people in the group. The United States has one of the most diverse populations of any country on earth, composed of hundreds of cultures. People here are guided by a variety of ethical principles and beliefs about right and wrong. This accounts for many of the disagreements that occur when the government tries to pass laws and make policy decisions that affect all citizens. The ongoing debate about abortion is an example of strongly held opposing beliefs in which each side believes it is right.

Even within a single ethical system, following one principle may appear to contradict another. This results in what is known as an **ethical dilemma**, a situation in which there is no clear answer. Table 3–1 contains examples of ethical dilemmas faced by Americans today.

Often, there simply is not a clear right answer that will satisfy everyone. Right behavior for some people results in wrong effects for others. Flight (2004), who writes about health care ethics, points out that realizing there may not be a "perfect" answer can prevent some of the agonizing that occurs when trying to make the "correct" decision.

ETHICS AND THE LAW

Ethics provides the general principles on which laws are based. Put another way, laws are a means of enforcing ethical principles. For example, if a society agrees that life is precious, its members pass laws that make murder a crime. The American legal system is based on the belief that everyone must take responsibility for his or her actions (Flight, 2004). Its purpose is to require people to act in the best interest of society as a whole. For example, the Occupational Safety and Health Administration (OSHA) was created to protect the health and safety of all workers. OSHA regulations

Table 3–1 Ethical Dilemmas Faced by Americans

Values	Action	Contradiction
Criminals should be punished for their crimes. ("An eye for an eye.") "Thou shall not kill."	Capital punishment for convicted murderers	If it is wrong to kill, can society justify killing anyone, even a criminal?
Freedom of speech is a human right. All people should be treated equally and be protected under the law.	Speeches on public grounds that contain hate messages directed toward minority groups	Should free speech be allowed if the messages encourage unequal treatment?
Citizens should have the right to own guns and protect themselves. Society must protect itself against criminals.	Criminals use guns to harm others.	Should gun sales be controlled if it results in limiting the rights of law-abiding citizens?

require employers to follow our society's ethical principle that human life and health are precious and should be safeguarded.

Laws, however, can conflict with the ethical and moral principles held by some members of society. The use of marijuana for medical purposes is an example. Marijuana has been found to relieve the nausea experienced by patients undergoing chemotherapy. Its use for this purpose is illegal in 29 states, however, because many people believe that it encourages inappropriate drug use, an unethical activity. At the same time, the citizens of 23 states and the District of Columbia have legalized its use, asserting it is unethical to allow human suffering when it can be prevented. Both groups believe they are doing the "right thing" for society.

Some well-intentioned laws do not succeed in bringing about justice. Others have harmful consequences that are not recognized until after the laws are in effect. For example, federal legislation requires hospital emergency rooms that accept Medicare to accept all patients who require care, regardless of their ability to pay. Many hospitals could not afford the financial losses of treating every patient who came for care. This resulted in many emergency rooms closing down, thus denying the entire community an important health care resource.

The third principle of the American Medical Association Principles of Medical Ethics addresses the issue of problematic laws:

> A physician shall respect the law and also recognize a responsibility to seek changes in those requirements, which are contrary to the best interests of the patient.

Acting in the best interest of patients is an important responsibility of health care professionals. At the same time, this can present difficulties if they become aware of laws, regulations, or policies that negatively affect patient welfare. For example, a facility policy may require that patients be given medications that are less effective than more expensive products in an attempt to control costs or conform to insurance company requirements.

It is *never* appropriate, however, to undermine a patient's trust in the care being given by discussing what the health care professional believes to be problems with the system. For example, it would be inappropriate for nurses to inform patients about the less effective medications. It is proper to listen to patients' concerns and then work to promote positive changes in the system. Professional organizations often provide opportunities to discuss these issues. Many groups represent their members in promoting legislation and policies that are beneficial for both patients and health care professionals.

ETHICS AND HEALTH CARE

The importance of ethics in the practice of health care has been recognized for thousands of years. Health care professionals have a significant impact on human life. The practice of health care involves life-and-death issues, which are often at the heart of ethical questions.

Recognition of the important role of health care professionals has existed since ancient times. Hippocrates was a Greek physician who lived about 2500 years ago. He was concerned with the ethical considerations of medicine. The Hippocratic Oath,

BOX 3–1

The Oath of Hippocrates

I swear by Apollo Physician and Aesculapius and Hygeia and Panacea and all the gods and goddesses, making them my witness, that I will fulfill according to my ability and judgment this oath and this covenant.

To hold him who has taught me this art as equal to my parents and to live my life in partnership with him, and if he is in need of money to give him a share of mine, and to regard his offspring as equal to my brothers in male lineage and to teach them this art—if they desire to learn it—without fee and covenant; to vie a share of precepts and oral instruction and all the other learning to my sons and to the sons of him who has instructed me and to pupils who have signed the covenant and have taken an oath according to the medical law, but to no one else.

I will apply dietetic measures for the benefit of the sick according to my ability and judgment; I will keep them from harm and injustice.

I will neither give a deadly drug to anybody if asked for it nor will I make a suggestion to this effect. Similarly, I will not give to a woman an abortive remedy. In purity and holiness, I will guard my life and my art.

I will not use the knife, not even on sufferers from stone, but will withdraw in favor of such men as are engaged in this work.

Whatever houses I may visit, I will come for the benefit of the sick, remaining free of all intentional injustice, of all mischief, and in particular of sexual relations with both female and male persons, be they free or slaves.

Source: Delmar's Comprehensive Medical Assisting *(4th ed.), by W. Lindh, M. Pooler, C. Tamparo, & B. M. Dahl, 2010, Clifton Park, NY: Delmar Cengage Learning.*

taken by physicians over the centuries, contains issues and ideas that are still being debated today. Read the Oath in Box 3–1 and look for the references to mercy killing, abortion, and sexual harassment. At the same time, the practice of medicine has changed over time—as with the use of surgery, which for centuries was not practiced by physicians.

Health care professionals today are confronted by more ethical problems than at any other time in history. Flight (2004) notes that, "Technology has progressed beyond society's readiness to deal with the ethical and legal issues it presents" (p. 235). Today we are able to prevent conception, prolong life, transplant organs, and perform lifesaving procedures to an extent never before imagined. In some cases, cures seem miraculous and add to human happiness. In others, society is confronted with difficult questions like the following:

- Anencephalic babies are born with only a partial brain. Most die shortly after birth. When this condition is diagnosed, usually at 18 weeks of pregnancy, should the mother be allowed to abort the child?
- Should life support be withdrawn from patients who are in coma and judged to have no chance of revival? After one year? After five years?
- Should painkillers be given in quantities sufficient to relieve extreme pain even if the patient might become addicted to them?
- If a patient is suffering from a painful form of terminal cancer, should his request to be assisted in dying "in a dignified manner" be honored?
- Should teenagers be given birth control information and products without their parents' knowledge?
- Should anyone be given birth control information and products?
- If immunizations must be rationed during an influenza pandemic, who should receive them?
- Should parents be required to vaccinate their children? (See Figure 3–1.)
- Should parents be required to get medical care for their children if this contradicts their religious beliefs?

Technological advancements have dramatically increased the price of health care. Spending for specialized training, equipment, and procedures continues to push costs up. As discussed in Chapter 2,

Fascinating Facts

Regulation of health care for the public good is not a modern idea. More than 4500 years ago, rules for physicians were included in the Code of Hammurabi. It contained a long list of do's and don'ts and penalties for not following the rules. It even included guidelines regarding the fees that physicians could charge.

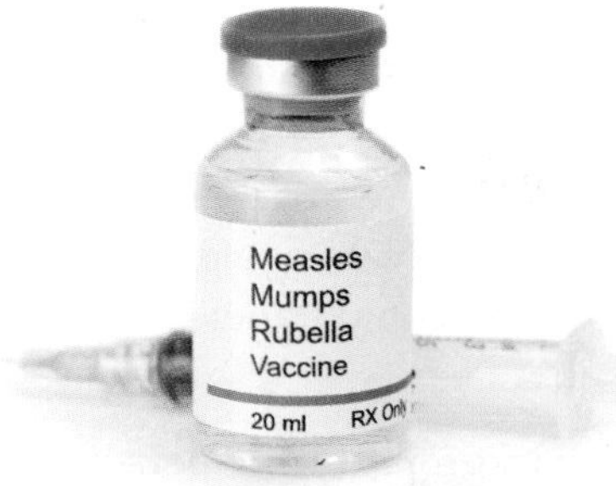

© Sherry Yates Young/Shutterstock.com.

FIGURE 3–1 Should parents who believe that vaccines will harm their children be required to have their children immunized to protect the health of others?

this has resulted in efforts to control these costs while attempting to maintain the quality of care provided. Decisions about how to distribute available health care dollars raise serious ethical questions about who receives care. Recently passed health care reform, discussed in Chapters 2 and 22, will put this belief into practice. It is hoped that the provisions in this sweeping legislation will improve the health care system and not result in the unintended consequence of long waits for service. Creating a sustainable system that ensures adequate care in a timely and cost-effective way for everyone who needs it remains a major challenge facing Americans today.

Professional Codes of Ethics

Health care professionals are guided by principles outlined in occupation-specific **codes of ethics** developed by professional organizations. While they vary in detail, the codes all share the same purpose: to set standards of professional conduct that promote the welfare of patients and ensure a high quality of care. Here are statements from three professional codes:

- The purpose of a professional code of ethics is to achieve the high levels of ethical consciousness, decision making, and practice by members of the profession. (Code of Ethics for Dental Hygienists)
- The American Occupational Therapy Association's (AOTA) Occupational Therapy Code of Ethics and Ethics Standards (2010) is a public statement of principles used to promote and maintain high standards of conduct within the profession. (American Occupational Therapy Code of Ethics)
- Position Statement, Item 1: To maintain the highest standards of professional conduct and patient care. (Association of Surgical Technologists)

The "ethical consciousness" mentioned in the dental hygiene code means being aware of the importance of, and the need for, standards in health care. You will likely encounter ethical issues throughout your professional life. It is your responsibility to read and understand the full text of the code of ethics for your occupation. You can obtain one by contacting your professional organization or locating it on the organization's website (see Appendix 1). See Box 3–2 for an example of a complete professional code of ethics.

The ethical problems encountered by health care professionals can be confusing and stressful. Although there are no simple recipes for handling difficult issues, ethical codes can provide guidelines when making important decisions about professional conduct.

Fascinating Facts

Technology has raised ethical issues no one would have imagined in the past. One example is email. Physicians now find email to be very effective for communicating with their patients. However, this brings a new set of ethical concerns regarding privacy and the need to maintain interpersonal contact with patients. Communication guidelines have been developed by the American Medical Association to handle these concerns.

Source: Available at http://www.ama-assn.org/ama/pub/physician-resources/medical-ethics/code-medical-ethics/opinion5026.page?

Personal Values

Values are the beliefs and ideals that provide the foundation for making decisions and guiding behavior. Individuals develop their personal values as they grow and mature. Values are influenced by factors such as family, religious teachings, education, and personal experience. They can be identified by thinking about what is important in life. For example, one person may place great importance on having material possessions; in comparison, another believes that enjoying close relationships with friends is more important. The first individual *values* possessions; the second *values* relationships.

Values are not necessarily right or wrong, but it is important to be clear about personal values. They may

BOX 3–2

Code of Ethics

The Code of Ethics of the American Association of Medical Assistants (AAMA) shall set forth principles of ethical and moral conduct as they relate to the medical profession and the particular practice of medical assisting.

Members of AAMA dedicated to the conscientious pursuit of their profession, and thus desiring to merit the high regard of the entire medical profession and the respect of the general public which they serve, do pledge themselves to strive always to:

A. render service with full respect for the dignity of humanity;

B. respect confidential information obtained through employment unless legally authorized or required by responsible performance of duty to divulge such information;

C. uphold the honor and high principles of the profession and accept its disciplines;

D. seek to continually improve the knowledge and skills of medical assistants for the benefit of patients and professional colleagues;

E. participate in additional service activities aimed toward improving the health and well-being of the community.

Source: Reprinted with permission of the American Association of Medical Assistants, Inc.

conflict with situations encountered on the job. Health care professionals, however, must support the decisions and practices of the facilities where they work. If this is impossible, it may be best to seek employment elsewhere. It is sometimes necessary to make personal adjustments to accommodate strongly held beliefs. The following example illustrates this type of situation:

> Hannah is one of eight children in a Catholic family. She attended Catholic elementary and high school and continues to attend Mass every Sunday. She believes that abortion is wrong and cannot be justified under any circumstances. Hannah recently graduated from a medical assisting program and is ready to seek employment. She realizes that she must support the desires and well-being of her patients and never judge them in any way. Therefore, Hannah has decided not to work in any facility where abortions are performed. In this way, she can avoid ethical conflicts between her personal beliefs and the needs of the patients.

Cultural background and personal values may influence the choice of a specific type of work, as in the following case:

> Karen Chin's parents emigrated from China to the United States in 1980. Her mother's parents came with the family and have always played an important part in Karen's life. She respects her grandparents' knowledge and experience and often turned to them for advice while she was growing up. Today, in spite of health problems and the inability to handle their daily needs, they remain in the family home, cared for by younger family members.
>
> Inspired by her home experience, Karen decided to do volunteer work in a nursing home. Karen's interest in caring for older patients increased. She has decided to specialize in geriatric nursing and devote her career to working with older patients. She wants to offer them the care and compassion that she believes older persons deserve.

GUIDING PRINCIPLES OF HEALTH CARE ETHICS

The discussion of health care ethics in this chapter is organized around eight guiding principles:

1. Preserve life
2. Do good
3. Respect autonomy
4. Uphold justice
5. Be honest
6. Be discreet
7. Keep promises
8. Do no harm

These principles are discussed in the following sections, along with examples of corresponding laws that support them. Refer to Table 3–2 for examples of how health care professionals apply ethical principles on the job.

Table 3–2 Applying Ethics on the Job

Ethical Principle	Examples of Health Care Professional Responsibilities
Preserve Life	• Provide all patients, including the terminally ill, with caring attention. • Become familiar with your state laws regarding organ donations.
Do Good	• Practice good communication skills. (See Chapters 15, 16, and 17.) • Treat every patient with respect and courtesy. • Serve as a positive role model and promote healthy living. • Learn about the stages of dying and grieving. (See Chapter 8.)
Respect Autonomy	• Be sure that patients have consented to all treatment and procedures. • Become familiar with the state laws and facility policies dealing with advance directives. • Respect the beliefs and values of various cultural groups.
Uphold Justice	• Treat all patients equally, regardless of economic or social background. • Know the rules for handling all categories of controlled substances. • Learn the state laws and your facility's policies and procedures for handling and reporting suspected abuse. • Follow all safety rules and OSHA guidelines to ensure the safety of yourself and others.
Be Honest	• Admit mistakes promptly. Offer to do what is necessary to correct them. • Refuse to participate in any form of fraud. • Document all procedures accurately. Perform coding accurately, if this is part of your responsibilities. • Give an "honest day's work" every day.
Be Discreet	• Never release patient information of any kind unless there is a signed release. • Do not discuss patients with anyone who is not professionally involved in their care. • Conduct necessary conversations about patients with other health care professionals in private areas. • Keep documentation out of the view of people who are not authorized to see it. (See Figure 3–2.) • Do not leave records or patient registers on the reception desk in plain sight of anyone who approaches the desk. • Keep phone conversations with or about patients private. • Protect the physical privacy of patients.
Keep Promises	• Be sure that necessary contracts have been completed. • Be very careful about what you say to patients. They may only hear the "good news." • Complete all tasks assigned by your employer.
Do No Harm	• Focus on providing excellent customer service. (See Chapter 23.) • Always work within your scope of practice. Never give information or perform duties you are not qualified to do. • Observe all safety rules and precautions. Keep areas safe from hazards and make the safety of patients a top priority. (See Figure 3–3.) • Perform procedures according to facility **protocols** (standard methods for performing tasks) listed in the policy and procedure manual or the employee handbook. Never take shortcuts. • Ask an appropriate person about anything you are unsure about. • Keep your skills up to date. See Chapter 14 for more information about continuing education. • Keep certifications current (cardiopulmonary resuscitation [CPR], first aid, professional certifications and/or licenses). • Stay informed about new laws that affect health care.

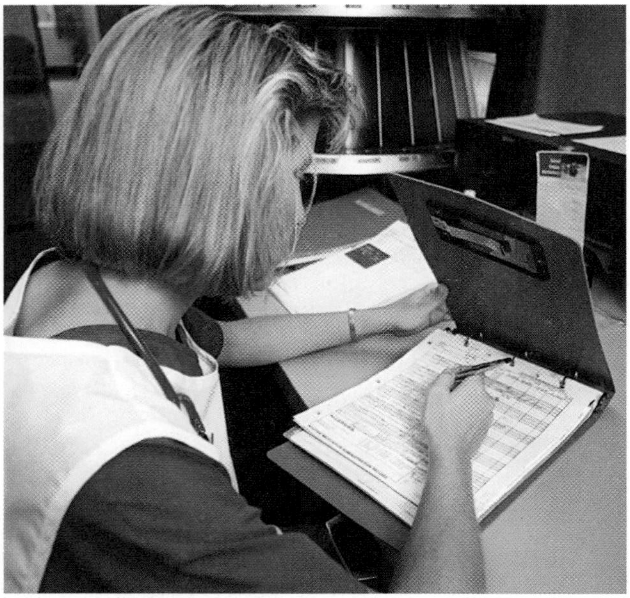

FIGURE 3–2 Always take care to protect the confidentiality of medical records.

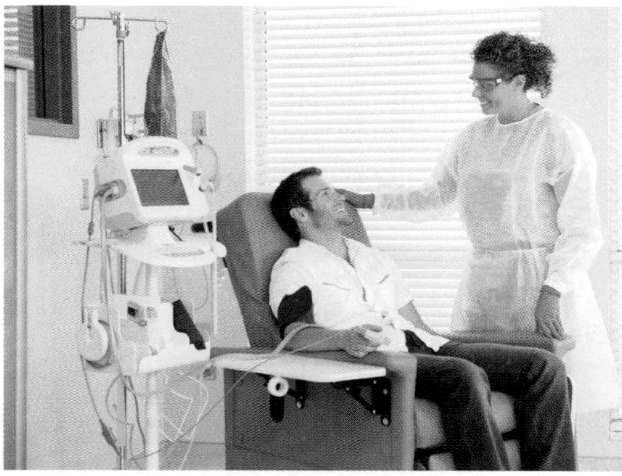

© Tyler Olson/Shutterstock.com.

FIGURE 3–3 Ensuring patient safety must be a high priority for health care professionals. For example, chemotherapy is often effective in treating cancer, but it must be monitored carefully.

Preserve Life

The basic guiding principle for health care professionals states that life is precious and that all possible means should be taken to preserve it. The Hippocratic Oath, which has influenced medical ethics for more than 2000 years, states: "I will neither give a deadly drug to anybody if asked for it, nor will I make a suggestion to this effect."

Thinking It Through

Juan Ruiz is a physical therapy assistant working in a skilled nursing facility. He loves his work and enjoys helping patients regain strength and range of motion through exercise. The amount of rehabilitation that patients may receive is limited by their insurance companies and Medicare. Juan is concerned that patients who could be regaining the full use of their limbs are not being given an adequate number of sessions. One of Juan's patients, on learning that he has only one more session with Juan, asks him if he has received "enough therapy." Juan believes that this person would benefit from at least five more sessions.

1. How should Juan respond?
2. What can he do to help the patient progress toward his full potential?
3. What can Juan do to help increase the funding allocated for rehabilitation services?

Difficulties arise when there is disagreement about the definition of "life." Advances in technology have made it possible to maintain life by artificial means, such as ventilators and feeding tubes. The argument has been made that patients suffering from terminal diseases and injuries are being forced to exist under cruel and unnatural conditions. Some suggest that a better description would take the quality of life into consideration. Is it worth prolonging a life, they ask, when the patient is:

- In severe pain that cannot be relieved?
- Suffering from a terminal condition?
- In a coma with no reasonable hope of regaining consciousness?
- Without brain function?
- Requesting that treatment be discontinued?
- Asking that life be terminated?

Withdrawing artificial means of supporting life has become widely accepted, as long as this is the desire of the patient or those who are authorized to make this decision. Withholding life support can be justified, some argue, because it simply allows an existing fatal condition to take its course. Artificial support merely delays a death that cannot be avoided. Others believe that life support should be sustained as long as possible. If a patient has not given instructions to the contrary through an advance directive (discussed later in this chapter), it may be impossible for health care providers to discontinue this support.

Euthanasia

Euthanasia, also called **mercy killing**, is performing an action that results in the death of a patient to alleviate suffering or when it is believed that there is no hope for recovery. Most physicians and health care professionals believe this to be contrary to their stated professional purpose. A well-known exception is Dr. Jack Kevorkian, a Michigan physician who assisted more than 100 patients to end their lives, believing that helping patients achieve a painless death is the kindest act a physician can perform. His actions were deemed illegal and in 1999, a jury convicted him of second-degree murder and he spent eight years in prison.

To date, five states have passed a physician-assisted life termination law: Montana, New Mexico, Oregon, Vermont, and Washington. The Oregon law was the first, passed in 1997. After its passage, it was successfully challenged by the U.S. Justice Department. However, in 2006, the U.S. Supreme Court upheld the law and it remains in force today.

Regardless of their personal beliefs about assisted dying laws, it is the duty of health care professionals to follow their state laws and dedicate themselves to maintaining as high a quality of life as possible for all patients. Respecting life means giving people attention during every phase of life, even in their final days. Many terminally ill patients report that they believe they receive less attention than those for whom "there is hope." These patients report that the loneliness experienced in the final days of their lives is worse than the idea of dying (Purtilo & Haddad, 2007). Some patients want to talk about their lives, fears, and approaching death. Health care professionals may find these topics uncomfortable and not know how to respond. Recognizing death as a natural part of life can help the health care professional listen and react honestly to patients who need consideration and understanding in dealing with their approaching death. Avoiding terminally ill patients or hurrying through their care is unethical.

Organ Transplantation

The ability of surgeons to successfully transplant organs has saved the lives of many who, without the procedure, had limited hopes for survival. At the same time, it created an ethical dilemma because not everyone agrees to have their own organs, or those of family members, donated at the time of their death. The following statistics show the extent of the problem:

- 123,351 people need an organ transplant at this time.
- 78,127 of these people are medically prepared for a transplant.
- 32,109 transplants were performed in 2014.
- 15,670 people were donors in 2014.
- 21 people die each day while waiting (http://optn.transplant.hrsa.gov).

While the organs from one person can save the lives of as many as eight others, it is illegal to take organs without the prior permission of the patient or, following death, his or her family members. Payment cannot be given to donors or to their survivors. To further prevent abuse, it is illegal for the physician who pronounces the donor's death to participate on the transplant surgical team.

Individuals who wish to be organ donors should make their wishes known to family members. Many states place symbols on driver's licenses indicating that the driver has consented to being a donor. Although signed donor cards and driver's licenses with an "organ donor" designation are legal documents, organ and tissue donation is always discussed with family members prior to the donation.

The allocation of donated organs is another ethical consideration. Who should get priority? People who are the sickest or those who have the greatest chance of surviving and achieving a long life? Should personal behavior, such as drug abuse, heavy smoking, or alcoholism that contributed to the organ failure, be considered? At present, the following are common considerations when choosing an organ recipient:

- Medical urgency
- Blood, tissue, and size match
- Time the patient has waited
- Proximity to the donor
- Age of the patient (children are sometimes given priority)

Organ transplantation presents difficult questions for which there are no easy answers (www.organtransplants.org).

Rationing Care and Resources

Rationing care has become an increasingly serious concern as the cost of health care rises. Some have argued that rationing has always existed because insurance carriers make decisions about which diagnostic tests and recommended treatments they will and will not cover. As a result, certain types of care are not available to patients who cannot pay for it themselves. Medicare and Medicaid, like private insurance companies, also have limitations on which services they cover. Medicaid, which helps low-income individuals and families pay for health care, is funded by the federal and state governments. Many states, dealing with thousands of new Medicaid recipients as a result of the Patient Protection and Affordable Care Act, are cutting benefits to prevent running out of funds. Examples of cuts include limiting hospital stays, not covering certain drugs, and not paying for vision and chiropractic care.

Access to health care itself is rationed to some degree. Because of low reimbursement rates to physicians, especially for Medicaid patients, many doctors are no longer accepting new patients who have Medicare or Medicaid. In spite of their desire to provide health care, they state that they cannot afford to run their practices if they have too many patients in these categories.

Do Good

Helping and promoting the welfare of others is a basic duty of the health care professional. The reasonable needs of a patient must be considered before the needs of self. Personal convenience is always secondary to patient welfare.

Working in the best interest of patients requires the following:

- Listening carefully to what they say
- Making an effort to understand their ethnic and cultural backgrounds
- Carefully assessing their needs
- Being aware of their ethical beliefs
- Explaining what you are doing as you perform tests, treatments, and other procedures
- Providing appropriate instruction
- Allowing the patient to feel comfortable enough to ask questions
- Answering all patient questions, or finding the answers if necessary

Part of the appeal of health care work is the potential to promote the well-being of the community. Health care professionals should serve as role models by being examples of healthy living practices. (See Chapter 12.)

Health care professionals are paid by their employer for their services and should never accept monetary tips from patients. "Doing good" includes the idea of performing one's job without the expectation of receiving anything extra.

Respect Autonomy

Americans value **autonomy**, which means self-determination. Patients have the right to make decisions about their health care, including whether or not they choose to receive treatment. They can choose who, if anyone, will treat them and what treatments they will receive. As much as possible, based on their physical and mental capabilities and age, patients should be involved in their own care.

Consent

Medical treatment cannot be carried out unless the patient gives his or her **consent** (permission). **Informed consent** is the process in which the patient receives information about treatment and gives his or her permission. Full informed consent consists of several elements:

- Explanation of the procedure
- Information about any alternatives
- Risks, benefits, and uncertainties of each alternative
- Assessment of patient understanding
- Acceptance of treatment by the patient (De Bord, 2014)

Touching a patient or performing a procedure without his or her permission can result in being charged with the crime of **battery**, which refers to any unauthorized touching of another person. If a patient feels threatened about receiving unwanted treatment, even if it is not performed, this can result in the crime of **assault**. Assault, in this case, is any threatened or implied act, whether carried out or not. (This use of the word should not be confused with an alternate definition of "assault" meaning a violent, physical attack.) It does not matter if the patient benefits from the treatment. The only difference between proper medical treatment and the crimes of assault and battery is whether the patient gives permission.

Thinking It Through

Dr. C. Everett Koop, formerly Surgeon General of the United States, presents the following situation. It involves a 5-year-old girl who has a type of childhood brain tumor that Dr. Koop has studied for many years. The child's original tumor was removed, but it has recurred in spite of all known treatment. Dr. Koop writes: "I know her days are limited and that the longer she lives the more likely she is to have considerable pain. She might also become both blind and deaf." He goes on to explain that the child is severely anemic and this causes her to be unaware of what is happening to her. If he treats the anemia, this may prolong her life. At the same time, it will increase her awareness of pain and ability to understand her situation. Anticancer drugs can be prescribed, but he knows these have no chance of curing the child. Dr. Koop poses the question "Would it be better to let this little girl slip into death quietly . . . or should we prolong her life?"

1. It can be argued that it is Dr. Koop's responsibility as a physician to treat all aspects of the child's condition, including the anemia. Do you agree? Explain your answer.
2. Should anyone else be involved in making the decision about how to treat this child? Explain why.
3. Discuss what you think should be done for this child.

An exception is emergency care administered when the patient is physically unable to give consent. This is discussed in Chapter 21.

Battery can also be charged if patients are handled more roughly than necessary. Flight (2004) describes a case in which a physician spanked a 4-year-old child who refused to lie still while he was removing her sutures (stitches). The spanking caused bruises that lasted for three weeks. The mother successfully sued the physician for assault and battery.

The patient's full consent must be obtained before performing any procedure. A resisted action, done "for the good of the patient," may be illegal and result in criminal charges or a lawsuit. Particular care should be taken when using any type of restraint, especially with an uncooperative patient. The health care professional must always use proper techniques when moving patients to prevent pulling on limbs or other unintended roughness.

Excessive persuasion is also a form of assault. A patient who feels "talked into" a procedure may charge assault and battery. For example, a woman who believes she was pressured into being sterilized by having her tubes tied, against her true wishes, may successfully sue. Patients who are worried about health problems or financial matters often feel afraid and confused. They may accept the advice of a health care provider, only to change their minds later.

There are two types of informed consent: implied and express. **Implied consent** is indicated by the patient's actions: showing up for a medical appointment, opening the mouth for the dentist to administer an injection, or participating in therapeutic exercises. **Express consent** is more formal, either oral or in writing, in which a patient gives permission to receive treatment. Express consent is required for many procedures, especially those that are invasive. (**Invasive procedures** involve punctures or incisions of the skin or insertion of instruments or foreign material into the body.) See Box 3–3 for a sample of a written consent form. Consent forms for complicated procedures, such as surgeries, will contain more information.

The conditions under which a consent form is signed are important. It is not sufficient that patients be given full information. They must understand it as well. If necessary, a translated written form or an interpreter, or both, must be provided. If patients do not understand English or are hearing impaired, means must be arranged to ensure that they completely understand all the required items listed previously for informed consent.

A written consent form does not protect the health care provider if the patient claims to have signed under pressure. It is essential that patients understand it is their right to refuse treatment and that signing is completely voluntary. It is legal for patients to refuse treatment, even if doing so may damage their health.

Consent forms can be signed legally by mentally competent adults (who are not impaired by medication). In most states, **adult** is defined as someone 18 years of age or older. **Emancipated minors** are individuals younger than age 18 who are financially independent, married, or in the military. They are considered to be legal adults and can sign consent forms on their own behalf for treatment. Individuals younger than age 18 who are not emancipated minors may require

BOX 3–3

Sample Consent for Treatment

Date ______________ Time ______________

I authorize the performance of the following procedure(s) ______________ on ______________ (name of patient) ______________ to be performed by (name of physician) ______________, MD.

The following have been explained to ______________ by Dr. ______________ (name of physician) ______________.

Nature of the procedure ______________ (describe procedure) ______________.

For the purpose of ______________

____

The possible alternative methods of treatment are ______________.

The risks involve the possibility of ______________.

The possible complications of this procedure are ______________.

I have been advised of the serious nature of this procedure and have been further advised that if I desire a more detailed explanation of any of the foregoing or further information about the possible risks or complications, it will be given to me.

I do not request a more detailed listing and explanation of the above information.

Signed ______________ Date ______________

(Patient/Parent/Guardian)

Witnessed by: ______________ Date ______________

a consent form signed by a parent or guardian before a procedure is performed. Many states allow non-emancipated minors as young as 14 to make decisions regarding their health care. Some states do not require parental permission for minors to receive birth control information, abortions, or drug counseling. It is essential that health care professionals learn the laws in the state where they work and keep up with changes to them.

A claim of **false imprisonment** can be charged if patients are held against their will, unless they are mentally incompetent or a danger to themselves. For example, a person cannot be kept in a hospital or clinic "for his own good" because he needs medical attention. Without the patient's consent, release is the only option. Patients may be asked to sign a statement that they are discontinuing care against medical advice. This may protect the facility and professional staff from damages (financial responsibility) if the patient suffers harm as a result of refusing treatment.

Advance Directives

Self-determination about health care decisions is possible through the use of **advance directives**. These are written instructions that outline individuals' desires regarding care should they become unable, as the result of illness or injury, to make these decisions. Two major forms of advance directives are described next:

1. **Designation of health care surrogate/representative**. In this document, sometimes called a "health care power of attorney," individuals designate specific people to act on their behalf if they become unable to make health care decisions. An individual can select anyone to be a surrogate; it is not necessary for the surrogate to be related. Each state has specific requirements and designation forms.
2. **Living will/health care instructions**. This document outlines an individual's wishes regarding the type and extent of care to be given. Some living wills allow the inclusion of specific directions about whether the individual consents to certain procedures, such as cardiac resuscitation, mechanical respiration, and feeding tubes. A "do not resuscitate" (DNR) request can be included. This means that CPR is not to be administered if the individual stops breathing. An exception is if the individual is not in a health care facility and emergency personnel cannot locate a DNR request. Living wills are regulated by state laws.

The Patient Self-Determination Act passed in 1991 is federal **legislation** (law) that requires hospitals, nursing homes, rehabilitation facilities, and hospices to have written policies regarding advance directives. They must provide adult patients with information about advance health directives upon their admission to the facility. Patients are not legally required to prepare advance directives, but they must be informed of their right to have them.

Problems can arise when patients do not indicate their wishes while they are competent to do so. Family members and physicians may disagree about the proper course of action. In some cases, the courts are called on to make the final decision. A well-publicized and very controversial case involved Terri Schiavo, a woman who, most physicians believed, was in a nonreversible vegetative state for 15 years. Her parents and husband disagreed about her state of awareness and wishes for care. After years of court battles, her husband's request to remove her feeding tube was granted and she died within two weeks. There are still many similar cases in the court system. Sometimes the conflict involves family members and health care providers. In March 2009, a New Jersey judge rejected a hospital's decision to remove the life support of a patient who had been in an unconscious state since suffering complications from surgery in January 2008. The family contested the hospital's decision and the hospital was required to reconnect a feeding tube, ventilator, and dialysis machine.

The growing number of older Americans has presented an increasing number of situations in which health care providers become involved in determining competency. Giving up one's home and independence can be extremely difficult and in many cases, individuals do not recognize that their safety and well-being are threatened by their living alone. Home care professionals are often faced with clients who do not use their walkers, as advised by their physicians; do not eat the meals delivered to their homes; and are unable to properly take their medications. In these cases, the need to provide additional care or to move the older adult to assisted living or a care facility conflicts with the principle of autonomy if the older adult is adamant about living alone or staying in the home. Sometimes a team approach that includes the physician, nurse, social worker, and family members must make difficult, but necessary, decisions regarding the client's welfare. Box 3–4 contains a list of other ethical issues that concern the care and welfare of older adults.

BOX 3–4

Ethical and Legal Topics of Concern Regarding Eldercare

- Management of chronic, intractable pain in aging patients
- Legislation impacting nursing home care
- Clinically validated tools that assess mental capacity in the elderly
- Recognizing and reporting physical and emotional abuse and financial exploitation of the elderly
- Management of geriatric patients with advanced illness when further active treatment is no longer desirable or feasible or not likely to improve the patient's quality of life

Source: National Conference on Medical, Legal and Ethical Issues of Eldercare (2007, September 28).

Uphold Justice

Justice refers to fairness. Justice requires that all patients, regardless of race, economic status, religion, nationality, or personal characteristics, receive the same level of care and consideration.

Illness and injury do not always bring out the best in human nature. Patients may experience fear and anxiety. Health problems shake self-confidence and upset otherwise stable lives. Patients can be unreasonable, unpleasant, and uncooperative. It is these very patients who are most in need of respect and consideration. To disregard or take advantage of them in any way is highly unethical.

Reporting Abuse

Justice also refers to the use of authority or power to uphold what is right or lawful. Our society encourages us to protect each other from harm. This principle supports the laws that require health care professionals, among others, to report suspected abuse. The Federal Child Abuse Prevention and Treatment Act was passed to require the reporting of physical, sexual, and mental abuse of children and to protect those who do the reporting. Patient confidentiality does not exist in cases of suspected abuse.

The health care professional must be aware of the signs of possible child abuse. These signs may be physical or behavioral and include the following:

- Bruises and welts
- Burns
- Lacerations and abrasions
- Skeletal injuries
- Head injuries
- Repeated injuries at a higher rate than normal for a child of the same age
- Different explanations for the cause of an injury given by the child and the parent
- Unusually compliant, fearful, or aggressive behavior of the child

Any suspected cases of child abuse should be reported immediately to the supervisor. In cases where this is not possible, most state laws have broad statutes that require "any person" to report, therefore enabling health care professionals themselves to report.

With the increasing number of older citizens, elder abuse is a growing problem. It is estimated that between one and two million people aged 65 and over are injured, exploited, or otherwise mistreated each year by someone on whom they depend for care (National Center on Elder Abuse, 2005). Abuse may be committed by a spouse, other family members (accounts for 90% of cases), or paid caregivers and can occur in various forms:

- Neglect and lack of proper physical care
- Taking financial and other resources without the permission or understanding of the older person
- Physical mistreatment
- Mental and emotional abuse
- Sexual abuse
- Abandonment

All states have reporting systems for elder abuse. The principal public agencies responsible for investigating elder abuse and providing treatment and protective services are Adult Protective Services, the area agency on aging, or the county department of social services. Most states have an elder abuse hotline. Current estimates of unreported cases of abuse range from one report to authorities for every five cases to one case in 14. Therefore, the actual number of cases may be between five and 14 *times* the number reported. The reasons the elderly do not report abuse is fear of retaliation, lack of physical or cognitive ability to report, or because they do not want to get the abuser into trouble (www.ncea.aoa.gov/Library/Data/).

Even if not required by law, it is the ethical duty of health care professionals to report suspected cases of elder abuse to their supervisors. Health care facilities have reporting procedures for handling all types of suspected abuse, including spousal abuse. Most states have mandatory reporting laws for health care providers when they know or reasonably suspect that their patient has been injured as a result of domestic abuse. (These laws are different from those covering child and elder abuse.) Some states list specific injuries and wounds that require reporting, such as firearm injury, battery, stabbing, and rape. A negative consequence of mandatory reporting is that some victims will not seek medical care for fear that the report to law enforcement will cause the abuser to retaliate. In these cases, health facilities are encouraged to address safety concerns and guide victims of violence through available options.

Health care professionals must be familiar with their state laws and the reporting procedures for their facility. (See Table 3–3 for a list of resources.)

Laws That Protect

Americans believe that government has an ethical obligation to protect all citizens. For example, employers may not take advantage of employees by exposing them to dangerous working conditions. The Occupational Safety and Health Act was established in 1970 by the federal government. The act requires employers to accept responsibility for the safety and health of their employees in the workplace. Health care employers are directed under OSHA to take

Table 3–3 Abuse Resources for Health Care Providers

Resource	Contact Information
Child Welfare Information Gateway	www.childwelfare.gov
The National Child Abuse Hotline	1-800-4-A-CHILD (1-800-422-4453)
List of state child abuse hotlines	www.nccafv.org/child_abuse_reporting_numbers_co.htm
Links to laws for each state	www.childwelfare.gov/topics/systemwide/laws-policies/state/
National Center on Elder Abuse (incudes list of state telephone numbers for reporting elder abuse)	www.ncea.aoa.gov
Eldercare Locator (referrals and information)	1-800-677-1116; www.eldercare.gov
Links to state domestic abuse laws	www.womenslaw.org

measures to prevent employees from contracting contagious diseases. Specifically, there must be a written plan that includes waste management procedures, personal protection methods, and employee training programs.

The prevention of behaviors that lead to individual and social harm is another responsibility that the government believes it has an ethical obligation to uphold. Drug abuse is an example of a behavior considered to be harmful to not only the individual, but to society as a whole. The Controlled Substances Act is a federal law regulated by the U.S. Drug Enforcement Administration (DEA) to help prevent the misuse of addictive substances. Drugs that have addictive potential are classified into five categories called schedules. (See Box 3–5.) Each group has specific guidelines for medical use, including prescribing and handling. Examples of drugs that fall under each of the five groups can be found at the Office of Diversion Control's website at www.deadiversion.usdoj.gov/schedules/. Violations of these laws are criminal acts and can result in fines and imprisonment. Not only is the illegal or overuse of drugs a criminal offense, it can lead to death as discussed in Chapter 2.

Be Honest

Good health care is based on honesty. Patients' trust in the health care professional is an important factor in their well-being, and trust is built on honesty. At the same time, it can be argued that telling a patient the truth may not be in his or her own best interest. For example, should a clinically depressed patient be told he has terminal cancer if it is believed this might lead him to attempt suicide?

Truth-telling is also critical among coworkers and with supervisors. This is not always easy. For example, if you make a mistake in performing a lab test, it is tempting to "forget" to mention it. Mistakes, however, can have serious consequences and must be admitted and corrected as quickly as possible.

Fraud is a form of dishonesty that involves cheating or trickery, and there are several forms that occur in health care:

- Submitting insurance claims for services not performed
- Charging different rates for insured and uninsured patients
- Selling treatments, drugs, and devices that have not been proven effective
- Claiming to have a degree, experience, or credentials that one does not have

Medical fraud can result in severe penalties, ranging from losing the right to bill Medicare to imprisonment.

The health care professional who dedicates time on the job serving the employer and patients is behaving honestly. Arriving late, using paid time to perform personal tasks, and socializing with coworkers rather than attending to patients are forms of dishonesty. Accepting payment to work in a health care position indicates agreement to do the tasks expected for that occupation. Conducting yourself honestly and ethically on the job means making work a priority and striving to do your best every day.

Thinking It Through

The Patient Protection and Affordable Care Act extends Medicaid coverage to millions of Americans, which may result both physician and funding shortages. One way to deal with this problem is to ration care.

1. Do you agree or disagree with the concept of basic coverage for everyone, if some treatments and procedures cannot be covered? Explain your reasons.
2. Who should decide which procedures will be paid for and which will not?
3. How would you rank medical procedures? Which ones should never be denied? Are there any that you believe patients should be required to pay for themselves?

Be Discreet

Being **discreet** means being careful about what you say, preserving confidences, and respecting privacy. In health care, this is not only one of the most important ethical principles, it is the law. Patients have a legal right to privacy concerning their medical affairs. This is referred to as **confidentiality**. Violating that right, even if well intentioned, can result in a lawsuit.

BOX 3–5

Schedules of Controlled Substances

1. Schedule I.
   A. The drug or other substance has a high potential for abuse.
   B. The drug or other substance has no currently accepted medical use in treatment in the United States.
   C. There is a lack of accepted safety for use of the drug or other substance under medical supervision.
2. Schedule II.
   A. The drug or other substance has a high potential for abuse.
   B. The drug or other substance has a currently accepted medical use in treatment in the United States or a currently accepted medical use with severe restrictions.
   C. Abuse of the drug or other substances may lead to severe psychological or physical dependence.
3. Schedule III.
   A. The drug or other substance has a potential for abuse less than the drugs or other substances in Schedules I and II.
   B. The drug or other substance has a currently accepted medical use in treatment in the United States.
   C. Abuse of the drug or other substance may lead to moderate or low physical dependence or high psychological dependence.
4. Schedule IV.
   A. The drug or other substance has a low potential for abuse relative to the drugs or other substances in Schedule III.
   B. The drug or other substance has a currently accepted medical use in treatment in the United States.
   C. Abuse of the drug or other substance may lead to limited physical dependence or psychological dependence relative to the drugs or other substances in Schedule III.
5. Schedule V.
   A. The drug or other substance has a low potential for abuse relative to the drugs or other substances in Schedule IV.
   B. The drug or other substance has a currently accepted medical use in treatment in the United States.
   C. Abuse of the drug or other substance may lead to limited physical dependence or psychological dependence relative to the drugs or other substances in Schedule IV.

Source: U.S. Drug Enforcement Administration, www.deadiversion.usdoj.gov/21cfr/21usc/812.htm

Thinking It Through

Carin is a medical assistant for Dr. Allen, a dermatologist who has been in practice for many years. During his first 20 years in practice, Dr. Allen had a registered nurse assisting him in the office. When speaking with patients, he often refers to Carin as "my nurse."

1. Do you believe that Dr. Allen is misleading his patients?
2. Why or why not?
3. What could be the consequences?
4. How should Carin handle this situation?

Patient information cannot be released to anyone without the patient's written approval. (See Box 3–6.) This includes relatives, friends, insurance companies, and others who may claim to have the "right to know." The only exceptions are disclosures and reports allowed or required by law, such as births, deaths, certain infectious and communicable diseases, abuse, and life-threatening injuries caused by violence. The exact requirements and methods for reporting vary, so health care professionals should become familiar with the laws in their location.

In 1996, Congress passed the Health Insurance Portability and Accountability Act, commonly referred to as HIPAA. Implemented in 2003, an important part of this law was to promote the creation of national

BOX 3–6

Sample Authorization to Release Health Care Information

Patient ______________ Date of Birth ______________

SSN ______________ Previous name ______________

I request and authorize ______________ to release health care information of the patient named above to:

Name ______________________________

Address ______________________________

This request and authorization applies to: (Please initial the appropriate box)

______________ Health care information **EXCLUDING** specific information relating to sexually transmitted diseases (including HIV/AIDS), alcohol or drug use, or visits related to psychiatric disorders or mental health.

______________ All health care information **INCLUDING** specific information relating to sexually transmitted diseases (including HIV/AIDS), alcohol or drug use, or visits related to psychiatric disorders or mental health. ________ Other: ______________

I understand that my express consent is required to release any health care information relating to testing, diagnosis, and/or treatment of HIV (AIDS virus), sexually transmitted diseases, psychiatric disorders/mental health, or drug and/or alcohol use. If I have been tested, diagnosed, or treated for HIV (AIDS virus), sexually transmitted diseases, psychiatric disorders/mental health, or drug and/or alcohol use, you are specifically authorized to release all health care information relating to such diagnosis, testing, or treatment. ______________
/ ______________

______________ ______________

Signature of patient or patient authorized representative — Relationship to patient's

____

Date

standards to protect patient privacy and personal health information, which many people believed could be compromised by the use of electronic medical records. Health care facilities have formulated policies to comply with HIPAA requirements, discussed in more detail in Chapter 19. The following paragraphs contain general guidelines for maintaining confidentiality, but it is essential that new health care professionals learn the specific policies of the facilities in which they work.

Health care professionals should not talk about patients with coworkers where they might be overheard by other people. They must remember that hospital cafeterias and clinic elevators are used by the public and are inappropriate locations for such discussions. Reports to friends and family about your work that include the mention of patients must be avoided. Even without giving the names of patients, there may be enough details revealed so that others can guess their identities. Friendly conversations that seem innocent may be serious breaches of confidentiality.

Disclosing unauthorized information can result in being charged with harming the reputation of another. This is known as **defamation of character**. When disclosed in written form it is called **libel**. In spoken form it is called **slander**. These are serious offenses and can result from innocent but careless behavior. For example, reporting a patient's acquired immunodeficiency syndrome (AIDS) test results within the hearing of others could result in charges of slander.

When working directly with patients, take care to protect their physical privacy. Shut the doors of occupied examination rooms, close curtains around hospital beds when performing procedures, and drape patients properly to ensure that there is no more exposure than necessary. If patients must move from one area to another, be sure they are covered properly and do not have to pass through a public area.

Individual rights to privacy sometimes conflict with the public's right to be informed about matters concerning its safety. An incident in Baltimore illustrates this dilemma. Firefighters assisted an injured woman and took her to the hospital. The hospital staff was aware that the woman had AIDS, but was forbidden by physician–patient confidentiality laws to inform the firefighters that they had been exposed to the virus (Flight, 2004). A more recent example is the arrival in the United States of patients from West Africa who had contracted the Ebola virus. HIPPA regulations prevented hospitals from reporting the

Thinking It Through

A nurse who worked at the Baltimore hospital, in the example referred to in the text, decided to tell the firefighters that they had been exposed to AIDS.

1. Do you believe that she did the right thing? Explain your answer.
2. Do you think that breaking the rules of confidentiality was justified in this case?
3. Do you think this nurse should be fired for her actions?
4. Did the nurse commit slander against the woman?
5. What might you do in a similar situation?
6. What consequences would you be willing to accept in order to carry out what you believe to be your ethical responsibilities?

names of patients who had been transferred for treatment. However, there were many who believed the public had a right to know because they viewed Ebola as a threat to public health.

Another difficult situation occurs when patients tell health care professionals information in confidence that, if not revealed, may result in harm to the patients themselves or to others. For example, if a patient discloses that she plans to use prescription drugs to end her life after her release from the hospital, the health care professional has a duty to inform the patient's physician. Health care professionals must reveal patient confidences to their supervisors *if* they believe serious harm is likely to result if they do not reveal the information.

Keep Promises

In everyday life, promises are an important part of our relationships with others. **Contracts** are formalized promises that are enforceable by law. They contain the agreements of people to do certain specified things. For example, a contract is formed when an orthopedic surgeon agrees to perform a knee replacement and the patient agrees to pay for the procedure. If one of the parties fails to fulfill his or her part of the agreement, this can result in a **breach of contract**. If this failure results in a loss for the other party, a court may award money to make up for this loss.

In order for a contract to be enforceable, it must contain three components:

1. *Offer*: This is the action that starts the process of forming a contract. Examples:
   - Mr. Nguyen visits the dentist because of a toothache. His attendance is considered a request for the dentist to enter into a contract to provide treatment.
   - Marcia Parsons is referred to a physical therapist. By making an appointment with the therapist, she initiates a contract.
2. *Acceptance*: This means that both parties—the patient and the health care provider—agree to enter into the contract. They each agree to do something. Examples:
   - The dentist agrees to treat Mr. Nguyen.
   - The physical therapist sets a time to see Ms. Parsons.
3. *Consideration*: Something of value must be exchanged by the parties. In health care this generally means that the professional provides a service and the patient pays for the service. Examples:
   - The dentist examines Mr. Nguyen, takes X-rays, and fills a cavity. The patient pays for the service before leaving the office.
   - The physical therapist teaches Ms. Parsons to perform a series of leg-strengthening exercises. The patient provides information about her medical insurance coverage and also agrees to pay for any portion not covered by the insurance plan.

In order for a contract to be enforceable, the people who enter it must be competent. The law defines competency by age and mental condition, as it does with consent. State laws govern who may legally enter into a contract. In addition, the actions agreed to must be legal. Suppose that a patient requests his physician to assist him in ending his life (committing suicide). In spite of the action being illegal, the physician agrees. If the drug given does not end the life of the patient as promised, he cannot legally sue the physician for breach of contract because the action agreed to was illegal. (The physician might be charged with a criminal action, however.)

Most contracts between health care providers and patients are **implied contracts**. This means that the actions of the parties create the contract. In the dental example earlier, the actions of visiting the dentist, filling the tooth, and paying for the service fulfill the requirements of an implied contract. Giving emergency treatment is also a form of implied contract.

An **express contract** is created when the parties discuss and agree on specific terms and conditions. The contract can be either written or oral. It is important for the health care professional to avoid making statements that might be interpreted as a contract. Although it is natural to want to reassure and encourage patients, this should never be confused with giving what might be understood as a guarantee or false hope. Being "too nice" as the result of good intentions can cause legal difficulties, as illustrated in the following example:

> A middle-aged man was worried after a consultation with a surgeon. "Looks like I'll have to have a heart bypass," the patient remarked to the assistant at the front desk.
>
> "Don't worry," she assured him, "the doctor is very good at that procedure. You won't have any trouble. I can promise you that."
>
> There were several complications during the surgery, and the patient died several weeks later. His family successfully sued the surgeon on the grounds that his assistant had made a promise that amounted to a warranty (Flight, 1998, p. 82).

The surgeon in this case was sued because the assistant was acting as his **agent**. An agent is someone who has the authority to represent another person. This case occurred a number of years ago. However, the fact that health care professionals are generally considered to be agents of the licensed professionals for whom they work remains true today and the principles still apply. Employers can be held liable (legally responsible) for the behavior and actions of their employees. This concept is known as **respondeat superior**, which means "let the master answer." The following examples illustrate this concept:

- A physician could be held liable for the consequences of a medical assistant administering the wrong medication.
- A patient suffering injuries from a fall caused by the incompetence of a physical therapist assistant could be awarded **damages** (money to compensate for an injury or loss). The supervising therapist could be financially responsible.

Do No Harm

An essential responsibility of health care professionals is to *do no harm*. They must work within their scope of practice, performing only those duties that they have been trained to do. It is critical that safety rules be followed and that medical advice never be given by a person who is not qualified to do so.

Harm can result from **negligence**. This is failure to meet the standard of care that can be reasonably expected from a person with certain training and experience. Negligence can result from an action performed incorrectly or from the failure to take a necessary action. People who are trained in health care are expected to have special knowledge and skills. Thus they are held to a higher standard of care than those who are untrained. There are various levels of standards within the health care professions:

- A physical therapist (PT) is held to a higher standard of care than a physical therapist assistant (PTA).
- The PTA is held to a higher standard than the PT aide.
- The PT aide is held to a higher standard than an untrained person.

Malpractice is the term for professional negligence. Malpractice lawsuits are filed by patients who believe they have received improper care. It is important to understand, however, that not all lawsuits are the result of actual malpractice. Leading causes of lawsuits are patient anger and the lack of a satisfactory personal relationship with the health care provider. Good interpersonal relationships are a key factor in preventing malpractice lawsuits. Most patients understand that positive treatment results cannot be guaranteed. But they want to be treated with dignity and to feel that everything possible has been done to help them. Patients who perceive a lack of attention, care, and respect are much more likely to sue than those who feel positive about their care. As Flight (2004) states, "anger is the thread running through the entire malpractice saga" (p. 113). Communicating well, especially listening, and treating patients with kindness and respect are the most effective ways to

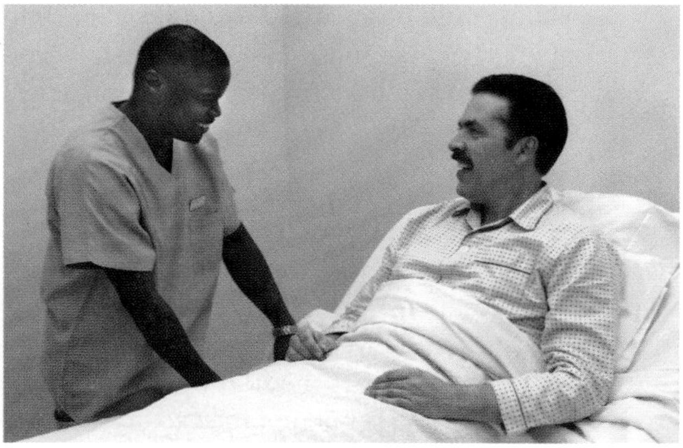

FIGURE 3–4 Communicating a sincere, caring attitude toward patients is the best defense against malpractice lawsuits.

reduce the risk of being sued. (See Figure 3–4.) See Chapter 23 for more information about providing good customer service.

Good Samaritan Laws

Good Samaritan laws have been passed by states to protect individuals, including health care professionals, from liability when they volunteer to give care in emergency situations. In order to be held liable, further injury must be caused intentionally or from extreme carelessness. Even in an emergency, it is important for health care professionals not to offer aid beyond their scope of training. Good Samaritan laws are discussed further in Chapter 21.

HANDLING ETHICAL DILEMMAS

The first consideration of the ethical health care professional is the well-being of patients. Illegal and unethical behavior can endanger patient welfare and cannot be tolerated. Observations of this behavior in others must not be ignored. Although it is difficult to confront a wrongdoer or "tell on" a coworker, doing what is right must override short-term discomfort. Accepting responsibility for making difficult decisions is part of health care work.

If the behavior observed in a coworker is illegal, it should be reported to the supervisor. For example, if a nurse observes a coworker using an illegal substance at the workplace, it should be reported immediately to the supervisor. If the behavior involves legal but ethically questionable behavior, such as "badmouthing" an employer, it may be best to first speak directly to the coworker.

Thinking It Through

Medical errors are a cause for growing concern. According to studies conducted by HealthGrades (2008), 238,337 Medicare patients died in the years 2004 through 2006 from potentially preventable, in-hospital errors. In 2000, President Clinton made an unsuccessful request for a law to require the public reporting of medical errors. Congress addressed the issue again in 2005, but no legislation was passed. People in favor of a reporting law believe it will improve the overall quality of health care. Those who are opposed, argue that it will result in increased attempts to cover up errors and thus prevent the follow-up needed to correct them. The Health Care Reform Act of 2010 reportedly does not require the reporting of medical errors.

1. Do you believe that medical errors should be reported publicly? Explain your answer.
2. How serious should errors be to require reporting them within the organization? Outside the organization?
3. Who should be responsible for tracking and handling medical errors?
4. What do you think might be the consequences if a law that required the reporting of medical errors were passed?

Source: Fifth Annual Patient Safety in American Hospitals Study, April 2008, HealthGrades. Available at www.healthgrades.com/media/dms/pdf/patientsafetyinamericanhospitalsstudy2008.pdf

WHO DECIDES?

When an individual or an organization is faced with a case that presents special ethical difficulties, there are several sources of help:

- The American Medical Association Council on Ethical and Judicial Affairs reviews situations and publishes opinions about current issues to provide guidelines for physicians.
- Hospitals and other large health care facilities have ethics committees composed of health care professionals and members of the community. These committees review individual cases and make recommendations.
- Clergy and counselors provide assistance to health care professionals in making decisions and dealing with personal feelings when coping with difficult situations.

- Conferences are held among the health care team members, the patient, and family members to explore possible actions.
- Many universities and medical colleges study ethical issues and share their findings.
- Some hospitals and clinics have a risk management department. Lawyers and specially trained health care professionals are charged with making ethical and legal decisions on behalf of the organization.

WORKBOOK PRACTICE

Go to your workbook and complete the exercises for this chapter.

SUGGESTED LEARNING ACTIVITIES

1. Locate articles on the Internet, in the newspaper, or in news magazines about ethical issues. Do you agree with the points of view presented?
2. Secure a copy of the code of ethics for your occupational area of interest. Can you find statements that correspond to the ethical principles presented in this chapter?
3. Explore your personal beliefs about ethical issues such as abortion, euthanasia, and individual privacy versus the public's right to know.
4. Contact the child protective unit of your state's department of social services (or their website) for information about reporting child abuse.
5. Visit the website of the National Center on Elder Abuse to learn more about this growing problem. Consider your role as a future health care provider working with elderly patients.
6. Contact a local health care facility and ask for a copy of their patient consent form.

WEB ACTIVITIES

American Hospital Association

www.aha.org

Enter "Patient Care Partnership" in the search box, then click on it to see the brochure. Which of the eight guiding principles of health care ethics discussed in this chapter are addressed in the brochure?

Department of Health and Human Services

www.hhs.gov

Enter "HIPAA" in the search box and click the search button. Then choose a topic to explore and write a short summary of what you learn.

National Library of Medicine—Medline Plus

www.nlm.nih.gov/medlineplus

Enter "medical ethics" in the search box. Choose a topic to explore (many links are available for the listed topics), and write a short essay describing the issue. Explain why it is considered to be an ethical issue.

REVIEW QUESTIONS

1. What is the purpose of ethics?
2. What is the purpose of a professional code of ethics?
3. How are ethics and laws related?
4. For each of the following ethical principles, explain its application to health care and give examples of actions health care professionals can take to support it.
   - Preserve life
   - Do good
   - Respect autonomy
   - Uphold justice
   - Be honest
   - Be discreet
   - Keep promises
   - Do no harm
5. Name four ethical challenges faced by today's health care providers.
6. What is the meaning of the following types of consent: informed, implied, and express?
7. What is the purpose of an advance directive?
8. List eight signs of child abuse.
9. What are the six forms of elder abuse?

10. Describe three actions that would violate patient confidentiality.
11. What is the difference between an implied contract and an express contract?
12. What is the meaning of negligence as it applies to health care?
13. What are six ways that health care organizations make decisions about ethical issues?

APPLICATION EXERCISES

1. Refer to the Case of the Missing Consent Form at the beginning of this chapter. Put together a list of the legal implications that might have resulted if the consent form was not signed.
2. You are working as a licensed practical nurse in a small urgent care center. You love the work. The physicians are excellent, and you have the opportunity to work with a variety of patients. You have become good friends with your coworkers and enjoy an especially close relationship with the administrative medical assistant, Amy. One day you observe Amy removing medication from the drug cabinet. You find this to be unusual because the administrative staff do not normally work with medications. While performing a routine inventory check later that day, you discover a shortage of a drug that is classified as a controlled substance. Explain what you would do in this situation.

PROBLEM-SOLVING PRACTICE

Maria has been working for a few weeks as a licensed practical nurse in a hospital. She has heard the other staff talking a lot about HIPAA and the many new rules, but she does not feel that she knows enough about these regulations. How can she use the five-step problem-solving process to become more informed?

SUGGESTED READINGS AND RESOURCES

Child Abuse. www.nlm.nih.gov/medlineplus/childabuse.html

De Bord (2014)

Edge, R. S., & Groves, J. R. (2006). *Ethics of health care: A guide for clinical practice* (3rd ed.). Clifton Park, NY: Delmar Cengage Learning.

Elder Abuse. www.nlm.nih.gov/medlineplus/elderabuse.html

Flight, M. (2011). *Law, liability, & ethics for medical office professionals* (5th ed.). Clifton Park, NY: Delmar Cengage Learning.

HG.org Legal Directories. Health—Guide to Health Law. www.hg.org/health-law.html

Judson, K., & Harrison, C. (2010). *Law & ethics for medical careers* (5th ed.). Boston: McGraw-Hill.

National Center on Elder Abuse. www.ncea.aoa.gov

Oregon Death with Dignity Act. www.oregon.gov/DHS/ph/pas/

Purtilo, R., Haddad, A., & Doherty, R. (2012). *Health professional and patient interaction* (8th ed.). St. Louis: Elsevier.

United States Department of Health and Human Services, Office of Civil Rights—HIPAA. www.hhs.gov/ocr/privacy/

University of Washington School of Medicine. Ethics in Medicine. http://depts.washington.edu/bioethx

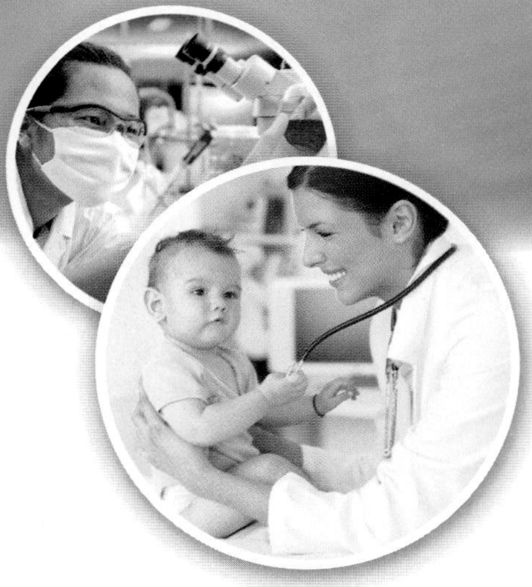

Unit 2

The Language of Health Care

This page intentionally left blank

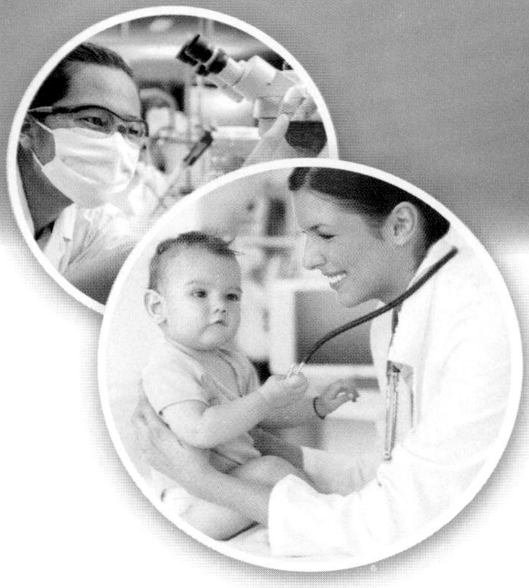

Chapter 4

Medical Terminology

OBJECTIVES

Studying and applying the material in this chapter will help you to:

- Understand the importance of being able to write, read, and communicate using medical terminology.
- Identify common word roots and combining forms, suffixes, and prefixes.
- Break down medical terms into their component parts and interpret the terms correctly.
- Use the spelling and pronunciation guidelines for medical terms derived from Greek and Latin.
- Define common abbreviations and interpret common symbols.
- Evaluate the features of a medical dictionary to determine its value as a reference for your specialty area.
- Approach the learning of medical terminology by using a variety of study techniques.

KEY TERMS

combining form
combining vowel
consonant
medical terminology
prefix
suffix
word part
word root

The Case of Where Is the Pain?

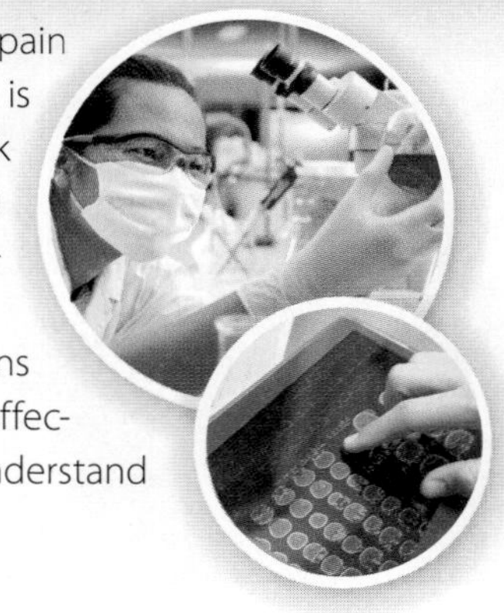

Dr. Chen states that Ms. Mitchell called yesterday complaining of *epigastric* (ep ih GAS trick) pain and requests that LaTonya, the medical receptionist, call her to follow up and find out if she is feeling any better. LaTonya calls Ms. Mitchell and says, "Dr. Chen has asked me to call and ask how the epigastric pain is today." Ms. Mitchell is confused and says, "I'm not sure what you mean. What is epigastric?" LaTonya does not know what "epigastric" means, and this has prevented her from restating the question in terms that the patient can understand.

Health care professionals must know medical terminology, such as this term (which means "over the stomach"). Failure to learn medical language prevents them from communicating effectively with other health care professionals and with patients. This chapter will help students understand this new language.

IMPORTANCE OF MEDICAL TERMINOLOGY

Understanding and correctly using **medical terminology** is essential to your career in health care. The study of medical terminology includes learning not only medical terms but also the associated abbreviations and symbols. Medical terminology is used during conversations with other health professionals, in medical charting and documentation, and in professional journals and texts. It adds necessary preciseness to professional communications. For example, when directions for procedures are described using exact language, there is less chance for confusion and error.

Patients can receive ineffective or even harmful treatment if words or abbreviations are misunderstood. For example, if the physician orders medication to be taken "a.c." (before a meal), a medication error will result if the health care professional interprets this to mean after a meal, which is written "p.c."

It is not always appropriate to use medical language. Most patients find the use of technical words confusing. They may be intimidated and will hesitate to ask for an explanation. When communicating with patients it is essential to first determine their level of understanding. Appropriate language can then be chosen to ensure clear communication. Patients cannot benefit from, and may even be harmed by, information they do not understand.

THE BUILDING BLOCKS OF MEDICAL LANGUAGE

Many health care programs include a more in-depth study of medical terminology than will be presented in this chapter. For those students with no prior study of medical terminology, this material will serve as an introduction to the subject. For other students, it will serve as a review.

Medical terms are composed of several parts, referred to as **word parts**. Each word part has its own meaning and location in the term. Like building blocks, they can be combined to create thousands of different words. Learning the meaning of commonly used word parts and applying this knowledge to decipher medical terms is much more efficient than trying to memorize each new word as it is encountered.

The four word parts that make up medical terms are a word root, combining form, prefix, and suffix.

Word Roots and Combining Forms

The **word root** is the part of the medical term that gives the main meaning. It usually, but not always, refers to the structure and function of the body. All medical terms have at least one word root. The following are examples of word roots:

- *gastr*—stomach
- *enter*—small intestine
- *cardi*—heart

Combining forms consist of word roots plus a vowel, usually the letter "o," separated from the word root with a slash mark:

- gastr/o
- enter/o
- cardi/o

The letter "o" is called the **combining vowel**. It links the word root to the next word part in the term, known as the suffix, if the suffix begins with a **consonant** (any letter *except* a, e, i, o, or u). (Suffixes are explained in the next section.) The combining vowel is always used when linking two word roots, even if the second one starts with a vowel. For example, *gastr/o* and *enter/o* are often combined when referring to both the stomach and the intestines. The combining form *gastr/o* is used even though *enter/o* begins with a vowel to form the word *gastroenterology*, which means "the study of the stomach and intestines." Note the word root *enter* is used because the next word part, *ology*, starts with a vowel. Medical word roots, when listed in the dictionary, appear as combining forms, and it is recommended that students learn them this way.

The vocabulary used by health care professionals differs from everyday language because, like the language of other sciences, many medical terms have their origins in Greek and Latin. Table 4–1 contains several examples.

There are thousands of word roots and combining forms that make up medical language. The complete list of combining forms each student must learn depends on his or her chosen occupation. Table 4–2 contains a list of commonly used combining forms that refer to the parts of the body.

Diagrams can be helpful when learning a new language. Many students find that illustrations provide visual clues for remembering new terms. Figure 4–1 illustrates some of the terms contained in Table 4–2.

Media Link

View the Combining Word Roots animation on the Online Resources for examples of joining word roots to form new terms.

Suffixes

Suffixes are word parts that are attached to the end of word roots and combining forms to add to or change their meaning. All medical terms have an ending, or suffix, unless the word root is a word itself. Some common meanings of suffixes include:

- Pathological (disease) conditions
- Diagnostic procedures
- Surgical procedures
- Pertaining to
- Produced by
- Resembling

Recall that the combining form is used when the suffix begins with a consonant, as in the following example:

cardi/o	+	megaly	=	cardiomegaly
heart	+	enlarged	=	enlarged heart

Notice that the slash mark is dropped when the suffix is attached to the combining form.

When the suffix begins with a vowel, it is attached to the word root, as in the following example:

gastr	+	itis	=	gastritis
stomach	+	inflammation	=	inflammation of the stomach

Each suffix can be added to many word roots. Knowing that *-itis* means "inflammation" enables the learner to know that the following words all indicate an inflammation of the body part indicated in the word root:

1. Appendicitis: Inflammation of the appendix
2. Arthritis: Inflammation of the joint
3. Gastritis: Inflammation of the stomach

Another common suffix is *-ectomy*, which means "surgical removal." Like *-itis*, it can be combined with many word roots. In each case, it means removal of the part indicated by the word root:

1. Appendectomy: Removal of the appendix
2. Gastrectomy: Removal of all or part of the stomach
3. Lumpectomy: Removal of a lump

Table 4–1 Origins of Medical Word Root Words

Original Word	Meaning	Modern Medical Combining Form
kardia (Greek)	heart	cardi/o
derm (Greek)	skin	derm/o
enteron (Greek)	small intestines	enter/o
bucca (Latin)	cheek	bucc/o
lumbus (Latin)	loin (lower part of the back)	lumb/o
vivere (Latin)	life	viv/o

Table 4–2 Common Combining Forms That Refer to Body Parts

Combining Form	Meaning	Combining Form	Meaning
adip/o; lip/o; steat/o	fat	lapar/o	abdominal wall
arteri/o	artery	laryng/o	voice box, larynx
arthr/o	joint	myel/o	spinal cord
axill/o	armpit	my/o; muscul/o	muscle
blephar/o	eyelid	nas/o; rhin/o	nose
cardi/o	heart	neur/o	nerve
cephal/o	head	ophthalm/o; ocul/o	eye
cerebr/o; encephal/o	cerebrum, brain	or/o; stomat/o	mouth
cervic/o	neck	oste/o	bone
cholecyst/o	gallbladder	ot/o	ear
col/o	large intestine	pancreat/o	pancreas
cost/o	rib	pharyng/o	throat
crani/o	skull	pneum/o; pneumon/o	lung
cyst/o	urinary bladder	ren/o; nephr/o	kidneys
cyt/o	cell	splen/o	spleen
derm/o; dermat/o	skin	thorac/o	chest
enter/o	small intestine	thyroid/o	thyroid gland
esophag/o	esophagus	trache/o	windpipe, trachea
gastr/o	stomach	ven/o; phleb/o	vein
hem/o; hemat/o	blood	vertebr/o	vertebra
hepat/o	liver		

When suffixes are listed in medical dictionaries and word lists, they are positioned alphabetically with other entries, preceded by a hyphen, and identified as a word part. Dictionary entries typically include the language of origin, as in the following sample dictionary entries:

- *-megaly* word part (Gr.) enlargement
- *-itis* word part (Gr.) inflammation
- *-ectomy* word part (Gr.) surgical removal

See Table 4–3 for a list of commonly used suffixes.

Prefixes

Prefixes are word parts that are attached to the beginning of word roots and combining forms to add to or change their meaning. Many, but not all, medical terms have a prefix. Some common meanings of prefixes include the following:

- Location
- Position
- Direction
- Time
- Number
- Negation, absence of
- Color

Just as with suffixes, the same prefixes can be attached to many word roots, resulting in thousands of variations. Knowing that the prefix *hyper-* means "abnormally increased" or "excessive" gives a clue to

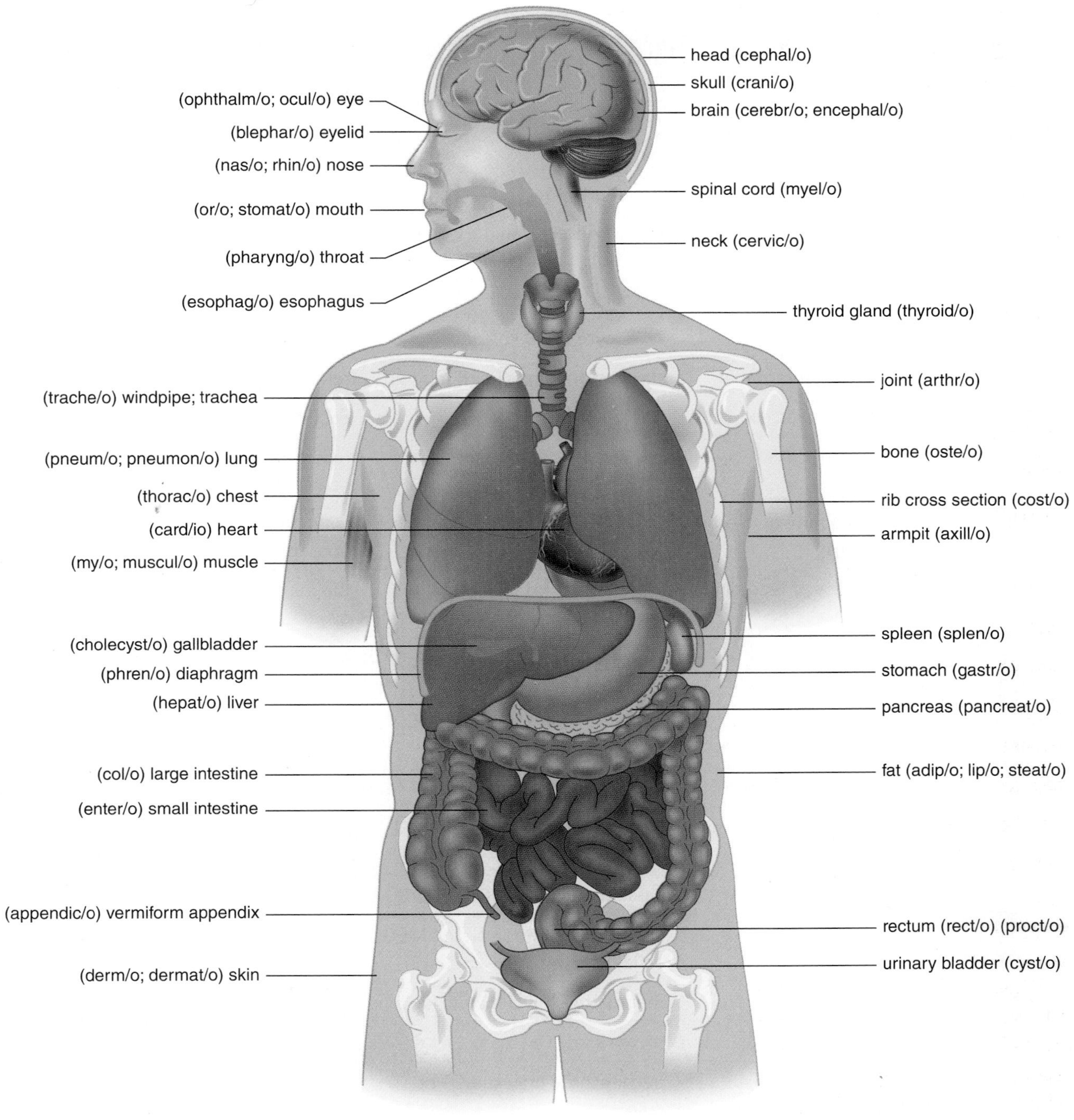

FIGURE 4–1 Medical terminology for body parts.

the meaning of the hundreds of words that contain this word part, including the following examples:

1. Hyperacid: Abnormally or excessively acidic
2. Hyperactive: Exhibiting abnormally increased activity
3. Hypertension: Persistently high blood pressure

In the same way, knowing that *poly-* means "many" or "much" helps decipher the following examples:

1. Polyatomic: Made up of many atoms
2. Polyglandular: Pertaining to or affecting many glands
3. Polyphobia: Irrational fear of many things

Table 4–3 Common Suffixes

Suffix	Meaning	Term	Meaning
-ac, -al, -ar, -ary, -eal, -iac, -ic, -ical, -ose, -ous, -tic	All of these mean "pertaining to"	cardi**ac** cellul**ar** psycho**tic**	pertaining to the heart pertaining to the cell pertaining to psychosis
-algia	pain	neur**algia** (new RAL jee ah)	pain along a nerve
-centesis	surgical puncture to remove fluid	amnio**centesis** (am nee oh sin TEE sis)	insertion of needle to withdraw sample of amniotic fluid
-cide	to kill, destroy	germi**cide** (JER mih side)	chemical substance that kills germs
-cyte	cell	leuko**cyte** (LOO koh cite)	white blood cell
-ectomy	surgical removal of	gastr**ectomy** (gas TREK toh me)	removal of part or all of the stomach
-emia	blood; blood condition	bacter**emia** (back ter EE mee ah)	bacteria in the blood
-gram	record	electrocardio**gram** (ee lek troh KAR dee oh gram)	record of the electrical activity of the heart
-graph	an instrument used to record	electrocardio**graph** (ee lek troh KAR dee ah graf)	instrument that records electrical variations in cardiac muscle activity
-graphy	process of recording	electrocardio**graphy** (*ee-lek-troh-kar-dee-AH-graf-ee*)	the making and study of electrocardiograms
-ia	condition, especially an abnormal state	tachycard**ia** (tak ee KAR dee ah)	condition of abnormal rapid heart rate
-ism	condition	hypothyroid**ism** (high poh THIGH roid izm)	condition created by less than normal levels of thyroid hormones
-itis	inflammation of	card**itis** (kar DYE tis)	inflammation of the heart
-lithiasis	presence of or formation of stones	chole**lithiasis** (koh lee lih THIGH ah sis)	presence of stones in the gallbladder
-logy	study of	cardio**logy** (kar dee OL oh jee)	study of the heart
-megaly	enlargement	hepato**megaly** (hep ah toh MEG ah lee)	enlargement of the liver
-oid	resembling	rheumat**oid** (ROO mah toyd)	resembling rheumatism
-oma	tumor	my**oma** (my OH mah)	tumor containing muscle tissue
-otomy	surgical incision	trache**otomy** (tray kee OT oh mee)	incision into trachea
-pathy	disease	encephalo**pathy** (en sef ah LOP ah thee)	disease of the brain
-plasty	surgical or plastic repair	rhino**plasty** (RYE no plas tee)	plastic surgery of the nose
-plegia	paralysis	hemi**plegia** (hem ee PLEE jee ah)	paralysis of one side (half) of the body
-pnea	breathing, respiration	a**pnea** (ap NEE ah)	temporary cessation of breathing

(continues)

Table 4–3 Common Suffixes (continued)

Suffix	Meaning	Term	Meaning
-rrhea	drainage, flow, discharge	rhino**rrhea** (rye no REE ah)	drainage from the nose
-scope	instrument used to view	oto**scope** (OH toh skope)	instrument used to examine the ear
-scopy	examination using a scope	sigmoido**scopy** (sig moy DOS koh pee)	examination of the sigmoid colon using a scope
-stasis	stoppage, controlling, standing	veno**stasis** (vee no STAY sis)	stoppage of blood in a vein
-stomy	surgically create an artificial mouth or stoma (opening)	colo**stomy** (koh LOSS toh me)	surgical opening into the colon to create a stoma

Prefixes can dramatically change the meaning of a word. For example, *systole* (SIS toh lee) means "contraction of the heart." The addition of the one-letter prefix *a*, which means "without," creates the word *asystole* (a SIS toh lee), meaning without contractions. This is a very different condition! Careful spelling is critical when using medical language. Illegible handwriting can also lead to errors. *Always make sure your spelling is correct and your writing is legible to others.*

When prefixes are listed in medical dictionaries and word lists, they are located alphabetically, followed by a hyphen, and identified as a word part, as in the following sample dictionary entries:

- *epi-* word part (Gr.) over; above; upon
- *hyper-* word part (Gr.) abnormally increased; excessive
- *poly-* word part (Gr.) many; much

See Table 4–4 for a list of commonly used prefixes.

Media Link

View the Word Parts Work Together animation on the Online Resources to see how word parts are joined to form complex medical terms.

DECIPHERING MEDICAL TERMS

Learning the meanings of commonly used word parts and understanding how they combine enable the health care professional to decipher thousands of medical terms. When confronted with a new term, start at the far right, with the suffix. Think of each word as a combination of building blocks, fitted together to create a precise meaning. (See Figure 4–2.) Work from right to left, identifying and defining each word part, as in the following examples:

Example # 1 cardiology

1. Starting from the right, find word part *-logy*
2. Determine meaning: study of
3. Moving left, find word part *cardio*
4. Determine meaning: heart
5. Combine word parts: study of the heart

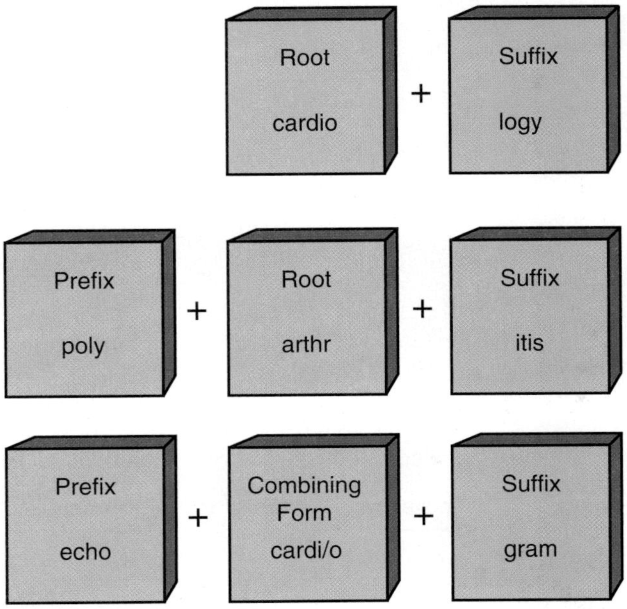

FIGURE 4–2 Think of the elements of medical terms as building blocks that can be used to construct new words.

Table 4–4 Common Prefixes

Prefix	Meaning	Term	Meaning
a-/an-	without, not, absence of	**an**uria (an YOU ree ah)	absence of urine formation
anti-	against	**anti**biotic (an tie buy AHT ick)	substance that inhibits growth of or destroys microorganisms
auto-	self	**auto**immune (aw toh ih MYOON)	disease that results in immune response to one's own body
bi-	two, double	**bi**furcate (BUY fur kate)	having two branches or divisions
brady-	slow	**brady**cardia (brad ee KAR dee ah)	slow heart rate
dys-	bad, difficult, painful, abnormal	**dys**pnea (disp NEE ah)	difficulty breathing
epi-	over, above, upon	**epi**gastric (ep ih GAS trik)	over the stomach
eu-	good, normal	**eu**pnea (oop NEE ah)	normal breathing
hemi-	half	**hemi**plegia (hem ee PLEE jee ah)	paralysis of one side or half of the body
hyper-	above, excessive	**hyper**tension (high per TEN shun)	high blood pressure
hypo-	less than, under	**hypo**tension (high poh TEN shun)	low blood pressure
inter-	between	**inter**costal (in ter COS tahl)	between the ribs
intra-	within	**intra**venous (in trah VEE nus)	within a vein
multi-	many	**multi**nodal (mul tih NO dahl)	having many nodes or knots
non-	not	**non**toxic (non TOK sik)	not poisonous
peri-	around, surrounding	**peri**anal (per ee A nal)	around the anus
poly-	many, much	**poly**uria (pol ee YOU ree ah)	excretion of large amounts of urine
post-	after, behind	**post**operative (post OP er ah tiv)	following a surgical procedure
pre-	before, in front	**pre**operative (pree OP er ah tiv)	before a surgical procedure
pseudo-	false	**pseudo**hematuria (sue doh hee mah TOO ree ah)	red pigment in the urine that makes the urine "falsely" appear to have blood in it
quadri-	four	**quadri**plegia (kwad rih PLEE jee ah)	paralysis of all four extremities
semi-	half	**semi**permeable (sem ee PER mee ah bull)	half permeable—a membrane that allows fluids but not the dissolved substance to pass through
sub-	under, below	**sub**sternal (sub STIR nail)	below the sternum
supra-	above, over	**supra**pubic (sue prah PEW bik)	above the pubic area
tachy-	fast, rapid	**tachy**cardia (tak ee KAR dee ah)	rapid heart rate
tri-	three	**tri**chotomy (try COT oh me)	division into three parts

Example # 2 polyarthritis

1. Starting from the right, find word part *-itis*
2. Determine meaning: inflammation
3. Moving left, find word part *arthr*
4. Determine meaning: joint
5. Moving left, find word part *poly*
6. Determine meaning: many, much
7. Combine word parts: inflammation of many joints

Example # 3 echocardiogram

1. Starting from the right, find word part *-gram*
2. Determine meaning: written, record
3. Moving left, find word part *cardi/o*
4. Determine meaning: heart
5. Moving left, find word part *echo*
6. Determine meaning: echo (reflections of sounds)
7. Combine word parts: recording of the heart using echoes (to determine position and motion)

SPELLING AND PRONUNCIATION

Accurate spelling is critical when using medical language. Some words look and/or sound similar and can be easily confused. (See Figure 4–3.) It is important to pay attention to the context (the surrounding words and facts) to determine the correct meaning. The following examples contain words that are often confused:

1. Ilium (ILL ee um): Part of the hipbone
   Ileum (ILL ee um): Part of the intestine
2. Alveoli (al VEE oh lie): Tiny air sacs in the lungs
   Areola (ah RE oh lah): Brown pigmented area around the nipple

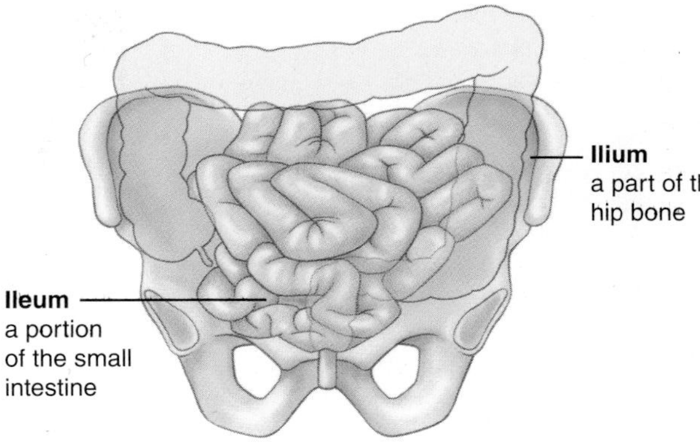

FIGURE 4–3 There is only one letter difference between ileum and ilium, but they are very different parts of the body.

As with nontechnical English words, which have their origin in many different languages, some medical terms are spelled differently from the way they are pronounced. Table 4–5 contains common examples. Many of the guidelines apply to familiar words as well and are taken for granted in everyday speech. For example, "ph" used as "f" in the words *philosophy, Philadelphia,* and *Phoenix.*

The plural forms of many medical words are created with the original Greek and Latin endings, instead of the familiar "s" used for many English words. (See Figure 4–4.) Table 4–6 contains guidelines for creating the plural forms of many medical terms.

Misspelled words can lead to treatment and medication errors. Take the time to learn the correct spelling when learning new word parts. Health care professionals cannot take the chance that others will guess correctly what they intended to write.

Table 4–5 Spelling and Pronunciation Guidelines

Letter	Sounds Like	Examples
c when followed by e, i, or y	S	cell, circulatory, cyst
ch	K	chronic
g when followed by e, i, or y	J	genetic, gingivitis, gyration
i when used to create plural	eye	bacilli (sing. bacillus)
ph	F	pharmacist
pn	N	pneumonia
ps	S	psychiatrist
x	Z	Xylocaine (pronounced "ZIE loh cane," this is an anesthetic applied to the skin)

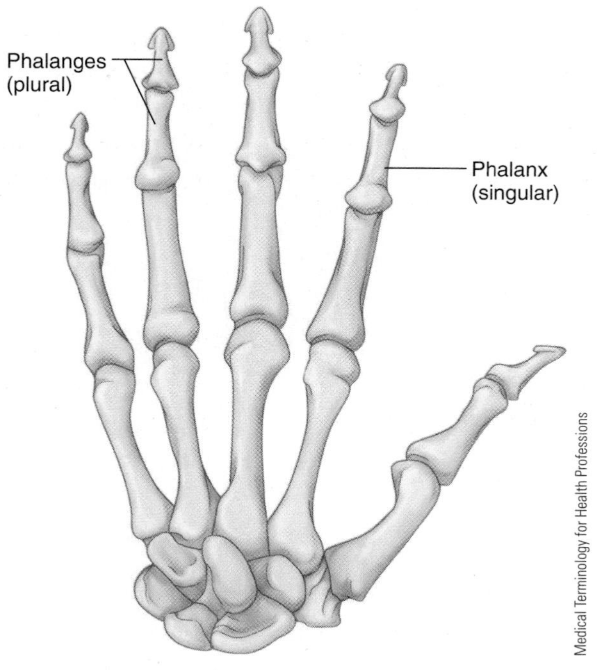

FIGURE 4–4 Singular and plural endings. A phalanx is one finger or toe bone. Phalanges are more than one finger or toe bone.

MEDICAL ABBREVIATIONS AND SYMBOLS

Medical abbreviations and symbols are the shorthand of medical language. Many of them have been standardized and are universally accepted. In addition, each health care profession, agency, and facility has its own list of approved abbreviations and symbols. Each medical office or facility should have a policy and procedure manual or an employee handbook that includes this information. It is important that the health care professional asks for a copy of and become familiar with the list. *Never* substitute personal versions of abbreviations and symbols for those on the list when preparing any type of written documentation that will be used by the facility. Using abbreviations or symbols not on the approved list is against state and federal regulatory guidelines. If misuse is discovered during an accreditation or licensing survey visit, the agency or facility can be cited for not following the guidelines. If there are common abbreviations or symbols missing from the list, the worker should notify the supervisor.

Table 4–6 Guidelines to Plural Forms

Guideline	Singular	Plural
1. If the term ends in **a**, the plural is usually formed by adding an **e**.	bursa vertebra	bursae vertebrae
2. If the term ends in **ex** or **ix**, the plural is usually formed by changing the **ex** or **ix** to **ices**.	appendix index	appendices indices
3. If the term ends in **is**, the plural is usually formed by changing the **is** to **es**.	diagnosis metastasis	diagnoses metastases
4. If the term ends in **itis**, the plural is usually formed by changing the **is** to **ides**.	arthritis meningitis	arthritides meningitides
5. If the term ends in **nx**, the plural is usually formed by changing the **x** to **ges**.	phalanx meninx	phalanges meninges
6. If the term ends in **on**, the plural is usually formed by changing the **on** to **a**.	criterion ganglion	criteria ganglia
7. If the term ends in **um**, the plural is usually formed by changing the **um** to **a**.	diverticulum ovum	diverticula ova
8. If the term ends in **us**, the plural is usually formed by changing the **us** to **i**.	alveolus malleolus	alveoli malleoli
If you are in doubt as to how a plural is formed, ***look it up*** *in a medical dictionary!*		

Source: *Medical Terminology for Health Professions* (7th ed.), by A. Ehrlich & C. L. Schroeder, 2013, Clifton Park, NY: Delmar Cengage Learning.

Refer to Tables 4–7 and 4–8 for a list of medical abbreviations and symbols. These are not complete lists but include examples of those that are frequently encountered in health care. Additional abbreviations and symbols will be encountered as learners take health care specialty courses. For example, a dental assistant will learn the standardized numbering system used for identifying each tooth.

Certain abbreviations, symbols, and dose designations have led to frequent errors due to misinterpretations. As a result of these reported errors, the Institute for Safe Medication Practices has created a list that is recommended never to be used in any medical communications. The Joint Commission has also developed a requirement that certain abbreviations must appear on an accredited organization's do-not-use list. (See Table 4–9.)

MEDICAL DICTIONARY

Students are encouraged to purchase a medical or specialty dictionary. It is a valuable resource not only when taking health care courses but also as

Table 4–7 Abbreviations

ad lib	freely, at will, as necessary	P	pulse
a.c.	before a meal	p.c.	after meals
ASAP	as soon as possible	PO, p.o.	by mouth
b.i.d., bid	twice a day	p.r.n.	as needed
BM	bowel movement	q.h., qh	every hour
BP	blood pressure	q.i.d., QID, qid	four times a day
c̄	with	R	respiration
CDC	Centers for Disease Control and Prevention	s̄	without
c/o, C/O	complains of	stat	immediately
h	hour	T	temperature
H_2O	water	t.i.d., TID, tid	three times a day
HTN	hypertension	TPR	temperature, pulse, and respiration
I&O	intake and output	Tx	traction or treatment
Lab	laboratory	URI	upper respiratory infection
NPO	nothing by mouth	UTI	urinary track infection
N&V	nausea and vomiting	VS, vs	vital signs
O_2	oxygen	wt.	weight
p̄	after	x	multiplied by, times

Table 4–8 Symbols

↑	higher, elevate, or up	°	degree
↓	lower or down	♀	female
#	pound or number	♂	male
′	foot or minute	Δ	change
″	inch or second		

Table 4–9 Examples of Abbreviations *Not* to Be Used

IU	International unit	Write "units." Could be mistaken as IV (intravenous) or 10 (ten).
q.d. or QD	every day	Write "daily." The period after q or the tail of the Q is mistaken for an "I," which is qid (four times a day).
q.o.d. or QOD	every other day	Write "every other day," Could be mistaken for "q.d." (daily) or "q.i.d." (four times a day) if the "o" is poorly written.
U or u	unit	Write "unit." Could be mistaken as the number 0 or 4 (e.g., 4U seen as "40" or 4u seen as "44." Also can be mistaken as "cc" (e.g., 4u seen as 4cc).

Thinking It Through

Mr. Fiacco is complaining of an irritation on his left arm where he had been applying a cream prescribed by the provider. You know that Mr. Fiacco has a skin condition and he was given a prescription for a cream he was to apply to his left arm q.d. for 10 days. You examine Mr. Fiacco's arm and note that the skin condition is gone, but now there is a red, irritated-looking area. You check the instructions on the prescription packaging and it says to apply the cream four times a day.

1. Is the patient applying the cream as originally intended?
2. Is there a reason for the newly reddened area on his left arm?
3. What does q,d. mean?
4. What is the abbreviation for four times a day?
5. Why do you think this problem occurred?
6. What should you do to correct the problem?

Thinking It Through

Charles Grant, LVN, is given Mr. Grover's chart and asked to take the BP and P stat. Charles reviews the notes and sees that Mr. Grover has hypertension and tachycardia and that the physician has ordered the patient to be NPO. The chart also states that he has polyuria, rhinorrhea, eupnea, and a history of cholelithiasis. When Charles greets Mr. Grover and informs him that he is going to take his BP and P, Mr. Grover requests a drink of water first, as he is feeling quite thirsty.

1. What are BP and P? Is there any urgency in doing these?
2. Noting that Mr. Grover has hypertension and tachycardia, do you expect the readings to be too high, normal, or too low? Explain.
3. What do polyuria, rhinorrhea, eupnea, and cholelithiasis mean?
4. Is it appropriate to give Mr. Grover a glass of water? Why or why not?

a handy reference in the work setting. The following features should be considered when selecting a dictionary:

- Clear, easy-to-understand definitions
- Explanations of medical procedures, conditions, disorders, and diseases
- Pronunciation hints
- Abbreviations and symbols
- Reference tables containing information such as laboratory values, units of measurement with conversion values, nutritional values of foods, and emergency resources
- Useful diagrams, charts, and tables
- Expanded explanations of topics of interest to the learner
- Application of information to patient care
- Extent of vocabulary coverage specific to learner's occupational area

It is very important to check the coverage of terms in the learner's specialty area. Some dictionaries are more inclusive than others.

MASTERING MEDICAL TERMINOLOGY

Learning to use medical language is challenging for many students. Many words come from languages, such as Latin, that are no longer spoken. The words look and sound strange and seem long and complex. Medical terminology, however, can be mastered. The keys are *study* and *practice*. The following suggestions have helped many learners:

- Study a few words each day. Avoid having to learn entire lists at the last minute just before test time.
- As word parts are learned, practice using them in new combinations.
- Use study techniques that correspond to individual learning styles, as discussed in Chapter 1. See the list of ideas in Table 4–10.
- Practice both the written and spoken forms as much as possible and in as many settings as possible.
- Learn new medical terms as they appear in this and other textbooks.
- Use a medical dictionary when unsure about how to spell or pronounce a word correctly.
- When working in a health care environment, accept help as needed from coworkers and supervisors to correct pronunciation and usage.

Having a strong understanding of the key concepts presented in this chapter will serve as a foundation for learning the material in subsequent chapters and throughout the entire health care educational program. The following are just a few of the subjects that depend heavily on knowledge of medical terminology:

- Anatomy (structure of the body)
- Physiology (function of the body)
- Pathophysiology (study of diseases and abnormal conditions)
- Medical insurance coding (assigning standardized codes to specific diagnoses and procedures)
- Pharmacology (therapeutic drugs)

The time initially spent learning the correct meaning, spelling, and pronunciation of medical word parts will save time later and prevent frustration when learning future subjects. Being proficient in the use of medical terminology is a mark of a competent health care professional.

Table 4–10 Suggested Study Techniques

Learning Style	Suggestions
Visual	• Write down medical terms that you hear during lectures. • Ask the instructor to write words on the board. • Create cartoons using medical terms. • Prepare flashcards with a word or picture on one side and the definition on the back. • Study word roots that refer to the body by studying drawings of the body parts. • Write words many times, using colored ink. • Visualize familiar images along with the new terms. For example, visualize the Queen of Hearts playing card for *cardi/o*.
Auditory	• Concentrate on terms when you hear them presented in lectures. • Read medical terms aloud to yourself. • Use commercially prepared tapes or make your own. • Take turns quizzing each other with another learner. • Create verbal rhythms; try setting them to music. • Create audio, "sounds-like" cues to remember definitions.
Kinesthetic	• Draw images, and even color them. • Create pairs of flashcards with the medical term on one card and the definition on the other. Then lay them out on a large table and move them around until you have them all matched correctly. • Touch the part of your body referred to in the term or point to where it is located if it is not on the surface. • Study the models of the body systems or build them from kits.

WORKBOOK PRACTICE

Go to your workbook and complete the exercises for this chapter.

SUGGESTED LEARNING ACTIVITIES

1. Start a list of new medical terms, with their definitions, as you encounter them. This can be a written list in your notebook or one on your computer.
2. Watch television programs that portray medical settings and listen for medical terms. Do the professionals on these programs use a different level of language when speaking among themselves than when speaking with patients? Do you recognize any of the terms used?
3. Watch and listen for "medical" prefixes and suffixes that are also used in everyday English (or Spanish!).
4. Using the examples of terms provided in Figure 4–5, create a few medical terms for the other body parts. Use the charts in this chapter and a medical dictionary.

WEB ACTIVITIES

MedLine Plus

www.medlineplus.gov/

Medline Plus is a service of the U.S. National Library of Medicine and the National Institutes of Health. It has an excellent medical dictionary and medical encyclopedia with illustrations.

MediLexicon International Ltd.

www.medilexicon.com/

MediLexicon is an online database of pharmaceutical and medical abbreviations. Use the search field to find definitions on five abbreviations and five medical terms. Record your findings.

Institute for Safe Medical Practices

www.ismp.org/

Review the "Error-Prone Abbreviation List" and identify 10 additional examples other than the samples presented in Table 4–9.

REVIEW QUESTIONS

1. Why is it important to know medical terminology?
2. What do the following terms mean: *word roots, combining forms, suffixes*, and *prefixes*?
3. What are the steps that should be followed to break medical terms into their component parts in order to interpret them correctly?
4. Provide five examples of medical terms that include a prefix and suffix. Give their meanings.
5. What are the guidelines for medical terms when the pronunciation differs from the spelling?
6. Provide five examples of abbreviations and five of symbols. Give their meanings.
7. What are the features of a medical dictionary? How do you determine which one will be the best for your specialty area?
8. What are the eight study suggestions for mastering medical terminology?

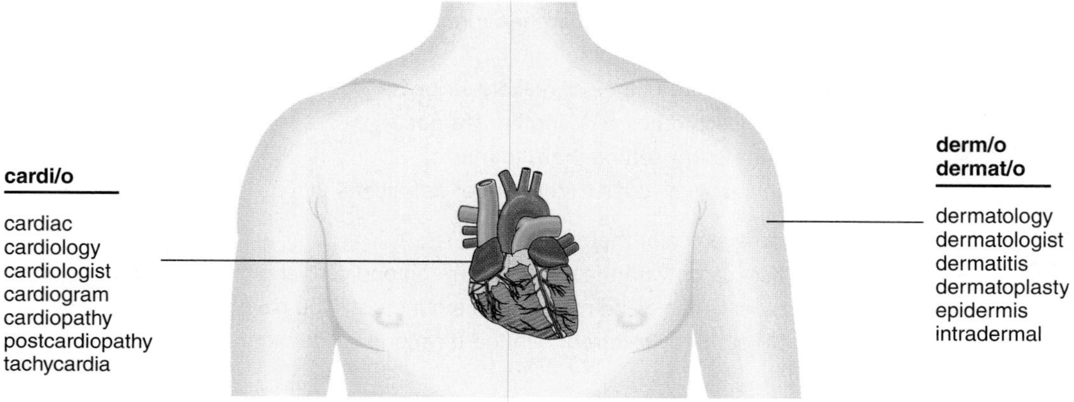

FIGURE 4–5 The combining form for each body part is the basis for many terms.

APPLICATION EXERCISES

1. Refer to The Case of "Where Is the Pain?" presented at the beginning of this chapter. What does *epigastric* mean? How would you respond to Ms. Mitchell's question, "What is epigastric?"
2. Kelly Cordeiro is a recent medical assisting graduate who is hired by a prominent ophthalmologist. She is excited about having the opportunity to work in this area. However, Kelly quickly discovers that there are many terms related to the anatomy of the eye, special procedures, eye surgery, and medications with which she is not familiar. She feels a little lost and is concerned about her ability to communicate effectively with the physician and maintain patient records appropriately.
   a. What references would you suggest for Kelly to learn the vocabulary she needs?
   b. Describe the techniques she can use to quickly learn the new vocabulary.

PROBLEM-SOLVING PRACTICE

Jason Lopez is currently taking a class in medical terminology. He studies hard and feels he knows the material well, but when he gets his test results back, there are several marked wrong that he says are correct. The instructor states that she could not read it clearly enough to be absolutely sure it was correct and refuses to change his score. Using the five-step problem-solving process, determine what Jason can do about his problem on the test.

SUGGESTED READINGS AND RESOURCES

Dorland's illustrated medical dictionary (32nd ed.). (2011). Philadelphia: W. B. Saunders Company.

Ehrlich, A., & Schroeder, C. L. (2011). *Medical terminology for health professions* (7th ed.). Clifton Park, NY: Delmar Cengage Learning.

Miller-Keane encyclopedia & dictionary of medicine, nursing, & allied health (7th ed.). (2013). Philadelphia: W. B. Saunders Company.

Quick reference for health care providers. (2005). Clifton Park, NY: Cengage Learning Delmar.

Stedman's medical dictionary for health professionals and nursing (7th ed.). (2011). Baltimore: Lippincott Williams & Wilkins.

Taber's cyclopedic medical dictionary (22nd ed.). (2013). Philadelphia: F. A. Davis.

This page intentionally left blank

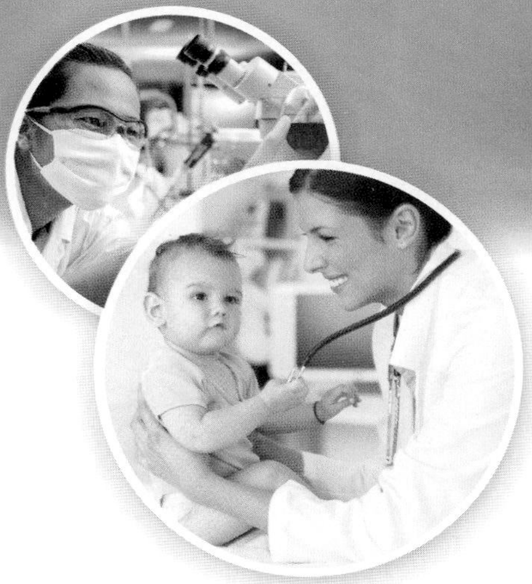

Chapter 5

Medical Math

OBJECTIVES

Studying and applying the material in this chapter will help you to:

- Understand how math anxiety prevents comfort and competence with calculations.
- Perform basic math calculations on whole numbers, decimals, fractions, percentages, and ratios.
- Convert between the following numerical forms: decimals, fractions, percentages, and ratios.
- Round off numbers correctly.
- Solve mathematical equivalency problems with proportions.
- Express time using the 24-hour clock (military time).
- Express numbers using Roman numerals.
- Estimate angles from a reference plane.
- Use household, metric, and apothecary units to express length, volume, and weight.
- Know equivalencies for converting among the household, metric, and apothecary systems of measurement.
- Convert between the Fahrenheit and Celsius temperature scales.

KEY TERMS

angles
apothecary system
Celsius (C)
decimal
degrees
estimating
Fahrenheit (F)
fraction
household system
improper fraction
math anxiety
metric system
military time
nomenclature
percentages
proportion
ratios
reciprocal
reference plane
Roman numerals
rounding numbers
whole numbers

The Case of Exactly How Much Does My Baby Weigh?

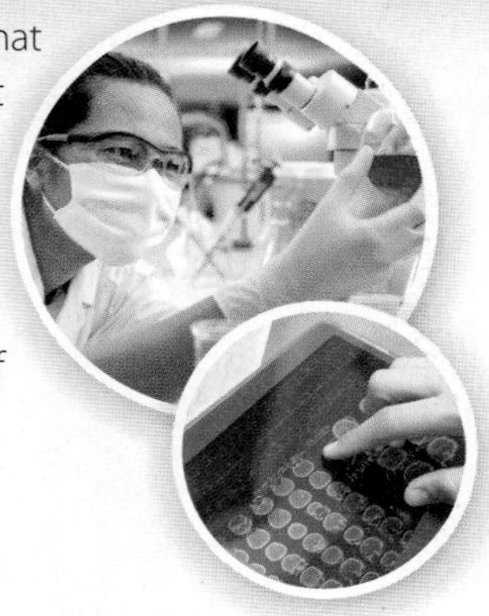

During a well baby checkup, Jamie Brown weighs Jessica Munoz and reports to the mother that her baby weighs 10 kilograms. The mother states her daughter weighed 20 pounds on the last visit and asks how much 10 kilograms is in pounds. Jamie explains that 10 kilograms is the same as 22 pounds, so there has been a 2-pound increase in weight.

Not knowing how to convert between kilograms and pounds would have prevented Jamie from answering the mother's question. This chapter will cover the math needed by the health care professional, including information about converting between commonly used systems of measurement.

IMPORTANCE OF MATH IN HEALTH CARE

Work in health care requires the use of math skills to measure and perform various types of calculations. There are applications in all types of occupations:

- Calculating medication dosages
- Taking height and weight readings
- Measuring the amount of intake (fluids consumed or infused) and output (e.g., urine, vomit)
- Performing billing and bookkeeping tasks
- Performing lab tests
- Mixing solutions

Errors in math can have negative effects on patients. For example, administering the wrong dosage of medication is a serious mistake and can harm the patient. Health care professionals must strive for 100% accuracy. *If there is any doubt, it is essential to ask your supervisor or a qualified coworker to double-check calculations.*

MATH ANXIETY

Millions of people experience a feeling of intimidation and fear when confronted with mathematics. This condition is called **math anxiety**, math avoidance, or math phobia. A person experiencing math anxiety is similar to the person experiencing stage fright. What stage fright entails is a feeling of something going wrong, of forgetting one's lines, or fear of going blank or of being judged. With math anxiety, there is the feeling of making mistakes, freezing up and going blank, or of being judged as a failure.

Math anxiety is an emotional reaction to mathematics based on a past unpleasant experience that harms learning. The good news is that a good experience learning math can overcome these past feelings and success with future achievement in math can be achieved.

Many learners suffer from math anxiety. Those who do are probably feeling dread at just the thought of reading this chapter. If you are unsure whether you suffer from math anxiety, take the math anxiety test listed in the Web Activities at the end of this chapter.

When a learner is experiencing math anxiety, it is impossible to actually test for math ability as the test-taker's anxiety will confound the results. Math anxiety can be felt so strongly that it prevents memorization, concentration, and the ability to pay attention, all of which are required for solving math problems.

Math anxiety is not inherent; that is, no one is born with it. Rather, it is a learned behavior that is often due to poor teaching and poor experiences in math. As such, math anxiety can be overcome. The first step is to recognize that it exists and be willing to do something about it. Many people who think they have a learning disability or just "can never do math" have found that it is the anxiety that causes the mental block and interferes with their ability to learn. Once this block is overcome, they are able to learn and perform the math necessary for their work. Table 5–1 addresses some common fear thoughts about math, which, if believed, set up mental blocks to learning.

Table 5–1 False Beliefs about Math

The Fear Thought	The Reality
I don't get math, never have and never will.	Math is a learned skill and requires practice.
Males are better at math than females.	Research has proven this to be false.
I am better with words than with numbers and you can't be good at both. I just will not ever get math.	People commonly show high capability on both mathematical and verbal testing.
There is only one right way to solve a problem.	The best way to do a math problem is the method that works for you.
It's bad to count on your fingers.	Most people find counting on their fingers helpful, and there is no reason to feel guilty. The Chinese have used an "abacus" for centuries. This is a sophisticated finger-counting machine that is fast and accurate.
Mathematicians do problems quickly, in their heads.	If anyone performs a skill quickly, it is because they have done it many times. Any unfamiliar process takes time and practice.
I don't have a good memory.	Understanding is superior to memorization. If you truly understand something, you will use reason to naturally arrive at the answer.
It is hopeless, and much too hard for the average person.	Once you overcome your emotional blocks and develop self-confidence by practice, you will be delighted to find that you also can do math.
There is a magic key to doing math.	There is no magic or any one approach you need to learn to do math well.

The constant fearful thoughts that a learner experiences can be thought of as "internal mental static." This static prevents clear thinking, rational thought, and recall of known information while causing other stress-related symptoms. Fighting it and trying to talk oneself out of it cannot decrease anxiety, but there are ways to diminish or eliminate this mental static. (See Table 5–2.)

If you are smart at any skill at all, you can be smart at math. Always remember that you are not as far behind as you think you are. It is never too late to catch up.

BASIC CALCULATIONS

The information presented on decimals, fractions, percentages, and ratios is included in this chapter as a review of the basics needed to perform many medical math applications. The purpose is to jog the learner's memory: "Yes, that's right, now I remember." For learners who cannot easily follow the review or believe they never learned the concepts, a refresher course or more extensive review is recommended. There are many excellent books and computer programs on basic arithmetic. Another option is to find out if your campus has a resource center that offers assistance to learners who need to review math.

Fascinating Facts

Quote from Albert Einstein (1879–1955)

"Do not worry about your difficulties in mathematics, I assure you that mine are greater."

To work safely in health care, it is essential to be able to add, subtract, multiply, and divide whole numbers, decimals, fractions, and percentages. Learners also need to understand equivalents when using decimals, fractions, and percentages. (See Figure 5–1.)

Many health care professionals use small calculators to assist them with calculations. During your health care studies, some instructors will allow the

Table 5–2 Overcoming Math Anxiety

What To Do	How This Helps
The first step is to identify that you have math anxiety.	Overcoming math anxiety calls for experiencing and being aware of your emotional responses to math.
Identify what you already know and what you need to learn.	This is less overwhelming than simply saying "I can't do math." It provides a starting point for learning.
Do not delay identifying and working on your weak areas in math.	Procrastination increases anxiety.
Say "I will keep trying" rather than "I can't do it."	As long as there is the willingness to continue trying, the mind will work on mastering new material.
Take breaks as needed to clear your mind.	When the mind lacks clarity, you will start going in circles. A break allows for a fresh start.
Maintain a positive and confident manner.	Doing math requires confidence and concentration; panic and anxiety make this impossible. Expecting the worse makes it hard to concentrate.
Accept that there are no secrets to be handed out.	Participation and engagement in the process is what is needed for success.
As with any new material, many repetitions will be needed to master the new material.	Some topics have to be read, heard, and/or discussed many times before they become clear. There is nothing wrong with this and it is part of the normal process of learning.
Monitor your thoughts and replace negativity with productive thoughts. For example, instead of thinking "This is just the kind of problem I can never solve," change it to "What is making this problem difficult for me, and what can I do to make it easier for myself?"	Those who do well in math are not necessarily smarter, but they seem to know themselves better. They can anticipate the difficulties they will have and know what questions and actions will give them the power and confidence to continue.
If you come across a formula or process that seems too complex, isolate it and examine it by breaking it down into little parts.	This will help you to overcome the fear of complexity and being overwhelmed.

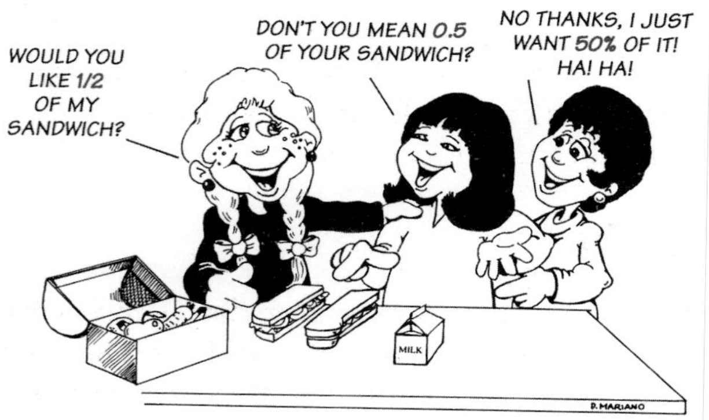

FIGURE 5–1 An easy way to remember how to convert decimals, percentages, and fractions is to think of this humorous cartoon.

use of calculators and others will not. It is always best to know how to do the basic functions by "longhand" (without a calculator), because calculators can quit working at any time during a test or at the workplace. Some professional exams required for licensure or certification do not allow the use of calculators.

Whole Numbers

Whole numbers are what we traditionally use to count (1, 2, 3, . . .). They do not contain fractions or decimals. For example, 30 is a whole number, whereas 30½ and 30.5 are not. Learners must be able to accurately add, subtract, multiply, and divide whole numbers.

- Add: 15 + 24 = 39 (verbal: fifteen plus twenty-four equals thirty-nine)
- Subtract: 54 − 15 = 39 (verbal: fifty-four minus fifteen equals thirty-nine)
- Multiply: 14 × 8 = 112 (verbal: fourteen times eight equals one hundred and twelve)
- Divide: 60 ÷ 12 = 5 (verbal: sixty divided by twelve equals five)

Decimals

Decimals are one way of expressing parts of numbers or anything else that has been divided into parts. The parts are expressed in units of 10. That is, decimals represent the number of tenths, hundredths, thousandths, and so on that are available. For example, 0.7 represents 7 of the 10 parts into which something has been divided. When reading decimals verbally, it is necessary to know the placement values for the decimals (digits to the right of the decimal point) and that the decimal point is read as "and." (See Figure 5–2.) For example:

- 0.5 is read "five tenths"
- 1.5 is read "one and five tenths"
- 1.50 is read "one and fifty hundredths"

Thinking It Through

Ms. Cree is a new graduate and has just been hired as a medical assistant in Dr. Albright's office. She is anxious about learning the new routines and doing a good job. She has always struggled with math calculations, but was able to develop her skills to pass her courses in school. However, when Dr. Albright orders a medication that needs to be calculated, Ms. Cree panics. She is unable to find her calculator, and even though she has been able to manually solve this type of problem in the classroom setting, she now becomes too afraid to trust her own skills. Where *is* that calculator? Ms. Cree is afraid of losing her job if she admits the problem, and yet she knows that if she makes a mistake, she could jeopardize the health of the patient.

1. What job-related factors are contributing to Ms. Cree's anxiety and panic?
2. What suggestions would you recommend to her?
3. What thoughts are going through her mind that may be adding to the problem?

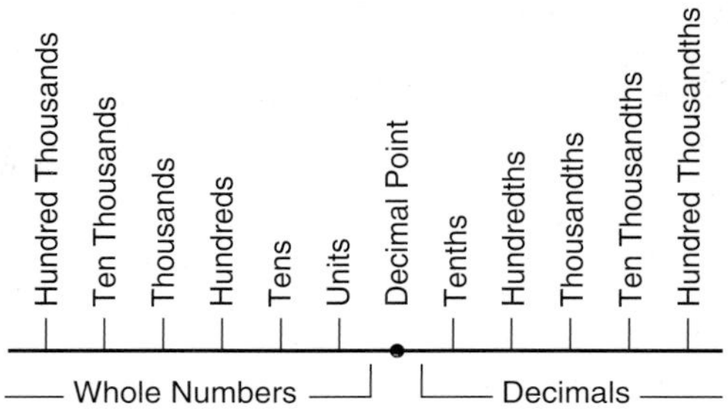

FIGURE 5–2 The position of the number to the left or the right of the decimal point is its place value. The value of each place to the *left* of the decimal point is *10 times* that of the place to its right. The value of each place to the *right* of the decimal point is *one-tenth* the value of the place to its left.

- 1.500 is read "one and five hundred thousandths"
- 1.5000 is read "one and five thousand ten thousandths"

See Table 5–3 for guidelines to practices that help reduce medication errors. The Joint Commission requires the following designations when writing decimals:

- Never use a trailing zero (e.g., write 1 mg, *not* 1.0 mg because the decimal point can be missed and read as 10 mg. This would result in a tenfold error in dosage.).
- Always use a leading zero if less than 1 (e.g., write 0.1 mg, *not* .1 mg because the decimal point can be missed and read as 1 mg. This would result in a tenfold error in dosage.).

Decimals are added, subtracted, multiplied, and divided in the same way as whole numbers. The most common mistake is incorrect placement of the decimal point. (See Table 5–4.)

Media Link

View Calculations with Decimals and Reading and Writing Decimals on the Online Resources to verify your understanding of working with decimals.

Fractions

Fractions are another way of expressing numbers that represent parts of a whole. A fraction has a numerator (top number) and a denominator (bottom number). An example of a fraction is 3/10, where the 3 is the numerator and 10 is the denominator. One way of looking at it is that the denominator (bottom number) defines how many parts make a whole and the

Table 5–3 Tips to Reduce Medication Errors

Avoid	Preferred Method	Rationale
~~u~~	units	Always write "units" *not* "u." The handwritten "u" after the dose is often read as zero, causing a potential tenfold overdose.
~~1.0~~ mg	1 mg	Never use a trailing zero. Do not follow a whole number with a decimal point and a zero. The decimal point is often not seen, causing a potential tenfold overdose.
~~.5~~ mg	0.5 mg	Always use a leading zero. Use a leading zero before a number with a decimal point. The leading decimal point alone is often not seen, causing a potential tenfold overdose.
~~cc~~	mL	Always write "mL" or "milliliter", *not* "cc." When handwritten, the abbreviation "cc" has been mistaken as "00" causing a potential one hundred-fold overdose.

Table 5–4 Working with Decimals

Function	Example	Key Points
Add (+):	1.5 + 2.25 3.75	1. Line up the decimal points. 2. Add the numbers. 3. Bring the decimal point straight down.
Subtract (–):	3.75 –1.25 2.50	1. Line up the decimal points. 2. Subtract the numbers. 3. Bring the decimal point straight down.
Multiply (×):	2.5 × 2.5 125 + 50 6.25	1. Multiply the numbers. 2. Count the total number of digits to the right of the decimal points in the numbers you are multiplying. 3. Count the same number of places in your answer. Start to the right of the last digit in your answer and move left that number of places. This is where the decimal point is placed.
Divide (÷):	2.5)50.5 25.)505.0 20.2 25)505.0 50 5 0 50 50 0	1. Move the decimal point to the right in the number you are dividing by (to make it a whole number). 2. Move the decimal point the same number of places to the right in the number being divided. Add zeros if necessary. 3. Divide the numbers. 4. Place the decimal point in the answer by moving it straight up from the number that was divided.

numerator (top number) is the actual number of parts of this whole. See Figure 5–3 for an illustration of this concept. The fraction 3/10 is read as "three tenths."

Although performing calculations with fractions is not difficult, it does require following a series of steps. These are described in Table 5–5. There are a few special considerations to remember when working with fractions. When adding and subtracting fractions, it is necessary to change all the denominators to the same number in order to perform the calculations.

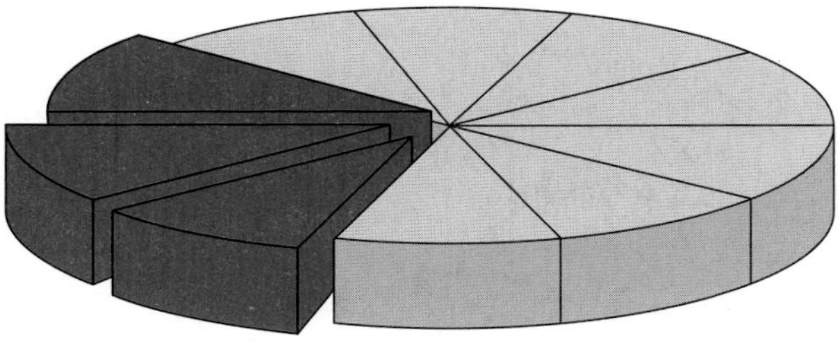

FIGURE 5–3 A fraction is a comparison of parts (numerator) to a whole (denominator).

This is known as "converting the fractions." To do this, find a number that each denominator can divide into evenly and then adjust the numerators to maintain an equivalent fraction. For example, to add $\frac{1}{2}$ + $\frac{1}{3}$, convert both fractions to sixths: $\frac{3}{6} + \frac{2}{6} = \frac{5}{6}$. (The denominators 2 and 3 both divide into 6 evenly; then the numerator is multiplied by the number of times the old denominator divides into the new denominator [2 divides into 6 three times, so 1 × 3 then creates the new fraction $\frac{3}{6}$; 3 divides into 6 two times, so 1 × 2 then creates the new fraction $\frac{2}{6}$]).

Multiplying fractions is straightforward. First multiply the two numerators and then the two denominators. For example, $\frac{1}{2} \times \frac{1}{2} = \frac{1}{4}$ (1 × 1 = 1 and 2 × 2 = 4).

Dividing fractions requires the dividing fraction to be inverted (turned upside-down). The new, upside-down fraction is called the **reciprocal**. The numerators and denominators are then multiplied to get the answer. For example, $\frac{1}{2} \div \frac{1}{2} = \frac{1}{2} \times \frac{2}{1} = \frac{2}{2}$ or 1.

Two processes are frequently used when working with fractions. Reducing the fraction to its lowest terms means finding a number that can be divided evenly into both the numerator and denominator. For example, the fraction $\frac{2}{4}$ can be reduced to the lower equivalent fraction of $\frac{1}{2}$ by dividing both the numerator and denominator by 2 (2 ÷ 2 = 1 and

Table 5–5 Working with Fractions

Function	Example	Key Points
Add (+):	$\frac{1}{5} = \frac{6}{30}$ $+\frac{1}{6} = +\frac{5}{30}$ $\frac{11}{30}$	1. If the denominators are not the same, find a number both denominators divide evenly into. 2. Multiply the numerators by the number of times the old denominators divide into the new denominator. 3. Add the numerators. 4. Place the new numerator over the denominator. 5. Reduce the fraction, if necessary.
Subtract (–):	$\frac{1}{5} = \frac{6}{30}$ $+\frac{1}{6} = \frac{5}{30}$ $\frac{1}{30}$	1. If the denominators are not the same, find a number both denominators divide evenly into. 2. Multiply the numerators by the number of times the old denominators divide into the new denominator. 3. Subtract the numerators. 4. Place the new numerator over the denominator. 5. Reduce the fraction, if necessary.
Multiply (×):	$\frac{1}{5} \times \frac{1}{6} = \frac{1}{30}$	1. Multiply numerators. 2. Multiply denominators. 3. Reduce the fraction, if necessary.
Divide (÷)	$\frac{1}{5} \div \frac{1}{6} = \frac{1}{5} \times \frac{6}{1} = \frac{6}{5} = 1\frac{1}{5}$	1. Invert the dividing fraction. 2. Multiply numerators. 3. Multiply denominators. 4. Reduce the fraction, if necessary.

$4 \div 2 = 2$). This process is also known as "simplifying the fraction."

Improper fractions have numerators that are larger than the denominators. To reduce these fractions, divide the denominator into the numerator. The result will be a whole number or a mixed number (whole number and a fraction). For example, the fraction $^{12}/_{4}$ would be reduced to the whole number 3 ($12 \div 4 = 3$); the fraction $^{11}/_{4}$ would be reduced to the mixed number $2\frac{3}{4}$ ($11 \div 4 = 2\frac{3}{4}$).

Media Link

View Fractions and Decimals, Converting Between Fraction Types, Calculations with Fractions, Calculate the Percentage of a Quantity, and Comparing the Values of Fractions and Decimals on the Online Resources to verify your understanding of working with fractions.

Percentages

Percentages are used to express either a whole or part of a whole. The whole is expressed as 100% (percent). Refer back to Figure 5–3 and imagine this as a hot apple pie sliced into 10 equal pieces. The 10 slices together equal the whole, or 100%, of the pie. One hundred divided by ten equals ten. Therefore, each slice represents 10% of the pie. If each slice is 10%, then three slices represent 30% of the pie.

When working with percentages, it is easier to convert the percentage to a decimal and then to perform the addition, subtraction, multiplication, and division. Converting percentages to decimals is explained later in this chapter.

Ratios

Ratios show relationships between numbers or like values: How many of one number or value is present in comparison to the other. Conversions between ratios and percentages are explained in the next section.

When working with liquids, it is necessary to look at the part compared to the whole quantity. For example, a 1:3 bleach to water solution is one part of bleach added for every three parts of water. The whole quantity in this case is four parts. To determine the strength of the bleach solution, the amount of bleach (1 part) is divided by the whole (4 parts). It can then be stated that this is a 25% bleach solution.

Converting Decimals, Fractions, Percentages, and Ratios

Decimals, fractions, and percentages all express parts of a whole. The cartoon in Figure 5–1 humorously portrays how they are related: The fraction $\frac{1}{2}$, the decimal 0.5, and the percentage 50% all represent the same amount of the sandwich. The steps involved in converting among these numerical forms are shown in Table 5–6.

Rounding Numbers

Rounding a number means changing it to the nearest ten, hundred, thousand, and so on. Deciding which to use depends on the size of the original number and the degree of accuracy required. Deciding whether to round up or round down depends on the digits (numbers) located to the right of the value chosen for rounding. The following examples illustrate how these rules are applied:

Example 1 When rounding to the nearest 10, look at the digit to the right of the tens place (the ones place). If the number is 5 or above, round up. If it is less than 5, round down.

88 rounds up to 90

83 rounds down to 80

Example 2 When rounding to the nearest 100, look at the digit to the right of the hundreds place (the tens place). If the number is 5 or above, round up. If it is less than 5, round down.

67 rounds up to 100

133 rounds down to 100

668 rounds up to 700

621 rounds down to 600

Example 3 When rounding to the nearest 1000, look at the digit to the right of the thousands place (the hundreds place). If the number is 5 or above, round up. If it is less than 5, round down.

7$\underline{7}$77 rounds up to 8000

7$\underline{3}$55 rounds down to 7000

Numbers of all sizes can be rounded. Review Figure 5–2 and study the examples in Table 5–7.

Table 5–6 Converting Decimals, Fractions, Percentages, and Ratios

Converting	Example	
Decimals to fractions	0.75 = 75/100 = 3/4	1. Drop decimal point. 2. Position number over its placement value (review Figure 5–2). 3. If necessary, reduce fraction.
Decimals to percentages	5.275 = 5.275 × 100 = 527.5	1. Move decimal point two places to the right because percentages are based on 100. This is the same as multiplying by 100.
	527.5%	2. Add percentage sign.
Fractions to decimals	3/5 = 3 ÷ 5 = 0.6	Divide numerator by denominator.
Fractions to percentages	7/8 = 7 ÷ 8 = 0.875	1. Divide numerator by denominator.
	0.875 × 100 = 87.5	2. Move decimal point two places to the right because percentages are based on 100. This is the same as multiplying by 100.
	87.5%	3. Add percentage sign.
Percentages to decimals	125.5% = 125.5	1. Remove percentage sign.
	125.5 ÷ 100 = 1.255	2. Move decimal point two places to the left because percentages are based on 100. This is the same as dividing by 100.
Percentages to fractions	5% = 5	1. Remove percentage sign.
	$\frac{5}{100} = \frac{1}{20}$	2. Place number over 100. 3. If appropriate, simplify fraction to lowest terms.
Percentages to ratios	75% = 75	1. Remove percentage sign.
	75:100	2. Create ratio using the former percentage and the number 100.
	3:4	3. Insert colon (:) between the numbers. 4. If appropriate, simplify ratio to lowest term.
Ratios to percentages	1:2 = 1/2 = 0.5 0.5 × 100 = 50	1. Divide number on left of colon by number on right of ratio sign. 2. Move decimal point two places to the right. Add zero(s) if necessary. This is the same as multiplying by 100.
	50%	3. Add percentage sign.

Media Link

View Rounding of Decimals on the Online Resources to verify understanding of rounding of numbers.

Solving Problems with Proportions

A **proportion** is a statement of equality between two ratios. For example, the proportion 2:6 = 3:9 means that 2 is related to 6 in the same way that 3 is related to 9. It is verbalized as "two is to six as three is to nine."

Proportions are useful for converting from one unit to another when three of the terms in the proportion are known. For example, you need $32.50, but only have quarters. How many quarters are needed? Three of the terms in the proportion are known:

1. $32.50
2. 4 (the number of quarters that are in $1.00)
3. $1.00

Table 5-7 Rounding Numbers

Round the Number 1234.5678 to the Nearest:	Result	Comments
Whole number	1235	The digit to the right of the whole number (1234) is 5, so you round up one number.
Tens	1230	The digit to the right of the tens place is 4, so you round down.
Hundreds	1200	The digit to the right of the hundreds position is 3, so you round down.
Thousands	1000	The digit to the right of the thousands position is 2, so you round down.
Tenths	1234.6	The digit to the right of the tenths position is 6, so you round up.
Hundredths	1234.57	The digit to the right of the hundredths position is 7, so you round up.
Thousandths	1234.568	The digit to the right of the thousandths position is 8, so you round up.
Ten thousandths	1234.5678	No change.

The proportion is set up as follows:

$$\frac{4 \text{ quarters}}{x \text{ quarters}} = \frac{\$1.00}{\$32.50}$$

The purpose of the proportion is to answer the question: "If four quarters equal one dollar, how many quarters are there in thirty-two dollars and fifty cents?" Or put another way: "4 quarters are to \$1.00 as 'x' quarters are to \$32.50." *Note that the two unit measurements on each side of the equation are the same* (quarters on the left and dollars on the right). The "x" stands for the number to be calculated.

To solve this problem, follow these steps:

1. Cross-multiply:

$$\frac{4 \text{ quarters}}{x \text{ quarters}} \quad \frac{\$1.00}{\$32.50}$$

$$1 \times x = 4 \times 32.50 = 1x = 130$$

2. Divide each side by the number in front of "x" (in this case each number is divided by one, and this does not alter the number).

$$1x \div 1 = x \text{ and } 130 \div 1 = 130$$

$$x = 130 \text{ quarters}$$

3. 130 quarters are needed to make a payment of \$32.50.

4. The completed proportion is:

$$\frac{4 \text{ quarters}}{130 \text{ quarters}} = \frac{\$1.00}{\$32.50}$$

Converting units of measure is another common application of proportions. For example, you want to know how many feet are in 29 inches. Again, three of the terms in the proportion are known:

1. 29 inches
2. 12 (the number of inches in 1 foot)
3. 1 foot

The proportion is set up as follows:

$$\frac{1 \text{ foot}}{x \text{ feet}} = \frac{12 \text{ inches}}{29 \text{ inches}}$$

To solve this problem, follow these steps:

1. Cross-multiply:

$$\frac{1 \text{ foot}}{x \text{ feet}} \quad \frac{12 \text{ inches}}{29 \text{ inches}}$$

$$12 \times x = 1 \times 29 = 12x = 29$$

2. Divide each side by the number in front of "x":

$$12x \div 12 = x \text{ and } 29 \div 12 = 2.42$$

$$x = 2.42 \text{ feet (rounded to nearest hundredth)}$$

3. The completed proportion is:

$$\frac{1 \text{ foot}}{2.42 \text{ feet}} = \frac{12 \text{ inches}}{29 \text{ inches}}$$

A common application of proportions in health care is to find the value of an unknown when converting medications from one form to another. For example, a physician orders a patient to have 50 grams of a medication. When the nurse checks, she notes that the medication is available only in 12.5-gram tablets. How many tablets should she give the patient?

$$\frac{1 \text{ tablet}}{x \text{ tablets}} = \frac{12.5 \text{ grams}}{50 \text{ grams}}$$

To solve this problem:

1. Cross-multiply:

$$\frac{1 \text{ tablet}}{x \text{ tablets}} \times \frac{12.5 \text{ grams}}{50 \text{ grams}}$$

$12.5 \times x = 1 \times 50 = 12.5x = 50$

2. Divide each side by the number in front of "x":

$12.5x \div 12.5 = x$ and $50 \div 12.5 = 4$

$x = 4$ tablets

3. 4 tablets are needed to equal 50 grams.
4. The completed proportion is:

$$\frac{1 \text{ tablet}}{4 \text{ tablets}} = \frac{12.5 \text{ grams}}{50 \text{ grams}}$$

Media Link

View Ratios, Converting Among Fractions, Decimals, Ratios and Percents; Comparing the Size of Fractions, Decimals, Ratios and Percents; and Calculate the Percentage of a Quantity on the Online Resources to verify understanding of converting between the various forms of expressing numbers.

ESTIMATING

Health care professionals must work carefully and thoughtfully when performing calculations. An important skill to help check work is anticipating the results. This involves **estimating**—calculating the approximate answer—and judging if the calculated results seem reasonable. If calculations are performed without thought and answers simply accepted, errors can go unnoticed. It is easy for mistakes to occur when you are working in a hurry. Numbers can be placed in the wrong order, decimal points misplaced, or operations carried out incorrectly. Knowing when an answer "just doesn't look right" serves as an alert to double-check the results. Working on "automatic pilot" is not acceptable when using math in the workplace.

Learning to estimate and detect incorrect answers takes practice and thought. Here are a few guidelines to make estimating useful:

- First, use rounding to get numbers that are easier to mentally compute. For example, when multiplying 47 times 83, round 47 up to 50 and 83 down to 80. 50 times 80 is much easier to mentally multiply than the original numbers.
- Second, watch place values carefully. In the 50 times 80 example, if 5 is multiplied times 8, two zeros must be added to the quick result of 40.
- Third, look at the size of the answer. Does it make sense? For example, when multiplying whole numbers, the answer should be larger than either of the numbers in the problem. When dividing, it should be smaller.
- Fourth, be careful about placing decimal points. Remember that everything to the right of the point is a fraction. Even 0.99999 does not equal 1.0.

MILITARY TIME

Military time is often used in health care to avoid the confusion created by the a.m. and p.m. used in the traditional system to designate the correct time. The problem with the traditional system is that if the a.m. or p.m. is omitted or misread, an error of 12 hours is made. Errors in recording times are unacceptable in health care. For example, accuracy is critical when entering data on a patient chart, reporting when medications are given, or signing off on physician orders.

When **military time** is the standard used, all time designations are made with the 24-hour clock. The twelfth hour is at 12 noon and the twenty-fourth hour is at 12 midnight. (See Figure 5–4.) When using the 24-hour clock, remember the following key points:

- Time is always expressed using four digits (e.g., 0030, 0200, 1200, 1700).

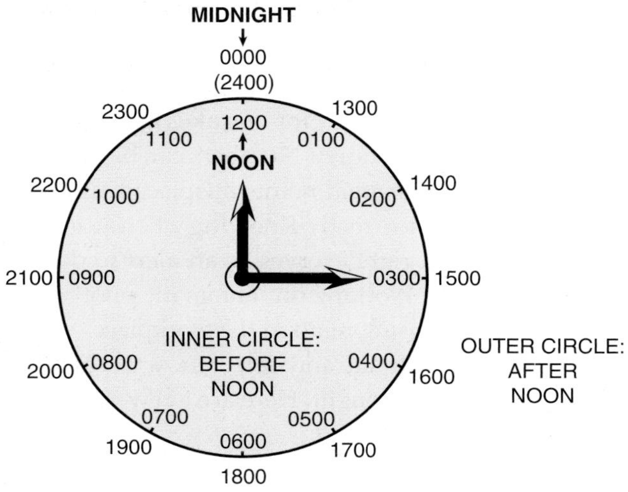

FIGURE 5–4 The military clock is based on a 24-hour day.

- The a.m. hours are expressed with the same numbers as the traditional clock:

  1 a.m.: 0100

  5:30 a.m.: 0530

  10 a.m.: 1000

- An easy way to convert the p.m. hours is to add the time to 1200. For example:

  1 p.m.: 1200 + 0100 (1:00 p.m. expressed in four digits) = 1300

  5:30 p.m.: 1200 + 0530 (5:30 p.m. expressed in four digits) = 1730

  10 p.m.: 1200 + 1000 (10:00 p.m. expressed in four digits) = 2200

- When times are verbalized, there is a specific way in which they are expressed:

  1300 = thirteen hundred hours

  1301 = thirteen oh one

  1730 = seventeen thirty hours

  2200 = twenty-two hundred hours

Study Table 5–8 to practice converting between traditional and military times.

Media Link

View Convert between Traditional and International Time on the Online Resources for an overview of this process.

Table 5–8 Military (24-Hour Clock) and Traditional Time Conversion Chart

Traditional	24-Hour Time	Traditional	24-Hour Time
12:01 a.m.	0001	12:01 p.m.	1201
12:30 a.m.	0030	12:30 p.m.	1230
1:00 a.m.	0100	1:00 p.m.	1300
2:00 a.m.	0200	2:00 p.m.	1400
3:00 a.m.	0300	3:00 p.m.	1500
4:00 a.m.	0400	4:00 p.m.	1600
5:00 a.m.	0500	5:00 p.m.	1700
6:00 a.m.	0600	6:00 p.m.	1800
7:00 a.m.	0700	7:00 p.m.	1900
8:00 a.m.	0800	8:00 p.m.	2000
9:00 a.m.	0900	9:00 p.m.	2100
10:00 a.m.	1000	10:00 p.m.	2200
11:00 a.m.	1100	11:00 p.m.	2300
12:00 noon	1200	12:00 midnight	2400

ROMAN NUMERALS

The traditional numbering system we use every day is referred to as Arabic numerals (1, 2, 3,...). In health care, it is necessary to know **Roman numerals** because they are used for some medications, solutions, and ordering systems. You may also see some files or materials organized using Roman numerals. When using Roman numerals, remember the following key points:

- All numbers can be expressed by using seven key numerals:

  I = 1

  V = 5

  X = 10

  L = 50

  C = 100

  D = 500

  M = 1000
- If a smaller numeral is placed in front of a larger numeral, the smaller numeral is *subtracted* from the larger numeral. For example: In IV, the 1 is placed before the 5, so it is subtracted (5 – 1 = 4).
- If a smaller numeral is placed after a larger numeral, the smaller numeral is *added* to the larger numeral. For example: In VI, the 1 is placed after the 5, so it is added (5 + 1 = 6).
- When the same numeral is placed next to itself, it is added. For example:

  III = 1 + 1 + 1 = 3

  XX = 10 + 10 = 20

  IXX: this has two of the same numeral preceded by a smaller numeral, but the rules still apply (10 + 10 – 1 = 19 *or* 10 – 1 + 10 = 19)
- The same numeral is not placed next to itself more than three times. For example:

  XXX = 30

  XL = 40 (XXXX is not correct)
- When Roman numerals are used with medication dosages, the lowercase (i, v, x, l, c, d, m) may be used rather than uppercase (capital letters). For example:

  ii = 2

  iv = 4

  ixx = 19

Table 5–9 Arabic and Roman Numeral Conversion Chart

Arabic	Roman	Arabic	Roman
1	I	23	XXIII
2	II	24	XXIV
3	III	25	XXV
4	IV	26	XXVI
5	V	27	XXVII
6	VI	28	XXVIII
7	VII	29	XXIX
8	VIII	30	XXX
9	IX	40	XL
10	X	50	L
20	XX	100	C
21	XXI	500	D
22	XXII	1000	M

Study Table 5–9 to practice converting between Arabic and Roman numerals.

ANGLES

Angles are used in health care when injecting medications, describing joint movement, and indicating bed positions. **Angles** are always defined by comparison to a **reference plane**, a real or imaginary flat surface from which the angle is measured. The distance between the plane and the line of the angle is measured in units called **degrees**. For example, if a flat stick is placed on a table (the reference plane), the angle is at 0 degrees. There is no distance between the plane and the stick. If the stick is lifted to stand straight up (perpendicular to the table), there is a 90-degree angle to the table. Moving the stick halfway between these two positions creates a 45-degree angle. Rotating the stick all the way around the arc and returning to the reference point creates a complete circle and represents 360 degrees. (See Figure 5–5.) The following examples illustrate how angles are used in health care:

Example 1 Angles for injecting needles vary, depending on the type of medication or procedure being performed. (See Figure 5–6.) Note that in this case the reference plane is the skin surface.

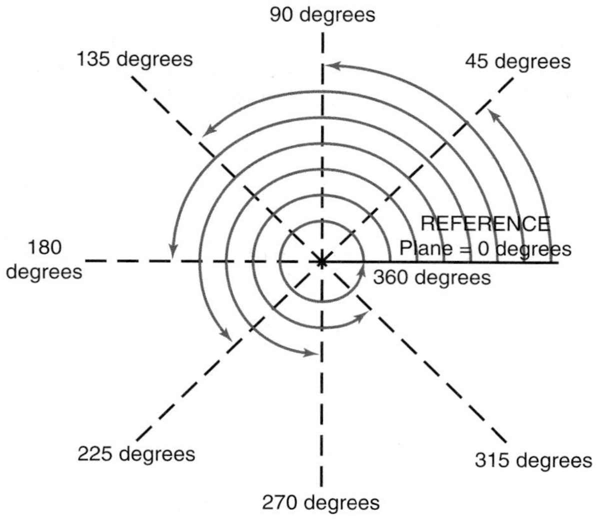

FIGURE 5–5 All angles are expressed in relation to a real or imaginary reference plane.

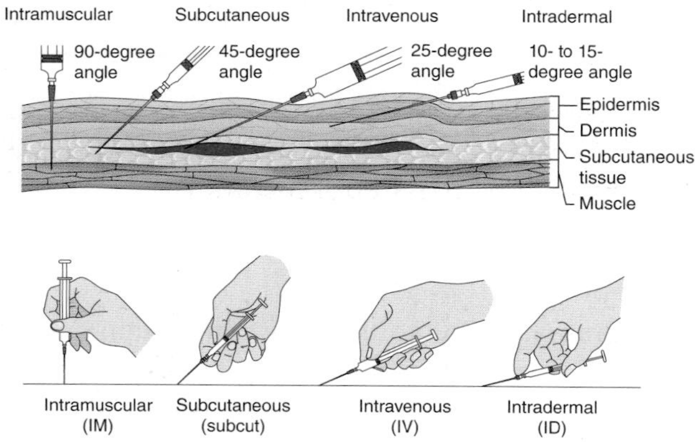

FIGURE 5–6 The correct angle must be used when inserting needles for administration of injections.

Example 2 When describing the angle of extremities (arms and legs), the body in a full upright position is the reference plane. (See Figure 5–7.) Each joint (e.g., elbow, knee, hip) in the body has a normal range it is intended to move within. Physicians assess the range of a patient's joint compared to this normal range to chart loss of function or progress of recovery.

Example 3 After surgery on a joint (e.g., hip or knee replacement), the physician will order that the joint not be moved more than a certain number of degrees to prevent the new joint from "popping" out of place.

Example 4 Sometimes the physician will order that the head of the bed be kept elevated by 30 to 45 degrees at all times. This is usually ordered to aid in

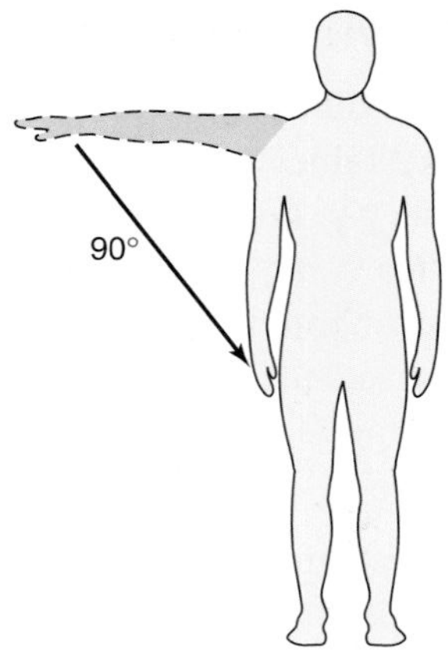

FIGURE 5–7 Body in full upright position with right arm lifted to 90-degree angle.

respiration or to prevent aspiration (stomach contents entering the lungs). In this situation, the bed in the flat position is the reference plane.

SYSTEMS OF MEASUREMENT

Basic skills in calculation are applied when learning and using the various systems of measurement used in health care. Each system has its own terminology for designating distance (length), capacity (volume) and mass (weight). Converting between these systems requires the use of the skills presented in this chapter. The three systems used in health care are household, metric, and apothecary. Each system has its own **nomenclature** (method of naming).

Household System

The **household system** is probably the method of measurement most familiar to learners who are educated in the United States. (See Table 5–10.) Note that "ounce" is used as both a measurement of capacity/volume and mass/weight. Health care professionals use both. Liquids, such as an 8-ounce glass of water, are measured in terms of capacity or volume. Determining mass or weight, such as with a 6-pound 12-ounce infant, is done by weighing with a scale. The various units of measurements in the household system relate to each other and conversions can be made within the system. For example, volume/capacity is measured in drops, teaspoons, tablespoons, ounces, cups, pints, quarts, and gallons. Knowing the equivalencies of these units enables you to calculate each one in terms of the others. (See Figure 5–8.)

Table 5–10 Household Measurement System

Type of Measurement	Nomenclature	Common Equivalents
Distance/Length	inch (″ or in)	12 in = 1 ft
	foot (′ or ft)	3 ft = 1 yd
	yard (yd)	1760 yds = 1 mi
	mile (mi)	
Capacity/Volume	drop (gtt)	60 gtts = 1 t
	teaspoon (t or tsp)	3t = 1 T
	tablespoon (T or tbsp)	2 T = 1 oz
	ounce (oz)	8 oz = 1 C
	cup (C)	2 C = 1 pt
	pint (pt)	2 pt = 1 qt
	quart (qt)	4 qt = 1 gal
	gallon (gal)	
Mass/Weight	ounce (oz)	16 oz = 1 lb
	pound (lb)	

When the basic equivalents are known, unknown measurements can be determined using proportions. Suppose that three tablespoons of a liquid are needed, but the only measuring device available is a cup marked in ounces (oz). How many ounces are in three tablespoons (3 T)? Knowing that 2T = 1 oz, the proportion would be set up as follows:

$$\frac{2T}{3T} = \frac{1\ oz}{x\ oz}$$

$$2x = 3\,oz$$

$$2x \div 2 = 3\,oz \div 2$$

$$x = 1.5\,oz$$

The next example involves measurement of height. If a patient is 63 inches tall and asks how many feet that is, the calculation would use the following proportion:

$$\frac{12\ inches}{63\ inches} = \frac{1\ feet}{x\ feet}$$

$$12x = 63$$

$$12x \div 12 = 63 \div 12$$

$$x = 5.25\ feet$$

$$x = 5.25\ feet = 5\ feet\ 3\ inches$$

$$(0.25\ feet \times 12\ inches = 3\ inches)$$

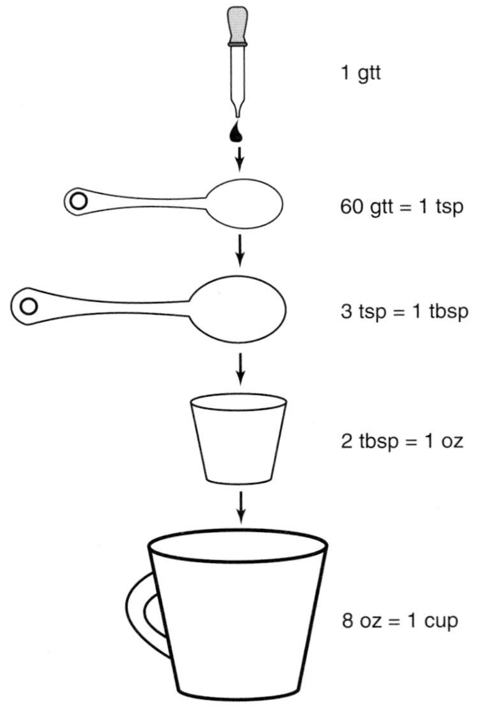

FIGURE 5–8 Common household measurements used in health care.

Media Link

View The Household System on the Online Resources for an overview of this system.

Metric System

The **metric system** will probably be familiar to learners who were educated outside the United States or have taken science classes. It is a more accurate system than the household system and also is easier to convert between numbers because everything is based on a unit of ten. The nomenclature for the metric units is as follows:

- Distance/length: meter (m)
- Capacity/volume: liter (l or L)
- Mass/weight: gram (g)

The meter, liter, and gram are modified by adding the appropriate prefix to express larger or smaller units. (See Table 5–11).

Being based on multiples of ten, conversions within the decimal system are calculated by multiplying by 10, 100, 1000, and so on:

- 1 *kilo*liter = 1000 × 1 liter = 1000 liters
- 1 *hecto*liter = 100 × 1 liter = 100 liters
- 1 *deca*liter = 10 × 1 liter = 10 liters
- 1 *deci*liter = 0.1 × 1 liter = 0.1 liter
- 1 *centi*liter = 0.01 × 1 liter = 0.01 liter
- 1 *milli*liter = 0.001 × 1 liter = 0.001 liter

A shortcut for performing these operations is to move the decimal point the number of places indicated by the prefix. Here are three examples:

Example 1 Multiplying 1 by 10 means moving the decimal point one place to the right. This may require adding one or more zeros.

Example 2 Multiplying 4.2 by 10 = 42

Example 3 Multiplying 4.2 by 100 = 420

Converting units within the metric system is accomplished by moving the decimal point. For example, if the physician orders 2000 milligrams of a medication and this needs to be converted to grams, the conversion is made as follows:

1. *Milli* is in the third place to the right of gram. Move the decimal point three spaces to the left *toward gram*: 2000 = 2.000, or 2.
2. Change unit name to grams: 2 grams.
3. The proper dose would be 2 grams, or two 1-gram tablets.

A second example involves converting 1000 centimeters to kilometers:

1. *Centi* is five decimal places to the right of *kilo*, so move the decimal point five spaces to the left *toward kilo*. Add zeros as needed: 1000 = 0.01.
2. Change unit name to kilometers: 0.01 kilometers.

See Figure 5–9 for a visual representation of decimal placement.

In addition to moving the decimal point the correct number of places, it is critical that it be moved in the correct direction. This can be confusing. The easiest

Table 5–11 Common Prefixes of the Metric System

Prefix	Meaning	Examples	Meaning of Examples
kilo	1000 times	kilogram	1000 grams
		kilometer	1000 meters
		kiloliter	1000 liters
hecto	100 times	hectogram	100 grams
deca (also "deka")	10 times	decaliter	10 liters
meter, liter, gram	Whole units of measurement		
deci	1/10	decigram	1/10 of a gram
centi	1/100	centimeter	1/100 of a meter
milli	1/1000	milliliter	1/1000 of a liter
micro	1/1,000,000	microgram	1/1,000,000 of a gram

PREFIX	KILO-	HECTO-	DEKA-	BASE	DECI-	CENTI-	MILLI-	DECIMILLI-	CENTIMILLI-	MICROMILLI-
Common Units	kilogram			gram liter meter		centimeter	milligram milliliter millimeter			microgram
Value to Base	**1000**	100	10	**1.0**	0.1	**0.01**	**0.001**	0.0001	0.00001	0.000001

FIGURE 5–9 Comparison of common metric units used in health care.

Thinking It Through

Part of Mrs. Cabinos's job as an admitting assistant in an ambulatory clinic is to ask all patients their height and weight and record it on a graph. When she asks Mr. Summerton, he reports that he is 6 feet tall and weighs 160 pounds and 8 ounces. The graph used at this clinic is in inches and pounds.

1. How many inches are in 6 feet?
2. How do you convert 160 pounds and 8 ounces to pounds only?

way is to determine if the answer should be a larger or smaller number and then just move the decimal point accordingly:

1. If converting from a larger to a smaller prefix (e.g., kilo to milli), the answer will be larger. It takes more of the smaller units to equal the larger units.
2. If converting from a smaller to a larger prefix (e.g., milli to kilo), the answer will be smaller. It takes fewer of the larger units to equal the smaller units.

Media Link

View The Metric System on the Online Resources for an overview of this system.

Apothecary System

The **apothecary system** is the oldest and least used of the three systems of measurement presented. (See Table 5–12.) This system is seldom seen in the modern health care environment. The Joint Commission has advised that the apothecary symbols and measurements should no longer be used, but has not yet added this system to its official "do-not-use" list.

Roman numerals can be used in conjunction with the apothecary system, and may be seen in uppercase

Table 5–12 Apothecary Measurement System

Type of Measurement	Nomenclature	Common Equivalents
Distance/Length	N/A	N/A
Capacity/Volume	minim (♏)	1 minim = 1 drop
	fluid dram (fl dr or f ʒ)	60 minims = 1 fl dr
	fluid ounce (fl oz or ℥)	8 fl dr = 1 fl oz
	pint (pt)	16 fl oz = 1 pt
	quart (qt)	2 pt = 1 qt
Mass/Weight	grain (gr)	
	dram (dr or ʒ)	60 gr = 1 dr
	ounce (oz. or ℥)	480 gr = 1 oz

or lowercase formats. If lowercase is used, the Roman numeral for "1" is written with a line and a dot. For example, "2" would be written as $\overline{\text{ii}}$. A commonly used abbreviation that originated with the apothecary system is $\overline{\text{ss}}$ which means "half." For example 2½ would be written as $\overline{\text{iiss}}$.

Media Link

View The Apothecary System on the Online Resources for an overview of this system.

Converting Systems of Measurement

Health care work sometimes requires that units from one system of measurement be converted to those of another. This requires knowledge of the equivalencies between the units of the systems. There are frequently no exact equivalents, so when converting between systems the answer is considered to be a close approximation. (See Table 5–13.)

Using the appropriate equivalencies, a proportion is then set up to identify and solve for the unknown quantity. The following steps are used for performing conversions:

1. Identify an equivalent between the two systems.
2. Set up a proportion so unit measurements on each side of the equation are the same.
3. Use "x" for the unknown value being calculated.
4. Cross-multiply.
5. Solve for "x."
6. Verify if the answer is reasonable.
   a. If converting from a smaller unit to a larger unit, the answer will be smaller. For example, when converting 2 quarters to dollars, the result will be smaller than 2 because a quarter is a smaller unit than a dollar. Because there are 4 quarters in 1 dollar, 2 quarters = 0.5 dollar.
   b. If converting from a larger unit to a smaller unit, the answer will be larger. For example, when converting 2 dollars to quarters, the result will be a larger unit than 2 because a dollar is a larger unit than a quarter. Because there is 1 dollar for every 4 quarters, 2 dollars = 8 quarters.

The following examples illustrate how to perform conversions:

Example 1 Convert 19 inches to centimeters:

1. Identify equivalency: 1 inch = 2.5 centimeters.
2. Set up a proportion with same units on each side of equation. Use "x" for the unknown.

$$\frac{1 \text{ in}}{19 \text{ in}} = \frac{2.5 \text{ cm}}{\text{x cm}}$$

3. Cross-multiply:

$$1\text{x} = 47.5 \text{ cm}$$

4. Solve for x:

$$1\text{x} \div 1 = 47.5 \div 1$$
$$\text{x} = 47.5 \text{ cm}$$

5. Verify if the answer is reasonable: It takes a larger number of centimeters (2½ times) to measure the same distance as 1 inch. Therefore, it makes sense that the answer is larger than 19.

Example 2 Convert 1.5 meters to inches:

1. Identify equivalency: 39.4 inches = 1 meter.
2. Set up a proportion with the same units on each side of equation. Use "x" for the unknown.

$$\frac{39.4 \text{ in}}{\text{x in}} = \frac{1 \text{ m}}{1.5 \text{ m}}$$

3. Cross-multiply:

$$1\text{x} = 59.1 \text{ inches}$$

4. Solve for x:

$$1\text{x} \div 1 = 59.1 \div 1$$
$$\text{x} = 59.1 \text{ inches}$$

Table 5–13 Approximate Equivalents between Measuring Systems

Distance/Length	Capacity/Volume	Mass/Weight
1 in = 2.5 cm	1 tsp = 5 mL	2.2 lb = 1 kg
39.4 in = 1 m	1 oz = 30 mL	1 grain = 60 milligrams (mg)
	1 qt = 1000 mL	15 grains = 1 gram (g)

5. Verify if the answer is reasonable: It takes many inches to measure the distance designated by 1 meter. Therefore, the answer 59.1 makes sense.

Example 3 Convert 5 teaspoons to milliliters:

$$\frac{1 \text{ tsp}}{5 \text{ tsp}} = \frac{5 \text{ mL}}{x \text{ mL}}$$

x = 25 mL

Example 4 Convert 75 milliliters to ounces:

$$\frac{1 \text{ oz}}{x \text{ oz}} = \frac{30 \text{ mL}}{75 \text{ mL}}$$

30x = 75 (note that in solving for x, each side is divided by 30)

x = 2.5 oz

Example 5 Convert 120 pounds to kilograms:

$$\frac{2.2 \text{ lb}}{120 \text{ lb}} = \frac{1 \text{ kg}}{x \text{ kg}}$$

2.2x = 120 (note that in solving for "x," each side is divided by 2.2)

x = 54.5 kg (rounded to nearest tenth)

Example 6 Convert 60 kilograms to ounces:

$$\frac{2.2 \text{ lb}}{x \text{ oz}} = \frac{1 \text{ kg}}{60 \text{ kg}}$$

This problem cannot be solved using this proportion, because the unit measurements on the left side of the equation are not the same size (pound and ounce). To solve this problem, pounds must first be converted to ounces. Refer back to the household system and Table 5–9: 16 ounces = 1 pound.

$$\frac{16 \text{ oz}}{x \text{ oz}} = \frac{1 \text{ lb}}{2.2 \text{ lb}}$$

x = 35.2 oz

Knowing that 2.2 pounds = 35.2 ounces = 1 kilogram allows the appropriate proportion to be set up:

$$\frac{35.2 \text{ oz}}{x \text{ oz}} = \frac{1 \text{ kg}}{60 \text{ kg}}$$

x = 2112 oz

Example 7 Convert 15 grains to milligrams:

$$\frac{1 \text{ gr}}{15 \text{ gr}} = \frac{60 \text{ mg}}{x \text{ mg}}$$

x = 900 mg

Example 8 Convert 2 g to grains:

$$\frac{15 \text{ gr}}{x \text{ gr}} = \frac{1 \text{ gm}}{2 \text{ gm}}$$

x = 30 gr

Media Link

View Approximate Equivalents on the Online Resources for an overview of converting between systems and the ratio method of solving problems.

MEDICATION SAFETY

The misidentification of alphanumeric characters in handwritten orders has been a long-standing problem and has led to medication errors resulting in severe problems and, in some cases, death. Fortunately computerized physician order entry can overcome most problems with poor handwriting. However, even typed or computerized physician orders may not help prevent all of them. Anyone familiar with email knows how easy it is to misidentify a computer-generated lowercase letter L (l) in an email address as the numeral one (1), or the letter O as zero (0)! It is also easy to confuse the uppercase letter Z with the number 2.

The Institute for Safe Medication Practices reports that the previously mentioned characters (l/1, O/0, and Z/2), plus the number 1, which can look like a 7, account for over 50% of the errors caused by character misidentification.

TEMPERATURE CONVERSION

Thermometers using **Fahrenheit (F)** as the measuring unit are more familiar to people living in the United States, though the **Celsius (C)** system (also known as centigrade) of measurement is frequently seen in medical practice. One way to start understanding the difference between the two systems is to compare how each one expresses the boiling and freezing points of water.

Boiling points: 212°F = 100°C

Freezing points: 32°F = 0°C

See Figure 5–10 for a comparison of Fahrenheit (F) and Celsius (C) thermometers, and Table 5–14 for a conversion chart. Health care professionals may have to convert between the F and C systems when a conversion chart is not available. Table 5–15 contains

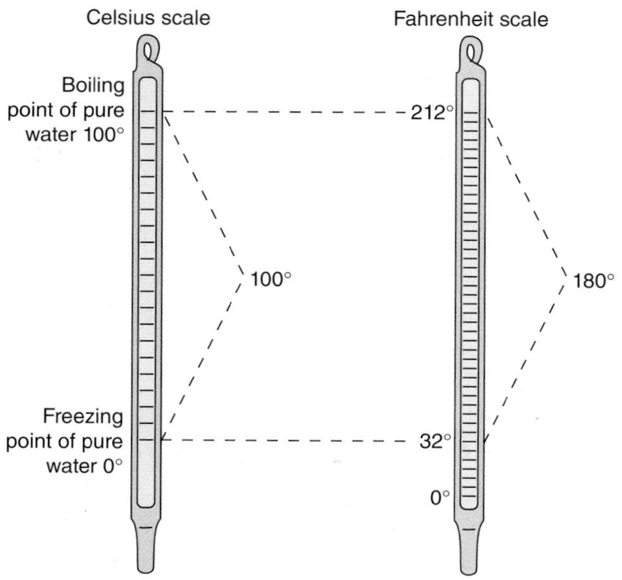

FIGURE 5–10 Comparison of Fahrenheit and Celsius temperature scales.

the formulas for conversion. A fraction and a decimal approach give the same results. Deciding which to use depends on whether you have stronger skills working with fractions or decimals. All the formulas include parentheses. These are used to indicate that the enclosed calculation must be performed first. For example the steps to solve the formula (°F – 32) × 5/9 = °C are to first subtract 32 from the value for F and *then* multiply that value by 5/9.

Table 5–14 Fahrenheit–Celsius Conversion Chart

Fahrenheit	Celsius
32 (freezing point)	0 (freezing point)
95	35
96	35.6
97	36.1
97.4	36.3
98	36.7
98.6	37
99	37.2
99.4	37.4
100	37.8
101	38.3
102	38.9
103	39.4
104	40
212 (boiling point)	100 (boiling point)

Media Link

View Convert between Celsius and Fahrenheit Temperature on the Online Resources for an overview of these calculations. Then, play an interactive game and complete the quiz for this chapter.

Table 5–15 Temperature Scale Conversion Formulas

Convert From:	Fraction Formula	Decimal Formula
Celsius to Fahrenheit	(°C × 9/5) + 32 = °F	(°C × 1.8) + 32 = °F
	Example: 37°C	Example: 37°C
	(37 × 9/5) + 32 = °F	(37 × 1.8) + 32 = °F
	333/5 + 32 = 98.6°F	66.6 + 32 = 98.6°F
Fahrenheit to Celsius	(°F – 32) × 5/9 = °C	(°F – 32) ÷ 1.8 = °C
	Example: 101°F	Example: 101°F
	(101 – 32) × 5/9 = °C	(101 – 32) ÷ 1.8 = °C
	69 × 5/9 = °C	69 ÷ 1.8 = 38.3°C
	345/9 = 38.3°C (rounded to nearest tenth)	(rounded to nearest tenth)

WORKBOOK PRACTICE

Go to your workbook and complete the exercises for this chapter.

SUGGESTED LEARNING ACTIVITIES

1. Consider the math anxiety section of this chapter. Do you feel you have math anxiety? If yes, identify available resources and create a plan to conquer the problem.
2. Cut a whole pie, cake, or paper plate into slices (you determine how many). Then practice by separating out some of the slices and expressing them as part of the whole in decimals, fractions, percentages, and ratios.
3. If you have a large wall clock, attach numbers cut out of paper to it to indicate military time. Or make a paper clock and put it up where you see it frequently. Practice telling time using the 24-hour format.
4. When you see numbers on street signs, practice converting them to Roman numerals.
5. Stand in front of a mirror and as you move your extremities try to estimate the degree of movement.
6. Practice, practice, practice using the systems of measurement until you can consistently use them accurately:
   - Weigh yourself in pounds and convert to kilograms.
   - Measure your height in inches and convert to meters.
   - Find various household measurement items (teaspoon, tablespoon, measuring cup) and convert them to the metric system.
   - Look at the strength of any medications you currently have in the house and convert them to another system of measurement (e.g., if the Tylenol or aspirin bottle has the strength listed in grains, convert to milligrams, or if listed as milligrams, convert to grains).
   - Take your temperature in Fahrenheit and convert to Celsius.
   - Exchange handwriting samples containing both alphabetic and numeric characters with another student. Look for any characters that are unclear or difficult to interpret. Exchange feedback.

WEB ACTIVITIES

Math.com
www.math.com/

Go to this site for a good review of math principles and examples. Review the information on fractions, decimals, and percents. Work with a buddy and each of you create five examples of fractions, decimals, and percents. When both of you have completed the math problems, compare your answers to see if they are the same. If you have any questions, seek out your instructor or another student to help solve the problems.

Math Anxiety
http://mathpower.com

Take the Math Anxiety Test and record your score. If you scored 20 points or higher, review the Ten Ways to Reduce Math Anxiety and develop a plan to decrease your math anxiety.

The Joint Commission
www.jointcommission.org

Find the "Do Not Use" list of abbreviations. Write down the items on the official do-not-use list and also the list of those being reviewed for possible inclusion.

REVIEW QUESTIONS

1. What is math anxiety, and what are the common fear thoughts that help create the anxiety?
2. What are the key points to remember when adding, subtracting, multiplying, and dividing decimals and fractions and when converting decimals, fractions, percentages, and ratios?
3. How does military time differ from the traditional system? What are the advantages?

4. How do Roman numerals differ from the traditional numbering system? What are the key points to remember when using Roman numerals?
5. Give three examples of how angles are used in health care.
6. What are the three systems of measurement currently used in health care? Within each system, what is the nomenclature used for length, volume, and weight?
7. What are the equations for converting between the three systems of measurement?
8. What are the equations for converting Fahrenheit to Celsius? Celsius to Fahrenheit?

APPLICATION EXERCISES

1. Refer to The Case of Exactly How Much Does My Baby Weigh? at the beginning of this chapter. Jaime explains that the baby also grew 2 inches. How many centimeters would this be?
2. Maria is working in the hospital and when taking vital signs, she discovers that a patient has a temperature of 37.6°C. When she checks the orders, she finds the physician has ordered Tylenol gr x to be given every four hours as needed for a temperature above 101°F. Maria notes it is 4 p.m. and the last dose was given at 1300 hours. The Tylenol tablets she has available are marked as 525 mg/tablet. She gives the patient two tablets and charts the time given as 1500.
   a. Assuming the last dose was given at 1300 hours, when would the next dose of Tylenol be due? If it is now 4 p.m., how much time has elapsed since the medication was given?
   b. Did Maria note the time correctly? If not, how is 4 p.m. expressed in military time?
   c. What would be the equivalent of 101°F in the Celsius system? Was the temperature elevated high enough to give the Tylenol as ordered?
   d. Was the correct amount of medication given? If not, was too much or too little given?

PROBLEM-SOLVING PRACTICE

Genevieve Foust has always dreamed of working in health care, but she is scared to death of taking math for Health Care Professionals next semester. She has always struggled with math and when she spoke with her parents about her fears they said, "It must be genetic as neither of us can do math either." Using the five-step problem-solving process, determine what Genevieve can do about her fear of the upcoming math course.

SUGGESTED READINGS AND RESOURCES

Kee, J. L., & Marshall, S. M. (2012). *Clinical calculations with applications to general and specialty areas* (7th ed.). Philadelphia: W. B. Saunders Company.

Simmers, L., et al. (2012). *Practical problems in math for health occupations* (3rd ed.). Clifton Park, NY: Delmar Cengage Learning.

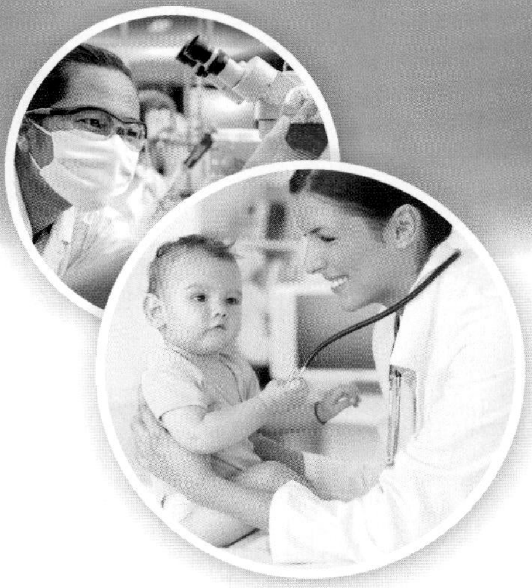

Unit 3

The Human Body

This page intentionally left blank

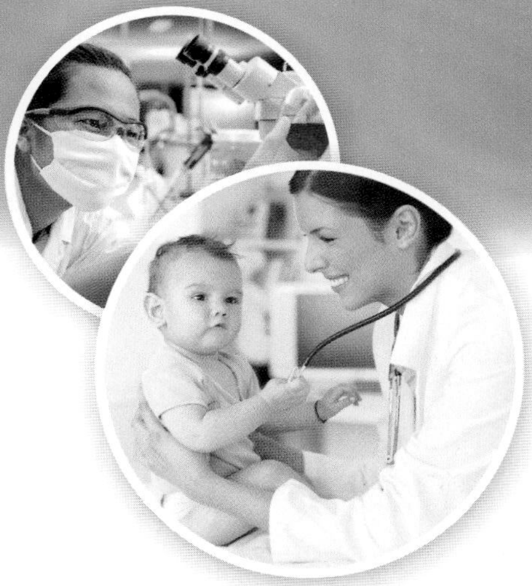

Chapter 6

Organization of the Human Body

OBJECTIVES

Studying and applying the material in this chapter will help you to:

- Explain the meaning of homeostasis.
- Name the levels in the structural organization of the body.
- Name and explain the functions of the main cellular components.
- Name and describe the four primary types of tissues.
- Describe the anatomical position.
- Identify and describe the location of the three directional body planes.
- Use directional terms to describe various locations on the body.
- Name the main body cavities and what structures are found in each.
- Identify the abdominal regions and quadrants.

KEY TERMS

abdominal cavity
anatomical position
anterior (ventral)
anterior body cavity
apex
base
body system
caudal
cell
cephalic (cranial)
cranial cavity
deep
distal
frontal plane
homeostasis
inferior
lateral
medial
midsagittal plane

(continues)

KEY TERMS (continued)

organ	posterior (dorsal)	spinal cavity	thoracic cavity
pelvic cavity	posterior body cavity	superficial	tissue
peripheral	proximal	superior	transverse plane

The Case of the Exact Location

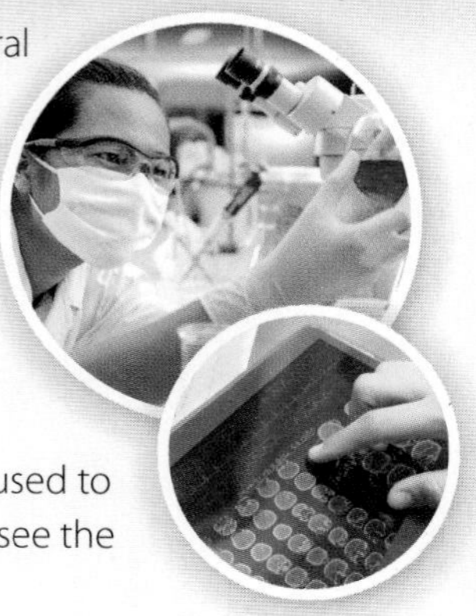

Paula Holland is seen in the urgent care center with complaints of pain in the left lower arm. Several bruises and cuts are also noted on the upper and lower areas of the same arm. Arlene Dealy is working at the center and charts: "Mrs. Holland has lower arm pain, with multiple bruises and cuts on the arm."

When the patient returns the following week because of complaints of pain in both her arms, Gary Heinz reads the notes made by Arlene and is unable to determine if the original visit was for pain in the left or right arm. He also questions how many, what size, and exactly where the bruises and cuts were located.

The material in this chapter will give the health care professional a medical language that is used to describe body locations, so other health care professionals will know where to check when they see the patient.

THE BASIS OF LIFE

The processes that maintain life are remarkable in their complexity and effectiveness. They can only be truly appreciated by studying all the structures and functions that make up the human body. Sormunen and Moisio (2009) express it well:

> Our bodies are marvelously intricate, delicate, and unique. Each part of the body has a purpose and function that fits into the total. Cells, tissues, organs, and systems are all part of the human anatomy.

The body is constantly working to keep itself in what is called a state of homeostasis. **Homeostasis** is the tendency of a cell or the whole organism to maintain a state of balance. To maintain this balance numerous tiny adjustments are made every second throughout the body. These occur without our conscious awareness.

The structural organization of the body can be described as a series of levels organized from the smallest to the largest. This text will not cover atoms, ions, and molecules. Our study will start at the smallest living structure in the body which is at the cellular level and will progress to the largest which is the human body as a whole. It can be summarized in the following order:

1. **Cells**: Smallest living structures in the body
2. **Tissues**: Cells with similar function grouped together
3. **Organs**: Two or more types of tissues combined to work together (examples: kidneys, lungs, heart, and liver)
4. **Body** (organ) **systems**: Two or more organs combined to provide a major body function (examples: respiratory, nervous, and urinary systems)
5. Human body as a whole

The human body is an amazing and complex organism. The cells themselves are complex living structures (see next section) that group together to form tissues. Different types of tissues work together to create body organs. When two or more of these body organs work together they create the major body systems that work in harmony to maintain a state of homeostasis for the human body.

The cells and tissues will be presented in this chapter, and the organs and body systems in the next. (See Figure 6–1.)

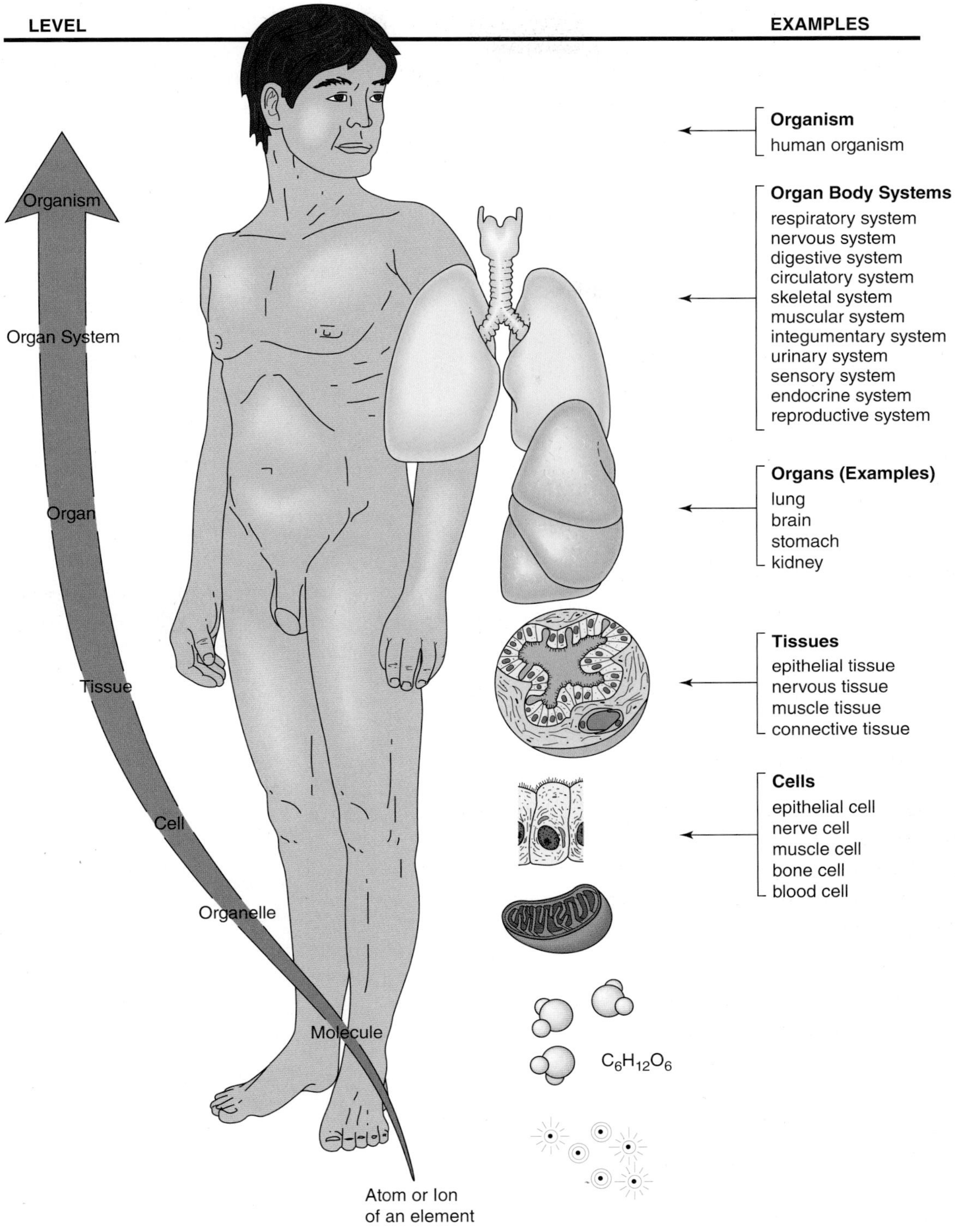

FIGURE 6–1 The structural organization of the body progresses from cells to the body as a whole.

Fascinating Facts

The largest cell in the human body is the female ovum (egg cell). The smallest cell is the male sperm. It takes about 175,000 sperm cells to equal the weight of a single egg cell.

Cells

Cells are the smallest structures that carry on all the fundamental functions of life. Many of them perform specialized functions, such as support (bone cells), communication (nerve cells), oxygen transportation (red blood cells), movement (muscle cells), and protection (skin cells). (See Figure 6–2.) Cells can reproduce, grow, and repair themselves. To perform these functions, they take in nutrients (food) and oxygen to create heat and energy. Cells can move, adapt to their environment, and eliminate waste products.

Cells generally contain the following components (Figure 6–3):

1. Cell membrane: The outer covering; it controls which substances enter and leave the cell
2. Cytoplasm (protoplasm): Gel-like liquid inside the cell that consists of water, proteins, carbohydrates, nucleic acids, lipids (fats), and salts
3. Organelles: Structures that have specialized functions
   - Nucleus: Controls the activity of the cell, reproduction; contains the 23 (normally) chromosomes that contain the genes that transmit hereditary characteristics
   - Mitochondrion: Produces energy used for cellular processes; called the "powerhouse"
   - Lysosome: Contain various enzymes that help to digest (break down) molecules
   - Ribosomes: Produce protein for the cell structures
   - Golgi apparatus: Produces, stores, and packages products for discharge from the cell (e.g., transports proteins made by the ribosomes)
   - Centrioles: Play a role in the division of the cell (reproduction)
   - Endoplasmic reticulum: Network of tubular structures to facilitate transport of materials in and out of the nucleus
   - Vesicles: Storage and transportation unit

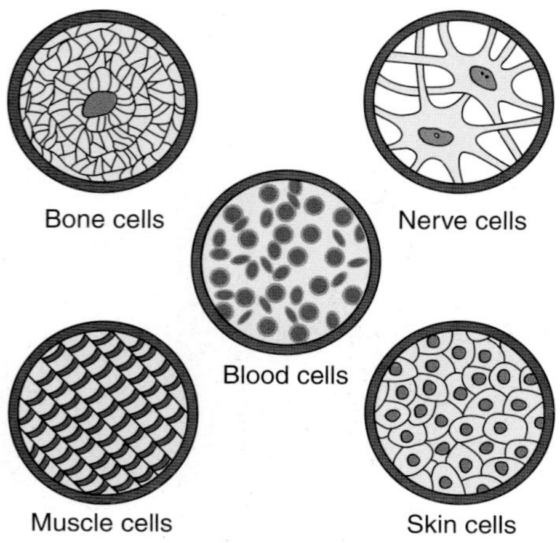

FIGURE 6–2 Cells vary in size, shape, and function.

Media Link

View the Anatomy of a Typical Cell animation on the Online Resources for a review of the components of the cell and their functions.

Tissues

Tissues are categorized into four primary types (Figure 6–4):

1. Epithelial: Covers the internal and external organs of the body; lines body cavities, vessels, glands, and body organs
2. Connective: Holds parts of the body in place; can be liquid (blood), fibrous (tendons and ligaments), solid (bone), fatty (protective padding), or cartilage (rings of the trachea)
3. Nervous: Transmits impulses throughout the body to activate, coordinate, and control many functions
4. Muscular: Contracts and relaxes to cause or allow movement; the three types are:
   - Skeletal: Attached to bone and causes movement of the skeleton
   - Smooth (visceral): Found in the walls of the hollow internal organs of the body (e.g., stomach and intestines), blood vessels, and lung airways
   - Cardiac: Makes up the muscular wall of the heart

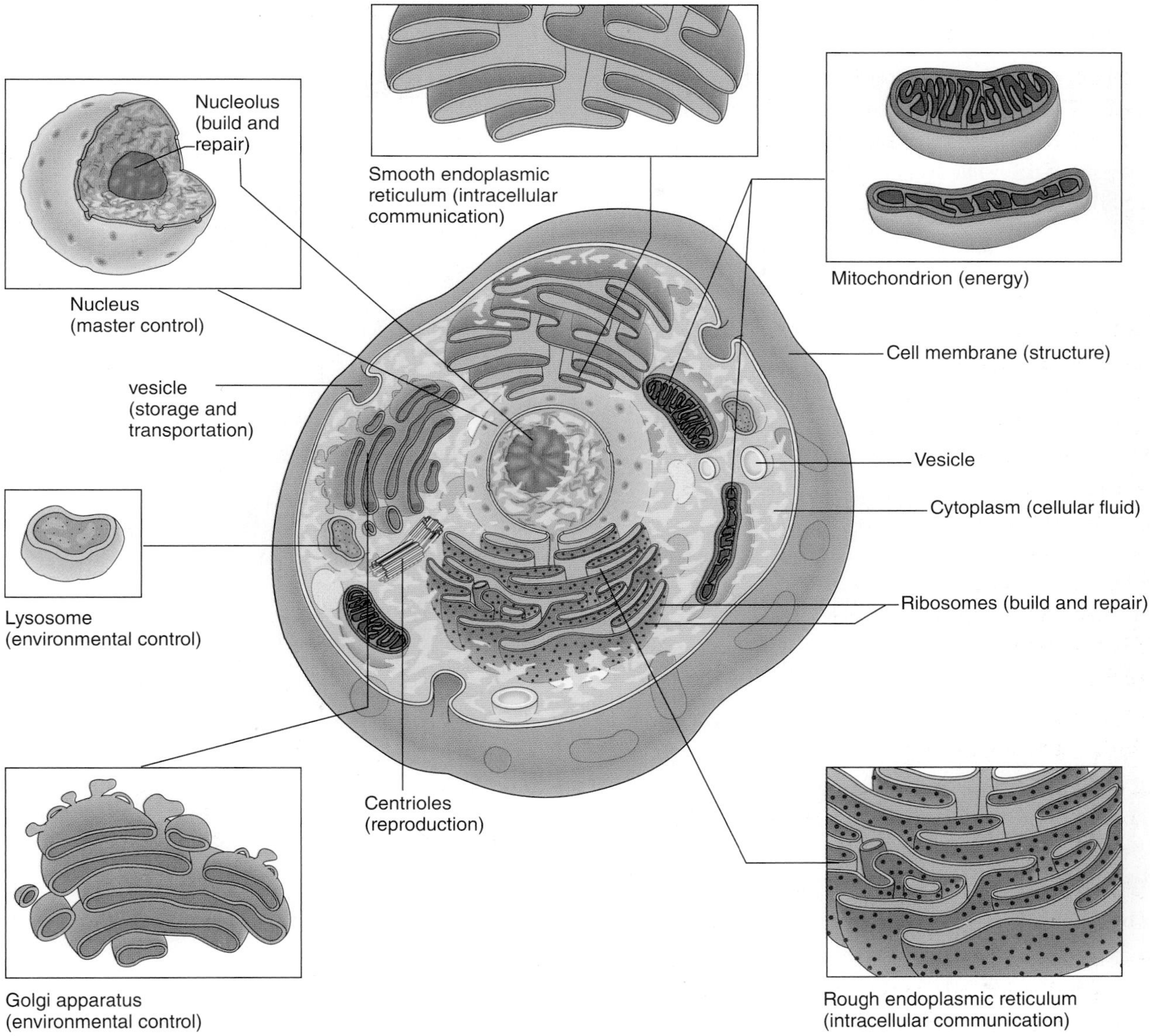

FIGURE 6–3 Major components of a typical human cell.

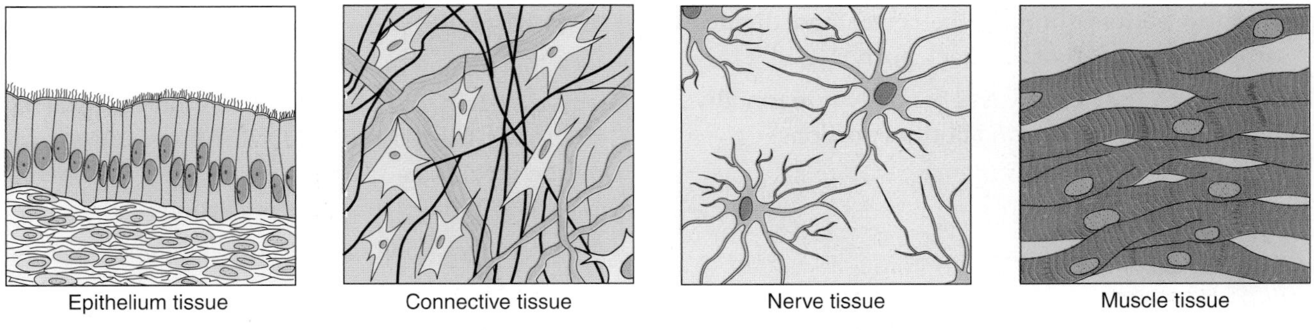

FIGURE 6–4 The four primary types of tissues found in the human body.

Fascinating Facts

There are approximately 75 trillion cells in the human body. They vary in shape and size, but most are microscopic and range from 1/3 to 1/13 the size of the period at the end of this sentence. Every human spent about half an hour as a single cell.

DESCRIBING THE BODY

Health care professionals need a language to use when speaking or writing about a particular location of a structure or area of the body. This language and special vocabulary describe body planes, directional terms, body cavities, and abdominal regions.

A mastery of these terms will allow you to accurately interpret descriptions written by other personnel and also to chart (document in writing) your findings in a way that others can understand.

The descriptive terms refer to the body as viewed in a full upright position (standing), with the arms relaxed at the side of the body, palms facing forward, feet pointed forward, and eyes directed straight ahead. This is called the **anatomical position**. (See Figure 6–5.)

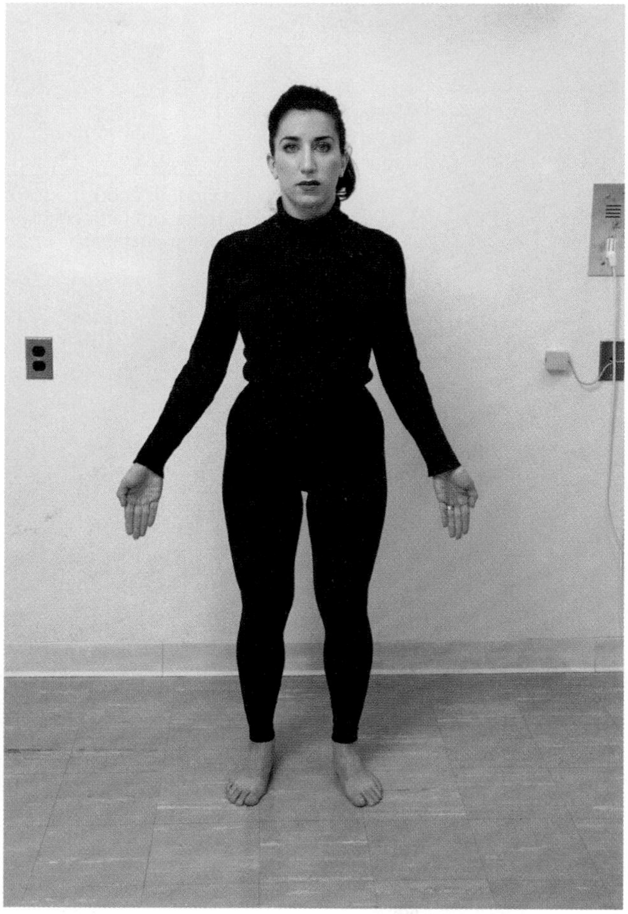

FIGURE 6–5 The anatomical position.

Body Planes

A body plane is an imaginary flat surface that cuts through the body either horizontally or vertically. Imagine the body divided up by a large pane of window glass. There are three primary planes (Figures 6–6a and 6–6b):

1. **Midsagittal** (median or midline) **plane**: Passes from top to bottom through the center of the body and divides it into equal right and left sides
2. **Frontal plane** (coronal): Divides the body from top to bottom through the center and divides the body into front and back portions
3. **Transverse plane**: Divides the body horizontally (crosswise) into top and bottom portions

Media Link

View the Body Planes animation on the Online Resources for a review of these terms.

Directional Terms

Using east, west, north, and south works well for traditional directions, but would be of no value when referring to the body. Directional terms for medical descriptions were created to solve this problem and are listed in Table 6–1. Also refer to Figures 6–6a and 6–6b.

The Body Cavities

Within the body there are interior spaces called cavities that contain and protect the internal organs. (See Figure 6–7.) The **posterior** (dorsal) **body cavity** protects the structures of the nervous system and has two parts (although the space is continuous):

1. **Cranial cavity**: Located in the skull and contains the brain
2. **Spinal cavity**: Located within the spinal column and contains the spinal cord

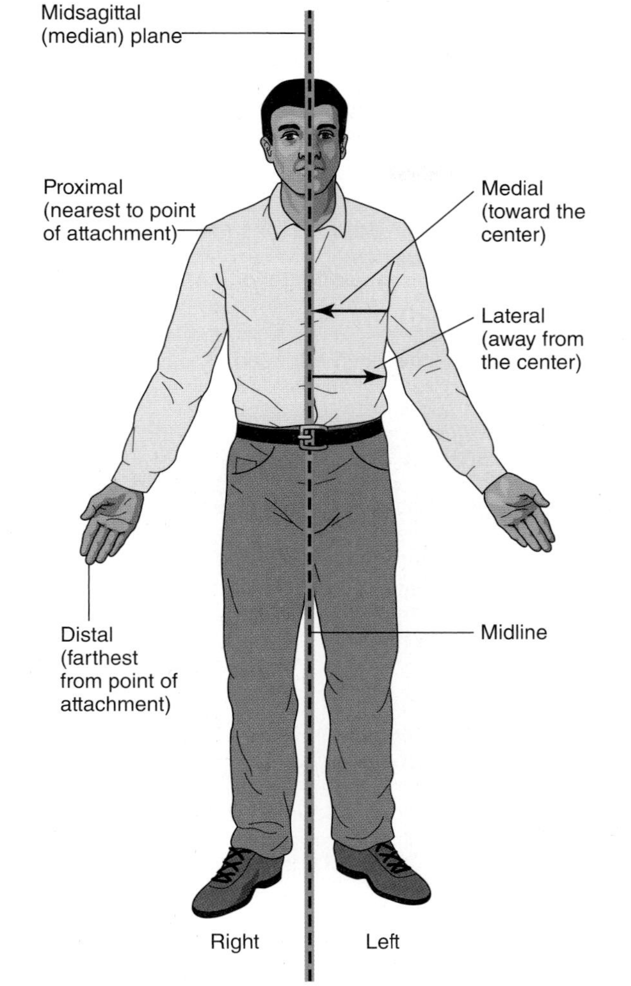

FIGURE 6–6a Sagittal plane. The midsagittal (median or midline) plane divides the body from top to bottom into equal left and right halves.

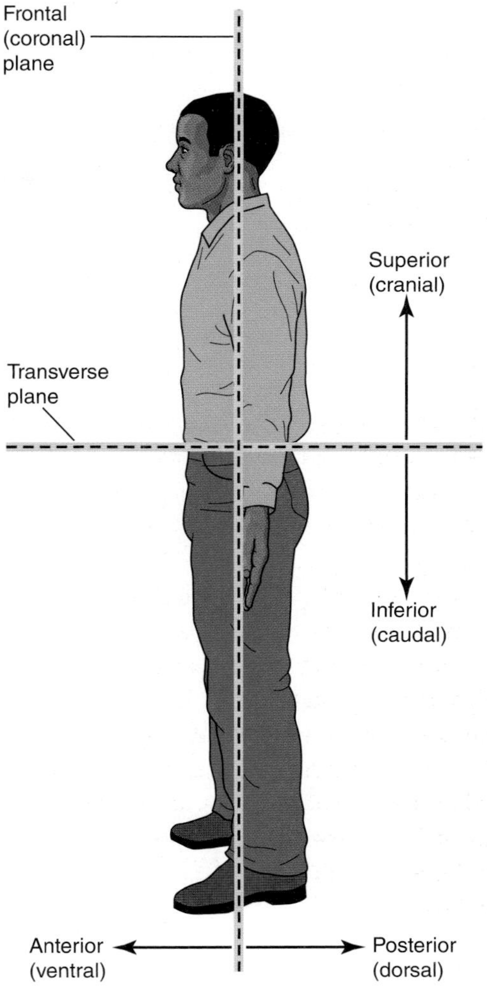

FIGURE 6–6b Frontal and transverse planes. The frontal (coronal) plane divides the body into front (anterior) and back (posterior) portions. It is located at right angles to the sagittal plane. The transverse plane divides the body horizontally into top (superior) and bottom (inferior) portions. This division can be at the waist or any other level across the body.

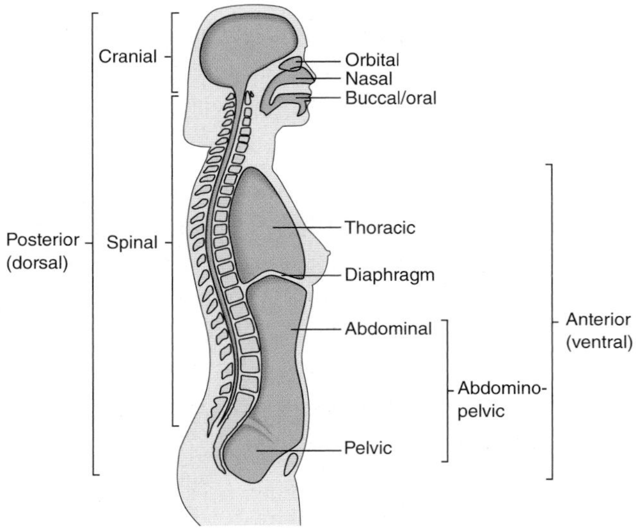

FIGURE 6–7 Cavities of the body.

Table 6–1 Directional Terms

Term	Meaning	Example
Lateral	Away from center of body (toward the sides)	The lateral ligament of the knee is located on the outer side of the knee.
Medial	Toward midline or center of body	The navel is on the medial line.
Anterior (ventral)	Toward the front of body	The breasts are on the anterior surface of the body.
Posterior (dorsal)	Toward the back of the body	The buttocks are on the posterior surface of the body.
Inferior	Below	The lungs are inferior to the head.
Superior	Above	The nose is superior to the mouth.
Caudal	Closer to the coccyx (lower back)	The hips are caudal to the waist.
Cephalic (cranial)	Closer to the head	The neck is cephalic to the shoulders.
Deep	Farther from the body surface	The accident victim had a deep laceration (wound or irregular tear) that exposed the muscle.
Superficial	Near or close to the body surface	There were only superficial scrapes on the skin.
Distal	Farther from the reference base point	The hand is distal to the elbow.
Peripheral	Away from the center	The patient had peripheral edema (excess fluid in the extremities—arms and legs).
Proximal	Closer to the reference point	The shoulder is proximal to the elbow.
Apex	At the top (highest point)	The top of the lung is called the apex.
Base	At the bottom (lowest point)	The bottom of the lung is called the base.

Source: Adapted from Essentials of Anatomy and Physiology *(4th ed.) by F. H. Martini & E. F. Bartholomew, 2008, San Francisco, CA: Benjamin Cummings Publishing.*

The **anterior** (ventral) **body cavity** protects the internal organs and has three parts:

1. **Thoracic cavity**: Located in the chest and contains the heart, lungs, and major blood vessels; the diaphragm separates this cavity from the abdominal cavity
2. **Abdominal cavity**: Located in the abdomen and contains the stomach, intestines, liver, gallbladder, pancreas, and spleen (the kidneys are located behind the abdominal cavity); the abdominal and pelvic cavities are continuous
3. **Pelvic cavity**: Located in the lower abdomen and contains the urinary bladder, rectum, and reproductive organs

Smaller cavities include the orbital, which contains the eyes and associated muscles, nerves, and ducts; the nasal, which contains the structures of the nose; and the buccal, which contains the teeth and tongue.

Abdominal Descriptions

The abdominal area is so large that it has been divided into nine regions so that specific areas can be described with greater accuracy. The nine regions include the lower portion of the thoracic cavity and the abdominal and pelvic cavities. (See Figure 6–8.)

These regions are:

- Epigastric ("over the stomach"): Located just below the sternum (breastbone)
- Right and left hypochondriac regions: Located below the ribs on either side of the epigastric region
- Umbilical: Located around the umbilicus (navel)
- Right and left lumbar regions: Extend anterior to posterior on either side of the umbilical region (a person will complain of lumbar or back pain)
- Hypogastric ("below the stomach"): Located over the pubic area

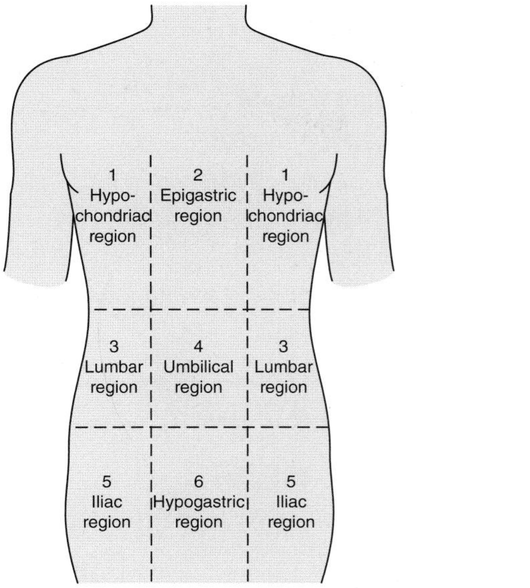

FIGURE 6–8 Regions of the lower thorax, abdominal, and pelvic cavities.

- Right and left iliac (hip bone) regions: Located on either side of the hypogastric region (also called right and left inguinal areas)

Another approach used in health care for describing the abdomen divides the region into quadrants. Imaginary lines are used to create four quadrants (Figure 6–9) that divide the abdominal area. All the

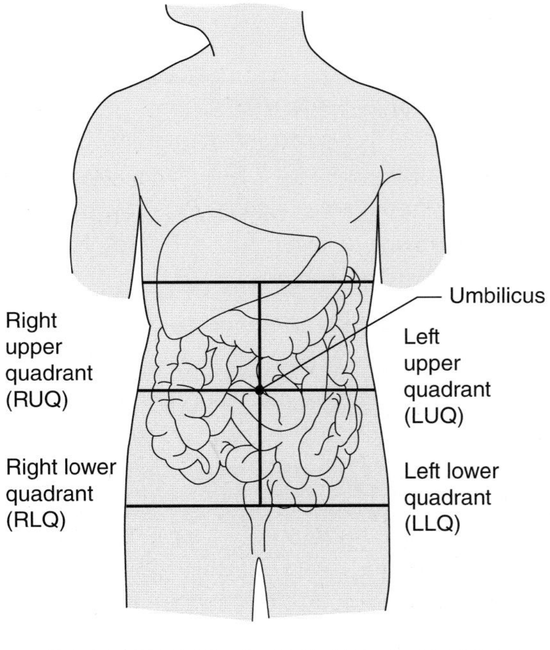

FIGURE 6–9 The abdomen divided into quadrants.

Thinking It Through

A patient arrives at the urgent care center to be seen for a recent laceration (cut) of the arm. Miss Heather Jones, a health care professional at the clinic, examines the arm and describes the injury as to size and location.

1. Examine the diagram below to visualize what Miss Jones observed.
2. Describe the size and location of the injury.

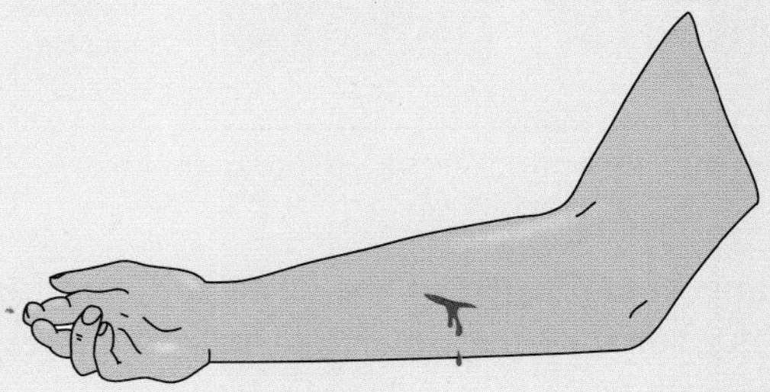

Thinking It Through

Esteban Valdez is a patient on a medical-surgical floor of a community hospital. He is experiencing some discomfort in the right buttock area and reports it to Martha Duarte, a licensed vocational (practical) nurse. The patient points to the area of discomfort, and Martha can see a small red dot but no other abnormalities. Martha notes that the location identified by the patient is on the upper lateral side of the right buttock and inferior to the waist. She thinks it may be tenderness due to a recent injection (shot) that was given to the patient and checks the medication record. The record shows that Mr. Valdez had an injection into the RUOQ (right upper outer quadrant) of the buttock.

1. RUQ, RLQ, LUQ, and LLQ do not apply only to the abdomen, but can be used to divide any area into four equal parts (See Figure 6–10). When giving an injection into the buttocks, the only correct sites would be into the upper outer quadrant of either buttock. Based on the description given, where was the small red dot located?
2. Do you agree with Martha's conclusion?

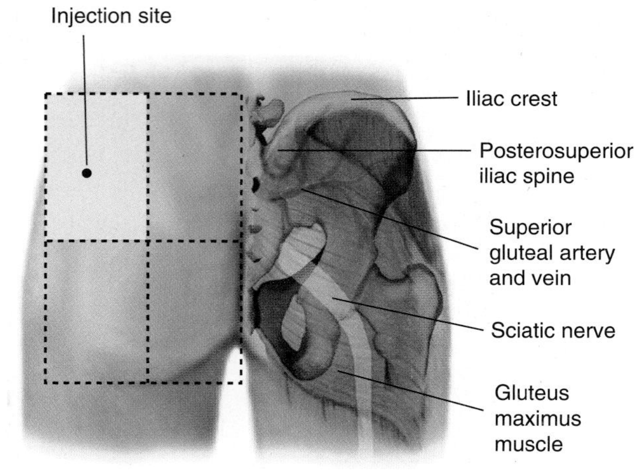

FIGURE 6–10 The buttocks divided into quadrants.

quadrants contain part of the large and small intestines, but some of the other internal organs can be identified within a particular quadrant.

1. Right upper quadrant (RUQ): Liver and gallbladder
2. Right lower quadrant (RLQ): Appendix and some of the female reproductive organs
3. Left upper quadrant (LUQ): Pancreas, stomach, and spleen
4. Left lower quadrant (LLQ): Some of the female reproductive organs

WORKBOOK PRACTICE

Go to your workbook and complete the exercises for this chapter.

SUGGESTED LEARNING ACTIVITIES

1. Draw and label the structures of the cell from memory.
2. Stand in front of a mirror in the anatomical position and visualize the midsagittal, frontal, and transverse planes of the body.
3. Point to any area of your body and describe its position using the directional terms.
4. Stand in front of a mirror and identify the abdominal regions and quadrants.

WEB ACTIVITIES

Seer's Training Website

www.training.seer.cancer.gov/

Do a search on "anatomical terminology." List the body cavities and which organs are located in each one. Also click on "Directional Terms" and "Planes of the Body" to review these topics.

REVIEW QUESTIONS

1. What is homeostasis?
2. What are the levels in the structural organization of the body?
3. What are the components of the cell, and what are their functions?
4. What are the four primary types of tissues?
5. What is the anatomical position?
6. What are the three body planes and how do they divide the body?
7. What are the main directional terms used for medical descriptions?
8. What are the primary body cavities and what structures are in each one?
9. What are the two methods used for describing the abdominal area?

APPLICATION EXERCISES

1. Refer to The Case of the Exact Location. If Arlene had used anatomical descriptions to identify Mrs. Holland's site of original pain, bruises, and cuts, what words would she have used?
2. A patient comes into the physician's office complaining of a lot of abdominal pain. You ask her to show you where the pain is located. She points to an area between her breasts and to another area to the right of the pelvic area. You then leave to report your findings to the physician.
   a. What abdominal descriptor would you use to describe the first location?
   b. What abdominal descriptor would you use to describe the second location?

PROBLEM-SOLVING PRACTICE

Moses Johnson is taking a course titled Introduction to Health Care. He has been studying hard and really pushing himself to learn each chapter completely. His goal is to get 100% on his tests and he has met this goal thus far. But when he starts to study the body planes, he finds himself feeling angry and discouraged. He cannot understand why top/bottom, back/front, and right side/left side cannot be used instead of learning more new terms that mean nothing to him. Every time he tries to memorize the new terms, he gets frustrated and continually confuses them. He fears he will not get them right on the upcoming exam. Using the five-step problem-solving process, determine what Moses can do about his problem.

SUGGESTED READINGS AND RESOURCES

Ehrlich, A. (2013). *Medical terminology for health professions* (7th ed.). Clifton Park, NY: Delmar Cengage Learning.

Scott, A. S., & Fong, E. (2014). *Body structures and functions* (12th ed.). Clifton Park, NY: Delmar Cengage Learning.

This page intentionally left blank

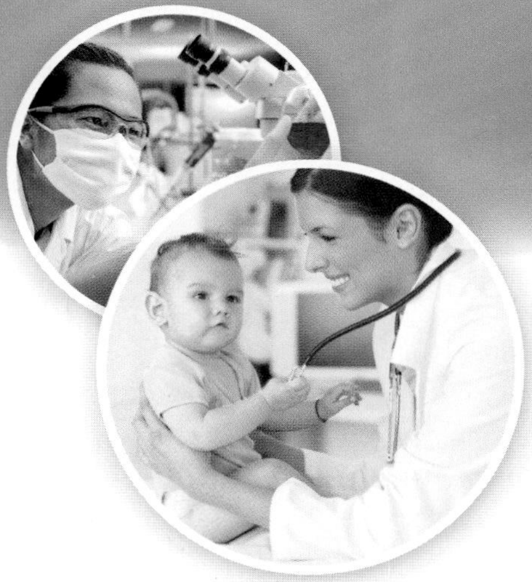

Chapter 7

Structure and Function of the Human Body

OBJECTIVES

Studying and applying the material in this chapter will help you to:

- Understand and explain the difference between anatomy, physiology, and pathophysiology.
- Define what determines a state of wellness as opposed to illness.
- Describe the primary anatomical features and physiological actions of the systems for movement and protection of the body.
- Name and demonstrate the movements made possible by joints.
- Describe the primary anatomical features and physiological actions of the systems for providing energy and for removing waste from the body.
- Describe the primary anatomical features and physiological actions of the systems for sensing and for coordinating and controlling the body.
- Describe the primary anatomical features and physiological actions of the systems for producing new life.
- Name common diseases or disorders associated with each system.
- Describe the behaviors and actions for each body system that promote health and prevent major diseases and disorders.

KEY TERMS

anatomy
diagnosis
diagnostic procedures
diseases
etiology
illness
objective
pathophysiology
physiology
prevention (of disease)
prognosis
signs and symptoms
subjective
syndrome
treatment

The Case of the Unfamiliar Diagnosis

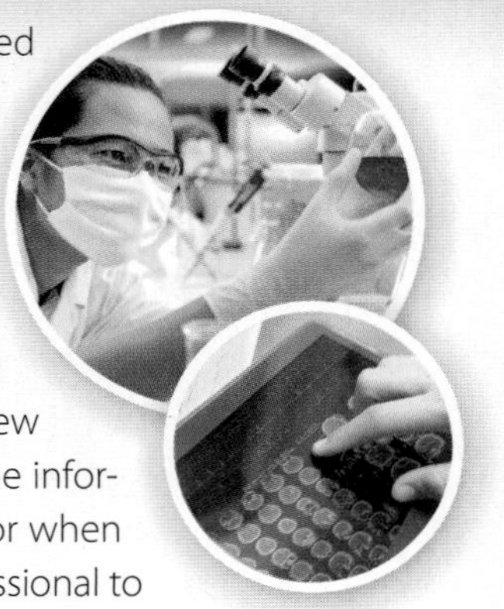

Janet Waring is an X-ray technician who works in a large medical center. Mr. Petersen is admitted with a diagnosis of red cedar disease, and a lung X-ray is ordered. Janet has never heard of this disease and decides to do some independent research. The reference she uses explains why and how this disease damages the lungs, what to watch for when caring for the patient, and what tests may be ordered. By understanding how to properly use reference materials, Janet is able to learn that this condition is a type of occupational asthma and can occur in loggers and sawmill workers when a high concentration of sawdust is inhaled, causing damage to the lungs. Janet knows the normal structure and function of the lungs and can now apply this new knowledge to determine what consequences the damaged lungs may have for her patient. The information she has accessed also clarifies why the chest X-ray was ordered and what to observe for when caring for the patient. Understanding the material in this chapter will assist the health care professional to understand the normal structure and function of the body.

THE IMPORTANCE OF ANATOMY AND PHYSIOLOGY

Many health care programs include a more in-depth study of anatomy and physiology than will be presented in this chapter. For those students with no prior study of anatomy and physiology, this material will serve as an introduction to the subject. For other students, it will serve as a review.

The study of anatomy and physiology (A&P) is fundamental to understanding the normal structure and function of the body. **Anatomy** is the study of the *form and structure* of an organism, such as the names and locations of the bones, muscles, and organs. **Physiology** is the study of the *functions* (how and why something works) of these structures. Examples include how bones and muscles produce movement, how organs assist in digestion, and how nerve impulses from the brain trigger the eyelids to blink.

The structure of the various body parts dictates the function of the body, thus understanding the normal structure and function of the body provides a base to help the health care professional recognize abnormal conditions. These abnormal conditions are called **diseases**. When an abnormality occurs it is referred to as a pathophysiological finding (*patho* means disease). **Pathophysiology** is the study of why diseases occur and how the body changes its function in reaction to the diseases. When studying pathophysiology, several other terms are used to provide a complete description of the disease process and related information. These terms are:

- **Etiology**: Study of the causes of diseases. Diseases have a variety of causes. Examples include bacteria, viruses, hazardous materials, and personal habits.
- **Signs and symptoms**: Signs and symptoms (S/S) are usually used as one phrase, but actually have separate meanings. Signs are **objective** evidence of an illness. This means that the health care professional can observe them. Signs include patient behaviors, visible marks on the body, and test results. Symptoms are **subjective**. They cannot be directly observed by the health care professional, but are reported by the patient. For example, a patient may report pain (subjective data), which cannot be observed directly. However, a behavior (objective data) such as a facial grimace or limp could be present that is an indication of pain. Another example is a patient who states that he has hypertension. This is subjective data and must be verified by taking the blood pressure to obtain objective data. Signs and symptoms serve as clues to the nature of underlying diseases or **syndromes** (not a precise disease, but a group of related signs and symptoms).
- **Diagnostic procedures**: Tests performed to determine the **diagnosis** (determination of a disease or syndrome). To arrive at a diagnosis, the signs and symptoms are evaluated by taking a thorough patient history, doing a physical exam, and ordering laboratory tests, X-rays, or other special tests. An accurate diagnosis is necessary

to determine the correct treatment and predict the outcome of the problem.

- **Treatment**: Medications or procedures used to control or cure the disease. Common treatments include surgery, exercise, and special diets.
- **Prognosis**: Prediction of the possible outcome of the disease and potential for recovery.
- **Prevention**: Behaviors that promote health and prevent diseases.

The state of wellness or illness of individuals is directly related to their body structure (anatomy), function (physiology), and underlying disease processes (pathophysiology). A state of wellness is experienced when the body maintains homeostasis. As explained in Chapter 6, homeostasis is the tendency of a cell or the whole organism to maintain a state of balance. A state of **illness** occurs when one or more of the body's control systems lose the ability to maintain homeostasis. All the cells of the body suffer when this occurs. A moderate dysfunction causes illness, and a severe dysfunction can lead to death.

There is an increasing focus on preventive measures as researchers learn more about the causes of diseases and injuries. Prevention is organized into three levels:

1. Primary: Prevent the initial occurrence of the disease or injury by maintaining homeostasis. Practicing good lifestyle habits (Chapter 12) and avoiding exposure to bacteria and viruses (Chapter 10) are examples of preventive measures.
2. Secondary: Treat conditions that do occur as quickly as possible to prevent further damage.
3. Tertiary: Rehabilitate to allow the person to regain as much function as possible and prevent further disability.

GENETICS

Genetics was previously discussed in Chapter 2 in relationship to research trends, and in Chapter 3 in regard to the ethical component. Genetics determines one's inherited characteristics, such as eye and hair color, height, and skin tone. The focus in this chapter is related to the impact of genetics on medical disorders that can be passed from parent to child. These inherited conditions can affect any of the body systems and are too numerous to include in this text. In the Web Activities section at the end of the chapter, a website is listed that describes various inherited conditions of each body system. A review of this site will provide an awareness of the prevalence of these conditions and the impact of disorders related to heredity.

> **Fascinating Facts**
>
> The adult human body on average contains enough iron to make a 3-inch nail, carbon to make 900 pencils, fat to make 7 bars of soap, phosphorous to make 2200 match heads, and water to fill a 10-gallon tank.

THE SYSTEMS OF THE BODY

Chapter 6 included a discussion about the function of cells and how cells that perform a similar function group together to form tissues. Recall that when two or more of the four primary types of tissues (epithelial, connective, nervous, and muscular) combine to work together, they form organs. When two or more organs combine to perform a major body function, it is called a body system. Examples of body systems include respiratory, nervous, and urinary. Review Table 7–1 for an overview of the organ systems covered in this chapter.

The systems work together in a very complex manner to maintain the body in a state of homeostasis or wellness. They are all interrelated and changes in one will affect others. A good practice when studying each system is to ask, "How does the function of this system affect all the other systems?" Some systems have a wide range of functions, and there are organs that actually belong to several systems and have more than one role.

Systems for Movement and Protection

The skeletal, muscular, and integumentary (skin) systems provide support, allow movement, and protect the body. Without bones and muscles, the body would be like an empty sack of skin without shape or the ability to move. The skin plays a critical role because it protects the body from hazards, prevents fluid loss, and helps control temperature.

Skeletal

The *skeletal system* is composed of the bones that provide a framework that:

- Gives shape to the body
- Provides places to which muscles can attach to produce movement
- Protects the internal organs
- Stores minerals
- Manufactures blood cells

Table 7–1 Organ Systems of the Body

	Organ Systems	Major Functions
Systems for Movement and Protection		
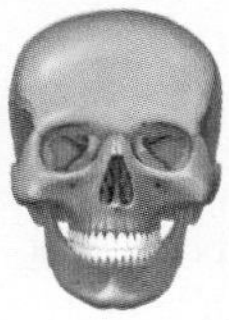	Skeletal	• Provide framework to support muscles, fat, soft tissues, and skin • Furnish locations for attachment of skeletal muscles • Protect internal organs • Store minerals • Help in the formation of red and white blood cells
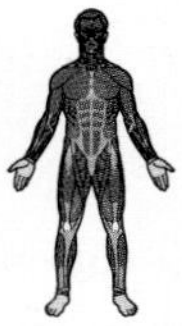	Muscular	• Enable locomotion (movement) • Give support to the body • Produce heat
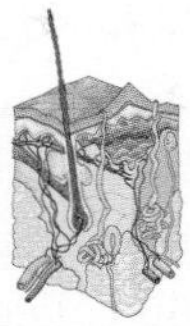	Integumentary	• Protect from environmental hazards • Control temperature
Systems for Providing Energy and Removing Waste		
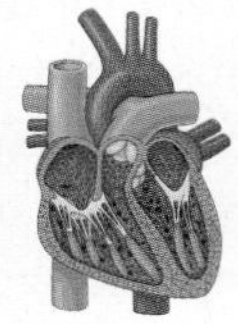	Circulatory (cardiovascular and lymphatic)	• Transport cells and dissolved materials, including nutrients, wastes, and gases • Provide defense against infection and disease • Maintain fluid balance • Remove waste products
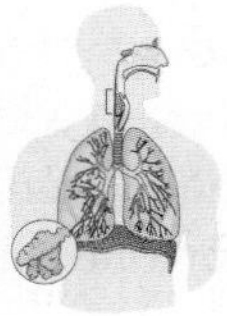	Respiratory (pulmonary)	• Deliver gases to sites where gas exchange occurs
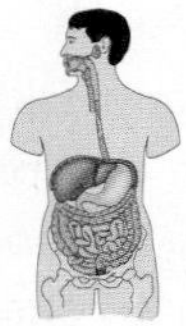	Digestive (gastrointestinal)	• Process food and absorb nutrients, minerals, vitamins, and water • Eliminate undigested food from the body
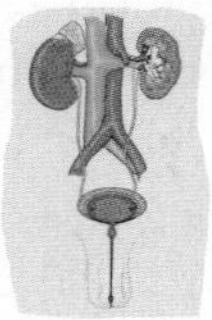	Urinary	• Eliminate excess water, salts, and waste products
Systems for Sensing, Coordinating, and Controlling		

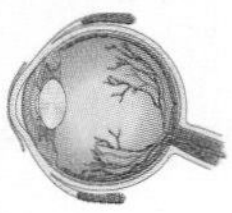	Sensory (eyes, ears)	• Collect visual and auditory information; note that the organs for the other three senses are covered in other systems:
		  • Smell (olfactory)—nose, discussed in respiratory
		  • Taste (gustatory)—tongue, discussed in digestive
		  • Touch—skin, discussed in integumentary

(continues)

Table 7–1 Organ Systems of the Body (continued)

	Organ Systems	Major Functions
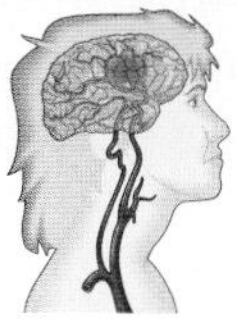	Nervous	• Direct immediate responses to stimuli, usually by coordinating the activities of other organ systems
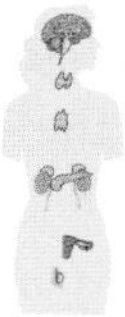	Endocrine	• Direct changes in the activities of other organ systems
Systems for Producing New Life		
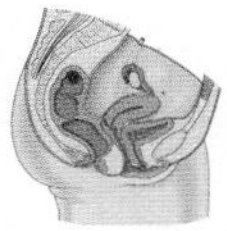	Female reproductive	• Produce sex cells and hormones necessary for female characteristics to develop and for pregnancy, delivery, and breastfeeding to occur
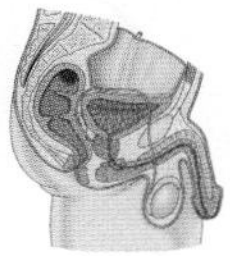	Male reproductive	• Produce sex cells and hormones necessary for male characteristics to develop and for production of semen for impregnation of female

Source: Adapted from Essentials of Anatomy and Physiology *(5th ed.), by F. H. Martini & E. F. Bartholomew, 2009, San Francisco, CA: Benjamin Cummings.*

Newborns have 270 bones. But as children grow, some of the bones fuse together, so adults have only about 206 bones. (The number of bones in the hands and feet can vary among individuals.)

Bones vary in shape and are classified as follows (Figure 7–1):

- Long bones: Longer than they are wide (arms: humerus, radius, ulna; legs: femur, tibia, fibula; fingers and toes: metacarpals, metatarsals, phalanges)
- Short bones: Similar in length and width (bones of the wrist and ankles, which are called carpals and tarsals, respectively)
- Flat bones: Two layers with space between them (cranium, ribs, shoulder blade [scapula], breastbone [sternum], pelvis)
- Irregular bones: Those that do not fit into the other categories (spinal column [vertebrae], facial bones, patella)

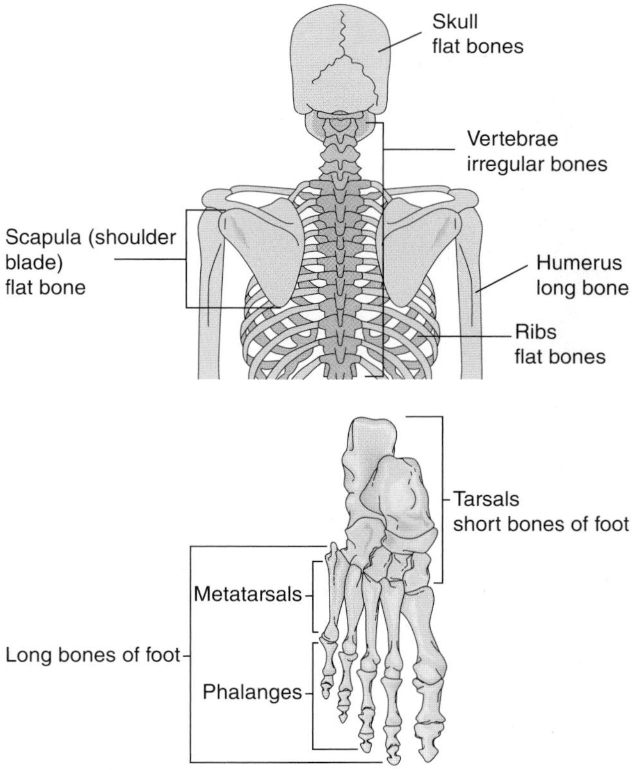

FIGURE 7–1 Bone shapes.

Bone Structure

It may be difficult to think of bones as organs, but they take in nutrients and oxygen and perform functions just like other organs. Bones do not consist of solid material, but contain layers that have different functions. The long bones have the following structure (Figure 7–2):

- Medullary cavity (canal): Center cavity containing *yellow marrow* (primarily fat cells); covered by a layer called *endosteum*
- Diaphysis: Portion that runs between the ends of the bone; also called the "shaft"
- Epiphyses: Ends of bone (proximal and distal)
- Periosteum: White, fibrous layer that covers the outside of bone; contains blood, lymph vessels, and nerves. Bone growth, repair, and nutrition occur in the periosteum. It also serves as an attachment for muscles, tendons, and ligaments.

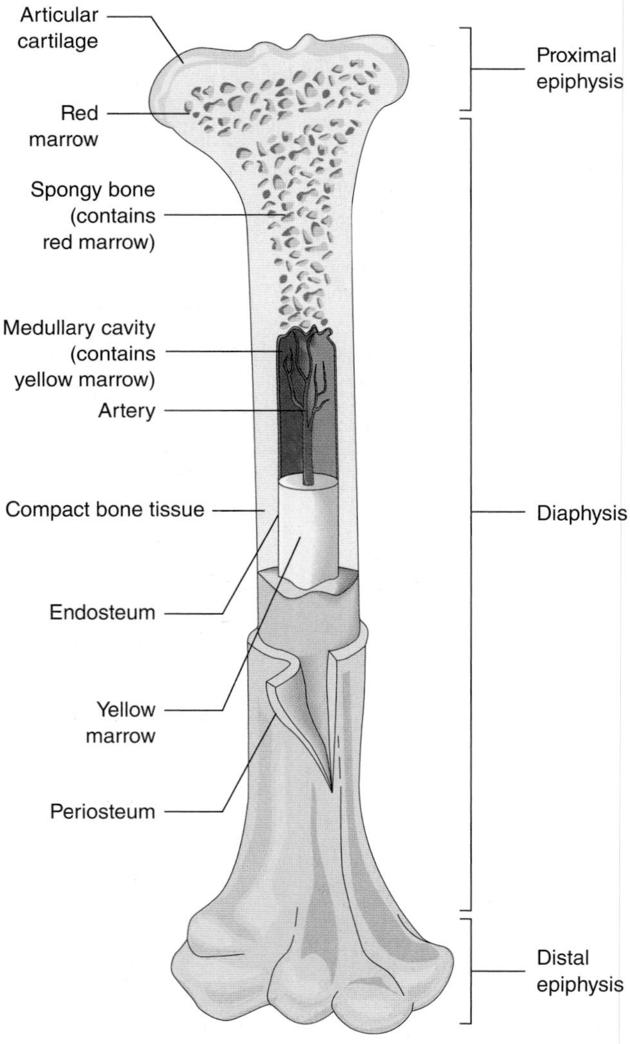

FIGURE 7–2 Structures of a long bone.

- Red marrow: Manufactures the red blood cells (RBCs), which carry oxygen, and the white blood cells (WBCs), which protect the body from infections. Red bone marrow is also found in other types of bones such as ribs (flat) and vertebrae (irregular).
- Cartilage: Elastic connective tissue that covers the end of the bones and functions as a cushion between bones. Cartilage also covers the surface of joints and forms the flexible parts of the skeleton, such as the ear lobes and the tip of the nose.

The skeletal system is divided into two major parts, known as the axial and the appendicular skeletons. The *axial skeleton* includes the bones of the:

- Skull
- Inner ear
- Hyoid (U-shaped bone lying at base of tongue)
- Spinal column
- Ribs
- Sternum (breastbone)

The *appendicular skeleton* includes the bones of the:

- Shoulders
- Arms
- Hands
- Pelvis
- Legs
- Feet

See Figure 7–3.

The 206 bones in the adult can be divided as follows into those of the axial skeleton and the appendicular skeleton.

Axial skeleton:

- Head: 29 bones (22 in the cranium, 3 in each inner ear, and 1 hyoid)
- Trunk: 51 bones (26 vertebrae in spine, 24 ribs, and 1 sternum)

Appendicular skeleton:

- Upper extremities: 64 bones in shoulders, arms, wrists, and hands
- Lower extremities: 62 bones in pelvis, legs, ankle, and feet

The Axial Skeleton

The *cranium* is composed of the skull and facial bones. (See Figure 7–4.) The skull may feel smooth to the

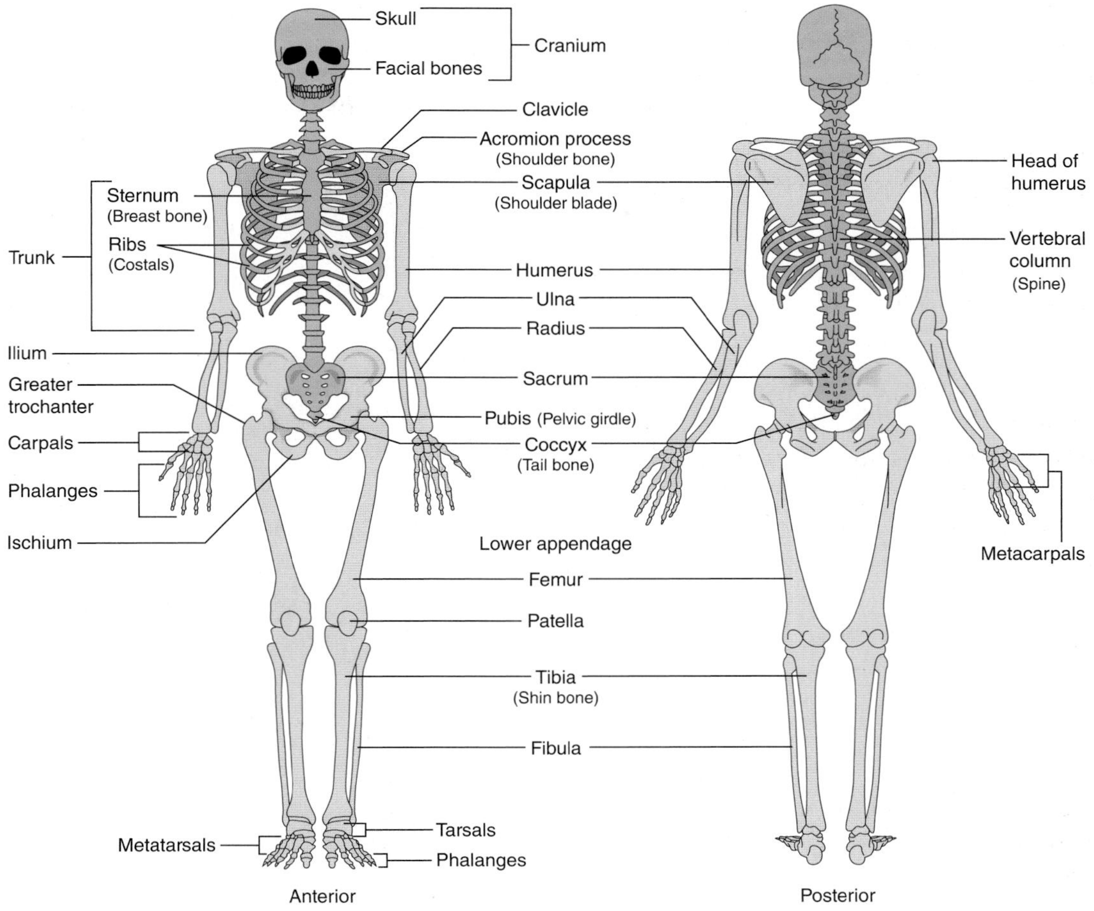

FIGURE 7–3 Bones of the skeleton (axial in blue, appendicular in tan).

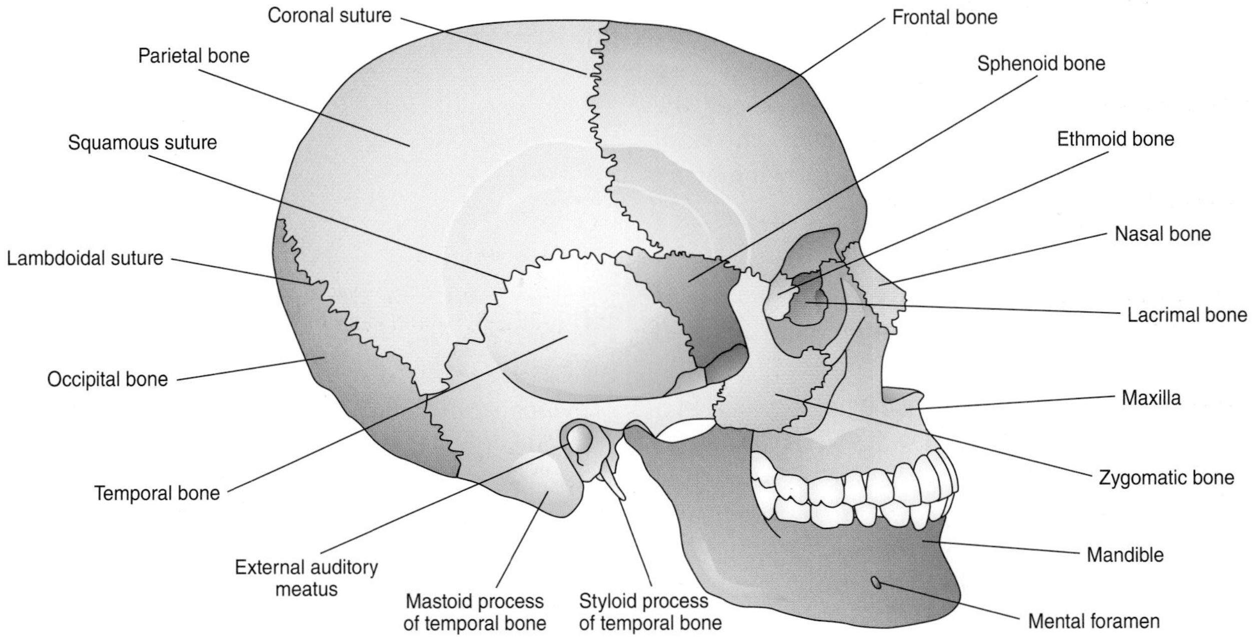

FIGURE 7–4 Bones of the cranium (skull and facial bones).

touch like one continuous bone, but it actually consists of eight bones:

- Temporal (2): Shapes the area around the ears
- Occipital (1): Shapes the base and back of the head
- Parietal (2): Shapes the top and sides of the head
- Frontal (1): Shapes the forehead
- Sphenoid (1): "Bat-shaped" bone that forms part of the cranial floor that acts as a bridge between the cranial and facial bones, and braces the sides of the skull
- Ethmoid (1): Located between the eyes and anterior to the sphenoid bone that forms part of the cranial floor, medial surface of the orbit of eyes, and the roof and sides of the nasal cavity.

The face consists of 14 bones:

- Nasal (5): Shapes the nose
- Lacrimal (2): Located in the inner corner of the eye (tear duct)
- Maxilla (2): Shapes the upper jaw
- Zygomatic (2): Shapes the cheeks
- Mandible (1): Shapes the lower jaw (only movable bone in the face)
- Palatine (2): Shapes the hard palate of the mouth

Other structures that are related to the cranium include:

- Suture lines: Areas where the cranial bones have joined together (e.g., lambdoidal, squamous, and coronal). This joining does not occur until after birth, usually by the end of the second year. During this period of rapid development, the "soft spots," called fontanelles, allow the skull to expand and accommodate the growing brain.
- Sinus: Air cavity within a bone that acts as a resonating chamber for voice quality.
- Foramina: An opening in the bone for blood vessels and nerves to pass through (e.g., mental foramen).

The spinal column consists of 26 *vertebrae* that serve to protect the spinal cord, support the head, and give shape to the back. The vertebrae are separated from each other and cushioned by *intervertebral disks* that are made of cartilage. (See Figure 7–5.)

Twelve pairs of *ribs* give shape to the chest wall and protect the internal organs. The first seven pairs of ribs are called "true ribs" because they attach to the sternum (breastbone) in the front of the body. The next five pairs are called "false ribs." The first three pairs of false ribs attach to the cartilage of the rib above. The last two pairs are called "floating ribs" because they do not attach to the front of the body. The small piece of cartilage at the bottom edge of the sternum is called the *xiphoid process*. Health care professionals become very familiar with the xiphoid process when they learn to perform cardiopulmonary resuscitation (CPR).

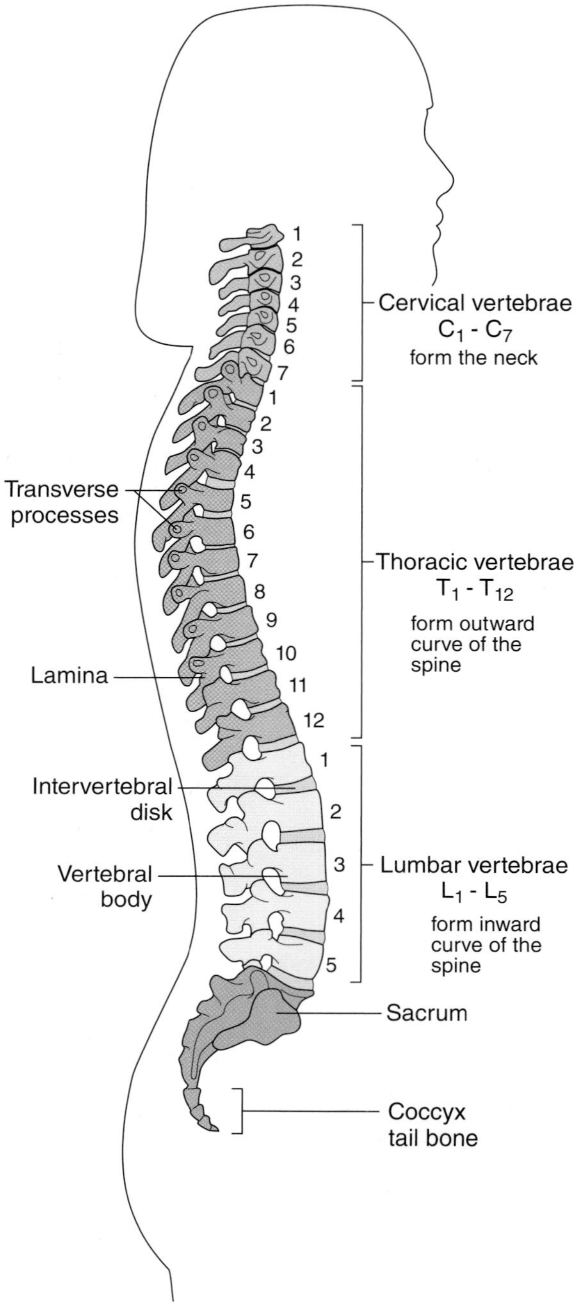

FIGURE 7–5 Lateral view of the spinal column.

Appendicular Skeleton

The upper extremities include the shoulder girdle, arms, wrists, and hands:

- Shoulder girdle: Two curved *clavicles* (shoulder bones) and the two triangular *scapulae* (shoulder blades).
- Arm: Long bone of the upper arm is the *humerus*, which is connected to the scapula by muscles and ligaments. The two long bones of the forearm are the *radius* (runs up thumb side) and *ulna* (proximal end forms the elbow that connects to the humerus).
- Wrist and hand: Eight bones in the wrist (*carpals*) form two rows of bones. The hands have five *metacarpal* bones (palm), and the five fingers have 14 *phalanges* (each finger has three except for the thumb, which has two). The hand, with its many bones, is truly an engineering marvel.

The lower extremities include the pelvic (hip) girdle, legs, ankles, and feet:

- Pelvic girdle: Serves as an area of attachment for the leg and to protect the internal organs of the lower abdomen. The girdle starts out as three bones (*ilium, ischium, and pubis*), which allows for growth. In adulthood these fuse to form the girdle. The bones fuse on the posterior side with the sacrum and in front by forming the *symphysis pubis*. The pelvis and pelvic inlet of the female are wider than those of the male to allow for childbirth.
- Leg: Long bone of the upper leg (thigh) is the *femur;* the femur is the longest bone in the body and fits into a cavity of the ilium known as the *acetabulum*. The two long bones of the calf are the *fibula* and *tibia*. The *patella* (kneecap) is found in front of the knee joint.
- Ankle and foot: Seven bones in the ankle (*tarsals*) provide a connection between the foot and leg bones. The foot has five *metatarsal* bones (forming the arch of foot), and the five toes have 14 *phalanges* (each toe has three except for the big toe, which has two).

> **Fascinating Facts**
>
> The ankles and feet account for one quarter of all the bones in the human body.

> **Media Link**
>
> View the Shoulder Injuries animation on the Online Resources for an overview of the movement of joints.

Joints

A joint (articulation) is the connection between bones that allows for movement. Joints are covered by a synovial membrane that produces a lubricating fluid called *synovial fluid*. This enables them to move freely and without discomfort. *Ligaments* are fibrous connective tissues that connect one bone to another and create the stability of the joint. Another structure that some joints (elbow, knee, and shoulder) have is a *bursa*, a small fluid-filled sac or cavity. A bursa serves as a cushion and prevents friction between moving parts, such as tendons and bones.

Joint types that enable a wide range of mobility are ball-and-socket (shoulder and hip) and hinge (elbow and knee). Not all joints have the structures that allow a lot of movement. For example, vertebrae move only slightly, and the bones of the cranium do not move at all, with the exception of the mandible (jaw), which is a hinge joint. Common movements made possible by joints are described in Figure 7–6 and Table 7–2.

Major Diseases and Disorders

- *Arthritis* is a group of diseases involving inflammation of the joints. Examples include *rheumatoid arthritis* (synovial membranes thicken), *gouty arthritis* (uric acid crystals build up in joints), and *degenerative joint disease*, also known as *osteoarthritis* (cartilage in the joints softens).
- *Back pain* is a common complaint that has many causes. The intervertebral disks sometimes press against nerves. Pain that runs down the leg is usually due to pressure on the sciatic nerve.
- *Carpal tunnel syndrome* is caused by pressure on a nerve in the wrist as a result of repetitive movement or trauma. This diagnosis has become quite common with the increased use of computers.
- Excessive *curvature of the spine* can occur in three directions.
  1. *Scoliosis* is a lateral (to the side) curvature.
  2. *Lordosis*, sometimes referred to as "swayback," is an inward curvature of the lumbar area.

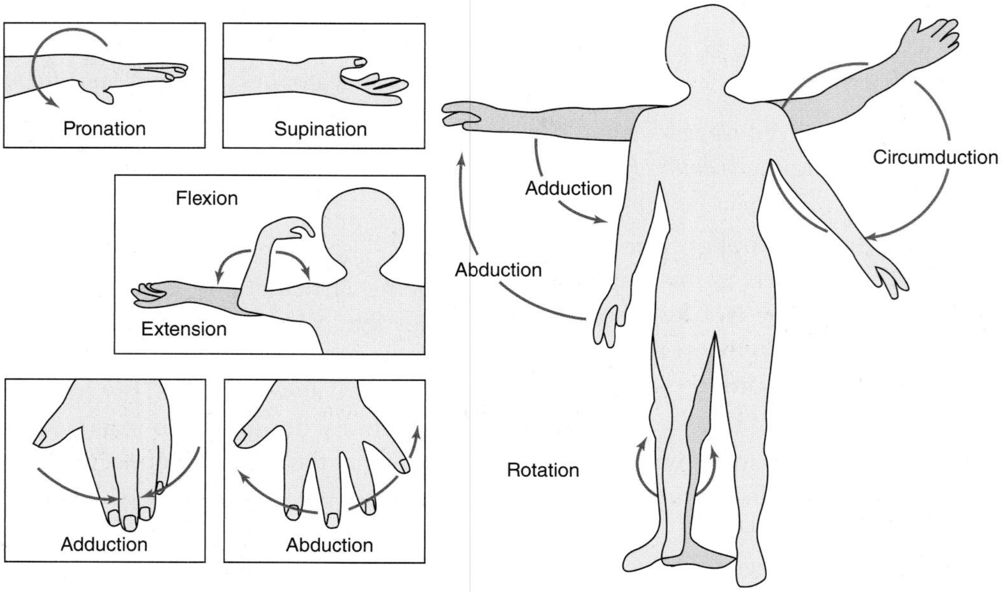

FIGURE 7–6 Movements of joints.

Table 7–2 Movement of Joints

Movement	Description
Abduction	Movement away from the median plane of the body
Adduction	Movement toward the median plane of the body
Circumduction	Movement in a circular direction
Extension	To straighten (increase the angle between the bones forming a joint)
Flexion	To bend (decrease the angle between the bones forming a joint)
Pronation	Turning the hand so the palm faces downward or backward (also refers to lying facedown)
Rotation	Motion around a central axis
Supination	Turning the palm or foot upward (also refers to lying face up)

3. *Kyphosis,* sometimes referred to as "hunchback," is rounded bowing of the thoracic area. (See Figure 7–7.)

- *Fractures* (broken bones) usually occur from some external injury to the body, but can also occur without injury if the bone is thin and brittle as a result of a disease (e.g., osteoporosis, Paget's disease). The fracture may be closed (skin not broken) or open (bone breaks through skin). The different types of fractures are shown in Figure 7–8.
- *Osteomyelitis* is an infection of the bone.
- *Osteoporosis* is a weakening of the bones caused by the loss of calcium in the bones.

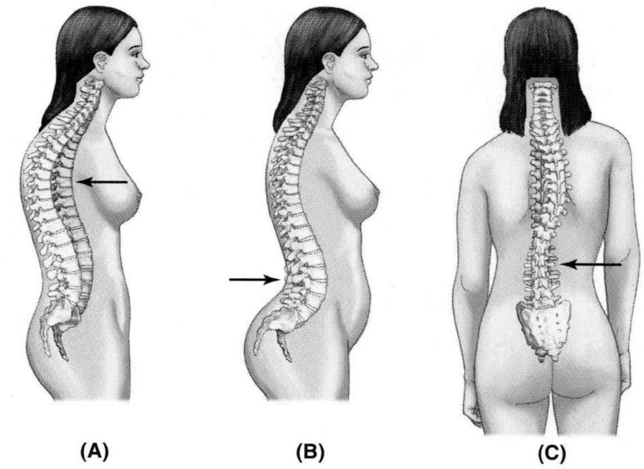

FIGURE 7–7 Abnormal curvatures of the spinal column: (A) kyphosis, (B) lordosis, (C) scoliosis.

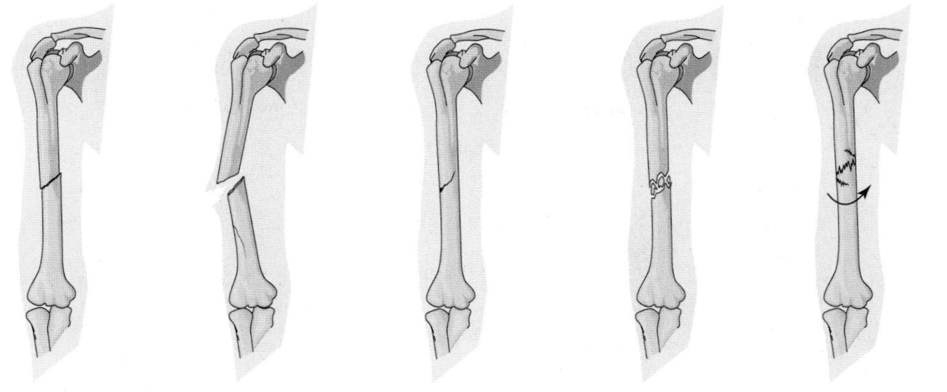

FIGURE 7–8 Types of fractures.

Preventive Measures

- Get adequate exercise, especially weight-bearing activities such as walking.
- Avoid overextension of joints.
- Eat properly and take in sufficient calcium and vitamin C.
- Do stretching exercises, especially before participating in other forms of physical activity.
- Maintain good posture (Chapter 9).
- Position the body properly when using a computer and other types of equipment (Chapter 9).
- Use proper lifting techniques (Chapter 9).
- Use protective equipment, such as seat belts when in a vehicle or kneepads and helmets when cycling and skateboarding.

Age-Related Changes: Skeletal System

- Decreased: Height, bone mass, flexibility
- Increased: Joint and cartilage erosion, thinning of vertebrae, demineralization of bones

Thinking It Through

Randolph Jenkins is brought by ambulance to the hospital emergency department after a serious automobile accident. His right arm and leg are broken, and he has a skull fracture above his right ear. Mr. Jenkins also complains of pain in the left upper and lower extremities, and Dr. Printz, the emergency department physician, is assessing function by asking Mr. Jenkins to move his left arm straight out from the side of his body and then back down, then to turn the left palm up toward the ceiling and then down toward the floor.

1. Does Mr. Jenkins have injuries to the axial or appendicular skeleton, or both?
2. What are the medical terms for the four movements the patient is requested to do with his left arm and hand?
3. From the description given for the location of the skull fracture, which cranial bone is most likely involved?

Muscular

The *muscular system* (Figure 7–9) consists of more than 600 muscles that produce movement, provide support, and produce heat to maintain body temperature. There are different types of muscles:

- Cardiac (heart): Located only in the heart. The pumping contractions and relaxations of the muscle occur with no conscious effort on the part of the individual (involuntary control).
- Skeletal: Attached to the bones, these require conscious effort to function (voluntary control). They are referred to as striated because they have alternating light and dark bands circling the muscle fibers. Any movement that is self-generated involves skeletal muscles (e.g., walking, chewing, and talking).
- Smooth (visceral): Located in the walls of internal organs (e.g., stomach, intestines, uterus, and blood vessels). Their movement is involuntary,

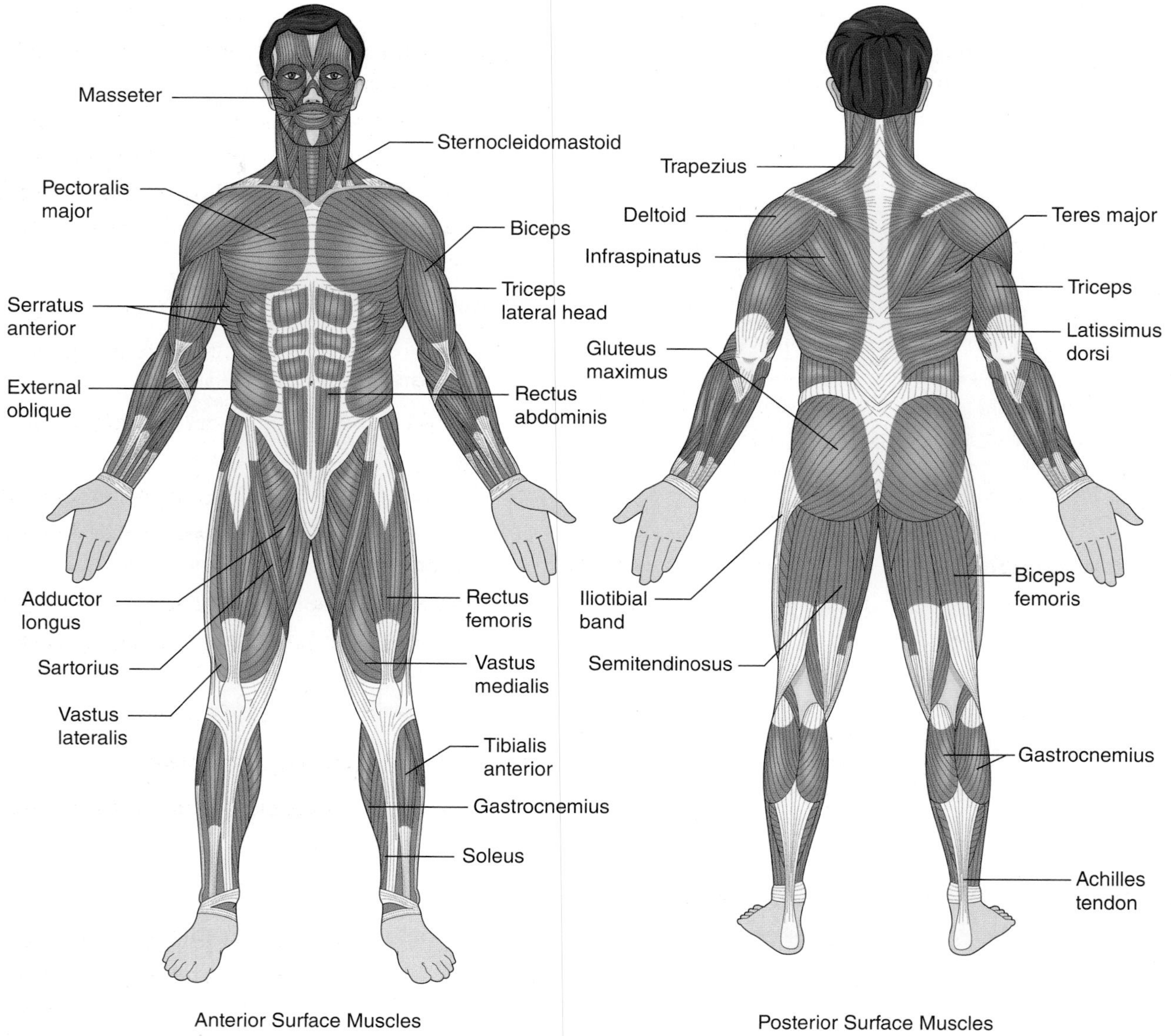

FIGURE 7–9 Muscles of the body.

they are nonstriated (no markings), and controlled by the autonomic (automatic) nervous system.

- Sphincter (dilator): A circular muscle that controls the opening and closing of a passageway, such as in the digestive (food passing into and out of the stomach) and urinary (urine passing out of the bladder) systems.

All muscles have the following four characteristics:

- Contractibility: Ability to be tightened, which makes the muscle shorter and thicker
- Excitability (irritability): Readiness to respond to various types of stimuli
- Extensibility: Ability to be stretched
- Elasticity: Ability to return to its original length when relaxing

Skeletal muscles are attached to the bones by bands of strong, tough connective tissues known as *tendons* or by a sheet-like membrane that covers, supports, and separates the muscles known as *fascia*. Tendons are like *ligaments* in being tough, flexible cords. But tendons differ from ligaments in that tendons extend from muscle to bone whereas ligaments go from bone to bone as at a joint. Skeletal muscles are attached to bones at two points: the *origin* and the *insertion*. The origin is the less movable bone; the insertion is attached to a more movable bone that will be affected by the action of the muscle. For example, the origin of the triceps muscle is toward the shoulder and the insertion is by the elbow. The *belly* is the central part of the muscle, seen most easily in the "bulges" developed by weightlifters.

Skeletal muscles work in pairs. The *prime mover* produces movement in one direction, and the *antagonist* produces movement in the opposite direction. The antagonist is the muscle on the opposite side of the joint and must relax to allow the prime mover to contract. Bend your elbow and you can feel the biceps (top of upper arm) contract and the triceps (back of upper arm) relax. Now extend your forearm and feel the biceps relax and the triceps contract. To demonstrate the need for opposing pairs of muscles, extend your arm partway, contract both the biceps and the triceps, and you will discover that movement is no longer possible.

Fascinating Facts

In a normal-weight average adult, the 600 muscles of the body comprise 40% of the body's weight.

The jaw muscles can exert about 200 pounds of force for the back teeth during chewing.

Muscle tone is a muscle's normal resistance to stretching caused by always being in a state of slight contraction. Loss of muscle tone can occur from illness, injury, or from lack of use. Too much tone is called *spasticity*. This, too, can be caused by illness or injury. Spastic muscles are too tight to move smoothly.

When the muscles are not used, they can *atrophy* (shrink in size and become weak) and appear floppy. Lack of use can also result in *contracture*, in which a shortened muscle holds the joint in a flexed position.

Major Diseases and Disorders

- *Contractures* occur when the muscle stays in a shortened position. If the joint is not moved regularly, it will lose its flexibility as ligaments and tendons shorten.
- *Gangrene* is caused by *Clostridium* bacteria, which kills muscle tissue.
- *Muscle spasms* (cramps) are sudden and painful involuntary muscle contractions.
- *Muscle sprain* is the result of torn ligament fibers that results in loosening of the joint.
- *Muscle strain* is the result of a sudden tearing of muscle fibers during exertion; also referred to as a pulled muscle.
- *Muscular dystrophy* is an inherited disease that causes progressive deterioration of the muscles.
- *Myasthenia gravis* is a chronic neuromuscular disease that causes gradually increasing muscle weakness.

Preventive Measures

- Perform warm-up exercises before engaging in physical activity.
- Remain active, engaging in walking or exercising every day.
- Receive therapeutic massage to relax stiff muscles.
- Practice relaxation exercises to relieve muscle tension (Chapter 12).
- Use proper lifting techniques.
- Do muscle-strengthening exercises, such as weight lifting.
- Eat adequate amounts of protein.

Age-Related Changes: Muscular System

- Decreased: Muscle mass, tone, and strength
- Increased: Risk of falls

Integumentary

The skin is the largest organ of the body; it accounts for about 15% of total body weight and has a surface area of about 25 square feet in an adult. The skin provides protection from environmental hazards, such as sunrays and bacteria. The nerve endings located in the skin are another protective feature. They respond to touch, heat, cold, pain, and pressure. (See Figure 7–10.) Without this warning system, individuals would not know when to move away from hazards. The skin participates in controlling body temperature through sweating and by widening and narrowing the blood vessels to control the entry and escape of heat. Finally, the skin acts as a waterproofing membrane. Without it, death would occur within minutes from *dehydration* (loss of water).

Fascinating Facts

There are 45 miles of nerves just in the skin of a human being.

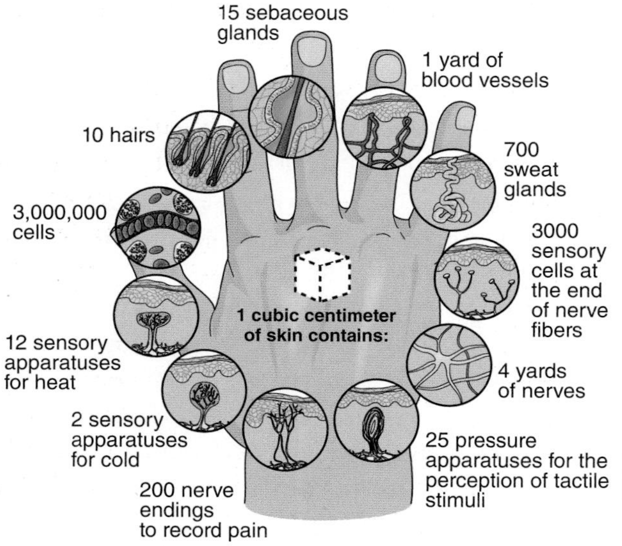

FIGURE 7–10 What is in the skin?

The *integumentary system* includes the skin and its appendages. (See Figure 7–11.) The *appendages* include hair, nails, and the sweat and oil glands.

Layers of the skin:

- Epidermis: This outer layer of the skin, consisting of five or six layers, contains no blood supply or nerves. The outermost layer is composed of cells (squamous) that have died from environmental exposure and are shed daily. These lost cells are then replaced with cells produced in the lower layers, a process that continues throughout the lifetime. About 500 million squamous cells are lost every day as we bathe, dry, dress, and move within our environment. Skin pigmentation is determined by the melanocytes that produce the pigment *melanin*. Melanin can be black or brown or have a yellow tint, depending upon racial origin. The amount of melanin (and other skin pigments such as carotene and hemoglobin) in the melanocytes determines the various shades of human skin. Patches of melanin are called freckles or, if related to damaged skin areas, "age spots." An albino is a person who has no skin pigmentation.
- Dermis: This is the second layer of skin, which contains involuntary muscles (arrector pili muscles that cause "goose bumps"), blood vessels, nerves, hair follicles, sudoriferous (sweat) glands, and sebaceous (oil) glands.
- Subcutaneous tissue: This is the innermost layer of the skin containing fatty and connective

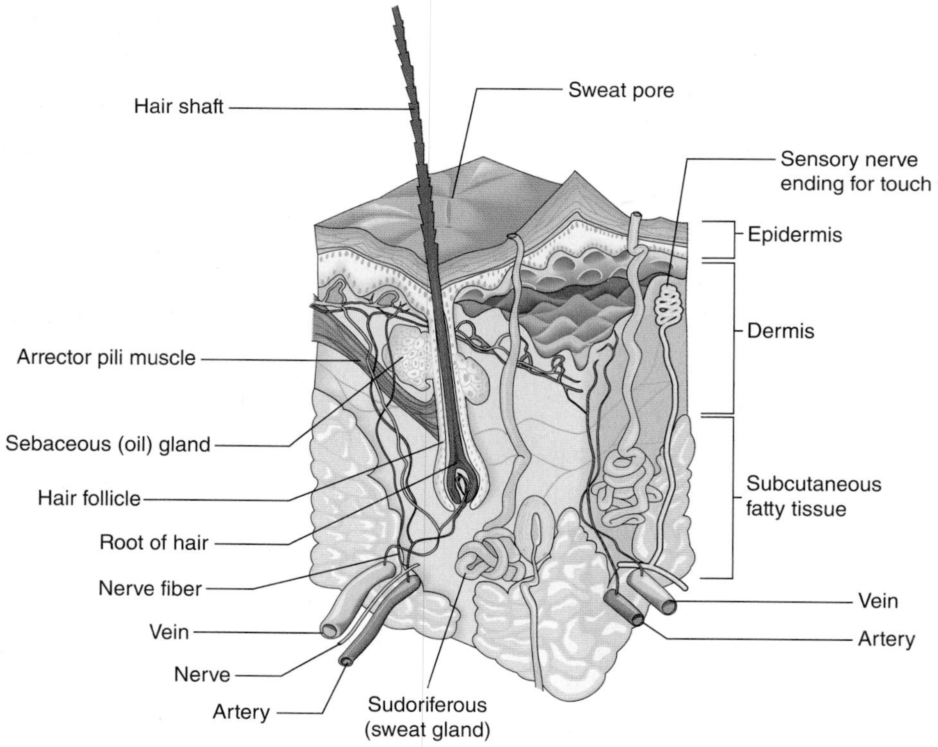

FIGURE 7–11 Structures of the skin.

tissue, which fastens the skin to the underlying muscles.

Fascinating Facts

A fingernail or toenail takes about six months to grow from base to tip.

Beards are the fastest growing hairs on the human body. If never trimmed, a beard could grow to 30 feet in length over the average lifetime.

The appendages:

- Hair: Each hair is encased within a hair follicle and ends in a root where new hair growth occurs. Hair is composed of a fibrous protein called keratin, which is a nonliving cell (a good thing, or haircuts would be very painful).
- Nails: Fingernails and toenails are also composed of keratin. The growth of the nail occurs at the base of the nail under the half-moon–shaped area. The function of the nails is to protect the fingers and toes.
- Sudoriferous (sweat) glands: During perspiration, water mixed with salt and waste products is excreted through the sweat glands. The function of the sweat glands is to excrete excess water and to assist the cooling of the body by the evaporation of water from the skin.
- Sebaceous (oil) glands: These excrete an oily substance (sebum) to lubricate and protect the skin. Sebum is slightly acidic, so it discourages the growth of bacteria.

Media Link

View the Skin animation on the Online Resources for an overview of this system.

Major Diseases and Disorders

- *Athlete's foot* is an infection of the skin caused by a fungus.
- *Boils (furuncles)* are a bacterial infection of the hair follicles or sebaceous glands.
- *Cancer of the skin* has three forms: basal cell, squamous cell, and melanoma. Basal cell is the most common and easiest to treat; squamous cell is more serious; melanoma is the most serious and can be life threatening.
- *Cellulitis* is a bacterial infection of the dermis and subcutaneous layers of the skin.
- *Pressure sores* (bed sores or decubitus ulcers) are areas of skin breakdown that occur over a bony prominence due to excessive and prolonged pressure that prevents adequate circulation to the tissues.
- *Dermatitis* is a general name for inflammation of the skin. *Contact dermatitis* is an allergic reaction to a substance that makes contact with the skin. *Eczema* is a generalized skin irritation usually caused by an irritant that appears as reddened areas on the surface of the skin.
- *Psoriasis* is a chronic, noncontagious, inherited skin disease in which too many epithelial cells are produced.
- *Warts* are caused by a viral infection of the skin.

Preventive Measures

- Practice good hygiene and keep the skin clean.
- Do not break open pimples or other growths on the skin.
- Do not scratch insect bites or other irritations.
- Avoid excessive exposure to the sun.
- Use sunscreen and wear a hat when in the sun.
- Have skin changes checked immediately.
- Protect skin from poisonous plants and insect bites.
- Get adequate amounts of vitamins A and C and niacin.

Age-Related Changes: Integumentary System

- Decreased: Elasticity of the skin, subcutaneous fat (insulation), and hair (head, face)
- Increased: Dryness, wrinkles, skin pigmentation, and susceptibility to irritation

Systems for Providing Energy and Removing Waste

These systems work together to provide energy for the body and to remove the products of waste. The circulatory system includes two powerful transportation systems—cardiovascular and lymphatic—these systems reach every area of the body and work closely together to maintain fluid balance and prevent infections and disease.

Fascinating Facts

Humans shed about 600,000 particles of skin every hour, which is about 1.5 pounds a year. By 70 years of age, the person will have lost 105 pounds of skin.

Humans shed and regrow outer skin cells about every 27 days. That totals almost 1000 new skins in a lifetime.

The respiratory system supplies oxygen, and the digestive system turns food into the fuel needed for energy and for the growth and repair of cells. This fuel is then delivered to the body cells via the cardiovascular system. The digestive and urinary systems excrete the waste by-products and help maintain fluid balance.

Circulatory

The cardiovascular and lymphatic systems are the two main transportation (circulatory) systems of the body. In the cardiovascular system, the heart pumps blood that circulates throughout the body and then back to the heart through a network of blood vessels. The lymphatic system does not have a central pumping station, but it does have an extensive network of lymphatic vessels similar in design to blood vessels. The two systems are in constant physical contact and work together to transport fluids, dispose of waste products, and fight infection.

Cardiovascular System

The cardiovascular system transports blood cells and dissolved materials, including nutrients and oxygen, to all areas of the body. The other important function of this system is temperature regulation. Human beings are warm-blooded animals and require a fairly narrow temperature range to maintain homeostasis. This temperature range is maintained by circulating the warmer blood from the center of the body to the surface of the skin where it is cooled. Regulation takes place by the blood vessels dilating to increase heat loss or contracting to reduce heat loss. On hot days the skin is pinker and warmer because the blood vessels are dilated to release heat. The opposite occurs when the outer temperature is cold because the blood flow is restricted. The skin appears pale and feels cool.

Fascinating Facts

Your fingerprints will grow in size during your lifetime, but unless your fingers are injured, the patterns of your fingerprints will remain the same. It is well known that fingerprints are unique, but did you know this is also true of your voice and tongue print?

The cardiovascular system consists of the heart and blood vessels. The blood vessels that carry blood away from the heart are called *arteries*, and the blood vessels that return blood to the heart are *veins*. Both arteries and veins are like branches on a tree, becoming narrower at each branching. The smallest of the branches are called *capillaries* and their diameter is less than the width of the period at the end of this sentence.

The heart is a strong pump composed of cardiac muscles. Its main function is to pump enough blood at a high enough pressure to supply every part of the body. A fully developed heart is about the size of an adult fist. It is located in the chest cavity, between the lungs, where it is protected by the ribs and sternum. The components of the heart include:

- Endocardium: Smooth layer that lines the inside of the heart
- Myocardium: Thick layer of muscle tissue that performs the pumping action
- Pericardium: Sac-like membrane that surrounds the heart
- Four chambers: Two for receiving blood (*atria*) and two for moving it out of the heart (*ventricles*). When blood is pumped out of the chambers, valves snap shut with a "thump-thump" (often referred to as "lub-dub"), which is the sound heard when listening to the heart. The valves prevent backflow of blood.

The blood arriving at the heart from the body takes the following path:

1. Arrives via the *inferior* and *superior vena cavae*
2. Enters the *right atrium* of the heart
3. Passes through a valve to the *right ventricle*
4. Passes through another valve into the right and left *pulmonary arteries*
5. Travels to the *lungs* to pick up fresh oxygen and drop off carbon dioxide

6. Returns to the heart by the *pulmonary veins* to the *left atrium*
7. Passes through another valve to reach the *left ventricle*
8. Leaves the *left ventricle* via the *aorta* to once again circulate throughout the body

Note: The pulmonary artery carries oxygen-poor blood to the lungs. The pulmonary vein carries oxygen-rich blood to the heart. In the rest of the circulatory system, arteries carry oxygen-rich blood to the body. Veins return oxygen-poor blood to the heart. (See Figure 7–12.)

The average adult heart rate is between 60 and 80 beats per minute. The heart rate is higher in children, gradually decreasing from its highest rate at birth until reaching its adult level. Athletes generally have lower rates because their heart muscle is stronger and pumps more blood with each beat. The heart rate varies to accommodate the body's needs. It speeds up during exercise to increase the flow of blood to skeletal muscles, after a meal to send extra blood to the digestive system, and during a fever so more blood flows to the surface of the body to release heat.

The heart has its own blood supply that wraps around its surface to provide it with nourishment and remove wastes. These are called the coronary arteries and veins. It is the blockage of coronary arteries that causes heart attacks. (See Figure 7–13.)

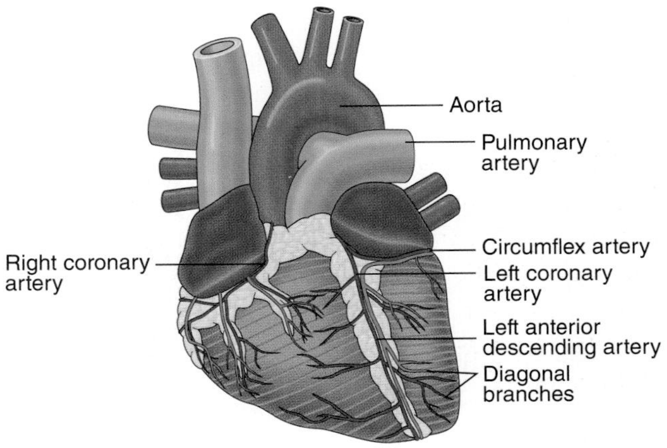

FIGURE 7–13 The coronary arteries.

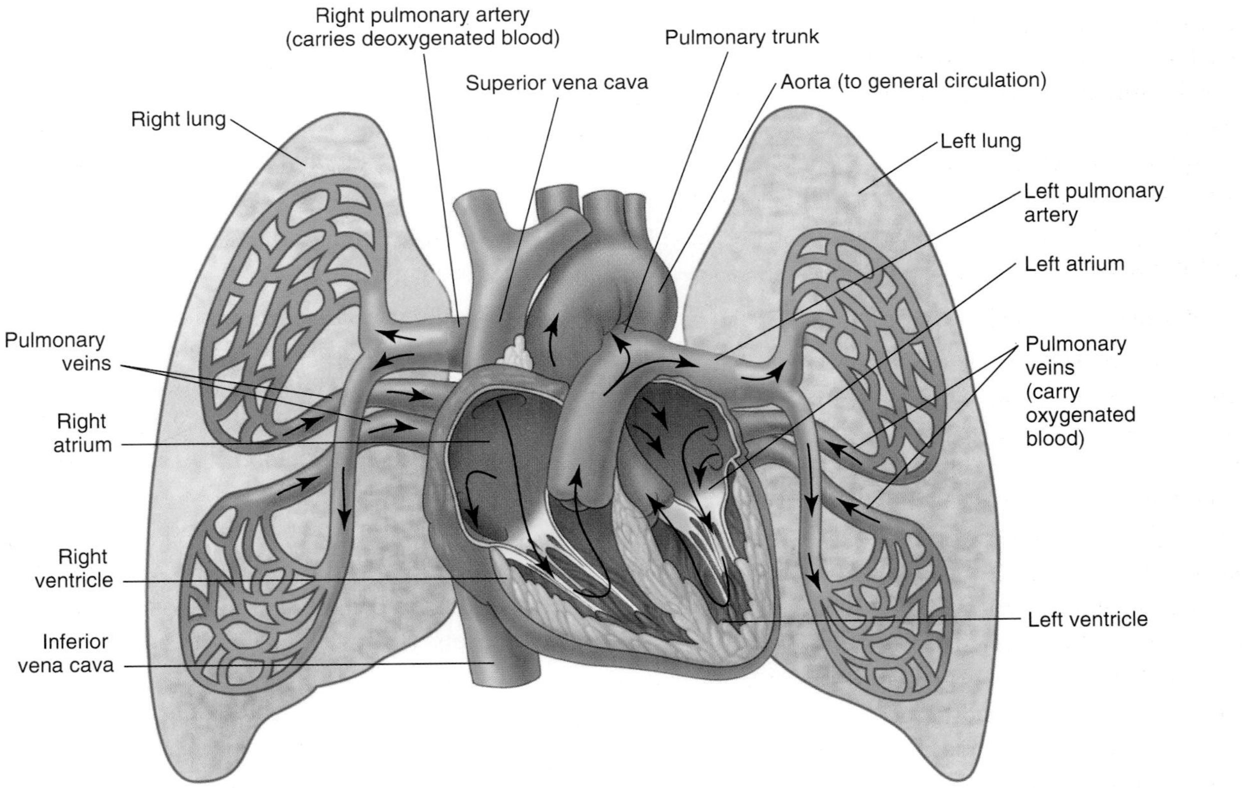

FIGURE 7–12 Cardiopulmonary circulation.

The heart also has its own electrical system that stimulates the cardiac muscle to contract and act as a pump. The electrical impulses, like the blood, follow their own set path through the heart:

1. An impulse originates at a cluster of nerve cells located in the upper right wall of the right atrium, called the *sinoatrial node (SA node).* This is the natural pacemaker of the heart, functioning to originate and regulate the heartbeat.
2. The SA node sends the impulse through a network of nerves that reaches all areas of both atria.
3. The right and left atria respond to the impulse by contracting and forcing the blood into the ventricles.
4. The impulse reaches another node, called the *atrioventricular node (AV node)* that is located between the atrium and ventricle.
5. The AV node sends the impulse through a network of nerve fibers called the *bundle of His* that splits into the *right* and *left bundle fibers* and then terminates in a diffuse network of nerve branches called the *Purkinje fibers.*
6. The right and left ventricles contract.

It is this electrical pattern that is measured during an electrocardiogram (ECG or EKG). The pattern gives information that is helpful in diagnosing heart problems. (See Figure 7–14.)

Media Link

View The Heart animation on the Online Resources for an overview of the electrical system.

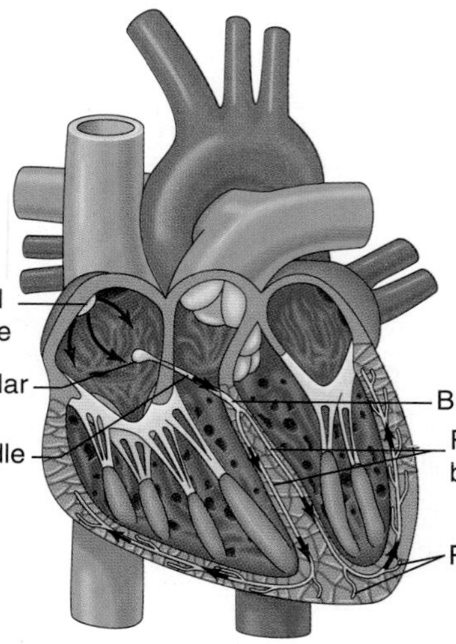

FIGURE 7–14 The electrical system of the heart.

Blood is carried throughout the body by means of a vast system of vessels, channels that carry fluid. As noted, there are three types of blood vessels: arteries, veins, and capillaries.

- Arteries carry oxygenated blood away from the heart and out to all areas of the body (recall that the pulmonary artery is the only artery that carries oxygen-poor blood, or what is called deoxygenated blood). The aorta, which receives blood pumped from the left ventricle, is the largest artery. On leaving the heart, it immediately begins to branch into smaller and smaller arteries. The smallest arteries are called *arterioles.* Arteries are muscular and elastic in order to handle the force of pumped blood. (See Figure 7–15.)
- Veins carry deoxygenated blood back to the heart from all areas of the body (recall that the pulmonary vein is the only vein that carries oxygenated blood). The farthest veins from the heart, *venules,* are also the smallest. The veins increase in size as they approach the heart. The largest veins are the *inferior* (carrying blood from lower body) and *superior* (carrying blood from upper body) vena cavae. These deliver the blood to the right atrium. Veins have one-way valves that prevent the blood from flowing in a backward direction and are thinner and less muscular than arteries. (See Figure 7–16.)
- Capillaries are the smallest blood vessels. They connect the arterioles with the venules. Their one-cell-thick walls allow substances to exit and enter the bloodstream. Nutrients and oxygen move from the blood into surrounding tissues. Waste materials and carbon dioxide are picked up for transport to the lungs and kidneys for removal from the body. (See Figure 7–17.)

The blood consists of red blood cells (RBCs), white blood cells (WBCs), platelets, and plasma:

- *Red blood cells* carry oxygen to the body cells. They pick up oxygen in the lungs and bind it to a substance called hemoglobin, then give up the oxygen when they reach the capillaries. An adequate intake of iron in the diet is essential for the production of hemoglobin to carry oxygen. RBCs have no nucleus so they cannot reproduce

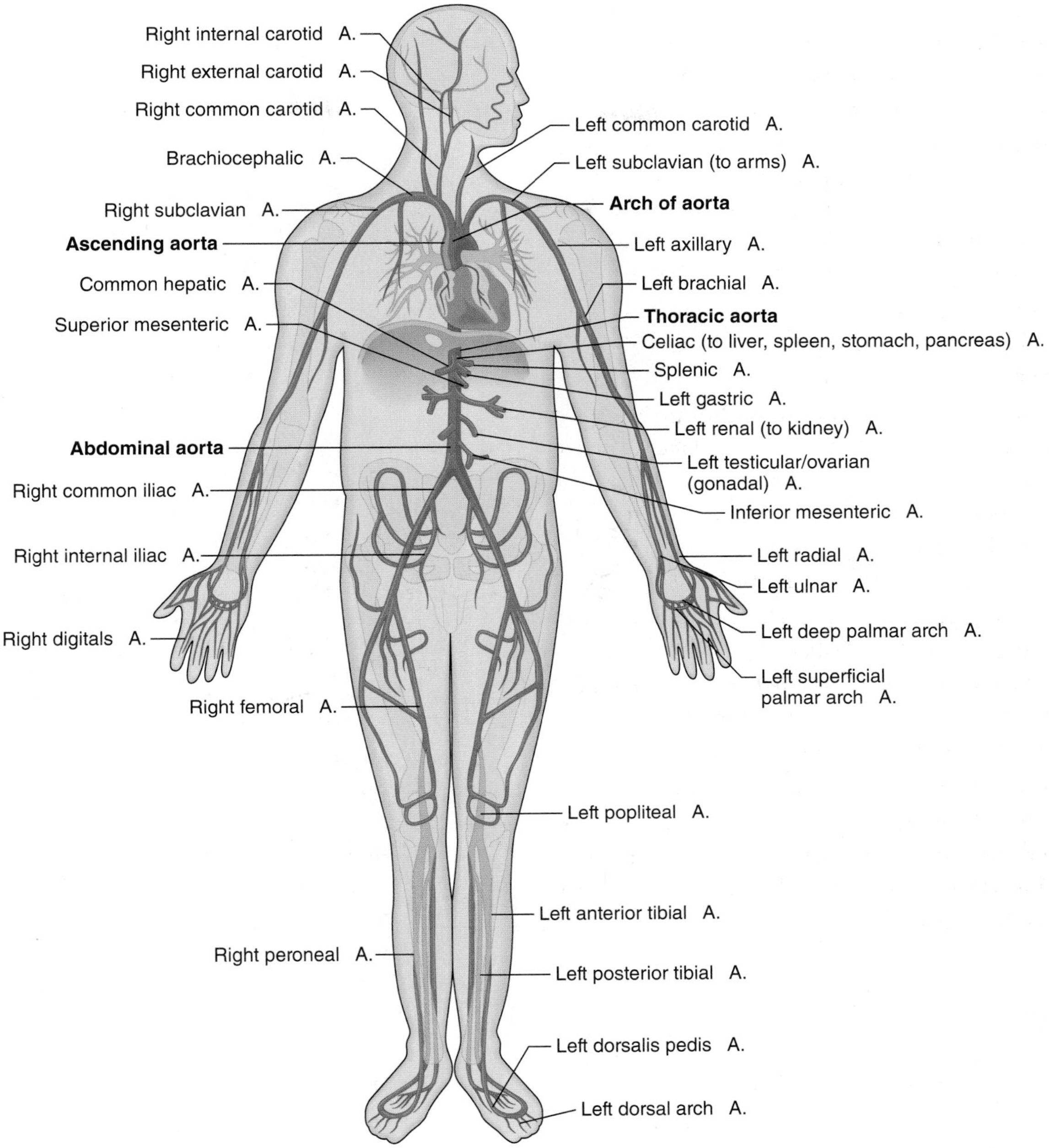

FIGURE 7–15 The major arteries.

themselves. They are primarily manufactured in the red bone marrow.

- *White blood cells* fight infections. They pass through the blood vessels to work in the tissues as needed. They function as scavenger cells that engulf and destroy infected cells (*phagocytosis*) and then remove wastes and dead cells. WBCs are manufactured in the bone marrow and the lymphatic system and can be produced on demand as needed by the body.
- *Platelets* clump together to form clots when a blood vessel is damaged and aid in preventing loss of blood. Platelets are manufactured in the bone marrow.
- *Plasma* is the liquid part of the blood, consisting mostly of water. Its purpose is to transport the other blood cells along with other nutrients and hormones. It also supplies the fluid needed inside and around the body cells.

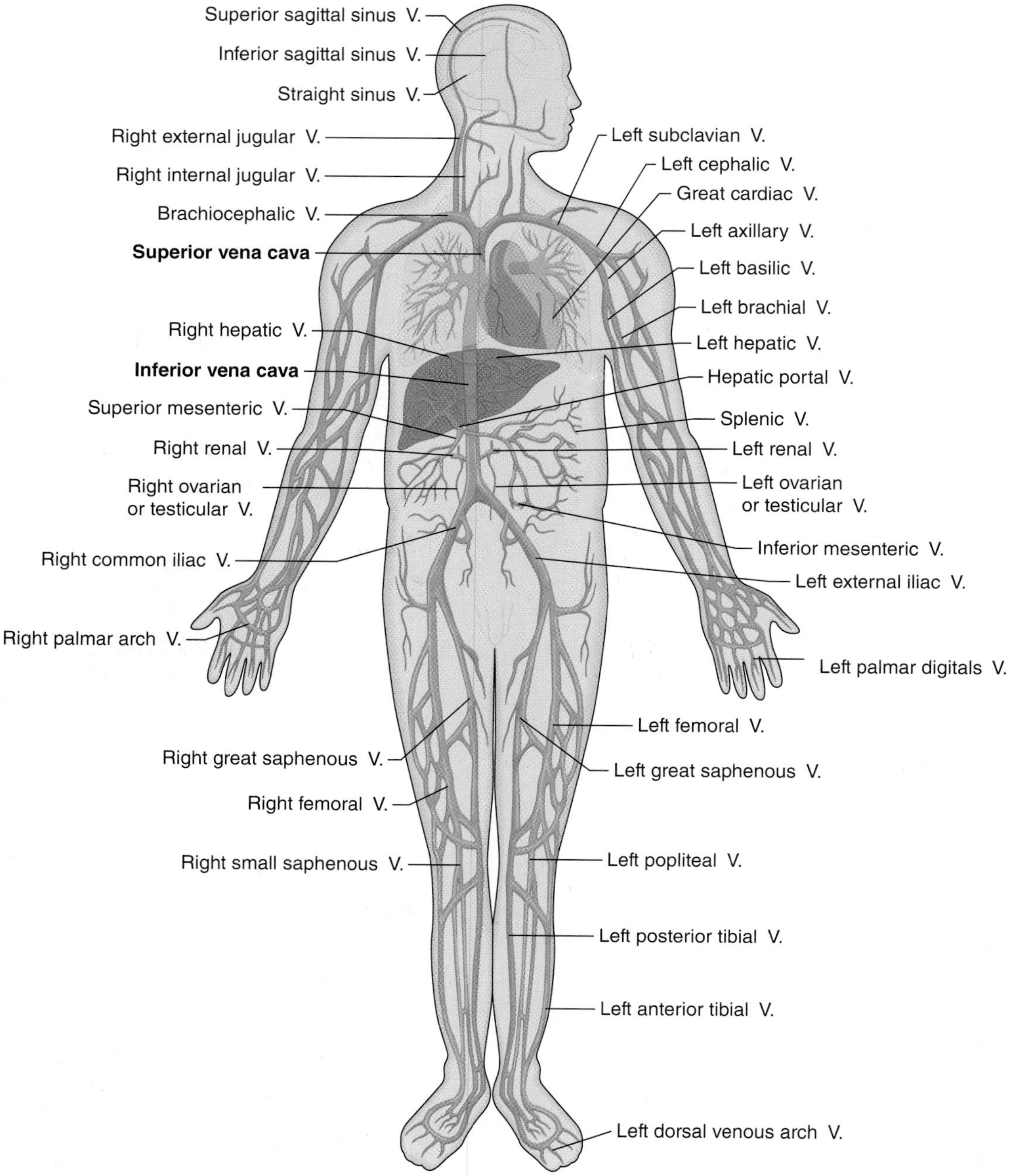

FIGURE 7–16 The major veins.

Media Link

View The Blood animation on the Online Resources for an overview of the components of the blood.

Lymphatic System

The second essential transportation system of the body is the *lymphatic system*. This network of fluid, called lymph, serves to defend against infection, maintain fluid balance, and remove waste products. Lymph is a straw-colored fluid that consists of water, waste products, digested nutrients, hormones, salts, and lymphocytes (special type of WBC). Lymph travels through vessels that are similar to blood vessels. Lymphatic capillaries combine to form increasingly larger vessels that eventually empty into two *lymphatic ducts*. The ducts, which are walled passageways, then empty into the superior vena cava, and the lymph joins the blood as it enters the right atrium.

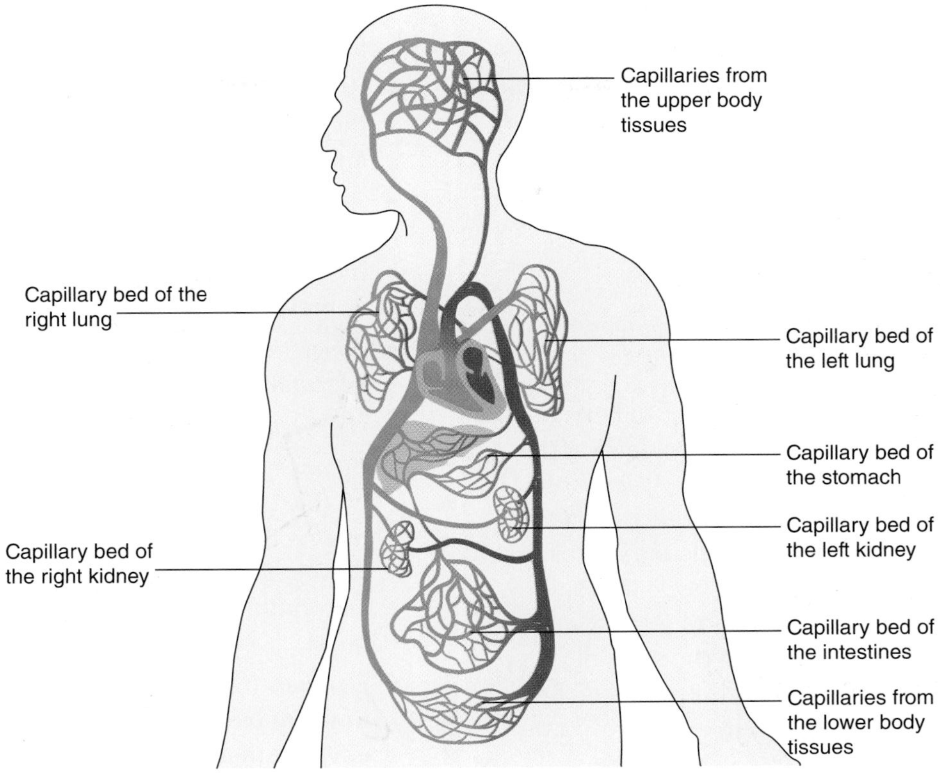

FIGURE 7–17 Examples of capillary beds.

As the lymph passes through the lymphatic vessels, it is filtered by oval-shaped *lymph nodes* made of specialized tissue. This tissue has the ability to remove substances, such as cancer cells, disease-causing organisms, and dead blood cells found in the blood. (See Figure 7–18.)

Lymphoid tissue is also found in the tonsils, adenoids, and the spleen. The *spleen* is located in the upper-left area of the abdomen just under the diaphragm. It filters blood instead of lymph fluid and has the following functions:

- Removes old, worn-out RBCs
- Removes iron from hemoglobin for reuse by the bone marrow
- Creates RBCs prior to birth (this function stops shortly after birth)
- Produces lymphocytes and antibodies to help the body fight infection
- Acts as a filter for foreign bodies
- Serves as a reservoir for blood that can be added to the cardiovascular system as needed

The lymphatic system also has a role in the immune response. The *immune response* occurs when

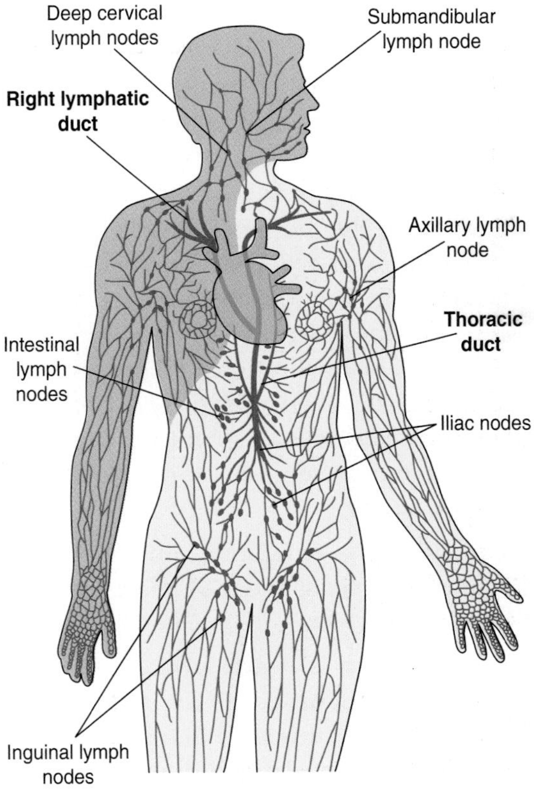

FIGURE 7–18 The lymphatic system.

something enters the body that it does not identify as its own tissue. Foreign substances are known as *antigens*. Examples include microorganisms, splinters, and poison. The body responds by producing antibodies to attack the antigen. The lymphatic system produces antibodies and lymphocytes. Signs that the immune system is fighting infection include fever, inflammation, and pus.

Fascinating Facts

If the heart beats at the average rate of 70 beats per minute, it will have beat about 2.5 billion times by the age of 70. To appreciate how hard your heart works, try this: let your hand imitate the squeezing action of your heart by fully opening and fully closing your hand at the same rate that your heart beats. Do this for five minutes without stopping. How do the muscles of your hand and forearm feel after five minutes? If your hand got tired, you could always switch to the other hand, but you only have one heart, so take good care of it.

Major Diseases and Disorders

Cardiovascular:

- *Anemia* results when the blood has an inadequate amount of hemoglobin, RBCs, or both. There are many different types of anemia, including *pernicious anemia* (RBCs not developed due to poor absorption of vitamin B_{12}), *iron-deficiency anemia* (inadequate hemoglobin due to iron shortage), and *aplastic anemia* (bone marrow destroyed by chemicals, radiation, or medications). There are also two genetic forms of anemia, *sickle cell anemia*, most common in people of African origin, and *thalassemia*, most often seen in people of Mediterranean origin.
- *Aneurysm* is a ballooning out of the arterial wall that weakens the wall and disrupts blood flow.
- *Angina pectoris* is heart pain caused by inadequate supply of oxygen to the heart by the coronary arteries. If this condition is severe enough, part of the heart tissue will die, resulting in a *myocardial infarction* (MI; heart attack). A common misconception is that men are more prone to heart disease than women, but it is the number one cause of death in women.
- *Arteriosclerosis* is a hardening or thickening of the arterial walls, resulting in loss of elasticity and contractility.
- *Atherosclerosis* occurs when fatty plaques are deposited on the walls of the arteries, narrowing the lumen (opening). The narrowing decreases or prevents blood flow.
- *Congestive heart failure* is a condition in which the heart fails as a pump.
- *Hypertension* is high blood pressure.
- *Inflammation of the heart* can occur at any of the three layers of the heart: *endocarditis* affects the inner lining of the heart and heart valves; *myocarditis* affects the cardiac muscle; *pericarditis* affects the sac that surrounds the heart.
- *Leukemia* (blood cancer) is an abnormal increase in white blood cells that are immature and less effective than mature cells in fighting infections. These immature cells become so prevalent that they replace the RBCs and cause anemia.
- *Septicemia* (blood poisoning) occurs when an infection enters the blood vessels.
- *Thrombosis* is a blood clot that forms in a blood vessel. If it breaks loose and travels through the body, it is called an *embolus*.
- *Varicose veins* are dilated veins filled with blood. Veins that lose their elasticity allow the blood to pool (stasis), and the result is decreased blood flow.

Lymphatic:

- *Acquired immunodeficiency syndrome (AIDS)* is caused by a virus and results in failure of the body's immune system.
- *Autoimmune diseases* occur when the body does not recognize its own tissue and initiates an immune response to destroy the tissue. Examples are *systemic lupus erythematosus*, which affects connective tissue, and *Hashimoto's disease*, which destroys the thyroid gland.
- *Hodgkin's disease* is a form of cancer that affects the lymph nodes.
- *Tonsillitis* is an infection of the tonsils caused by the large number of microorganisms they are filtering through their lymph tissues.

Fascinating Facts

Laughing lowers levels of stress hormones and strengthens the immune system. Six-year-olds laugh an average of 300 times a day. Adults only laugh 15 to 100 times a day.

Preventive Measures

- Practice good nutrition.
- Avoid being overweight.
- Get adequate exercise.
- Check blood pressure regularly (hypertension does not have symptoms).
- Treat cuts in the skin promptly to prevent infection.
- Do not smoke.
- Do not cross the legs for long periods.
- Develop coping skills for handling stress (Chapter 12).
- Practice safe sex habits.
- Follow standard precautions, specific techniques and practices to prevent the transmission of diseases. Chapter 10 contains a detailed explanation of standard precautions.

Age-Related Changes

Cardiovascular system:

- Decreased: Arterial elasticity, efficiency of heart valves, cardiac contractility, cardiac output
- Increased: Narrowing of the arteries due to plaque buildup

Lymphatic system:

- Decreased: Inflammatory response, effectiveness of vaccines
- Increased: Susceptibility to viral and bacterial infections

Respiratory

The *respiratory system* consists of the nose, pharynx, larynx, trachea, bronchi, and lungs. (See Figure 7–19.) The main function of the system is to deliver air to sites where gas exchange can occur between the air and the circulating blood. The cardiovascular and respiratory systems function together and are sometimes referred to as the *cardiopulmonary system*. The lymphatic system also works closely with the respiratory system to transport excess fluid from the tissues and to destroy any particles that have escaped the filtering systems and traveled deep into the lungs.

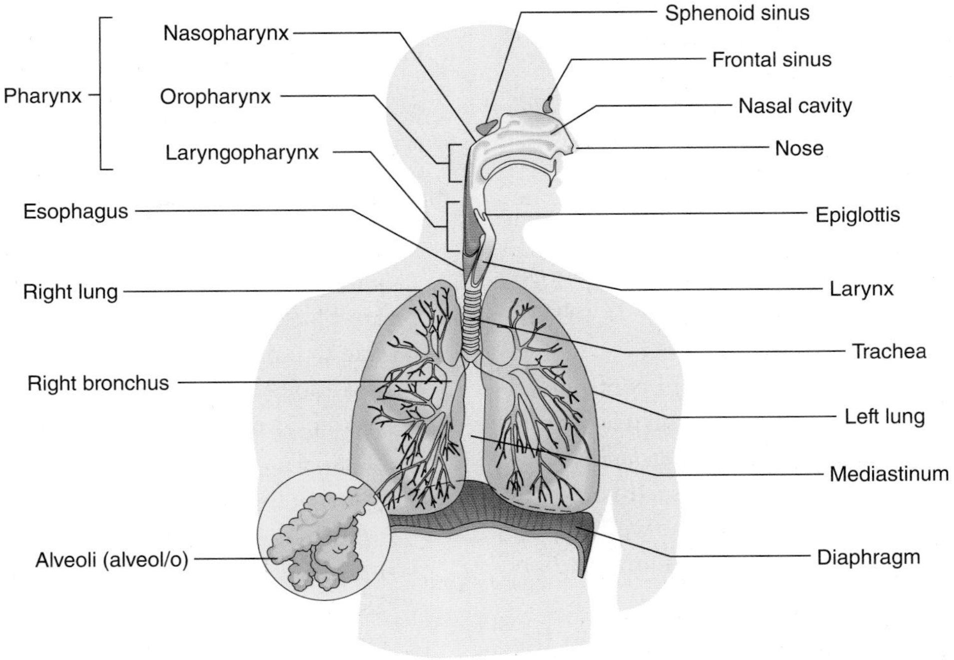

FIGURE 7–19 Structures of the respiratory system.

Fascinating Facts

Half a liter of water a day is lost through breathing. This is the water vapor you see when you breathe onto glass.

- Nose: The sensory organ for smell (olfactory). It is also important in the respiratory system. The nose is the first filter for the incoming air. Hairs and bony ridges in the nasal cavity trap the larger particles, while the nasal cavity has a *mucous* membrane that produces *mucus* to trap smaller particles. (Note that mucous and mucus sound the same, but are spelled differently.) The nose also humidifies and warms the air as it passes through with moisture from the mucus, sinuses, and tear ducts. *Sinuses* are cavities filled with air that are located around the eyes and nose. Lined with mucous membrane, they also create a resonance to the voice. (The change in the voice during a nasal cold is due to the blockage of sinuses.)
- Pharynx: The throat. Located behind the nasal cavities, it is the passageway for food and liquids, along with air. To prevent swallowed items from entering the passageway to the lungs, there is a flap-like structure called the *epiglottis* that closes off the larynx automatically during swallowing. The soft palate, at the upper rear of the roof of the mouth, blocks food and liquid from entering the nose.
- Larynx: The voice box containing the vocal cords. These are usually relaxed and open. Sounds, such as speech and singing, are produced when the cords are tightened at the same time that air is passed out of the lungs.
- Trachea: The windpipe, which serves as a passageway for air. At its distal end, it splits to form the right and left bronchi.
- Bronchi: The right and left bronchi continue to branch into smaller and smaller airways until they become the thin-walled *bronchioles*. The bronchioles terminate into tiny, sac-like structures called *alveoli*. It is through the walls of the alveoli that the exchange of oxygen and carbon dioxide takes place.
- Lungs: The right lung has three lobes and the left has two lobes, each containing a branch of the bronchi with its system of airways. The lungs are soft, elastic, spongy, and very light. Each is surrounded with an airtight covering called the pleura. Lungs have no muscles of their own and depend on the muscles around the chest cavity to do their work.
- Diaphragm: A sheet of muscle that separates the chest from the abdomen and stretches from the spine to the front of the rib cage. It provides a movable floor for the lungs. As the diaphragm contracts, it moves downward. This causes the air pressure in the lungs to decrease, which pulls air into the lungs (called inhalation). As the diaphragm relaxes, it moves up, raising air pressure in the lungs and forcing air out (called exhalation). The diaphragm is the major muscle involved in respiration, but there are also some small muscles between the ribs that sometimes help, especially when taking a deep breath.

Important protective structures built into the respiratory system in addition to the mucous membranes are the small, hair-like structures called *cilia*. They sweep mucus upward toward the nose and mouth so that trapped debris can be swallowed, coughed up, and sneezed or blown out. Coughing removes harmful particles that irritate the lining of the throat, trachea, or bronchial passages. Sneezing removes particles from the nasal cavity.

Media Link

View the Respiration animation on the Online Resources for an overview of this system.

Major Diseases and Disorders

- *Atelectasis* occurs when the alveoli are either partially or totally collapsed. Common causes are blockage in the lung, not breathing deeply due to pain or injury, and inability to cough up secretions.
- *Chronic obstructive pulmonary disease (COPD)* is a general term that refers to chronic diseases that obstruct airflow. For example, *asthma* causes the bronchial tube walls to spasm, which narrows the passageway for airflow. The narrowing prevents an easy exhalation of air and the patient experiences a sense of suffocation. *Chronic bronchitis* is an inflammation of the bronchi and bronchial tubes. *Emphysema* causes the alveoli to become

stretched out, which prevents them from efficiently exchanging oxygen and carbon dioxide.

- *Lung cancer* is the growth of tissues in the lung that destroy or block the flow of oxygen to the healthy lung tissue. This results in the entire body being deprived of oxygen.
- *Pneumonia* is an inflammation of the lungs that can be caused by bacteria, viruses, or fungi.
- *Pneumothorax* is the collapse of a lung due to air in the chest cavity. The lung can develop an internal leak or air can enter through a hole from the outside, such as a gunshot or stab wound.
- *Tuberculosis* is a disease that damages the lungs and is caused by the tubercle bacillus (*Mycobacterium tuberculosis*). It is transmitted from person to person through the air.
- *Upper respiratory infection (URI)* is any infection of the upper respiratory structures. For example, *rhinitis* is an inflammation of the nasal mucosa resulting in a runny nose or congestion; *sinusitis* is an inflammation in the sinuses and can cause headache or pressure, congestion, discharge, and change in voice quality; *pharyngitis* (pharynx) causes a sore throat; *laryngitis* (larynx) is inflammation of the vocal cords and can result in hoarseness or loss of voice; *tonsillitis* is a painful inflammation of the lymph nodes. A URI includes the symptoms usually referred to as a common cold.

Preventive Measures

- Do not smoke.
- Use a protective mask when working around dust, toxic fumes, paints, cleaners, and so on.
- Maintain good posture.
- Take deep breaths occasionally.

Age-Related Changes: Respiratory (Pulmonary) System

- Decreased: Lung elasticity, lung expansion, functional alveoli, vital capacity, ciliary action, sense of smell
- Increased: Respiratory rate, diameter of chest (barrel chest), rigidity of lungs

Digestive

The *digestive system* provides energy for the body by processing food. All the cells require nutrients to do the work of building, repairing, and controlling body systems. Carbohydrates, proteins, and fats are taken in and converted into glucose, amino acids, and fatty acids that are distributed throughout the body through the capillaries. Minerals and vitamins do not require digestion, but can be absorbed directly by the capillaries. The body requires adequate amount of water to maintain and support functions. Undigested food products are eliminated by the digestive system. The entire digestive system consists of a long tube called the alimentary canal. This canal is about 30 feet long and extends from the mouth, where food is taken in, to the anus, where waste products are eliminated.

The digestive system uses both mechanical and chemical means to process food. Mechanically the food is chopped, mashed, and mixed. Chemically, food is broken down by digestive enzymes that are produced within the system or added by other organs. Enzymes break down food into absorbable nutrients.

The digestive system is often referred to as the *gastrointestinal system*. The main structures that participate in the digestion of food include the mouth, esophagus, stomach, small intestines, and large intestines. (See Figure 7–20.)

- Mouth: Food enters the mouth, where its taste triggers the saliva glands to produce digestive enzymes, which begin the breakdown of carbohydrates. The teeth chop and grind and the tongue mashes the food against the hard palate, mixing it with saliva. The mouth cools or warms the food to body temperature. The tongue moves the food to the back of the throat to be swallowed.
- Esophagus: A strong, muscular tube that connects the pharynx to the stomach. It lies behind the trachea and in front of the spinal column. It is composed of layers of muscle that contract to move the food. This action, called *peristalsis*, is controlled by the autonomic nervous system. Food passes into the stomach through the *cardiac sphincter*, which prevents the acidic content of the stomach from backflowing into the esophagus.
- Stomach: A muscular, elastic bag that fits under the diaphragm on the left side of the abdomen and is protected by the lower ribs. Food usually remains in the stomach for two to four hours while its muscles contract to mix it well with digestive juices. The glands in the stomach release hydrochloric acid to kill bacteria, pepsin

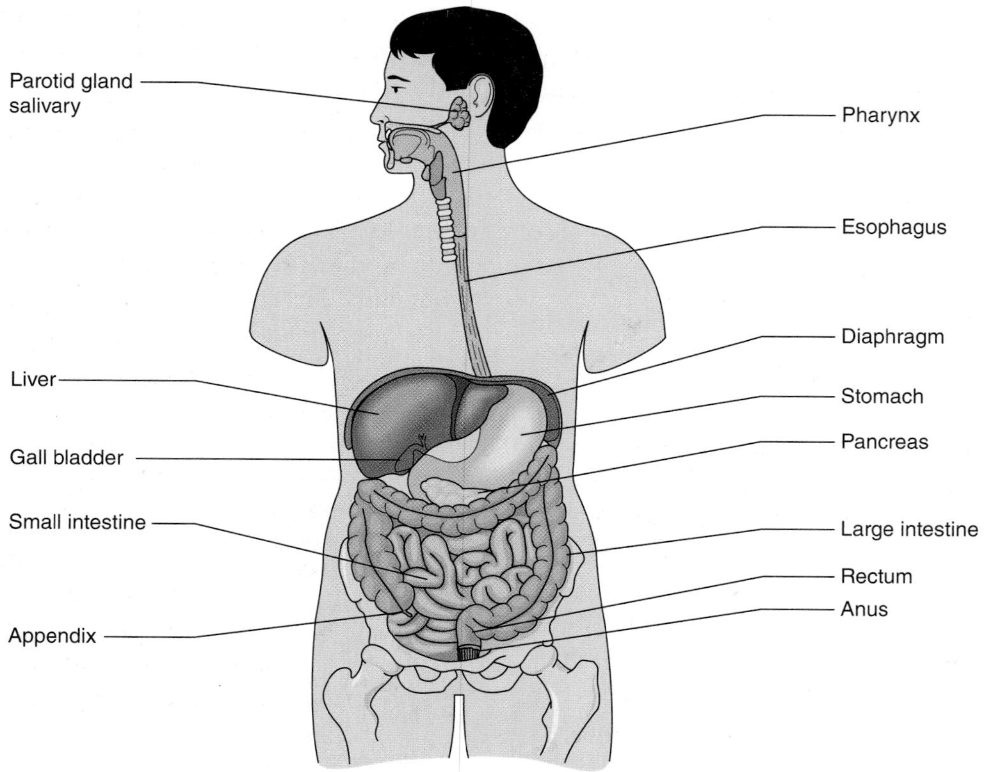

FIGURE 7–20 Structures of the digestive system.

to break down protein, and mucus to protect the stomach wall from the acidic gastric juices. When the partially digested food leaves the stomach, it goes through the pyloric sphincter and enters the small intestine.

- Small intestine: Also known as the small bowel, it consists of three parts: duodenum, jejunum, and ileum. Once the food passes into the small intestine, additional intestinal juices are added, including bile from the liver and pancreatic juice from the pancreas. Digestion continues, but absorption also begins to occur through a network of small, finger-like projections called *villi* that line the small intestine. Each villus contains a network of blood and lymph capillaries; the lymph system absorbs the fatty acids and the blood capillaries absorb the amino acids and simple sugars. Vitamins and minerals pass unchanged from the small intestine into the blood and lymph. The material leaving the small intestine normally consists only of indigestible substances, waste material, and excess water. This passes through the *ileocecal valve* into the large intestine.
- Large intestine: Also known as the large bowel. Nutrients and water not absorbed in the small intestine are absorbed here. The large intestine contains bacteria that work on the undigested substances and synthesize vitamin K (essential for blood clotting), as well as some of the B-complex vitamins (promote various body functions). The *appendix*, located just below the *ileocecal valve* in the lower right quadrant of the abdomen, has no known function. The last portion of the digestive system serves as a storage and elimination structure for indigestible substances.

Fascinating Facts

A sneeze can exceed the speed of 100 mph.

Every day, the average person produces about a quart of mucus. That comes to a total of over 25,000 quarts in a lifetime (calculated using 70 years), which is enough to fill two swimming pools. What happens to the mucus if it is not coughed out? It is swallowed! Typically, you swallow a quart of mucus every day.

Accessory organs:

- Liver: Located in the upper right quadrant under the diaphragm; produces thick, green liquid, called bile. Bile breaks down lipids (fat) into fatty acids for absorption. The liver has many other vital functions: maintaining blood sugar levels; filtering out and destroying old RBCs, saving the iron to be used again; storing vitamins; producing prothrombin, necessary for blood clotting; and filtering out harmful toxins (poisons) that have been swallowed, including alcohol and many drugs.
- Gallbladder: Small green organ located on the inferior side of the liver; stores bile made by the liver until it is needed for the digestion of fats.
- Pancreas: Located posterior to the stomach; excretes pancreatic digestive enzymes into the duodenum of the small intestine. These enzymes help digest proteins and fat. The pancreas also functions as an endocrine gland, which will be discussed under the endocrine system presented later in the chapter.

Major Diseases and Disorders

- *Appendicitis* is an inflammation of the appendix from unknown causes. The only treatment is surgical removal (appendectomy).
- *Ascites* is not a disease, but a general term used to describe the abnormal accumulation of fluid in the peritoneal cavity (space between the layers of the membrane that lines the abdominal and pelvic cavities). Cirrhosis, cancer, and advanced congestive heart failure can cause this condition.
- *Cirrhosis* is a group of chronic diseases that involve scarring of liver tissue, which decreases the ability of the liver to perform its functions.
- *Cholelithiasis* is the presence of stones in the gallbladder. *Cholecystitis* is an inflammation of the gallbladder.
- *Colon cancer* involves an abnormal growth in the large intestines that damages tissue and can cause a blockage of the digestive system.
- *Constipation* is the inability to pass feces, the body's waste that is passed through the anus. The most common causes are lack of dietary fiber, inadequate fluids, certain medications, and lack of exercise. It causes abdominal distension and discomfort.
- *Diarrhea* is the passage of frequent and watery stools. It can be caused by certain diseases, stress, medications, and diet.
- *Diverticulosis* is the weakening of the colon wall leading to an outpouching in the wall (diverticula). These diverticula can trap digestive material and become infected. *Diverticulitis* is an inflammation of the diverticula.
- *Gastroenteritis* is an inflammation of the mucous membranes that line the stomach and intestines. Causes include food poisoning, infection, and toxins. *Gastritis* is when the lining of the stomach becomes inflamed and can be caused by spicy foods and certain medications.
- *Heartburn* occurs when the gastric juices back up through the cardiac sphincter and irritate the lower end of the esophagus (the esophagus does not have a protective mucous membrane like the stomach does to protect it against the acidic juices).
- *Hemorrhoids* are painful, dilated veins in the lower rectum or anus.
- *Hepatitis* is an inflammation of the liver caused by a virus or poison.
- *Pancreatitis* is an inflammation of the pancreas that can be caused by a variety of factors.
- *Peritonitis* is a condition in which the lining (peritoneum) of the abdominal cavity becomes inflamed.
- An *ulcer* is an open sore in the lining of the digestive system. Pain occurs when the protective lining is damaged and the acidic juices come into contact with the delicate tissues underneath. A *peptic ulcer* can occur in the stomach or duodenum. Stomach ulcers are also called *gastric ulcers*. *Ulcerative colitis* is a severe inflammation of the colon with the formation of ulcers and abscesses (collection of pus in a cavity).

Age-Related Changes: Digestive (Gastrointestinal) System

- Decreased: Peristalsis; control of external sphincter; taste; saliva production; liver size, weight, and efficiency; gastric acid secretion; intestinal movement; appetite
- Increased: gum disease, constipation, indigestion

Preventive Measures

- Eat an adequate amount of fiber.
- Drink plenty of water.
- Avoid excessive alcohol.
- Follow standard precautions (Chapter 10).
- Avoid large amounts of high-fat foods.
- Avoid fad diets and other extreme eating habits.
- Avoid pushing hard during bowel movements (avoid constipation).
- Do not rely on the regular use of laxatives.
- Make routine dental appointments for examination and cleaning of teeth.
- Have flexible sigmoidoscopy or colonoscopy performed at the age and frequency recommended by your health care provider.

Fascinating Facts

In a lifetime, each individual spends about six years eating about 700,000 meals, which includes 60 tons of food. And don't forget the fluid—on the average, a person drinks 16,000 gallons of fluids.

Urinary

The *urinary system* eliminates excess water, salts, and waste products from the body. It consists of the kidneys, ureters, urinary bladder, and urethra. (See Figure 7–21.)

- Kidneys (2): Located behind the peritoneum (lining of the abdominal cavity) and on either side of the spinal column, below the diaphragm. The kidneys clean the blood and regulate the amount of water in the body. The artery that enters the kidney divides into a network of blood vessels that terminate in a grouping of capillaries called a *glomerulus*. Each glomerulus is surrounded by a kidney tubule that forms a capsule called *Bowman's capsule*. This intertwining of the blood capillaries and the kidney tubules is called a *nephron* and is where the real work of the kidney occurs: retaining waste products while returning most of the water, glucose, amino acids, and salts to the body. The nephrons, numbering more than 1 million per kidney, are located in the cortex (outer layer) of the kidney. The waste products flow into the *medulla* (inner layer) of the kidney, where water is returned to the body. The average daily fluid

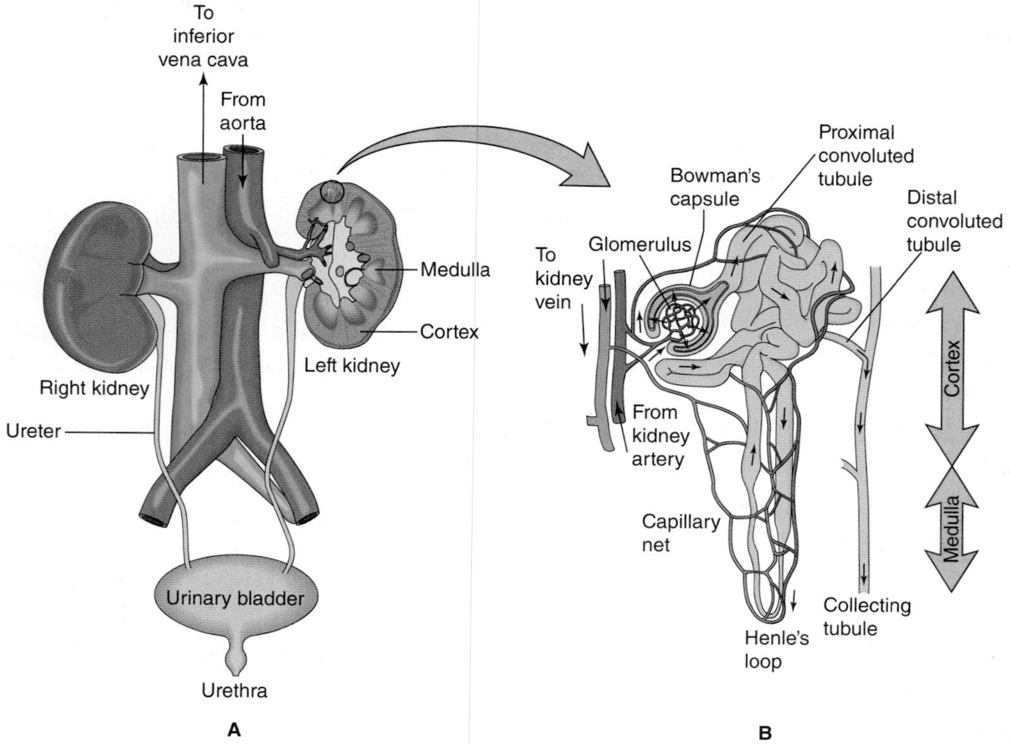

FIGURE 7–21 A. Structures of the urinary system. B. Nephron and related structures.

output of urine is about 1500 mL (1½ quarts), but varies with fluid intake.

- Ureters (2): The ureters connect the kidneys with the bladder, forming passageways for the urine.
- Urinary bladder: Stores urine, expanding and contracting its smooth-muscle walls as needed. When the bladder wall is stretched by a large amount of urine, the nerves in the wall send a message to the brain conveying the need to urinate. The opening to the urethra is kept closed by two sphincter muscles, one of which is under voluntary control.
- Urethra: The tube through which urine is passed to the outside of the body. Passage requires relaxation of the voluntary sphincter.

Media Link

View The Lymphatic System animation on the Online Resources for an overview of this system.

Major Diseases and Disorders

- *Edema* is not a disease but a general term used to describe the abnormal accumulation of fluid in the tissues. Kidney failure, congestive heart failure, and many other conditions can cause edema.
- *Kidney (renal) failure* occurs when the nephrons are unable to filter liquid waste from the blood. The buildup of waste products in the blood is called *uremia*. To sustain life, toxins are removed by regular *dialysis* treatments. Hemodialysis is a procedure in which the blood is passed through a device that functions as an artificial kidney.
- *Kidney (renal) calculi* are kidney stones and are usually composed of uric acid or calcium crystals.
- *Urinary incontinence* is the inability to control urination. *Urinary retention* is the inability to urinate when the urge is felt or the bladder is full. These conditions have many causes.
- *Urinary tract infection (UTI)* is an infection of the lower urinary structures. *Urethritis* is an inflammation of the urethra and *cystitis* is an inflammation of the bladder.
- *Kidney infections* include *nephritis* or *glomerulonephritis*, which refers to an inflammation of the glomerulus (nephrons). *Pyelonephritis* is an inflammation of the kidney tissue and renal pelvis (collecting part of the kidney that narrows into the ureter).

Preventive Measures

- Drink adequate amounts of water (eight glasses per day).
- Use proper toilet hygiene to prevent bladder infections.
- If you have hypertension or diabetes, manage it closely because both are primary contributors to renal failure.
- Be aware of and take cautiously any medications that can damage the kidneys. Never take illegal drugs.
- When taking antibiotics, increase your intake of water to prevent crystals from forming in the kidneys.

Fascinating Facts

The kidney is only about 4 inches long, 2 inches wide, and 1 inch thick, but it filters approximately 200 liters (quarts) of blood every day, removing two liters (quarts) of toxins, wastes, and water. It accomplishes this with a system of filters and tubes that stretch 140 miles.

Age-Related Changes: Urinary System

- Decreased: Glomerular filtration rate, renal blood flow, renal mass, functional nephron units, bladder capacity, sphincter muscle control
- Increased: Frequency and urgency of urination, nocturia (need to urinate during the night)

Systems for Sensing, Coordinating, and Controlling

The five senses (seeing, hearing, smelling, tasting, and touching) provide the brain with input from the external environment. The nervous system, in turn, interprets this input into sights, sounds, odors, flavors, or sensations of touch.

Eyes and Ears

The *eye* is often compared to a camera. It receives visual information from light rays through a transparent layer called the *cornea*. The light then enters an opening called the *pupil*, the round, black center of the eye. The *lens* projects the light rays on the *retina*, the innermost layer of the eye. (See Figure 7–22.) An upside-down image is produced, which is then converted to electrical signals and transmitted by the *optic nerve* to the brain, which "sees" it as right side up. A series of muscles attached to the eye coordinate movement so the eyes can focus.

The eye has three layers, the sclera, the choroid, and the retina (Figure 7–23):

- Sclera: The "white of the eye" is tough, fibrous tissue that serves as a protective shield. It contains the *cornea*.

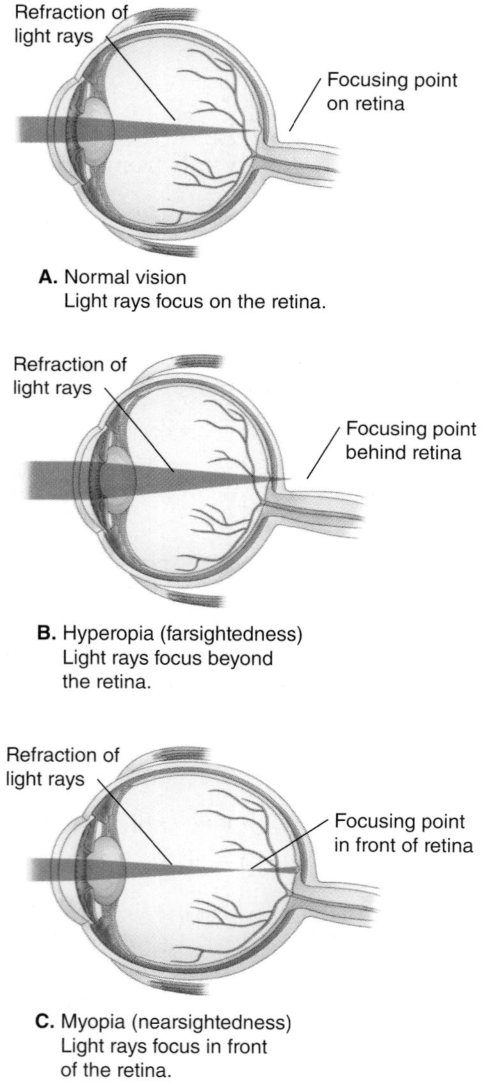

FIGURE 7–22 Normal vision occurs when the light rays are focused on the retina. An eyeball that is too long or too short prevents the proper focus.

- Choroid: Containing many blood vessels to nourish the eye, it includes the iris, pupil, and lens. The *iris* is the colored part, usually shades of blue, brown, or green and what people refer to when they say you have blue, brown, or hazel eyes. It is a sphincter muscle that controls the size of the pupil opening. In low light the iris relaxes, allowing the pupil to dilate and more light rays to enter for a better image. In bright light it contracts to protect the eye from too much light. Behind the pupil is the *lens* that is attached by ligaments to the *ciliary muscles*, which adjust the shape of the lens to ensure that a sharp image is projected on the retina.
- Retina: Thin membrane attached to the back of the eye on which images are projected. It contains two types of light-sensing receptors called *rods* and *cones*. The rods are responsible for seeing in dim light and the cones for seeing colors and in bright light.

A number of structures provide protection for the eye:

- Orbit: Skull bones that form protective cavities for the eye.
- Eyelids, eyelashes, and eyebrows: Eyelids help distribute moisture over the eye and remove small particles that get into the eye. They also automatically close when an object suddenly comes toward the eye. The eyebrows and eyelashes catch moisture and particles to prevent them from falling into the eye.
- Conjunctiva: Membrane that lines the underside of each eyelid and extends to the cornea on the surface of the eye.
- Lacrimal glands: Produce tears for cleaning and moisturizing the eye.
- Aqueous humor: A clear, watery fluid in the anterior chamber of the eye that bathes the iris, pupil, and lens.
- Vitreous humor: A clear, jelly-like fluid in the posterior chamber that maintains the shape of the eyeball and bends light rays.

Media Link

View the Digestion animation on the Online Resources for an overview of this system.

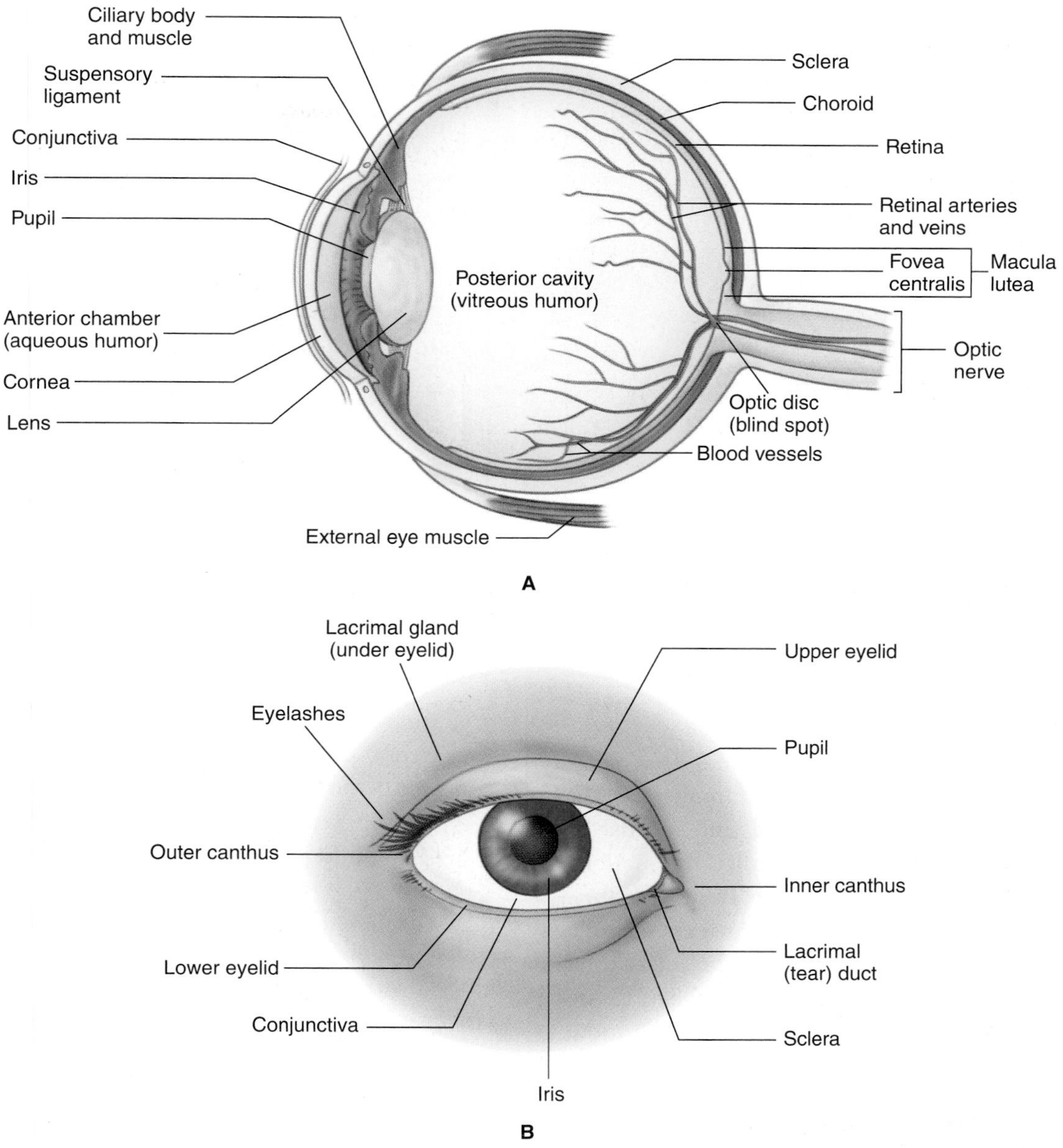

FIGURE 7–23 A. Internal view of the eye. B. External view of the eye.

The *ears* have both auditory (hearing) and balance organs. The outer ear collects sound waves, which are directed through a canal to the *eardrum*. When sound waves hit the eardrum, they set up a vibration that travels through the middle and inner ear chambers. From the *inner ear*, the vibration is converted to electrical signals and transmitted by the *auditory nerve* to the brain, which "hears" it as sounds, such as words and music.

The ear can be divided into three areas: the external (outer) ear, middle ear, and internal (inner) ear. Each has its own structures and functions (Figure 7–24):

Outer ear:

- Auricle: The outer, visible projection of the ear. Designed to direct sound waves into the ear canal.
- External auditory canal: The canal that extends from the outside to the eardrum. Earwax (cerumen) is produced by ceruminous glands to prevent foreign bodies from entering the ear.
- Eardrum (tympanic membrane): Located at the end of the external auditory canal, it separates the outer and middle ears. The membrane vibrates when hit by sound waves, which are then transmitted to the middle ear.

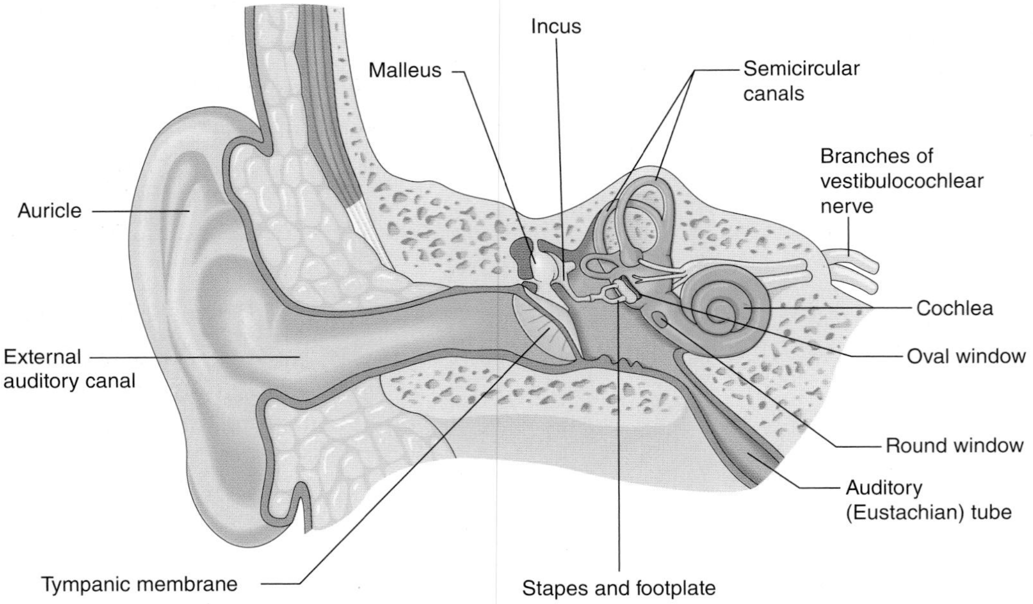

FIGURE 7–24 Structures of the ear.

Middle ear:

- Ossicles: Three tiny, delicate bones that form a chain to carry and amplify (make louder) sound vibrations from the eardrum. Because of their shapes, these bones are called the malleus (*hammer*), incus (*anvil*), and the stapes (*stirrup*). The malleus connects to the eardrum on one side and the incus on the other; the incus then connects to the stapes, which is attached to the *oval window* on its other side. The oval window separates the middle and inner ears.
- Eustachian tubes: Connect the nose and throat to the middle ear to equalize pressure. The uncomfortable sensations sometimes experienced in airplanes and under water are caused by sudden pressure changes. Chewing gum is recommended in airplanes because it helps open the tubes so that pressure is equalized.

Inner ear:

- Cochlea: A spiral-shaped, bony structure filled with fluid. The vibrations amplified in the middle ear set the fluid in motion. This movement of fluid then starts a wave-like motion in tiny, hair-like receptors, signals that the auditory nerve sends to the brain.
- Semicircular canals: These are the organs of balance (equilibrium). They contain receptor cells that report movements of the head. There are three canals: one is parallel to the ground; a second parallel to the side of the head; a third is parallel to the face. Dizziness experienced after spinning around rapidly is caused by movement of the fluid in these canals.

Media Link

View the Hearing animation on the Online Resources for an overview of this system.

Major Diseases and Disorders

Eyes:

- *Cataract* is the condition in which the lens of the eye loses its transparency, preventing light from reaching the inner eye.
- *Conjunctivitis* is an inflammation of the eyelid lining caused by bacteria or irritation from a particle of debris in the eye. It is sometimes referred to as "pink eye."
- *Glaucoma* occurs when the pressure within the eye increases. This pressure can cause deterioration of the optic nerve.
- *Macular degeneration* is a disorder of the retina that results in dimming and/or distortion of vision.
- *Visual impairments* include a number of very common problems that require corrective lenses.

For example, *myopia* (nearsightedness) occurs when the eyeball is longer than normal and cannot focus clearly on faraway objects. *Hyperopia* (farsightedness) occurs when the eyeball is shorter than normal and results in the inability to focus clearly on nearby objects. *Astigmatism* is an imperfect curvature of the cornea that results in blurred vision. *Presbyopia* is farsightedness caused by the loss of lens elasticity that occurs as part of the normal aging process. This is why many people over 40 need to wear "reading" glasses. (See Figure 7–22.)

Ears:

- *Hearing loss* is classified as either conductive or sensory. *Conductive hearing loss* occurs when the sound waves do not reach the inner ear (e.g., wax plug, ruptured eardrum, infection, or obstruction in ear). *Sensory hearing loss* results from damage to the inner ear or auditory nerve. Many cases of hearing loss can be treated with amplification devices (hearing aids), corrective surgery, or cochlear implants (a device that does not restore normal hearing, but allows the individual to hear sounds that can be interpreted for meaning).
- *Labyrinthitis* is an inflammation of the inner ear.
- *Otitis externa* is an inflammation of the external auditory canal. For example, *swimmer's ear* occurs in this part of the ear.
- *Otitis media* is an infection of the middle ear.
- *Ruptured eardrum* can occur as a result of infection, a sudden blow to the ear, or a violent change in air pressure such as occurs with an explosion or from an object placed in the ear. Ruptures usually heal without treatment, but massive or repeated injury can cause scar tissue to form and impair hearing.
- *Tinnitus* is not a disease but a medical term for ringing in the ears. It can only be heard by the patient (subjective) and can occur when there is wax buildup in the ear or an ear infection or as a result of an overdose of certain drugs (e.g., quinine or aspirin).

Preventive Measures

Eyes and ears:

- Wear UV-protective sunglasses when in the sun.
- Wear and clean contact lenses only as instructed.
- Get regular eye tests for glaucoma.
- Use eye protective devices around machinery and other hazards.
- Protect the ears from loud noises.
- Do not insert objects into the auditory canal.
- Use earplugs when swimming.

Age-Related Changes: Sensory System

Eyes:

- Decreased: Peripheral (side) vision, night vision
- Increased: Difficulty in reading small print and seeing objects at a distance, time to adjust from light to dark, sensitivity to glare

Fascinating Facts

Eye—Unlike cones, rods are able to detect light at a much lower level. This is why we see only black and white in dimly lighted rooms or while out viewing a star-filled night sky. *Ear*—The whole area of the middle ear is no bigger than an M&M.

The Maabans, an African tribe, live in such a quiet environment that they can hear a whisper from across the length of a baseball field, even when they are very old.

A busy urban street, diesel truck, or food blender are examples of 90 dB noises and cause hearing damage after eight hours. Thunderclaps or live rock music are 120 dB sounds and start to damage hearing after only seven and a half minutes. Earphones at a high level are 140 dB, and the eardrum ruptures at 150 dB.

Ears:

- Decreased: Ability to hear high-frequency sounds (e.g., telephone ringing, doorbell)
- Increased: Difficulty hearing when there is background noise (e.g., music or other people talking)

Nervous

The *nervous system* consists of the brain, spinal cord, and nerves. It detects sensations from all parts of the body and controls all the body's actions. It is also responsible for thoughts, emotions, and memories. A complex network of nerves constantly collects information from both inside and outside the body. This information is then transmitted by electrical stimuli through the spinal cord to the brain for interpretation. The information is stored, and if any response is required, such as pulling the hand away from a hot stove, direction is immediate and usually accomplished by coordinating the activities of other organ systems. In the case of the hot stove, communication would be with the muscles.

As learners read this paragraph, their nervous systems are performing numerous functions:

1. Directing the eyes to move across the page
2. Recognizing the images as letters and combining them to form words and sentences
3. Storing some of the ideas as memories
4. Recalling previous memories to help in understanding the new information
5. Directing skeletal muscles to maintain a sitting position
6. Causing the eyes to automatically blink to stay moist and clean
7. Controlling the heart rate, blood pressure, and respiration to keep fresh oxygen supplied to the brain to keep them alert
8. Sending sensations of tiredness or hunger after a few hours of studying

These eight examples are just a small fraction of what the nervous system is actually doing at any given moment. It is amazing how complex this system is and how well it works.

The brain makes up only about 2% of the body's weight, but uses 20% of the energy produced. It requires a constant supply of glucose (sugar) and oxygen to function. Low blood sugar causes the brain to partly shut down, resulting in feelings that begin as hunger and irritability and then progress to a weak, faint feeling. The brain is even more sensitive to the lack of oxygen, and brain cells begin to die within five minutes when they are deprived of oxygen.

Central Nervous System

The *central nervous system (CNS)* includes the brain and the spinal cord. The brain consists of the cerebrum, cerebellum, diencephalon, and brain stem. (See Figure 7–25.)

- Cerebrum: Two large hemispheres that control the higher brain functions. Their many folds (*convolutions*) greatly increase the brain's surface area and thus the storage capacity of the brain. The hemispheres are joined by bands of nerve fibers, including the *corpus callosum* that help the hemispheres communicate. Each hemisphere has a core of white matter surrounded by a layer of gray matter called the *cerebral cortex*. The cerebral cortex controls voluntary actions, including physical action (e.g., running, walking, and chewing), mental activity (e.g., learning,

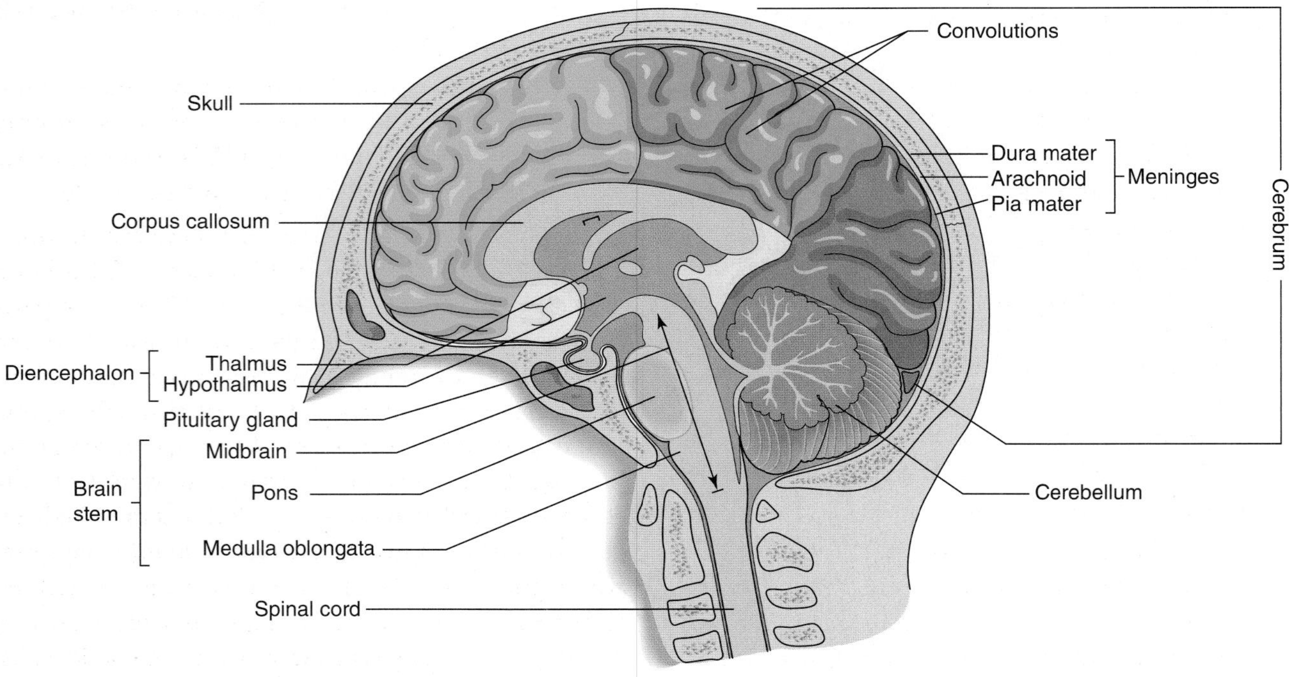

FIGURE 7–25 Cross-section of the brain.

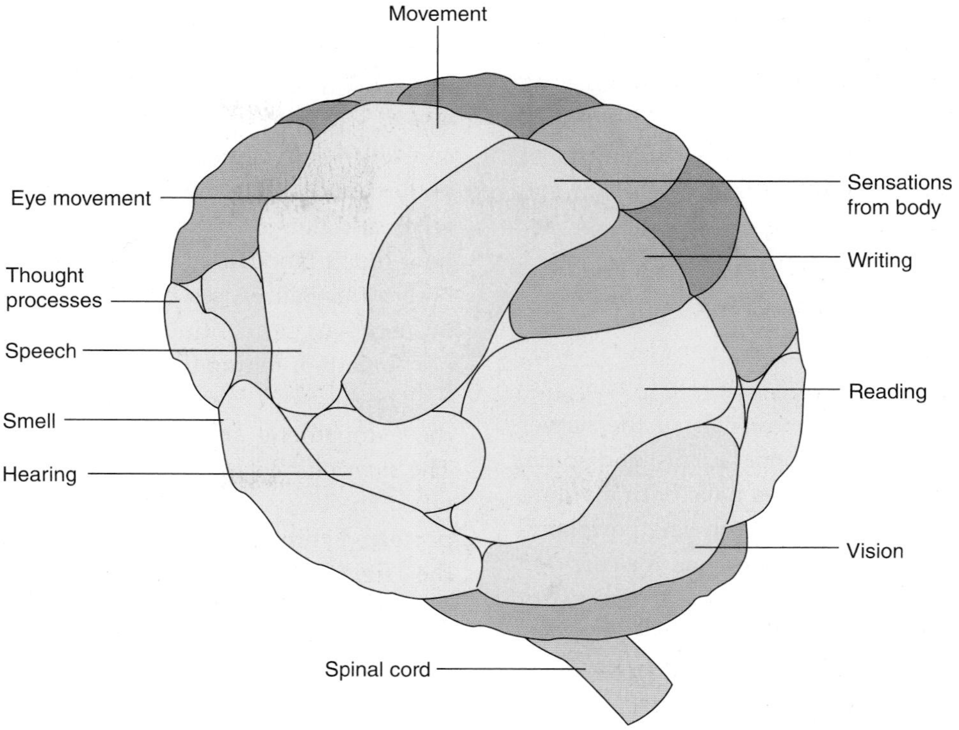

FIGURE 7–26 Functions of the cerebral cortex.

judgment, decision making, and creativity), conscious body sensations (sense of pleasure to what we see or how we are touched), and some emotions. (See Figure 7–26.) It is surprising to note that one hemisphere of the cortex controls the opposite side of the body. That is, the right hemisphere controls the left side of the body and vice versa. For example, a stroke that occurs on the right side of the brain can cause paralysis of the left arm and leg. The left hemisphere is generally responsible for learning academic subjects such as speech, reading, writing, math, and logic. The right hemisphere generally affects how an individual learns and the learning of the arts (enjoyment of music, artistic ability, creativity), and how an individual experiences emotions. When people refer to themselves as either right-brained or left-brained, they are describing their interests and abilities in these areas.

- Cerebellum: Located at the back of the brain between the cerebrum and brain stem. Working in conjunction with the cerebrum by fine-tuning and coordinating messages for muscular movement, it is also involved in balance, posture, and muscle tone.
- Diencephalon: Contains the *thalamus* and *hypothalamus*. The thalamus relays sensory stimuli to the cerebral cortex. The hypothalamus initiates and controls many involuntary body functions necessary for living, such as water balance and body temperature.
- Brain stem: Consists of the midbrain, pons, and medulla oblongata. It serves as a pathway between the spinal cord and brain and regulates respiration, blood pressure, and heart rate.

The *spinal cord* carries messages between the brain and other parts of the body. It is attached to the brain and is encased in the spinal column. Thirty-two pairs of nerves branch out from the cord, passing between vertebrae and extending to the various parts of the body. Once the nerves branch off from the spinal cord, they are part of the peripheral nervous system.

Besides carrying messages to and from the brain, the spinal cord also serves as a reflex center. Reflexes are automatic responses that do not require any communication with the brain. For example, the jerking that occurs when the doctor taps the knee, elbow, or wrist during a physical exam is an automatic reflex action. Also, when a finger touches a hot surface, a reflex occurs to pull it away. The reason pain is not felt until after the finger is removed from the hot surface is that the sensation must travel through the spinal cord to the brain for interpretation as pain.

The brain and spinal cord are protected not only by bone (skull and vertebrae), but also by membranes and a fluid cushion. Wrapped around the brain and spinal cord are three layers of protective membranes called *meninges*. The two innermost meningeal layers form a space where *cerebrospinal fluid (CSF)* flows around the brain and spinal cord.

Peripheral Nervous System

The *peripheral nervous system* consists of the nerves that emerge from the brain (*cranial nerves*) and spinal cord (*spinal nerves*). These nerves have both a voluntary and an involuntary component. The peripheral nerves contain two types of fibers, one for carrying messages to the central nervous system (sensory fibers) and another for carrying messages from the central nervous system to the skeletal muscles (motor fibers). (See Figure 7–27.)

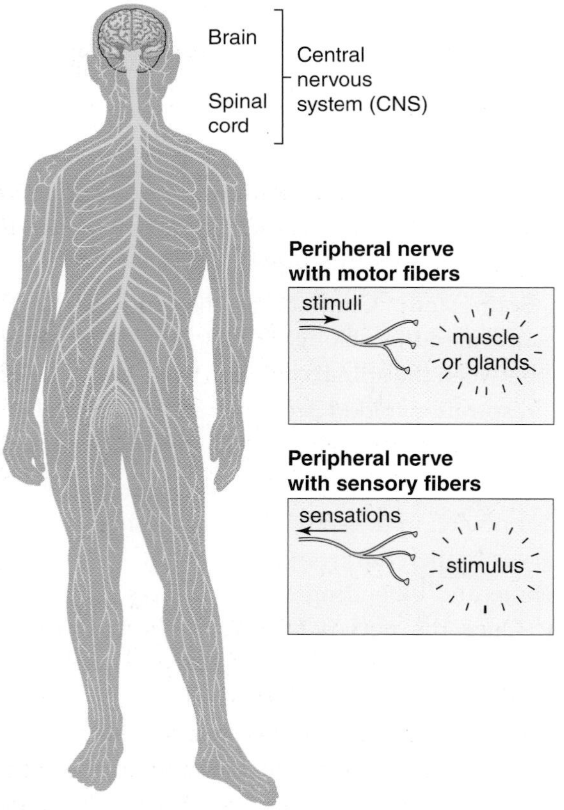

FIGURE 7–27 The peripheral nervous system connects the CNS to the structures of the body. When the peripheral nerve contains both motor and sensory fibers, it is called a mixed nerve.

The *involuntary nerves* of the peripheral nervous system contain fibers leading to and from the internal organs. These nerves belong to the *autonomic nervous system*, which means the individual has no voluntary control over the actions involved. For example, the body cannot be told when and how to digest food, when and how much urine to produce, or where and how much blood to circulate. It is a good thing the body's internal processes are automated or it would be necessary to continually think about taking the next breath or telling the heart to beat.

The autonomic nervous system can be divided into the sympathetic and the parasympathetic systems. The *sympathetic system* is activated in times of stress when the body senses the need to get away from a perceived threat or danger, commonly referred to as the "fight or flight" reaction. The sympathetic nervous system can make the difference between life and death. For example, in a crisis this system has enabled people to perform amazing feats of strength during rescues. But the body cannot tolerate prolonged stress without suffering physical or mental harm. The *parasympathetic system* maintains normal function on a day-to-day basis. (See Table 7–3.)

The autonomic nervous system works closely with the hormones produced by the hypothalamus. This will be discussed in the section on the endocrine system.

Neurons

There are billions of *neurons* (nerve cells) in the body, the majority of them located in the brain. Neurons grow rapidly before birth, and then stop reproducing after birth. When a person learns a new skill, new brain cells are not being produced. Rather, the neurons are trained to connect in a new way. New ideas come from new connections between neurons. When people who have brain damage are relearning to speak or walk, they are working to establish new connections between the neurons they had at birth. Damaged cells may be able to repair themselves, but dead ones cannot be replaced.

The neuron consists of a *cell body*, from which branch several dendrites and one axon. The *dendrites* are short fibers that bring electrical signals to the cell body, and an *axon* is a long fiber that carries the signal away from the cell body. Some of the neurons are covered in a fatty material called *myelin*. (See Figure 7–28.) Myelin-covered fibers can transmit impulses much faster than uncovered fibers. The myelin gives a

Table 7–3 Actions of the Sympathetic and Parasympathetic Nervous Systems

System or Organ	Sympathetic System (to cope with emergencies) "fight or flight"	Parasympathetic System (normal daily functions) "rest and digest"
Heart	Increases rate and force of contraction, which enhances blood flow to skeletal muscles	Decreases rate and force of contraction
Lungs	Dilates airways (bronchioles) to take in more oxygen for body	Constricts the diameter of the air passages (bronchioles) when the need for oxygen has diminished
Arteries	Constricts arteries, thus raising blood pressure	Dilates arteries to lower blood pressure
Gastrointestinal	Diverts blood flow away from the gastrointestinal (GI) tract and skin via vasoconstriction. This results in a slowing of peristalsis and digestive activity to send more blood to the brain and skeletal muscles	Dilates blood vessels leading to the GI tract, increasing blood flow. Speeds peristalsis, increases salivary gland production and digestion to aid in absorption of nutrients
Urinary	Relaxes bladder	Constricts bladder, thus encouraging urination
Eye muscles	Dilates pupils and relaxes the lens, allowing more light to enter the eyes	Constricts pupils and lens
Sweat glands	Increases secretion to prevent overheating of body	Decreases secretion
Hair muscles	Contracts muscles and causes piloerection (goose bumps)	Relaxes muscles, causes hair to lie flat

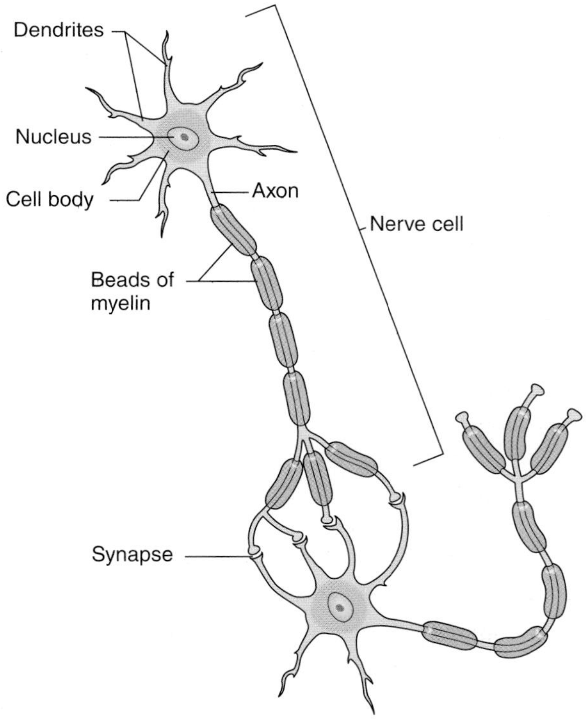

FIGURE 7–28 The neuron.

white appearance to the neurons. For example, the white matter of the cerebrum is covered with myelin, and the gray matter (cerebral cortex) is not.

The neurons do not actually touch each other when impulses are transmitted. When the axon of one cell reaches a dendrite of another cell, they are separated by a gap, called a *synapse*. The electric impulse crosses the synapse with the help of chemicals called *neurotransmitters*. For a summary overview of the nervous system, see Figure 7–29.

Major Diseases and Disorders

- *Cerebral palsy* is caused by brain damage and results in a lack of control over the voluntary muscles.
- A *cerebrovascular accident (CVA)* involves the brain and its blood supply and is commonly referred to as a "stroke." A CVA can be caused by a block in the blood flow (e.g., emboli) or result from a ruptured vessel. The disruption of blood flow to the brain can cause tissue damage or even death. The signs and symptoms

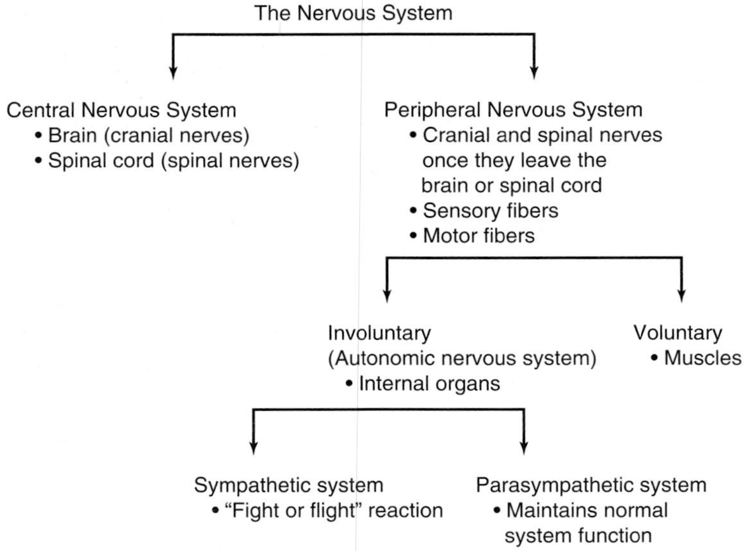

FIGURE 7–29 Overview of the nervous system.

will depend on what part of the brain has been damaged. Common results are paralysis of one side of the body (*hemiplegia*) and difficulty in or inability to communicate through speech, writing, or signs (*aphasia*). *Transient ischemic attacks (TIAs)*, called "ministrokes," occur when blood flow is only temporarily impaired. TIAs may be warning signs of a future CVA.

- *Dementia* is a loss of memory and impairment of intellectual function. *Alzheimer's disease* is only one of several diseases that cause dementia. *Senile dementia* refers to dementia when it occurs in the elderly.
- *Encephalitis* is an infection of the brain.
- *Epilepsy* is a disorder of the brain resulting from abnormal electrical impulses in the neurons. Seizures can range from very mild (petit mal) to generalized severe seizures (grand mal). Anticonvulsant drugs are very effective in controlling epilepsy.
- *Meningitis* is the inflammation of the protective covering (meninges) of the brain and spinal cord.
- *Multiple sclerosis* is a chronic, progressive, disabling condition resulting from a defect in electrical transmission of the neurons, which is caused by degeneration of the myelin sheath.
- *Neuritis* is the inflammation of a nerve. *Neuralgia* is nerve pain.
- *Parkinson's disease* is a chronic, progressive condition involving degeneration of brain cells because of a decrease in a neurotransmitter (dopamine). It is characterized by tremors, shuffling walk, muscle rigidity, and loss of facial expression.
- *Shingles (herpes zoster)* is caused by a virus. Blisters appear on the skin following the nerve pathways. It is very painful, and even after the blisters heal, pain can be experienced for years along these nerve pathways.
- *Spinal cord injury* results in a loss of sensation and voluntary movement. The location of the injury determines the amount of impairment. If the injury is in the lower portion of the spinal column, only the lower half of the body is affected. This is called *paraplegia*. If the injury is in the upper portion of the cord, all four extremities can be affected. This is called *quadriplegia*.

Fascinating Facts

Nerve impulses in your body travel at various speeds. A nerve impulse to signal removing a hand from a hot stove may travel as high as 330 feet (100 meters) per second. Intellectual pursuit impulses travel much slower, at 70 to 100 feet (20 to 30 meters) per second.

Preventive Measures

- Do not use illegal drugs.
- Avoid excessive alcohol.
- Continue learning new things throughout life.
- Use protective devices such as helmets and seat belts.
- Get sufficient sleep.

Age-Related Changes: Nervous System

- Decreased: Response and reaction time, number of brain cells, amount of neurotransmitters, ability to sleep, balance and coordination, cerebral blood flow
- Increased: Awakenings during sleep, muscle tremors

Endocrine

The *endocrine system* consists of glands that manufacture hormones. A *hormone* is a chemical substance secreted by a gland in one part of the body that travels via the bloodstream to direct changes in the activities of other organ systems. There are many different hormones, and each has its own function.

The nervous and endocrine systems work closely together to coordinate and control the body's functions. For example, recall that the sympathetic nervous system is stimulated in times of crisis. This is caused by a hormone secreted by the adrenal glands, part of the endocrine system.

There are two types of glands: exocrine and endocrine glands. *Exocrine* glands do not produce hormones, but rather produce liquids that flow through a duct (small tube) to reach a body cavity or to the surface of the skin. Examples of exocrine secretions are sweat, saliva, mucus, and digestive juices. The pancreas has the unique characteristic of being both an exocrine (secretes digestive enzyme) and an endocrine gland (produces the hormone insulin).

The hypothalamus is attached to the brain and spinal cord by many nerves. This organ links the autonomic nervous system and endocrine system. It plays an important role in the regulation of most of the involuntary mechanisms of the body and regulates the work of the pituitary gland.

The pituitary gland is often called the "master gland" because it secretes hormones that stimulate other endocrine glands to produce their own hormones. An important feature of the endocrine system is the *feedback mechanism*. This mechanism is similar to the thermostat that controls the temperature in a house. The thermostat measures the internal temperature and then turns heat or air conditioning off or on as needed to maintain the desired temperature. In a similar way, the pituitary determines if there is enough of each hormone circulating in the bloodstream and turns the stimuli to produce hormones on and off. Study Figure 7–30 and Table 7–4 to learn more about each of the endocrine glands, the hormones they produce, and the actions of the hormones. The ovaries and testes are part of the endocrine system, but will be discussed with the female and male reproductive systems.

Major Diseases and Disorders

Adrenal glands:

- *Addison's disease* is caused by inadequate hormone production by the adrenal cortex. It causes excessive skin pigmentation, decreased sugar and salt in the blood, and decreased blood pressure.
- *Cushing's syndrome* is caused by excessive hormone production of the adrenal cortex triggered by oversecretion of adrenocorticotropic hormone (ACTH, from the anterior lobe of pituitary). This results in a redistribution of fat to create a more rounded face (*"moon face"*) and a hump below the back of the neck (*"buffalo hump"*). It also causes increased blood pressure; unusual hair growth, called *hirsutism*; and easy bruising.

Pancreas:

- *Diabetes mellitus* is caused by inadequate insulin production. This results in *hyperglycemia* (too much glucose in the blood). The signs and symptoms are *polydipsia* (unusual thirst), *polyuria* (increased urine output), and *polyphagia* (unusual hunger).

Parathyroid glands:

- *Hyperparathyroidism* is caused by excessive parathormone that results in an increased calcium blood level. The excessive calcium levels cause stone formation in the urinary system and elsewhere. The bones are also robbed of their calcium, and this makes them vulnerable to fractures.
- *Hypoparathyroidism* is caused by inadequate parathormone and results in a decreased calcium

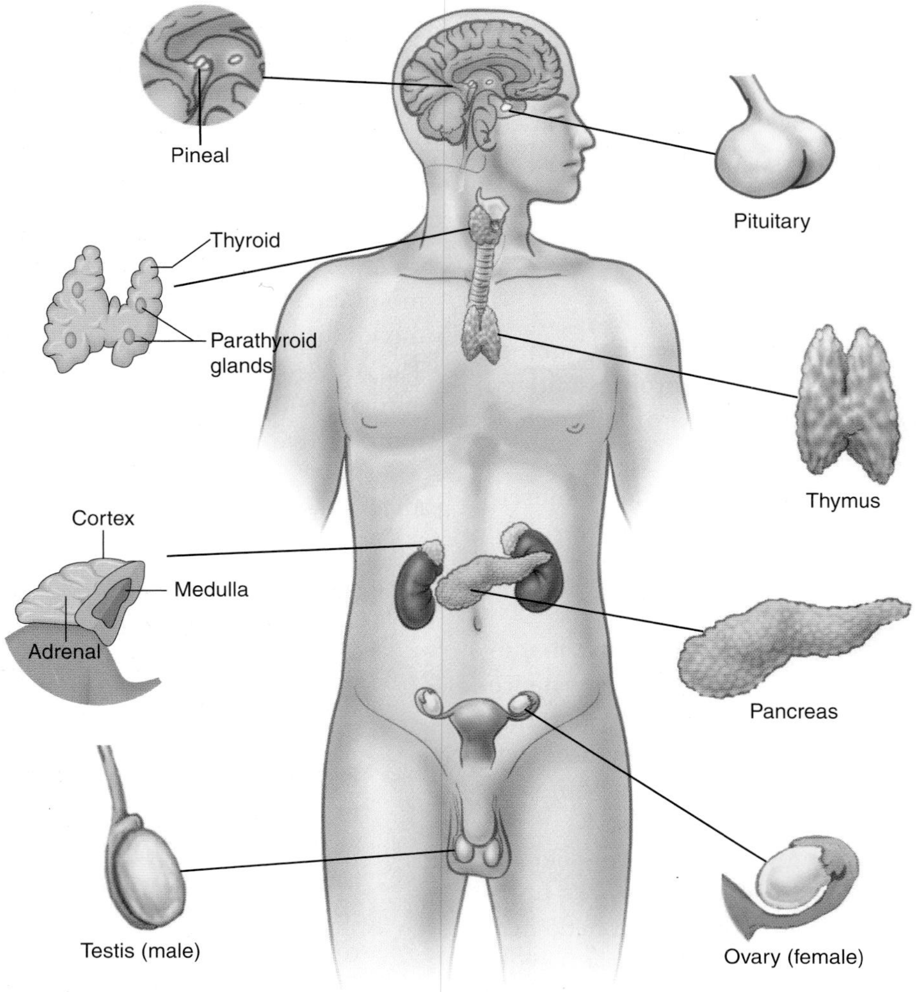

FIGURE 7–30 Locations of the endocrine glands.

Table 7–4 Hormones and Their Actions

Gland and Location	Hormone	Actions
Pituitary (cranium)		
Anterior lobe:	GH—growth hormone	Directs normal growth of body tissues
	ACTH—adrenocorticotropic hormone	Stimulates cortex of adrenal gland
	TSH—thyroid-stimulating hormone	Stimulates thyroid gland
	MSH—melanocyte-stimulating hormone	Stimulates production of melanin, which causes skin pigmentation
	FSH—follicle-stimulating hormone	Promotes egg development in the female and sperm production in the male
	LH—luteinizing hormone	Stimulates ovulation and production of female hormones (estrogen and progesterone)

(continues)

Table 7–4 Hormones and Their Actions (continued)

Gland and Location	Hormone	Actions
	ICSH—interstitial cell-stimulating hormone	Stimulates production of male hormone (testosterone)
	LTH—lactogenic hormone or prolactin	Promotes development of breast tissue and production of milk in females
Posterior lobe:	ADH—antidiuretic hormone, or vasopressin	Acts on kidneys to concentrate urine and conserve fluid in the body; also constricts blood vessels
	Oxytocin (pitocin)	Causes contraction of uterus during childbirth; stimulates milk flow
Pineal (cranium)	Melatonin	Controls onset of puberty; affects wake/sleep cycle
Thyroid (neck)	Thyroxine (T_4) and triiodothyronine (T_3)	Controls metabolism and stimulates physical and mental growth
	Calcitonin	Moves calcium from the bloodstream into the bones for storage
Parathyroid (neck)	PTH—parathormone	Promotes absorption of calcium from the intestines, decreases calcium excretion by the kidneys, and moves calcium from the bones to the blood (opposite effect of calcitonin)
Thymus (chest beneath sternum)	Thymosin	Stimulates production of antibodies in early life
Adrenals: (one on top of each kidney)		
Cortex:	Mineralocorticoids (aldosterone)	Regulates the balance of electrolytes (chemicals that, when dissolved in water, can conduct electrical current) by stimulating the kidneys to retain salt (sodium) and excrete potassium
	Glucocorticoids (cortisone)	Aids in metabolism of proteins, fats, and carbohydrates; provides resistance to stress; depresses immune responses (anti-inflammatory)
	Gonadocorticoids (androgens)	Sex hormone, produced by both males and females; function is unclear
Medulla:	Epinephrine (adrenaline) and norepinephrine	Activates sympathetic nervous system in times of stress; increases blood pressure by constricting blood vessels
Pancreas (mid-abdomen under stomach)	Insulin	Regulates the transport of glucose (sugar) from the blood into the body cells
	Glucagon	Increases the amount of glucose in the blood by stimulating the liver to convert glycogen (stored form of glucose) to glucose (type of sugar that is the main source of energy to cells)

blood level that interrupts the normal function of nerves. This causes a condition called *tetany*, convulsive muscle twitching, and can lead to death if the respiratory muscles are affected.

Pituitary gland:

- *Acromegaly* is caused by excessive growth hormone (anterior lobe of pituitary) in adults. It causes an enlargement in the bones of the hands, feet, and jaw.
- *Diabetes insipidus* is caused by a decrease in antidiuretic hormone (posterior lobe of pituitary). It causes an increase in urine production that can lead to dehydration and electrolyte imbalances.
- *Dwarfism* can be caused by inadequate secretion of growth hormone as a child develops. The body does not develop to an average adult size.
- *Gigantism* is caused by excessive secretion of growth hormone as a child develops. This causes elongation of the long bones and results in excessive height.

Thyroid glands:

- *Hyperthyroidism* is caused by excessive thyroid hormones. It results in nervousness, increased pulse rate, weight loss, irritability, sensitivity to heat, and increased blood sugar.
- *Hypothyroidism* is caused by inadequate thyroid hormones. Hypothyroidism results in edema (excessive fluid in tissues), obesity, lethargy (extreme fatigue), decrease in heart rate, decreased mental function, cold sensitivity, and thinning of the hair.

Media Link

View the Urine Formation animation on the Online Resources for an overview of this system.

Preventive Measures

- Maintain healthy weight.
- Avoid excessive refined sugars.
- Take children for checkups to monitor growth and development.
- Avoid the use of steroids unless prescribed (never use for purposes of muscle building during weight training programs).

Age-Related Changes: Endocrine System

- Decreased: Thyroid gland function, basal metabolic rate (energy needed to maintain body functions), adrenal gland function, insulin release, ability to break down glucose to provide energy for the body
- Increased: Incidence of hyperglycemia (increase in blood sugar) with ingestion of sugar

Systems for Producing New Life

Reproduction is one of the most fundamental functions common to all living organisms. The reproductive system allows the creation of a new human being who is both like and unlike each of the two parents. Reproduction is essential for the continuation of human life on the earth.

Female Reproductive

The *female reproductive system* can be divided into the internal and external reproductive organs (Figure 7–31).

Internal reproductive organs:

- Ovaries: There are two ovaries, one on each side of the uterus, which is located in the lower abdomen. They produce the hormones *estrogen* and *progesterone*, which determine the female characteristics (body shape, hair patterns, and breast development) and are necessary for pregnancy

Thinking It Through

Mary Steward recently retired after 40 years of teaching high school. Since her retirement, she has noticed that she is increasingly tired, sleeping much more than usual, and seems to feel cold all the time. She loved her job and at first thought that her tiredness was just part of adjusting to retirement and that feeling cold was from lack of exercise. But the symptoms have become more severe, and she made an appointment with her family physician. After an examination and blood work, Mrs. Steward is informed that she has hypothyroidism.

1. What is the function of the thyroid gland?
2. Based on the symptoms, does Mrs. Steward have too much or too little thyroid function?
3. Is the thyroid an exocrine or endocrine gland? Why?

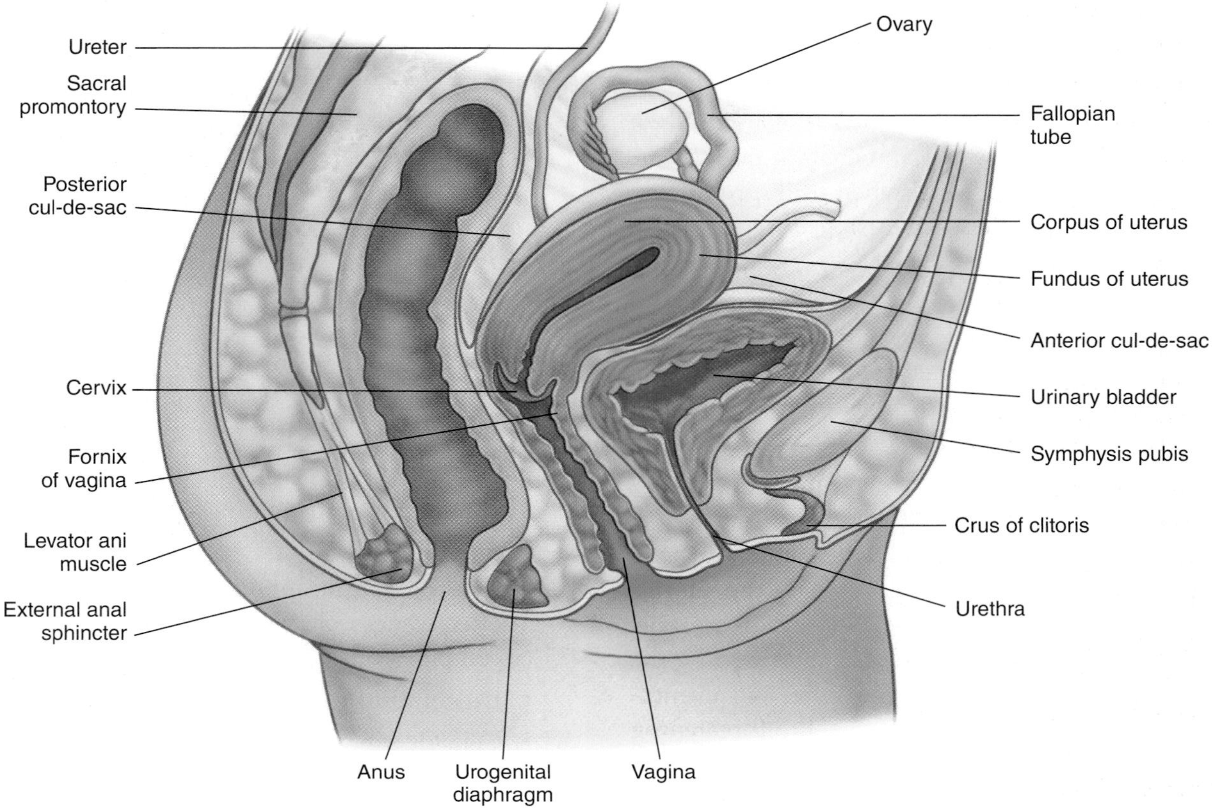

FIGURE 7–31 Cross-section of the female reproductive organs.

and subsequent childbirth to occur. Within each ovary are tiny sacs called *graafian follicles*, each of which contains one *ovum* (egg). The ovum is the female sex cell.

- Fallopian tubes: Arise from the upper portion of the uterus and end in finger-like projections (*fimbriae*) that draw the ovum, released from an ovary, down into the tube. Sperm (male sex cells) travel up into these tubes, which is where fertilization takes place. Once fertilized, the ovum moves down into the uterus.
- Uterus (womb): A muscular, hollow organ located behind the urinary bladder and in front of the rectum. It has three parts: the *fundus* (upper portion where fallopian tubes attach), the *corpus* (body or middle section), and the *cervix* (narrow, bottom area that attaches to the vagina). When the fertilized ovum reaches the uterus, it implants itself into the wall and grows and develops into a fetus. If a fertilized ovum is not implanted, the lining of the uterus is shed and menstruation occurs.
- Vagina: Opening that connects the outside of the body to the uterus. Made of smooth muscle and lined with a mucous membrane, it is capable of expanding to allow for childbirth and then contracting back to original size.

External reproductive organs (*genitalia*):

- Labia majora: Large fleshy folds of fat tissue that surround and protect the opening of the external female genitalia. They are covered with hair on their outer surfaces.

Media Link

View the Female Reproductive System animation on the Online Resources for an overview of this system.

- Labia minora: Smaller fleshy folds that lay inside the boundaries of the labia majora for further protection.
- Clitoris: Located at the top junction of the labia minora, this is a very sensitive organ composed of erectile tissue similar to that of the male penis.

- Bartholin's glands: Located on each side of the external opening of the vagina, these produce mucus secretions that lubricate the vagina.

The *breasts (mammary glands)* are composed of connective and fatty tissues and contain milk ducts. The female hormones signal when milk production (*lactation*) is needed after childbirth.

Major Diseases and Disorders

- *Menstrual disorders* can result from hormonal imbalances, structural deformities, excessive exercise or stress, and nutritional imbalances. *Amenorrhea* is the absence of menstruation. *Menorrhagia* is excessive bleeding. *Dysmenorrhea* is painful menstrual cramps.
- *Ectopic pregnancy* occurs when the fertilized ovum becomes implanted outside the uterus. The most common site is in the fallopian tube. As the embryo develops, pain is caused by the distension of the tube. The tube will eventually rupture, which creates a life-threatening situation if excessive internal bleeding occurs.
- *Endometriosis* is the growth of endometrial tissue (which lines the uterus) outside the uterus. The tissue can be transferred from the uterus by the fallopian tubes, blood, lymph, or during surgery.
- *Fibroid tumors* are tumors in the uterus. They are usually benign (not cancerous) and often produce no symptoms.
- *Pelvic inflammatory disease (PID)* is an inflammation of all the pelvic reproductive organs and causes scarring of the fallopian tubes. This can lead to an increased occurrence of ectopic pregnancies and infertility. Sexually transmitted diseases are often the cause of PID.
- *Premenstrual syndrome (PMS)* is a general term for a variety of symptoms that occur prior to the beginning of bleeding (menses). They include irritability, depression, impaired concentration, headache, and edema. PMS may be related to hormonal, biochemical, or nutritional imbalances.
- *Sexually transmitted disease (STD)* or venereal disease is a general term that refers to any disease transmitted through sexual contact. Examples include gonorrhea, syphilis, chlamydia, scabies, pubic lice, genital herpes, genital warts, trichomoniasis, and AIDS.
- *Vaginitis* is a nonspecific infection of the vagina.

> **Fascinating Facts**
>
> All of the graafian follicles that a woman will ever have are present in the ovary at birth. During ovulation, typically only one will mature and be released.

Preventive Measures

- Practice safe sex if sexually active (Chapter 12).
- Use good toilet hygiene.
- If menstrual irregularities occur or PMS is severe, have your health care provider perform an evaluation.
- Have early and routine examinations during pregnancy.
- If using contraception, be informed about the effectiveness of the method and any potential complications.
- Do not routinely perform douches.
- Consult a health care provider if sexual intercourse is uncomfortable or painful.
- Do monthly self-examination of the breasts. Report any lumps or irregularities to your health care provider for further evaluation.
- Have Pap smears and breast examinations (including mammograms) at the age and frequency recommended by your health care provider.
- Report any sores or growths on labia and any unusual vaginal discharge or itching.

Age-Related Changes: Female Reproductive System

- Decreased: Vaginal lubrication
- Increased: Susceptibility to vaginal infections

Male Reproductive

Most parts of the male reproductive system are located outside the body because sperm are heat sensitive and would not survive normal body temperatures (Figure 7–32):

- Testes (testicles): The two testes are encased in a sac-like structure known as the scrotum and manufacture sperm (spermatozoa), the male sex cell. Once sperm is manufactured, it is stored in the epididymis, a coiled duct along the back part of the testes. During ejaculation (expulsion of the semen from the body), the sperm travels

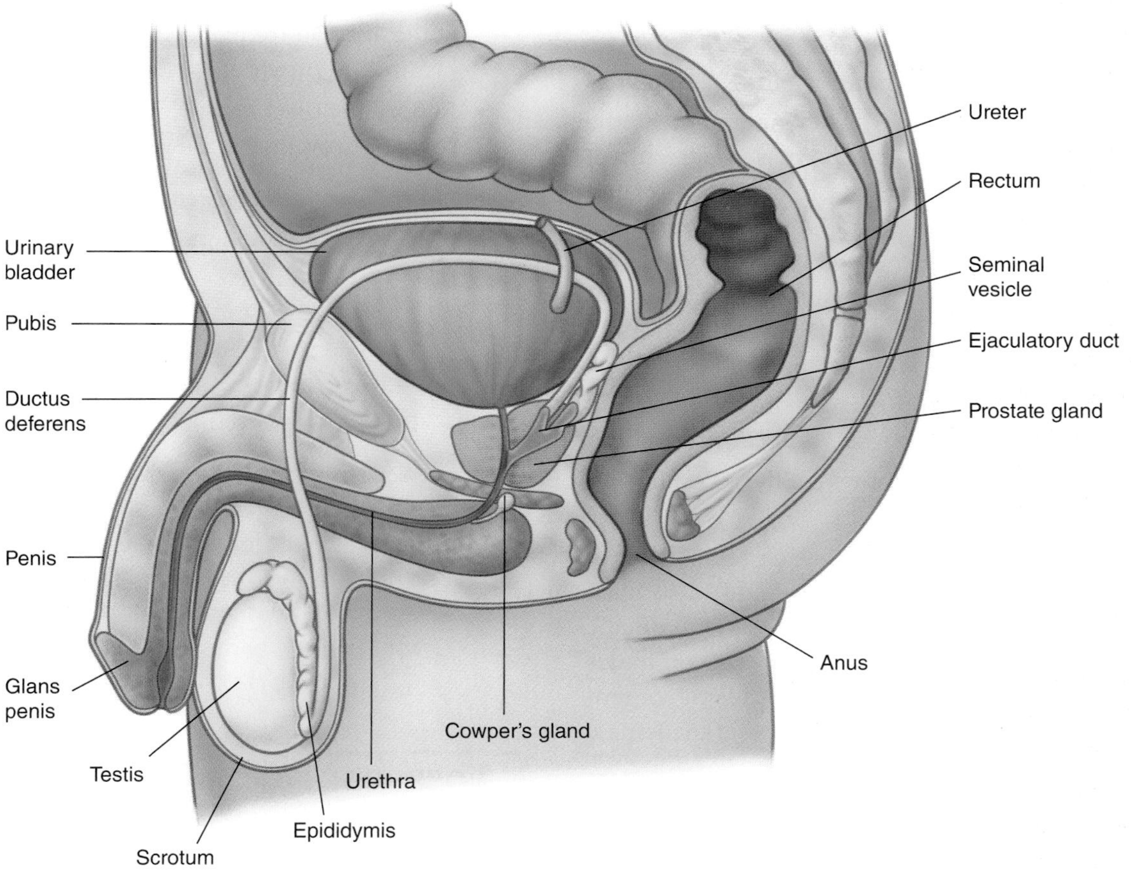

FIGURE 7–32 Cross-section of the male reproductive organs.

through a small tube (vas deferens) that enters the lower pelvic area, goes around the urinary bladder, and back down to join the urethra. The testes also produce a male hormone called testosterone, which aids in the maturation of sperm and is responsible for the development of male characteristics (body and facial hair, large muscles, and deep voice).

- Seminal vesicles: These glands join at the final portion of the vas deferens to form the ejaculatory duct. They produce a thick, yellow secretion that nourishes the sperm.
- Prostate gland: Secretes an alkaline fluid into the ejaculatory duct to aid in the movement of sperm (motility) and neutralize the acidity of the vagina. It contracts during ejaculation to propel the semen forward and to close off the urethra to prevent urine from passing at the same time.
- Penis: Composed of erectile tissue that when aroused fills with blood and becomes erect. At the distal end of the penis is an enlarged area known as the glans penis that is covered with a prepuce (foreskin). The foreskin is sometimes removed in a surgical procedure called circumcision.
- Urethra: Connects to the urinary bladder, passes through the penis, and exits at the end of the penis through an external opening called a meatus. It serves as a dual passageway for both urine from the urinary bladder and semen from the reproductive tubes.
- Cowper's (bulbourethral) gland: Produces a thick, white, alkaline secretion to lubricate the urethra and decrease the acidity of urine residue in the urethra.

Media Link

View the Vision animation on the Online Resources for an overview of this system.

Major Diseases and Disorders

- *Epididymitis* is an inflammation of the epididymis. It causes intense pain, swelling, and fever.
- *Prostatic hypertrophy* is an enlargement of the prostate that causes symptoms as a result of pressing on the urethra. It can be an age-related condition known as *benign prostatic hypertrophy (BPH).* It can also be caused by an inflammation, change in hormonal activity, benign (noncancerous) tumor, or malignant (cancerous) tumor.
- *Orchitis* is inflammation of the testes. It causes swelling of the scrotum, pain, and fever. It can lead to atrophy of the testes and cause sterility.
- *Phimosis* refers to a tightness of the foreskin over the end of the penis.
- *Sexually transmitted diseases*—see section under female reproductive diseases and disorders. Some of the diseases listed are asymptomatic (have no symptoms) in males. However, males can be carriers of the disease-causing organism and require treatment to prevent the female from being infected.

Preventive Measures

- Practice safe sex if sexually active (Chapter12).
- Use good toilet hygiene.
- Male contraceptive methods are limited to five options (abstinence, condoms, outercourse, vasectomy and withdrawal). Research may provide other options in the future. As with any contraceptive that may be used, always be informed about the effectiveness of the method and any potential complications.
- If a decrease in libido or ability to obtain an erection develops, discuss this with the health care provider because both physical and emotional factors can be involved. Medications (e.g., antihypertensives, which decrease blood pressure) can also cause this to occur and can be discussed. Do not take medications to increase libido (e.g., Viagra) until there is a thorough examination to detect risk factors and potential complications.
- Consult a health care provider if orgasm or urination is uncomfortable or painful.
- Report any lumps or irregularities of the breasts to your health care provider for further evaluation.
- Have prostate gland examinations performed at the age and frequency recommended by your health care provider.
- Report any discharge from the urethra, and any sores or growths on the genitalia.

Age-Related Changes: Male Reproductive System

- Decreased: Production of sperm and seminal fluid, size of testes
- Increased: Size of prostate gland

Fascinating Facts

The average sperm count is approximately 60 million per milliliter. This number has been decreasing in the past several decades by 1% to 2%. An amount over 20 million is considered normal. Every time a male ejaculates, he releases, on the average, 1 to 6.5 milliliters of semen. An amount of 2 milliliters or more is considered normal.

WORKBOOK PRACTICE

Go to your workbook and complete the exercises for this chapter.

SUGGESTED LEARNING ACTIVITIES

1. Think of the last time you were ill. Identify the system that was involved (e.g., respiratory for head colds, digestive for stomach flu) and review its anatomy and physiology. Identify the pathophysiological changes that occurred with this illness. What was the etiology of the illness? What were your signs and symptoms? Did you have any diagnostic procedures done? What was the treatment for this illness? What was the prognosis? Are there any preventive measures you can take to avoid a reoccurrence of the problem?
2. Think about the physiological changes your parents or grandparents have experienced. Can you describe these changes to them in everyday language?
3. Locate and name as many bones and muscles as you can in your own body by pressing on the surface of your skin.

4. Move your extremities to demonstrate the various positions made possible by your joints.
5. If you have a stethoscope, listen to your heartbeat and identify what is happening in the chambers, with the valves, and in the electrical system of the heart when you hear the "thump-thump" or "lub-dub" sound.
6. Take in a deep breath of fresh air and review the path that will be taken until the oxygen reaches the level of the individual body cell. What physiological actions occur along the way?
7. Next time you have a meal, review the path the solid food and the liquids will take through your body until they are excreted. What physiological actions occur along the way?
8. Change the italicized phrase in the following saying to its correct medical equivalent: "Don't shoot until you see the *whites of their eyes*!"
9. Think of the last time you were very frightened ("fight or flight" reaction) and identify the physiological changes that the sympathetic nervous system would have initiated.
10. Review all the conditions that must be present for pregnancy to occur (remember to include the endocrine system).

WEB ACTIVITIES

Human Anatomy Online

www.innerbody.com

Choose a body system and draw a schematic to detail the structure and function of the system.

National Human Genome Research Institute

www.genome.gov

Search for "Genetic Disorders." Choose one of the conditions listed and write a one-page report on the selected condition.

REVIEW QUESTIONS

1. What are the definitions for the terms *anatomy*, *physiology*, and *pathophysiology*?
2. What is the key difference between wellness and illness?
3. What are the primary anatomical features and physiological actions of the systems for movement and protection of the body?
4. What are the names of the movements made possible by joints?
5. What are the primary anatomical features and physiological actions of the systems for providing energy and for removing waste from the body?
6. What are the primary anatomical features and physiological actions of the systems for sensing and for coordinating and controlling the body?
7. What are the primary anatomical features and physiological actions of the systems for producing new life?
8. What are the common diseases or disorders associated with each body system?
9. What are three preventive measures for each body system?

APPLICATION EXERCISES

1. Now that you know the normal anatomy and physiology of the lungs, what signs and symptoms can you anticipate that Mr. Petersen may experience as a result of red cedar disease, discussed in The Case of the Unfamiliar Diagnosis?
2. Kelly Alexico comes into the office and states he was recently diagnosed with diabetes. Wanda Hector, the health care professional, asks him if he is referring to diabetes mellitus or diabetes insipidus. He responds by saying, "I don't know for sure, all I know is that I was peeing a lot."
   a. Is this adequate information to determine if it is diabetes mellitus or diabetes insipidus?
   b. What other questions could the health care professional ask him to determine which type of diabetes is most likely the diagnosis?

c. If it is diabetes mellitus, what can Wanda tell him about the anatomy and physiology of the related system? What is the pathophysiology of this diagnosis?

d. If it is diabetes insipidus, what can Wanda tell him about the anatomy and physiology of the related system? What is the pathophysiology of this diagnosis?

PROBLEM-SOLVING PRACTICE

1. Terrance Pompei is currently taking a class in anatomy and physiology. He enjoys the class and is learning the material easily. Another student in his class is struggling with the material and has asked him to study with her. She states that the instructor speaks too fast and she is unable to grasp the material. Using the five-step problem-solving process, determine what Terrance can do to help his classmate.

SUGGESTED READINGS AND RESOURCES

American Cancer Society. www.cancer.org

American Diabetes Association. www.diabetes.org

Arthritis Foundation. www.arthritis.org

Ehrlich, A. (2013). *Medical terminology for health professions* (7th ed.). Clifton Park, NY: Delmar Cengage Learning.

Epilepsy Foundation. www.epilepsyfoundation.org

Kapit, K., & Elson, L. M. (2013). *Anatomy coloring book* (4th ed.). New York: Addison-Wesley.

Muscular Dystrophy Association. www.mda.org

National Kidney Foundation. www.kidney.org

National Parkinson Foundation. www.parkinson.org

Scott, A. S., & Fong, E. (2014). *Body structures and functions* (12th ed.). Clifton Park, NY: Delmar Cengage Learning.

Sickle Cell Disease Association of America. www.sicklecelldisease.org

Tamparo, D. D., & Lewis, M. A. (2011). *Diseases of the human body* (5th ed.). Philadelphia, PA: F. A. Davis Company.

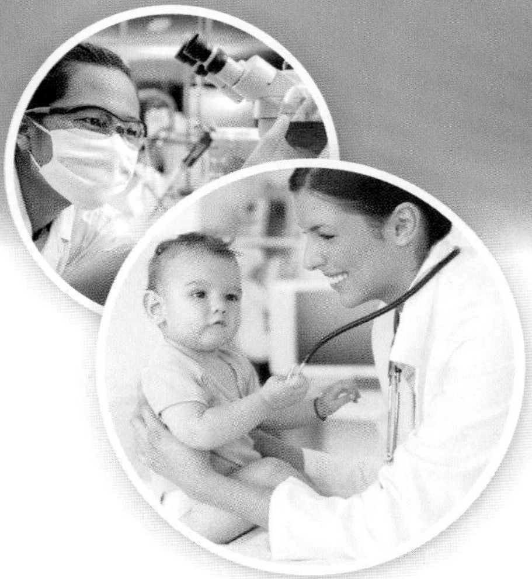

Chapter 8

Growth and Development

OBJECTIVES

Studying and applying the material in this chapter will help you to:

- Explain the differences between *physical, cognitive*, and *psychosocial* as they relate to growth and development.
- Identify the nine life stages according to the theory of Erik Erikson and the corresponding age span for each.
- Discuss the physical, cognitive, and psychosocial changes that occur at each life stage according to the theory of Erik Erikson.
- Identify the psychosocial developmental tasks to be accomplished according to the theory of Erik Erikson.
- Implement specific approaches to care at each life stage based on a knowledge of growth and development.
- Discuss the main concepts of the developmental theories of Piaget, Kohlberg, and Gilligan.
- Identify and describe the five stages of the dying process.

KEY TERMS

chronic illness
cognitive development
development
Erikson's stages of psychosocial development
Gilligan's stages of the ethic of care
growth
Kohlberg's moral stages
life review
physical development
Piaget's cognitive stages
psychosocial development
stages of dying
terminal illness

The Case of the Curious 4-Year-Old

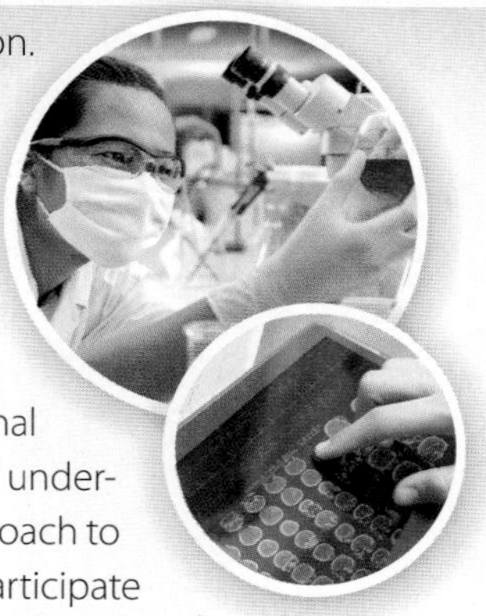

Paul, a 4-year-old child, is brought to the physician's office by his mother for a routine examination. Heathrow Wilson, the medical assistant, directs them to the room and begins to ask the mother routine questions and to take Paul's vital signs (blood pressure, temperature, heart and respiratory rate). Heathrow finds the tasks impossible to accomplish as the child wiggles, tries to pick up or touch everything, and asks continual questions. The mother becomes increasingly frustrated as she repeatedly tells the child to be quiet and sit still.

This may seem like a simple situation that has been observed many times, but there is a deeper dynamic being portrayed. The material in this chapter will help the health care professional to understand that Paul's tremendous curiosity and activity are normal for his age. As a result of understanding the stages of growth and development, the health care professional could alter his approach to constructively deal with Paul's behavior by implementing a strategy that will allow the child to participate (e.g., engaging the child by giving him something to do to help, asking questions directly of the child, or first letting Paul listen to his heart with the stethoscope). An age-appropriate response will prevent frustration and allow the child to meet his needs for this stage of development.

KNOWING YOUR PATIENT

From before human beings are born until they die, all individuals go through a series of stages in which they develop physically and mentally. Becoming a person happens over time. The study of growth and development is about these stages in life and what is accomplished in each. **Growth** refers to the physical changes that take place in the body. Examples of physical changes include:

- Increases in height
- Increases in weight
- Motor sensory adaptation
- Development of the sex organs

Development refers to the increase in mental, emotional, and social capabilities of the individual. Examples include increases in:

- Intellectual (cognitive) ability
- Variety in expression of emotions
- Ability to cope with complex situations
- Social and interpersonal skills

The following terms describe key concepts in human growth and development:

- **Physical development**: Growth of the body, including motor sensory adaptation. Monitoring growth is an important task in health care. The health care professional may be responsible for measuring and recording height, weight, and head circumference for infants and children. The Learning Activities at the end of this chapter cite the address for the government website that publishes the norms for weight, height, body mass, and head circumference according to percentiles. It is important for the physician to be notified if the measurements fall outside the norms because it may be an indication of a problem that can be addressed before it worsens.
- **Psychosocial development**: Includes both psychological and social development. Psychological refers to the emotions (love, hate, joy, fear, anxiety), attitudes, and other aspects of the mind. Social refers to an individual's interactions and relationships with other members of society.
- **Cognitive development**: Cognitive refers to intellectual processes and includes thought, awareness, and the ability to rationally comprehend the world and determine meaning. Seeking new information and applying it to make judgments and solve problems in positive, productive ways helps develop cognitive ability. For example, using the problem-solving model presented in Chapter 1 is a way to work on mental development. The information presented in each chapter of this text and the decision-making applications incorporated into the Thinking It Through exercises are designed to develop cognitive ability.

Human needs vary as individuals move through the life span. It is important for health care professionals to understand the developmental milestones of each stage of life, because they may provide care to individuals of all ages. The study and application of growth and development along with individual patient assessment will guide the health care professional in age-appropriate communication and care. It is also important to realize that there are always exceptions and that no one follows the stages exactly. Generalizations cannot take the place of considering each patient as a unique individual.

LIFE STAGES

The study of growth and development across the life span has been categorized into time frames. Certain changes and needs characterize each. There are a number of variations of these time frames in terms of the months or years that they cover. The age ranges listed in Table 8–1 are commonly used. They start with conception (when an ovum is fertilized) and proceed through infancy, childhood stages, adolescence, and adulthood. A study of the life span includes the final stage, that of dying.

The psychosocial aspects of each life stage are based on **Erikson's stages of psychosocial development.** (See Table 8–1.) Erik Erikson, an immigrant from Germany who taught at Yale and Harvard, studied the influence of society and culture on human development. He studied human responses to life's events to gain an understanding of how attitudes and behaviors change throughout the life span. He based his theory, first published in 1950, on the belief that psychosocial development occurs as the result of resolving specific types of conflicts encountered at each stage. Resolving these conflicts, at least in part, allows the individual to advance successfully to the next stage. Erikson's developmental tasks are explained in the discussions of each stage later in this chapter.

Although failing to complete a stage can delay the psychosocial growth of the individual, it does not necessarily prevent the successful completion of the stage at a later date. It is also important to understand that transitions are gradual between stages: They do not begin and end abruptly at exact ages. An individual under stress, such as during an illness, may regress (return) to the behaviors characteristic of a previous stage. Erikson did not assign specific beginning and ending ages to each stage, but he emphasized that they occur in the same order for each individual. Researchers and writers have assigned different age ranges to his stages. The ranges chosen for Table 8–1 are representative of the life span of today's adult.

Note that in Table 8–1, the later adulthood stage is expanded to identify three subdivisions. Erickson's original stage of later adulthood included ages 65 to death. With the increasing number of individuals living into their 80s, 90s, and even 100s, using only one

Table 8–1 Life Stages and Erikson's Stages of Psychosocial Development

Life Stage	Age	Erikson Stage
Prenatal	Conception to birth	
Infancy	Birth to 1 year	Trust vs. Mistrust
Toddler	1 to 3 years	Autonomy vs. Shame/Doubt
Preschooler	3 to 6 years	Initiative vs. Guilt
School-Age Child	6 to 12 years	Industry vs. Inferiority
Adolescence	12 to 20 years	Identity vs. Role Confusion
Young Adulthood	20s and 30s	Intimacy vs. Isolation
Middle Adulthood	40 to 65 years	Generativity vs. Stagnation
Later Adulthood:		Ego Integrity vs. Despair
Young–Old	65 to 74 years	
Middle–Old	75 to 84 years	
Old–Old (the frail elderly)	85 years to death	

category is no longer reflective of our society. Our country now commonly sees healthy, active adults age 65 and older who are still making major contributions to society. This is the most rapidly expanding part of the population, which means that the age gap between the health care professional and the patient will increase. It is critical that health care professionals have a respect for and an understanding of the medical, psychological, and cognitive needs of this segment of the population, since this is the primary population seeking medical care today.

Older adults have previously been stereotyped as one group. However, there is a wide difference within the broad category of those who are 65 and older. To compare a person who is 65 years old with someone who is 95 years old would be similar to including a 5-year-old with someone who is 35 years old. The changes that occur in this 30-year period are as significant at the later life span as they are at the younger life span.

Fascinating Facts

Many symptoms experienced by the older person are thought of as normal for aging, such as falling, weight loss, incontinence, dizziness, or mental impairment. These are not normal aging processes. They are a result of a disease process.

The baby boomers are the generation born post–World War II and encompass the 79 million babies born in the United States between 1946 and 1964. This is an average of 4 million babies each year. Prior to this time, an average of 2.5 million babies were born each year. This large group by its sheer mass has impacted every aspect of life as it has moved through society. In 2006, the oldest baby boomers turned 60 years old. The boomers are healthier, more active, better educated, more affluent, and working longer than the generations that preceded them. Many boomers do not silently go into retirement, but still believe that it is possible to make the world a better place. As a result they are making significant contributions by setting up various enterprises to assist others, getting involved in community projects, or volunteering at nonprofit organizations.

A word of caution to the health care professional: Do not rely on age alone as an indicator of the patient's needs. Assessment of the individual and his or her needs is at the center of good health care. For example, even though the current trend is to break down the 65 and older group into three subdivisions, this does not dictate how to care for them. One 65-year-old may be very frail and suffering from severe chronic illnesses, whereas an 80-year-old may leave you behind on a hiking trail.

Prenatal

The *prenatal* period begins with conception (fertilization of an ovum by a sperm) and ends with birth. The cell formed when the two reproductive sex cells join is called a *zygote*. The zygote contains all the genetic information from both parents that will determine gender and physical characteristics, such as eye color, hair color and texture, and skin pigmentation. Many other areas are not completely determined by genetics. For example, personality, intellect, and other mental characteristics are influenced by many other factors, such as:

- Family relationships
- Cultural customs
- Religion
- Education
- Physical health

Physical growth is affected by factors such as adequate supplies of appropriate food, opportunities for exercise, and access to health care. Individuals are not simply combinations of genetic material, but unique combinations of both genetic and environmental influences.

Human growth and development begin the moment fertilization occurs. The fertilized ovum is implanted into the uterine wall, and rapid cell division and multiplication occur. The period from the second to the eighth week after fertilization is called the *embryo stage*. From 8 weeks until birth, the embryo is called a *fetus*.

Rapid prenatal growth and development make the developing human especially vulnerable to environmental factors. Congenital anomalies (birth defects) can occur if the mother inhales toxins or consumes alcohol, drugs, or nicotine. Therapeutic drugs, beneficial for the mother, can cause harmful side effects in the fetus. Therefore, all over-the-counter (OTC) and prescription medications must be reviewed by the physician to determine whether they are safe to take during pregnancy.

The speed of prenatal growth is illustrated in Table 8–2.

Table 8–2 Prenatal Development

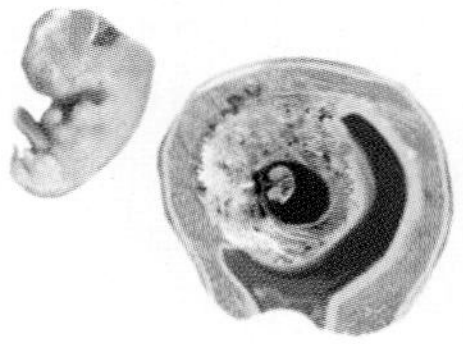 4 Weeks	By end of 1 month: • Half the size of a pea • Heart is beating
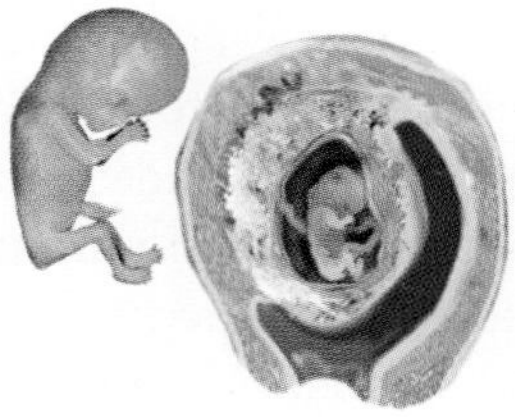 8 Weeks	By end of 2 months: • Approximately 1 inch in length • Resembles human being • All body organs have begun forming
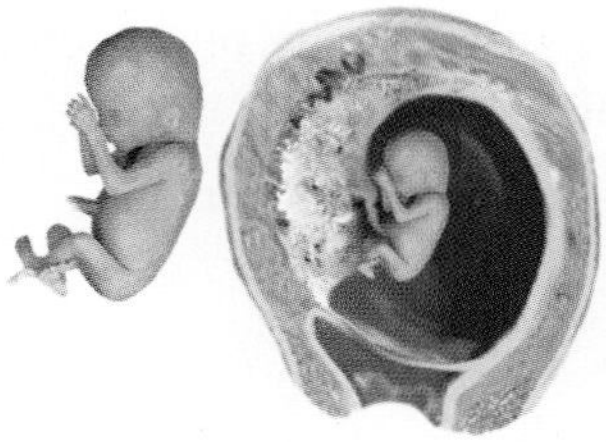 12 Weeks	By end of 3 months: • 2 ½ to 3 inches long • Fully formed • Can swallow and kick (mother cannot usually feel kicks until fourth month) • External genitalia formed and male or female can be distinguished
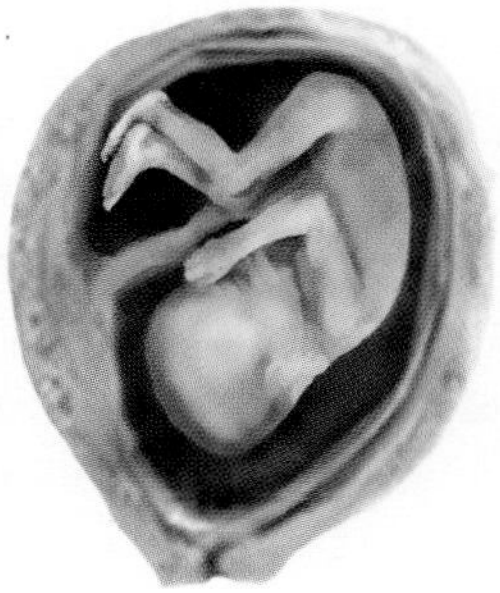 24 Weeks	By end of 6 months: • Weighs 1 ½ to 2 pounds • Eyelids can now open and eyes can move up, down, and sideways • Eyebrows, eyelashes, and taste buds present • Can hear mother when she talks or sings
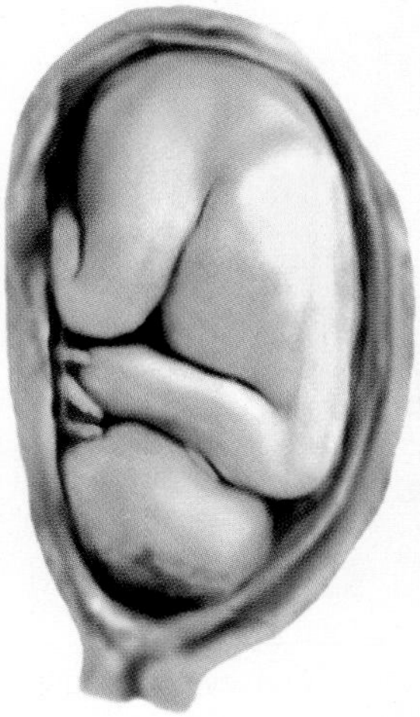 40 Weeks	By end of normal term (40 weeks): • Fetal development is complete • Weighs 6 to 8 pounds • Length is 19 to 22 inches

Infancy

During the first month of life, the newborn is often referred to as a *neonate*. (See Figure 8–1.) In this text, *infant* is used to describe the time frame from birth to 1 year of age.

This is a period of tremendous physical growth. The birth weight triples or quadruples to 21 to 27 pounds by age 1. Length will increase to between 29 and 30 inches. Teeth erupt between ages 8 and 12 months.

The muscular and nervous systems develop rapidly. At first, movements are primarily reflexive rather than being purposefully made by the infant. Over time, infants develop the ability to raise their heads, and then move on to turning and rolling over. They increase their ability to focus their eyes. By 1 year many infants crawl, stand alone, and walk with assistance.

Cognitively, vocalization progresses to several words. Infants learn by imitation. During the first few months of life, they learn to manipulate objects, recognize familiar objects and persons, and obey simple commands. It has been proven that infants must receive adequate tactile stimulation (e.g., touching, cuddling, and hugging) to have normal physical and mental development.

Erikson's psychosocial stage for the infant is *trust versus mistrust*. Infants are dependent on others for their physical and emotional survival. Those who receive consistent loving care that satisfies the need for food, warmth, and other physical comforts will develop trust in their caregivers. Inconsistent and inadequate care leads to mistrust of others.

Toddler

The *toddler* stage is from 1 to 3 years of age. (See Figure 8–2.) Physical changes occur as the body grows and proportions change. The characteristic protruding abdomen is still present, but the head no longer looks as oversized for the body as it does in the infant. By 3 years of age, approximately 20 teeth are present, and many toddlers, especially females, have achieved bowel and bladder control.

The motor sensory ability progresses from walking independently to running, jumping, and climbing. This is a very difficult time for the parents, because the activity of the toddler is directed toward continually investigating and searching out new experiences. Keeping the toddler safe and away from hazards requires "child-proofing" the environment and maintaining constant surveillance of the child, as in the following examples:

- Placing breakable items out of their reach
- Locking cabinets
- Using gates to prevent access to swimming pools and other hazards
- Locking away all poisonous substances
- Ensuring that they cannot leave the house by themselves
- Preventing access to any item that can be used for climbing

Cognitive skills develop rapidly as toddlers acquire language skills and begin to speak in sentences. They can understand simple instructions

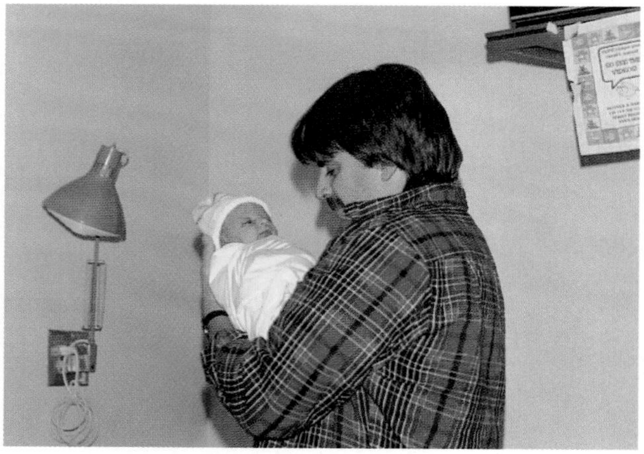

FIGURE 8–1 It is important that the parents bond with the newborn because this will initiate a loving and trusting relationship.

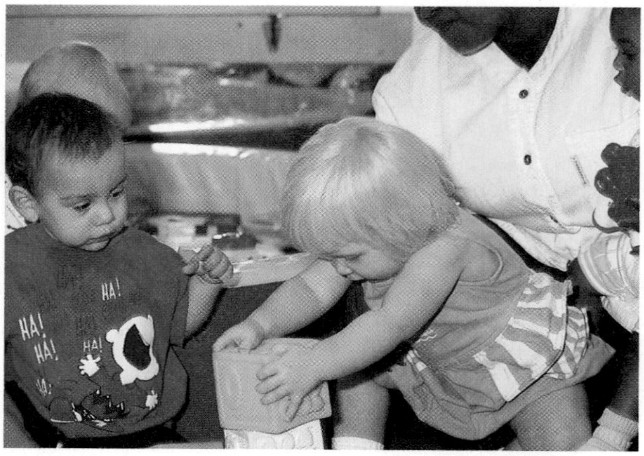

FIGURE 8–2 Toddlers develop motor sensory and cognitive skills as they manipulate and investigate items in their environment.

and requests, but their attention span is very short. Toddlers begin to learn ideas, attitudes, and values, but at the same time, they also believe that their point of view is the only one. This belief, combined with an emerging sense of independence, can lead to temper tantrums.

Erikson's psychosocial stage for the toddler is *autonomy versus shame and doubt*. Toddlers will develop confidence in their ability to care for themselves (autonomy) when they receive encouragement to explore their environment and learn independent skills such as dressing, feeding, and toilet training. Parents who are overly protective or have unrealistic expectations, may initiate the development of doubt and shame in their toddler. This can lead to a sense of general inadequacy.

Preschooler

The *preschooler* stage ranges from 3 to 6 years of age. (See Figure 8–3.) Physically, preschoolers become taller and thinner than toddlers. Self-care skills increase, and they progress to being able to independently dress themselves.

Continuing motor sensory development leads to an improved sense of balance. This allows toddlers to skip and jump in a coordinated manner and enables them to learn skills such as jumping rope and skating.

Cognitively, they can now speak quite well in sentences. They have also developed an awareness of other people who are not in their immediate environment. They still assume that everyone thinks as they do. They have short attention spans. They are able to count, recite the alphabet, and recall their address and phone number.

Erikson's psychosocial stage for the preschooler is *initiative versus guilt*. Preschoolers can build on the confidence developed as a toddler to initiate their own learning. They seek out new experiences and knowledge and strive to understand new activities. If their parents severely restrict this initiative, criticize, or scold them for their attempts, a sense of guilt will develop. This feeling of guilt will diminish the preschooler's natural enthusiasm for learning new motor and language skills. As a consequence, they can become hesitant to take on new challenges.

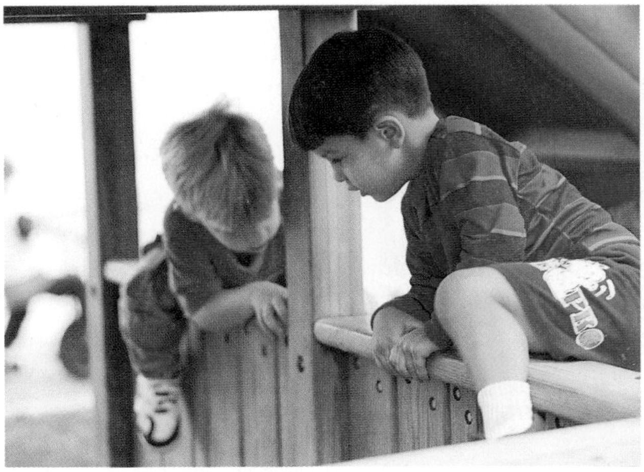

FIGURE 8–3 Preschoolers develop confidence as they succeed at new activities. Socialization skills are also practiced by interacting with their peers in group events.

School-Age Child

The *school-age child* stage ranges from 6 to 12 years of age. (See Figure 8–4.) The physical growth of the

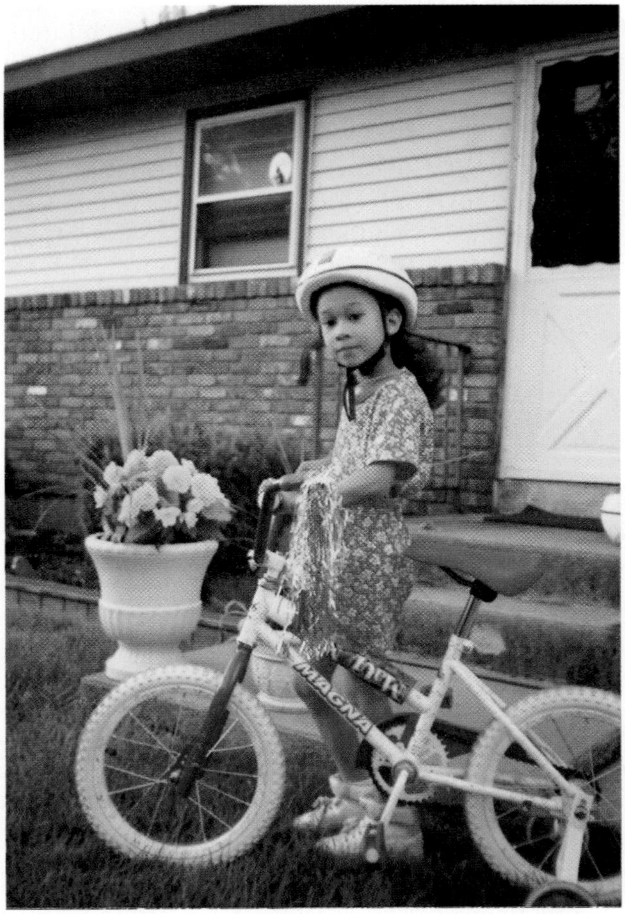

FIGURE 8–4 A school-age child has the motor sensory skills to master activities that require coordination and agility. Protective equipment, such as a helmet, plays an important role in keeping the child safe.

body continues with a more pronounced development between 10 and 12 years with the beginning of puberty (the period in life when boys and girls become functionally capable of reproduction). The permanent teeth also begin to erupt at this stage of growth.

The motor sensory skills become well coordinated, and the child develops grace and agility. School-age children can assist with household duties and show more responsibility in assigned tasks. They have a desire for both quiet time and intense physical activity.

Cognitive development has progressed to logical thinking and the ability to see things from different perspectives. The attention span has increased, and pride is taken in personal accomplishments. Children at this state reason, problem solve, learn to follow rules, and develop a sense of morality (right and wrong) to guide their behavior.

Erikson's psychosocial stage for the school-age child is *industry versus inferiority*. School-age children experience pleasure from the successful completion of projects and anticipate recognition for their accomplishments. They prefer friends to family and are influenced by the approval of their peers. If school-age children are not accepted by peers or cannot meet the expectations of family, a sense of inferiority and lack of self-worth may develop.

Adolescence

Adolescence is the stage ranging from 12 to 20 years of age. (See Figure 8–5.) There are dramatic physical changes as maturation of the reproductive systems occurs.

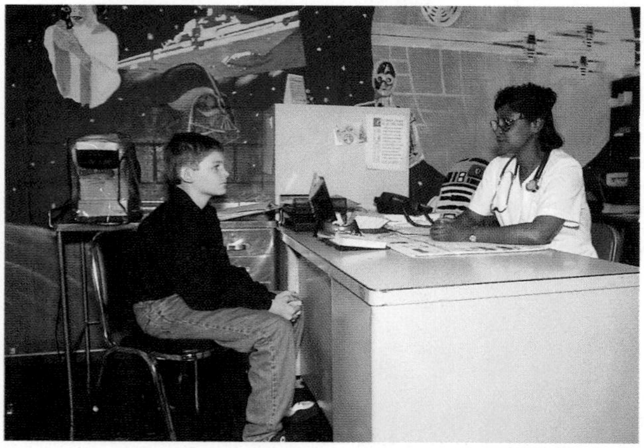

FIGURE 8–5 Adolescents need adults they can easily talk with to share their concerns and to help them understand how their mental and physical health is affected by the decisions they make.

The fine motor skills improve, but awkwardness in the gross motor skills is evident. The adolescent may easily become fatigued with activity and requires adequate rest and sleep.

Cognitive abilities greatly increase. Adolescents are able to acquire large quantities of knowledge and are able to use reasoning skills. They have the capacity for introspection and start to develop their philosophy of life and create their future occupational identity. Adolescents are also more prone to stress than those at the other life stages.

Erikson's psychosocial stage for adolescence is *identity versus role confusion*. They are interested in the tremendous changes taking place in their bodies, but are also confused about identities as they move through the transition from child (dependent) to adult (independent). Mood swings are quite common as a result of the hormonal changes. Adolescents may try different roles, including rebellion, in the search for their identity as they work through who they are and who they will become. They may be critical of parents and resent the advice offered or criticism given. Peers continue to exert a significant influence on their behavior, because of strong concerns about how they are perceived. If adolescents are unable to determine their identity and direction, they will lack a sense of who they are. This is known as "role confusion."

Young Adulthood

Young adulthood includes the 20s and 30s. (See Figure 8–6.) Physical functioning peaks at about 30 and then starts to slowly diminish as aging continues. For example, after 30 the skin begins to lose moisture, gastrointestinal secretions diminish, and problems with weight gain may begin.

Motor sensory skills also peak during this time and then begin to decline. Muscular strength peaks in the 20s and 30s and then begins to decline after the mid-30s. The visual and auditory senses also start to decline.

Fascinating Facts

The rate of decline does not accelerate with age. It is the same rate of 1% per year, every year, starting at age 30. Therefore, there is a decrease of function by 1% per year whether the person is 35 or 95 years of age.

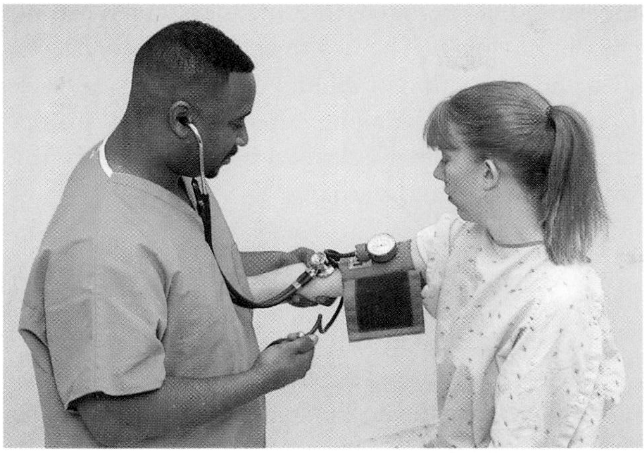

FIGURE 8–6 Young adults can feel a great deal of stress as they attempt to succeed at the many roles they have at this stage. When caring for young adults it is important to maintain an open communication that allows them to discuss and problem solve these concerns.

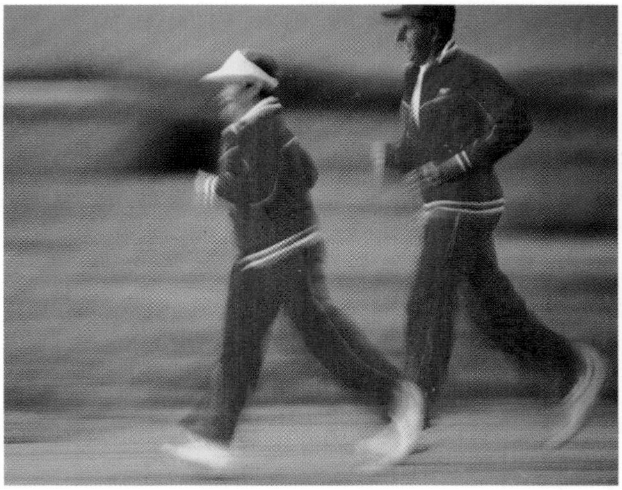

FIGURE 8–7 Middle adulthood leads to more physical challenges. Keeping active adds to the adult's health, vitality, and longevity.

Young adults experience optimal cognitive functioning. Their problem-solving skills and creativity are excellent. This is a period of maximum potential.

Erikson's psychosocial stage for young adulthood is *intimacy versus isolation*. The task of young adults is to complete the transition from dependency to responsibility, to make commitments to others, and to establish themselves in society. The responsibilities of this time are usually great: form an intimate relationship, have and raise children, obtain advanced education, and establish a career. A fear of making commitments to others may result in isolation and loneliness.

Middle Adulthood

Middle adulthood includes the years 40 to 65. (See Figure 8–7.) The physical abilities continue to decline. For example, bone and muscle mass, physical strength, and endurance decrease. At the same time, the skin loses some of its elasticity, wrinkles begin to develop, and major body systems begin to decline. Middle adults may begin to have concerns about their physical health. Although a **chronic illness** (health problem of long duration in which the disease or condition shows little change or slowly gets progressively worse) may begin at any time, it is during this stage that it is more likely to begin to appear.

The motor sensory skills diminish. The reflexes, muscles, and joints respond more slowly. There is decreased balance and coordination and a more prolonged response to stress. The visual, auditory, and gustatory senses diminish.

Cognitive abilities are still quite strong, although learning may take longer. Problem solving and memory remain consistent until the late middle years. Creativity may increase during this stage.

Erikson's psychosocial stage for middle adulthood is *generativity versus stagnation*. This is a time of shifting concerns from the self to the next generation, as well as toward an increased involvement with friends and community. There is a desire to make a contribution of value. It is a time of self-assessment and evaluation of the accomplishment of goals. There may be many adjustments if children leave home, health issues develop, and concerns arise about retirement. This is the period when many individuals face what is referred to as a "midlife crisis." This may be brought on by the recognition of limitations and unmet goals. If individuals are unable to establish their worth or recognize their contribution to the world, stagnation may occur. This can result in self-absorption and becoming obsessed with health concerns.

Later Adulthood

Later adulthood encompasses age 65 through death. (See Figure 8–8.) Physical decline continues to occur, with loss of muscle and bone and atrophy of the reproductive organs. The cardiac, renal, and immune systems decline. Decreased peripheral (arms and legs) circulation leads to less tolerance for heat and cold.

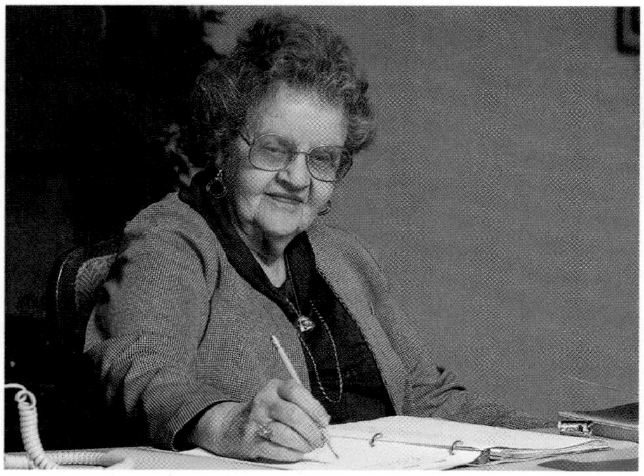

FIGURE 8–8 Keeping involved and active during later adulthood adds greatly to the enjoyment of life.

The motor sensory abilities also continue their decline. The visual, auditory, gustatory, and olfactory senses diminish. The ability to tolerate pain decreases, physical responses are slower, and some motor skills decline.

Erikson's psychosocial stage for later adulthood is *ego integrity versus despair*. The many challenges are a continuation of changes that began in middle adulthood: retirement, loss of spouse and friends, new family roles (becoming in-laws and grandparents as children marry), and increasing concerns about health. As individuals face their mortality, they review the events of their lives and the related successes and failures. If they experience a sense of satisfaction and pleasure from the events of their lives, a sense of ego integrity will be experienced. In contrast, if the review is interpreted as a series of failures and disappointments, there is a sense of sadness and despair.

The life span has increased in the past several decades, and people are living longer than ever before in history. Many older adults maintain active, productive lives. It is no longer uncommon to see adults working into their 90s. Older persons are able to make various kinds of valuable contributions to society. Americans' views of what it means to be "old" will continually adjust as this segment of the population increases.

As noted in Tables 8–1 and 8–3 and discussed earlier, the later adulthood stage can be broken into three subdivisions. The important point to emphasize here is this: *Do not stereotype any person*. It is particularly important not to presume that an older person is frail, weak, and helpless. The health care professional will find a wide variation of mental ability, physical ability, and health status among adults in this age group. Using your assessment skills will help identify the health level of the individual.

Fascinating Facts

Many young people think that creativity and contributions diminish as one ages. Read the following examples, and evaluate this assumption.

- Sarah Bernhardt (1844–1923) was a famous American actress. She lost a leg in her early 70s but continued acting until her death at age 78.
- Mahatma Gandhi (1869–1948) successfully completed negotiations with Britain to grant India's independence at the age of 77.
- Frank Lloyd Wright (1867–1959), America's most famous architect, designed the Guggenheim Museum in New York City at 91.
- Eleanor Roosevelt (1884–1962), the wife of President Franklin D. Roosevelt, was very active in social causes and chaired the United Nations Commission on Human Rights from ages 62 to 67. She wrote her autobiography, titled *On My Own* at the age of 74.
- Alfred Hitchcock (1899–1980) directed the movies *Psycho* and *The Birds* in his 60s and *Frenzy* at 73 years of age.
- Nelson Mandela (1918–2013) was inaugurated as president after South Africa's first free election at the age of 75. This was after he had spent 27 years of his life in prison for his political beliefs.
- George Burns (1896–1996), comic and actor, was still appearing in public and telling jokes with perfect timing when he was 100.
- Grandma Moses (1860–1961), the famous American painter whose real name was Anna Mary Robertson, started her art career when she was in her 70s.

CARE CONSIDERATIONS

Each life stage is characterized by its own physical, cognitive, and psychosocial challenges. The advantage of studying general categories is that it assists health care professionals in their understanding of areas to focus on during patient assessment and for determining age-appropriate approaches to care. The danger of using generalizations is that it is possible to make false assumptions about people and lose sight of the unique individual needs of each patient.

All patients at all times need respectful, compassionate, and empathetic care. Families and friends are also involved in and affected by the health of the patient, so the same consideration must be extended to them. A routine question to always ask is if the family members have any concerns, problems, or questions they would like to discuss. When talking with family or friends, the patient's right for confidentiality must always be respected. No information can be shared with anyone else without the consent of the patient. Examples of specific care considerations as they relate to each life stage are presented in Table 8–3. Some considerations apply to most stages, such as involving patients in decisions regarding their care and adapting education and instructions to the learning style of the patient. They are included in the chart when they are considered to be primary considerations for that stage.

Table 8–3 Care Considerations for the Health Care Professional

Life Stages	Care Considerations
Prenatal (Conception to birth)	• Emphasize care of mother to ensure a normal pregnancy • Address unhealthy habits • Assist mother in developing strategies to make healthy changes • Always ask if any over-the-counter medications or products from health food stores are being used. Commonly used medications and products can have harmful effects on unborn babies • Inquire about mother's nutrition • Educate the mother about the need for adequate nutrition and fluids
Infancy (Birth–1 year)	• Involve parents in care • Provide for safety • Do not allow the infant to play with objects that have moving or removable parts • Cuddle and hug infants • Obtain height, weight, and head circumference measurements to track growth patterns
Toddler (1–3 years)	• Use a firm, direct approach • Distract and use a game approach to improve cooperation • Give only one direction at a time and state it simply • Involve toddlers in their care by allowing them to make choices when possible • Prepare them for procedures with simple explanations • Set limits and maintain safety
Preschooler (3–6 years)	• Explain procedures and unfamiliar objects prior to performing or using them • Encourage verbalization skills • Praise good behavior • To improve acceptance of painful procedures, allow them to make choices when possible (injection site); give a token of bravery, such as a colorful sticker; and use distraction (have them recite alphabet or sing their favorite song)
School-Age Child (6–12 years)	• Explain procedures and equipment using correct terminology, but in words they understand • Provide for privacy and some personal control • Define and enforce behavior limits • Encourage independence • Educate with clear, simple visual aids

(continues)

Table 8–3 Care Considerations for the Health Care Professional (continued)

Life Stages	Care Considerations
Adolescence (12–20 years)	• Give explanations along with the rationale • Encourage questions • Involve them in the decision-making process • Determine how they learn best and adapt an approach for their needs, including visual aids and written materials • Provide privacy • Do not talk about them where they can overhear the conversation
Young Adulthood (20s and 30s)	• Involve significant other as appropriate • Watch body language for clues regarding feelings • Assess them for stress resulting from the multiple roles and responsibilities of this stage • Involve them in the decision-making process • Provide teaching according to their learning style
Middle Adulthood (40–65 years)	• Involve them in the decision-making process • Encourage self-care • Explore their concept of illness as it relates to body image and career • Provide teaching according to their learning style • Encourage lifestyle changes, such as quitting smoking, improving nutrition, and increasing exercise to help lessen the effects of natural age-related decline
Later Adulthood Young–Old (65–74 years)	• If still working, encourage discussion about work plans, activities, and accomplishments • If retired, encourage social activity with peers (e.g., volunteer, participation in community organizations or clubs) • Encourage active learning, thinking, and use of memory skills • Assist with adjustment to new roles (e.g., grandparent, widower, balancing independence and dependence)
Middle–Old (75–84 years)	• Explore support systems • Encourage them to talk about their feelings of loss, grief, and achievements • Provide support for coping with any impairments • Provide a safe, comfortable environment • Be alert to overmedication and sensitivity to medications
Old–Old (frail elderly; 85 years to death)	• Encourage independence by providing physical, mental, and social activities • Support end-of-life decisions by providing information and resources • Assist with self-care • Involve family members in caregiving • Be sensitive to sensory impairments • Provide care to maintain skin integrity and regular bowel movements

OTHER DEVELOPMENTAL THEORIES

Erickson's stages of psychosocial development offer a classic approach to development that remains the most frequently used theory today. But other theories have also contributed to the field of life stages and personal development. A few of these will be presented next.

Jean Piaget

Piaget's cognitive stages is concerned with children, rather than all learners. According to this psychologist, children progress through four cognitive stages of development. Each stage is marked by how children understand the world. Piaget believed that children are like "little scientists" and they actively try to explore and make sense of the world around them.

Through his observations, Piaget developed a theory of intellectual development that included four distinct stages, as listed in Table 8–4. To Piaget, cognitive development was a progressive reorganization of mental processes as a result of biological maturation and environmental experiences. Children construct an understanding of the world around them, then experience discrepancies between what they already know and what they discover in their environment.

Lawrence Kohlberg

Moral development in humans is the focus of **Kohlberg's moral stages**. He emphasized that human beings develop philosophically and psychologically in a progressive fashion. He identified six stages that are classified into three levels, as seen in Table 8–5. Kohlberg believed that a person could only progress one stage at a time, not "jump" stages, and that most moral development occurs through social interaction. Kohlberg's scale is about how people justify behaviors and his stages are not a method of ranking how

Table 8–4 Piaget's Cognitive Stages

Cognitive Stage	Age	Comments
Sensorimotor	Birth to 2 years	Infants and toddlers acquire knowledge through sensory experiences and manipulating objects. See Figure 8–9.
Preoperational	2 to 7 years	Children learn through pretend play, but still struggle with logic and being able to take the point of view of other people. See Figure 8–10.
Concrete operational	7 to 12 years	Children begin to think more logically, but their thinking can also be very rigid. They tend to struggle with abstract and hypothetical concepts.
Formal operational	12 years to adulthood	Involves an increase in logic, the ability to use deductive reasoning, and an understanding of abstract ideas.

Table 8–5 Kohlberg's Moral Stages

Stage/Level	Social Orientation
1. Preconventional	Obedience and Punishment • Generally found at elementary school level • One must behave according to socially acceptable norms as told by some authority figure (parent or teacher) • Obedience is compelled by threat or application of punishment
2. Preconventional	Individualism, Instrumentalism, and Exchange • View that right behavior means acting in one's own best interests
3. Conventional	"Good Boy/Girl" • Characterized by an attitude that seeks to do what will gain approval of others
4. Conventional	Law and Order • One is oriented to abiding by the law and responding to obligations of duty
5. Postconventional	Social Contract • Understanding of social mutuality and genuine interest in welfare of others
6. Postconventional	Principled Conscience • Respect for universal principle and demands of individual conscience

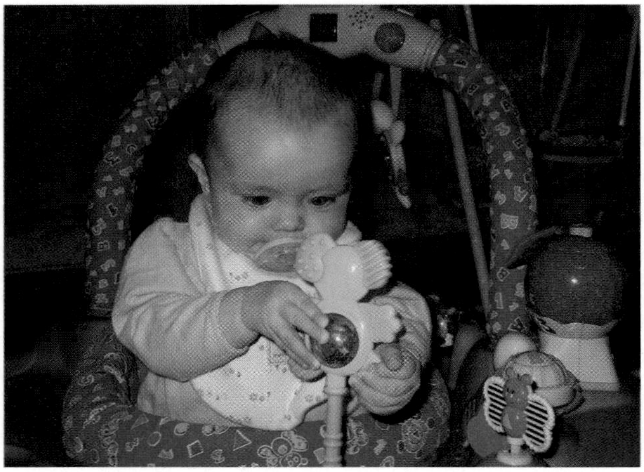

FIGURE 8–9 Infants develop their sensorimotor skills by sucking on and manipulating objects.

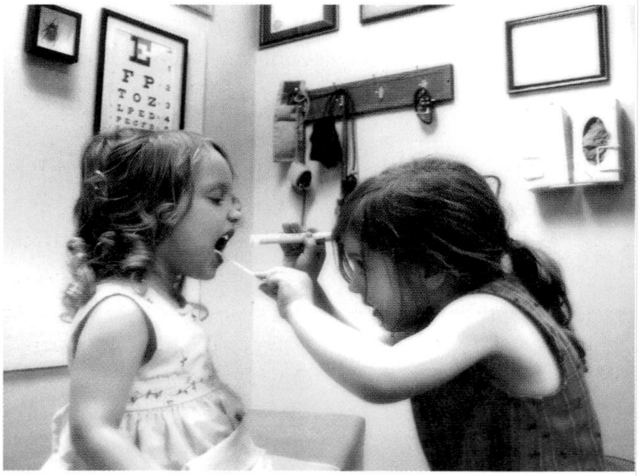

FIGURE 8–10 Children begin to use representational thought through pretend play.

moral someone's behavior is. He also felt that stage 3 was not reached by the majority of adults.

Carol Gilligan

Gilligan worked with Lawrence Kohlberg on his theory of moral development (see previous section), but eventually began to criticize Kohlberg's work. She noted that Kohlberg only studied "privileged, white men and boys," resulting in a biased perspective that overlooked aspects of women's lives. Women's development in terms of their caring effect on human relationships was given less significance than some of the male characteristics of rights and rules. Gilligan observed that as women progress through stages of development, they must learn to address their own interests *and* the interests of others, and that women hesitate to judge because they see the complexities of relationships. Her work outlined features specific to female moral development. **Gilligan's stages of the ethics of care** is divided into three stages of moral development, as seen in Table 8–6.

FUTURE TRENDS

William H. Thomas is a Harvard-educated physician with a special interest in revolutionizing long-term care communities. His book *What Are Old People For? How Elders Will Save the World* (2007) discusses how, with the older population projected to double in the next few years, sweeping changes will be seen. Older people are healthier, more active, and more verbal than ever before in history, and this will change the way aging is experienced in the United States.

Thomas breaks the life span into five groupings, but does not assign specific ages to the groups. He views the aging process as a cycle that begins with

Table 8–6 Gilligan's Stages of the Ethics of Care

Stage	Goal	Orientation
1. Preconventional	Individual survival	Care only for themselves in order to ensure survival (normal in children)
2. Conventional	Self-sacrifice is goodness	More responsibility shown for other people (seen in the roles of mother and wife), but sometimes carries on to ignore needs of self
3. Postconventional	Principle of nonviolence: Do not hurt others or self	Acceptance of care for self and others; transition is from goodness to the truth that she is a person too Some people never reach this stage

a state of "being," transitions through "doing," and ends with "being":

- Infant—the purest example of *being*.
- Adolescent—a time of transition to adulthood. This is not an easy passage and is fraught with complexity and turbulence. The individual transitions from the joyfulness of play to a clear preference for *doing* over *being*.
- Adult—the focus is on *doing*. The most frequent question asked between two adults is "What do you do?"
- Senescence—a time of transition to elderhood. As in adolescence, this is not an easy passage. Dr. Thomas states, "Sheltered for decades by energy and vitality, adults are utterly convinced of the rightness and goodness of their family and their chosen work. The first sign that you are preparing to grow out of adulthood is the dawning awareness of the heavy toll taken by things that you 'have to do'" (2007). This awareness starts gradually and grows as the individual's insight grows. The senescent person begins to realize that his or her life is not as unique or significantly important as once imagined. Rather, the person begins to understand that his or her family and job are much like those of millions of others who love their families and have contributed significantly in their work. These painful insights lead to the desire to put aside the *have to do* and explore the mysteries of *want to do*. Dr. Thomas states, "It is the beginning of ripening, just as adolescence is the beginning of maturation" (2007).
- Elderhood—this stage completes the cycle and returns the individual back to being. There is a clear preference to put aside the *have to do* for the *want to do*; this is a gift of great value.

Aging is gradual, ongoing, and unstoppable. There are no surprises as we see the process occurring all around us. It does not happen overnight, but it does happen to all of us. An awareness and respect for this process will make you a better and more compassionate health care professional.

DEATH AND DYING

Death is the natural end to life. It is, in a sense, the last stage of human development. Health care professionals may work with patients and their families during this last phase of the life process. To help understand dying, many turn to the classic work of Swiss physician Elisabeth Kübler-Ross. She earned her medical degree at the University of Switzerland in 1957 and her degree in psychiatry from the University of Colorado in 1963. After years of study and research, she published her first book, *On Death and Dying*, in 1969. She was the first person to study and write about death in a way that brought it to public attention. Kübler-Ross conducted extensive interviews with people who knew they were going to die and made notes about the process they followed as they struggled to put their lives in perspective. These studies encouraged general discussion of what had previously been a taboo topic. Her research findings and subsequent books have provided the information that health care professionals and the general public need in order to become more informed about this area.

Based on her research, Kübler-Ross developed a model called the "stages of dying" or "stages of grief." According to the model, people who are dying go through five stages when they learn that they have a **terminal illness** (a condition or disease that because of its nature can be expected to cause the patient to die). The five **stages of dying** are summarized as follows:

- Denial: When first learning about a terminal illness, the individual may feel numb and in a state of disbelief. The belief is that this cannot be happening or that a mistake has been made. Common reactions are inability to focus, feeling a sense of it as unreal, hysteria or passivity, or the contemplation of suicide.

Thinking It Through

Calvin Bell is a dental hygienist in an urban dental clinic. His patients range in age from toddlers to older persons. On one busy day, he saw patients in the following stages: preschooler (3), school age (9), adolescent (15), young adult (26), and later adulthood (83).

1. Explain how his behavior might change to be most appropriate with each patient (hint: refer to Table 8–3).
2. What would be the most likely dental health care concerns for each patient?
3. What might be the most effective patient education techniques to use with each?

- Anger: Once the reality of death hits, intense anger may be experienced. It is common for the individual to ask, "Why me?" It seems unfair, and there is envy of those with good health. Acute rage is experienced at the prospect of the upcoming loss. This rage may be directed only toward the illness, but it is also commonly directed toward everyone and everything.
- Bargaining: In this stage the person bargains for the one thing not possible—more time. Dying individuals want time to complete unachieved goals, see their children reach a certain level of maturity, have grandchildren, or travel to unseen parts of the world. The bargaining is often done with whomever they consider to be the higher being who has authority over life and death. They make promises to be better people, to change bad habits, and to live an exemplary life if only given more time.
- Depression: This is a profound sadness felt over the prospect of no longer being alive and not being able to change the course of events. There is a turning inward as they consider all the time that was wasted, the things left undone, and the joys that will not be experienced. Younger individuals feel particularly deprived of a long healthy life and feel they should have had the opportunity to live up to their potential.
- Acceptance: When this stage is reached, there is a dramatic change. Individuals experience a sense of peace with themselves, family, friends, and community. They now accept that they are dying and can focus on tying up any loose ends they perceive need to be resolved in preparation for death. This is referred to as "completing any unfinished business." For example, they may want to talk to certain friends or family to express their feelings or resolve issues or complete any necessary financial arrangements. Another important component of this stage is the need to do a life review. The **life review** involves telling the events of their lives to those close to them (including health care professionals). Part of the process is the desire to put one's life in perspective by performing a self-evaluation. This leads to a sense of closure. During this stage, dying individuals may be very open to talking about their feelings about death. As the time of death approaches, however, withdrawal often occurs.

Thinking It Through

Veronica Johnson, age 77, is a home health patient with a terminal illness. She lives in her home and is cared for by her husband. Josephine Mitchell, a hospice nurse, visits Mrs. Johnson on a regular basis to determine if the patient's needs are being met, to educate her husband on how to care for his wife, to offer emotional support, and to help resolve any difficulties that may arise. Mrs. Johnson states, "I am dying. I have known this for some time. I know it will not be much longer now, but I have had a full life and I am not afraid." But she also states, "I want to tell my daughter how much I love her, but I don't know how to do this as there seems to be a distance between us. I am also afraid I will begin to cry and not be able to stop." Ms. Mitchell speaks with the daughter and determines that the daughter also wishes to talk with her mother to say goodbye, but is reluctant to do so because she is also afraid of starting to cry and not being able to stop.

Mrs. Johnson asks Ms. Mitchell to be present when her daughter arrives to visit her. When the daughter arrives, both mother and daughter repeat their concerns about starting to cry and not being able to stop. Ms. Mitchell then says with humor, "Don't worry about it, I will start mopping up if it gets too deep." At that point, the daughter rushes to her mother's bedside, and a very loving conversation takes place.

1. What stage of the dying process is Mrs. Johnson in?
2. Mrs. Johnson is in which life stage? According to Erik Erikson's stages of psychosocial development, what is the conflict to be met at this life stage? Does it sound as if she has successfully met this challenge or not? Why?
3. Should the hospice nurse have been present during the meeting between the mother and daughter?
4. Was the humor used by the hospice nurse appropriate?
5. What outcome would you anticipate to occur as a result of the daughter and mother openly sharing their feelings?

It is as if the external world is no longer important. It is also possible that they do not have the energy to try to communicate with others who do not have the same understanding of life as the dying have now achieved.

During the acceptance stage of dying, it was stated that patients often feel the need to do a life review. This same behavior is also commonly noted in the elderly when no specific terminal illness has been diagnosed. As a health care professional, it is important to take the time to hear (or hear again) these stories because they represent a significant step in the patient's developmental process. You may note that some patients tell their life stories with acceptance of past events, others with bitterness, guilt, or anger. Sometimes the events will be told in a glorified manner. At other times, the telling of stories may be more dispassionate. Another approach is to phrase past events in such a way as to pass on the individual's wisdom or cultural heritage. There is no one right way, and the health care professional can be of most help by showing interest and allowing patients to express themselves in the manner most comfortable to them.

Dying patients do not always go through all these stages, nor do they go through them in an orderly and sequential manner. One of the criticisms of Elisabeth Kübler-Ross's theory is that the stages are too rigid. Theorists who followed her have confirmed these stages, but note that not all people experience all of them, or go through the same sequence, or complete the stages. In addition, tremendous differences are caused by gender, class, and culture.

This model has been presented as it applies to the dying patient, but there is a wider application that will also assist the health care professional. It can be applied to any form of loss. When any loss is perceived, there is suffering and a grieving process is initiated. There are many types of loss:

- Failure to achieve an important goal
- Loss of a job, resulting in a change of social identity
- Divorce
- Death of a pet
- Accident
- Injury
- Upcoming surgery
- Moving away from friends and family
- Grieving about the impending or recent death of a loved one
- Financial setbacks, such as bankruptcy, foreclosure on home, or loss of savings

Helping patients—and others with whom they have contact—handle loss is a valuable skill for health care professionals. Providing caring concern in times of need promotes patient welfare, eases the dying process, and helps others come to terms with their losses.

WORKBOOK PRACTICE

Go to your workbook and complete the exercises for this chapter.

SUGGESTED LEARNING ACTIVITIES

1. Go to the website www.cdc.gov/growthcharts/ to find the growth charts published by the government for the purpose of monitoring normal physical growth. Then answer these questions: What is the normal range in inches and centimeters for the head circumference of a 12-month-old girl? What is the normal weight range in pounds and kilograms for a 15-year-old boy?
2. Observe family members and friends who fit into each of the life stages from infancy to later adulthood and relate the information given for each stage. How does it compare? What can you identify in terms of physical, cognitive, or psychosocial behaviors?
3. What life stage are you currently in? Can you relate your current activities and focus to the life stage?
4. Think of an older person you currently know or have known whom you admire. What did you learn from this person? What was his or her attitude toward life? Where does or did this person's strength of character come from? What are some other reasons you admire this individual?
5. Sit in a relaxed position with no external distractions, close your eyes, take some deep breaths, and clear your mind. Now imagine that you are 85 years old. Once you can settle quietly into this process, mentally start to ask yourself questions: Where do you live? What is your health like? Who

are your friends? What activities do you enjoy? What is important to you? Are you peaceful about the aging process or frightened by it? When you have completed the activity, open your eyes and discuss the experience with other classmates.

WEB ACTIVITIES

Worldometers

www.worldometers.info

Look at the figures under "World Population" and calculate the estimated percentage growth in the world population this year.

Tufts University Child and Family Web Guide

www.cfw.tufts.edu

Find a topic of interest on this site and write a report of your findings.

Elisabeth Kübler-Ross

www.ekrfoundation.org

Learn more about the woman who researched death and dying to bring to the nation an awareness of this process.

REVIEW QUESTIONS

1. What do the terms *physical, cognitive*, and *psychosocial* mean, as they relate to growth and development?
2. What are the nine life stages? What age group does each stage represent?
3. What are the primary physical changes that occur at each of the life stages?
4. What are the challenges of each stage according to Erik Erikson's psychosocial development theory?
5. What specific care considerations would relate to each of the life stages that would address age-appropriate communications and care?
6. What are the main theoretical points of Piaget's cognitive stages, Kohlberg's moral stages, and Gilligan's stages of the ethic of care?
7. List the five stages of grief and give an example of behaviors that may be observed during each stage.

APPLICATION EXERCISES

1. Refer to The Case of the Curious Four-Year-Old. What life stage is Paul in, and what are the unique challenges of this stage? What are the possible psychosocial ramifications if his initiative is restricted and he is severely criticized and scolded for his attempts to explore and question his environment? What are the potential positive outcomes if the time is taken to answer his questions and engage him in his care?
2. Ed Klein has been diagnosed with terminal cancer. He has elected to stay at home with his wife, who is his principal caregiver. They also have regular visits from various hospice health care professionals who assist with pain management, bathing, and any problems that arise. The hospice nurse, Sandy Johnson, visits three times a week. She notes that Mr. Klein frequently mentions what he will do as soon as he gets better. Sandy also notices that Mrs. Klein is reluctant to enter the room when she is working with Mr. Klein. On her third visit, Sandy decides to ask Mrs. Klein to come in and assist her with Mr. Klein's care. During the procedure, he acts very angry with his wife and criticizes everything she does to help.
   a. What stage(s) of dying does Mr. Klein demonstrate?
   b. Why do you think the wife was reluctant to enter the room?
   c. Do you think Mr. Klein truly does not know he has a terminal illness?
   d. What type of care assistance do you think this couple needs?

PROBLEM-SOLVING PRACTICE

1. Your grandmother just arrived at your house to celebrate her 75th birthday. When she drives up, someone in the family comments, "We had better have her stop driving—she is too old to be safe on the road." This idea is upsetting because you know her independence would be greatly curtailed and you are not sure if it is even appropriate.

You do some research and discover that crash rates begin to rise at age 70 and continue to rise as age increases. However, older drivers have the lowest crash rate per licensed driver, but the highest fatality rate per vehicle mile driven (older drivers have a high fatality rate because they are more physically fragile than their younger counterparts). Using the five-step problem-solving process, identify what you can do to determine if your grandmother should still be driving or not.

SUGGESTED READINGS AND RESOURCES

National Council on the Aging. www.ncoa.org

National Association of Child Care Resource and Referral Agencies. www.naccrra.org/

Thomas, W. H. (2007). *What are old people for? How elders will save the world*. Acton, MA: VanderWyk & Burnham.

This page intentionally left blank

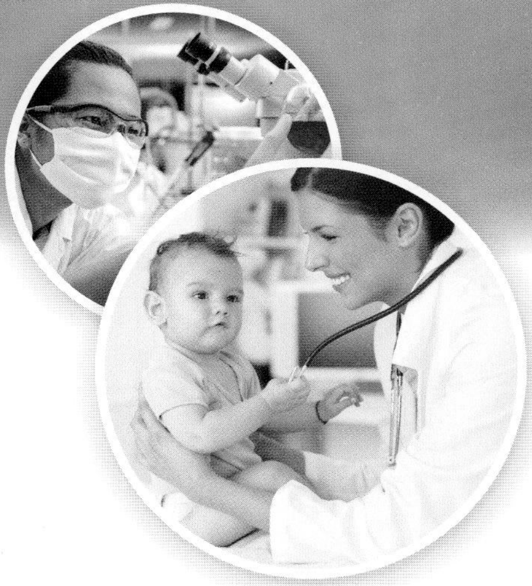

Unit 4

Personal and Workplace Safety

This page intentionally left blank

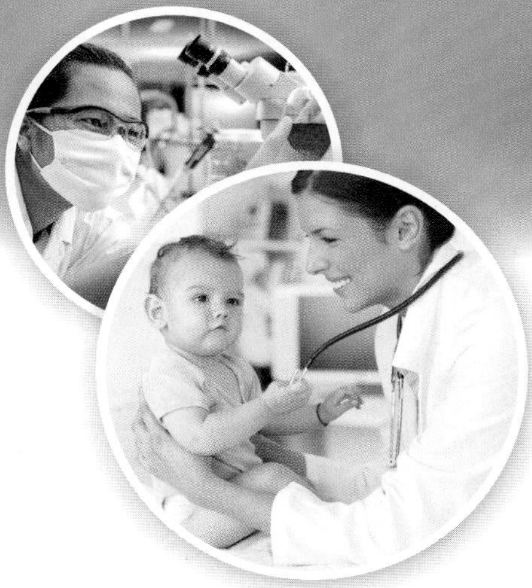

Chapter 9

Body Mechanics

OBJECTIVES

Studying and applying the material in this chapter will help you to:

- Understand and explain the importance of practicing good body mechanics and ergonomics at all times to prevent injury.
- Explain how repetitive injuries occur and how to prevent them.
- Demonstrate proper methods of sitting when working to prevent injury.
- Demonstrate proper methods of walking and standing at work to prevent injury.
- Demonstrate proper methods of lifting to prevent injury.
- Demonstrate proper methods of working at the computer to prevent injury.
- Properly use special adaptive devices to reduce the risk of workplace injuries.

KEY TERMS

body mechanics
ergonomics
repetitive motion injury (RMI)

The Case of Broken Dreams

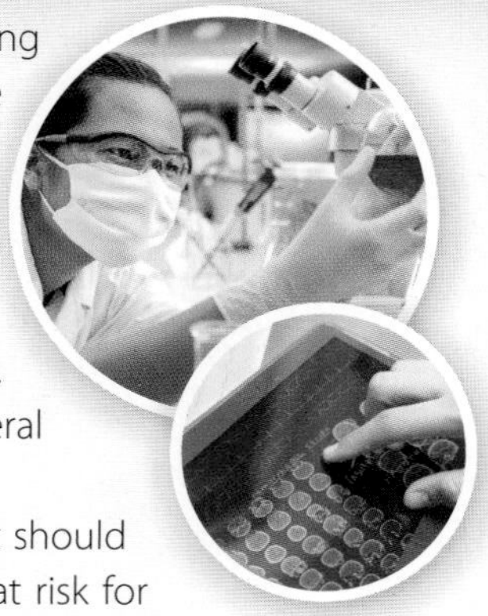

Rene Alvarez has dreamed of a career in health care for many years. She is thrilled about graduating next month and anticipates that the large medical center where she has been hired will be the fulfillment of her dreams. She has decided to move into a new apartment that is closer to her new employer and only has the weekend to get everything moved, in addition to studying for an important exam. Rene packs quickly and with the help of family and friends starts to load the truck rented for the move. In her haste, Rene forgets to follow proper body mechanics and lifts a box that is very heavy. She feels a tearing sensation in her back, followed by severe pain. She is rushed to the emergency department and is told that she will need to stay in bed for several weeks and surgery may be required if the bed rest provides her no relief.

This chapter will cover the basic principles of good body mechanics and ergonomics that should be followed at all times to prevent personal injury. Health care professionals are particularly at risk for injury because their daily job duties often include lifting equipment, supplies, and patients. Other health care professionals may not lift as much in their jobs but may have long periods of sitting, standing, or working with computers and other tabletop equipment.

THE IMPORTANCE OF PREVENTION

Health care professionals perform a number of mechanical movements with their bodies that can lead to injury. Following safety guidelines reduces the chance of injury and prevents unnecessary pain and suffering. Injuries are usually the result of poor practices over time that involve the repetition of improper movements. In other words, it is not the one-time incident that leads to the greatest number of injuries, but rather the same mistakes repeated over time. As one ages, it is especially important to follow sound practices. As flexibility decreases and recovery time increases, the chance of sustaining injuries is greater.

Certain risk factors increase the likelihood of injury. These include:

- Poor posture
- Poor body mechanics
- Low level of fitness
- Obesity
- Stress, both mechanical and psychological

The best preventive practices are simple and commonsense:

- Use good posture and body mechanics during all activities.
- Stay fit by exercising regularly.
- Maintain flexibility with stretching exercises.
- Stay trim by eating correctly.
- Reduce mental stress through good lifestyle habits (see Chapter 12).

Most injuries are cumulative, and so it is habitual activity repeated over years that determines the future risk of injury. Health care professionals should build good habits and safe practices into everyday life. Although the focus of this chapter is on workplace injuries and their prevention, the same principles apply to activities at home, at play, and even at rest.

Body mechanics and ergonomics are two terms used when discussing the prevention of injury. **Body mechanics** refers to the correct positioning of the body for a given task, such as lifting a heavy object or typing. **Ergonomics** is the science of designing and arranging things in the working and living environments for maximum efficiency and maximum health and safety. An ergonomic environment provides the highest possible comfort level and efficiency while limiting possible exposure to discomfort or potential injury. Developing the habit of following proper body mechanics and working in an ergonomically correct workplace are vital to decreasing the chance of injury to the worker.

GENERAL GUIDELINES

Numerous activities done every day at work and play can cause injuries. Workplace examples include:

- Nurses lifting patients
- Insurance coders sitting and working at the computer for long periods

- Surgical technicians standing during long operations
- Medical transcriptionists keyboarding for many hours each day
- Laboratory technicians bending over microscopes for prolonged periods

Injuries commonly suffered by health care professionals involve the musculoskeletal or nervous systems. Strained back muscles and inflamed tendons are common examples.

Repetitive motion injuries (RMIs) encompass many different injuries, but they are all based on the overuse of one part of the body. Motions that are repeated over time eventually put undue stress on muscles, tendons, nerves, blood vessels, or joints and cause inflammation, swelling, and pain. It is estimated that 50% of all industrial injuries in the United States are attributable to RMIs. Most of these injuries involve the hands, arms, neck, and shoulder area. RMIs are commonly thought of as work related, but they can occur as a result of academic, leisure-time, or household activities as well.

The symptoms of RMIs include:

- Pain. The pain is typically felt as an aching sensation that gets worse as the affected joint or limb is moved or used.
- Paresthesias. Paresthesia refers to an abnormal sensation or pricking, tingling, or burning in the absence of an external stimulus.
- Numbness, coldness, or loss of sensation
- Clumsiness, weakness, or lack of coordination
- Impaired range of motion or locking of the joint
- Popping, clicking, or crackling sound in the joint
- Swelling or redness in the affected area

Common RMIs suffered today include carpal tunnel syndrome, thoracic outlet syndrome, and tendonitis. (See Table 9–1.)

The following general principles help prevent injury to the musculoskeletal and nervous systems:

- Practice proper posture by maintaining the three normal curves of the back (e.g., avoid hunching over the desk or computer). (See Figure 9–1.)
- Warm up and stretch before and after activities that are repetitive, static (lacking movement), or prolonged.
- Use the largest joints and muscles to do the work (e.g., squat down to lift a box because this uses your legs and not your back).
- Avoid static positions for prolonged periods. Muscles fatigue faster when they are held in one position. Take a break and move around every 20 to 30 minutes when it is necessary to maintain a sustained position. This is also a good time to stretch stiff muscles. Alternately contract and relax muscles to increase blood circulation. (See Box 12–3 in Chapter 12 for muscle relaxation exercises.)
- Change positions or stop whenever activities cause pain.
- Use splints and wrist supports only upon recommendation of a physician or therapist. Be sure to follow instructions on the proper use of equipment.
- Seek treatment early if problems arise. Do not delay and simply hope the problem will go away.

Table 9–1 Most Common RMIs

Condition	Etiology (Cause)	Signs and Symptoms
Carpal tunnel syndrome	Repeated hand motions cause inflammation and swelling, which pinch nerves that pass through a tunnel of bones and ligaments in the wrist	• Tingling, numbness, and pain in the hand • Inability to make a fist • Loss of strength in hand
Thoracic outlet syndrome	Repeated motion causes bones or disks to compress nerves in the neck	• Tingling, numbness, and pain in the neck, shoulder, arms, or hands • Poor blood circulation in the hands and fingers • Weakness in arms and hands
Tendonitis	Repeated motion in a joint inflames tendons	• Swelling, tenderness, or weakness in the tendons of the shoulders, elbows, or hands

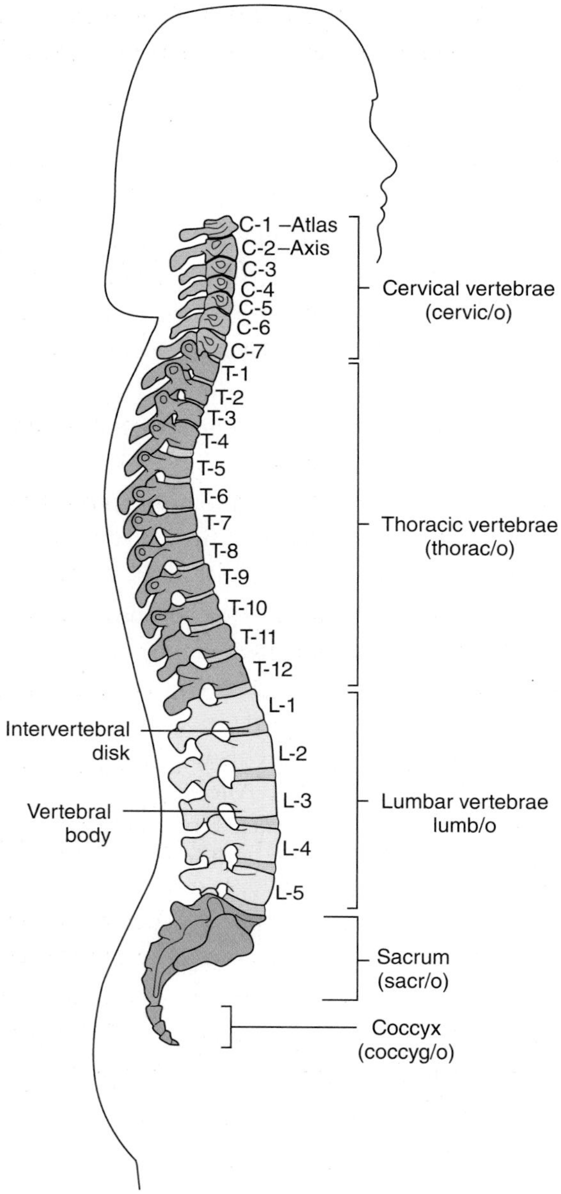

FIGURE 9–1 Normal curves of the spinal column.

- Learn to cope with psychological stress. People who are worried, afraid, or angry often carry their tension in their back, neck, or shoulder muscles. This tension reduces blood circulation in the affected tissues.

The treatment of RMIs varies with the severity of the injury. It may be possible to manage the injury with conservative measures, but surgical intervention is sometimes required. Physical and occupational therapists are an important part of the treatment team, advising about proper use of the injured body part and developing a home exercise program.

Thinking It Through

Dan McGregor has built model constructions since childhood. His other passion is computer games. Dan admits he spends too much time sedentary as both of these activities require little or no movement. He is very excited about his career path, which is to become a surgical technologist. He realizes this will require him to stand, bend, stoop, or sit for long periods in one location with minimal or no breaks. He will also be expected to manipulate instruments, supplies, and equipment with speed, dexterity, and good eye–hand coordination. Dan feels he is a perfect match for these job skills as they are similar to the activities he prefers and utilizes in his main hobbies.

1. Why might Dan have potential problems with RMIs?
2. Should Dan choose a different career option?
3. What might he do to avoid developing RMIs?

Psychotherapy may also be appropriate if the injury is related to job dissatisfaction or when an occupation or favorite activity must be given up due to the injury.

Fascinating Facts

Emotional stress has been shown to influence people's perception of physical pain. Workers who are unhappy in their jobs are more likely to seek treatment for work-related disorders.

Once the diagnosis is made, a treatment plan will be developed for the individual. Below are some common conservative treatment measures:

- Resting the affected part; complete rest should last no longer than two to three days as range of motion can be lost
- Applying ice packs or gentle heat
- Oral medications (mild pain relievers, anti-inflammatories)
- Corticosteroid injections can be injected into joints to reduce inflammation.
- Splinting is most commonly used for hand and wrist injuries and can be custom molded by an occupational therapist.

- Ergonomic corrections can be made in the home or workplace.
- Transcutaneous electrical nerve stimulation (TENS); TENS involves the use of a patient-controlled portable device that sends mild electrical impulses through injured tissues via electrodes placed over the skin. It is reported to relieve pain in 75% to 80% of patients treated for RMIs
- Acupuncture can reduce pain related to injury.
- Sports massage, Swedish massage, and shiatsu encourage improved blood circulation and relaxation of muscles.
- Yoga and tai chi result in a gentle stretching that helps to improve blood circulation and maintain range of motion without tissue damage.
- The Alexander technique is an approach to body movement that emphasizes correct posture, particularly the proper position of the head with respect to the spine.
- Hydrotherapy (warm whirlpool baths) improves circulation and relieves pain in injured joints and soft tissue.

Recovery from an RMI may take only a few days of rest or modified activity, or it may take several months when surgery is required. RMIs are treated with surgery only when conservative measures fail to relieve the patient's pain after a trial of 6 to 12 weeks. The most common surgical procedures performed include nerve decompression, tendon release, and repair of loose or torn ligaments. Rehabilitation programs are tailored to the individual patient and the specific disorder involved.

The prognosis for recovery from RMIs depends on the specific disorder, the degree of damage, and the patient's compliance with the recommended exercises and activity. Most patients experience adequate pain relief from either conservative measures or surgery. Some, however, will not recover full use of the affected part and must change occupations or give up the activity that produced the original injury.

Fascinating Facts

The Bureau of Labor Statistics reports that 75.2% of all occupational injuries and illnesses occur in service-providing industries.

Study Boxes 9–1, 9–2, and 9–3. They include specific information about proper sitting, standing, walking, and lifting.

BOX 9–1

While Sitting:

1. Use a chair that supports the normal curves of the back (use a lumbar support if needed). Avoid sitting on stools. Don't slouch in chairs or on couches.
2. Keep head and shoulders aligned over hips. Avoid bending neck forward for long periods.
3. Avoid pressing the back of the knees against the edge of the chair seat.
4. Minimize twisting and bending motions. Position equipment and work so that the body is directly in front of and close to them.
5. When turning is necessary, pivot entire body in unison or use a swivel chair.
6. Change positions frequently. Get up and move around and stretch at regular intervals.
7. Position your chair so work is at eye level and feet are flat on floor or on a footrest.
8. When using the telephone frequently or for extended periods, use a speakerphone or headset.
9. When not using your hands, keep your upper arms close to your body, elbows at a 90- to 100-degree angle, forearms neutral (thumbs toward ceiling), and wrists straight.

BOX 9–2

While Standing and Walking:

1. Be aware of your posture. Maintain the three normal curves of the back.
2. Keep your neck in a neutral position (avoid jutting the chin forward or slouching).
3. Wear cushioned shoes with good support if work requires standing or walking a lot.
4. When standing, shift your weight often.
5. If standing in one place for long periods, use a footstool. Alternate placing one foot up on the stool to take the strain off the back.

BOX 9-3

While Lifting:

1. Move in close to the object to be lifted.
2. Be aware of your posture. Maintain the three normal curves of the back. (See Figure 9–1.)
3. Increase the base of support by positioning your feet 6 to 8 inches apart. (See Figures 9–2 and 9–3.)
4. Squat down (bending hips and knees), maintaining normal curves of the back. (See Figure 9–4.) When picking up objects, bend at the knees rather than at the waist.
5. Position your hands underneath the object to be lifted.
6. Take a deep breath and tighten your abdominal muscles prior to lifting. This increases intra-abdominal pressure to increase the support for the spine and back muscles.
7. Lift the load with the legs (not with the back). Use the large muscles of the legs to lift load. (See Figure 9–2.)
8. Always ask for assistance from other health care professionals when needed. (See Figure 9–2)
9. Use two hands to lift rather than one, even with light objects. (See Figure 9–3.)
10. Carry objects close to body at waist level. (See Figure 9–3.)
11. When turning, move your entire body in unison (avoid twisting). To change directions, use the feet rather than the back: Move and turn the feet instead of twisting the spine while the feet are planted in one position. (See Figure 9–2.)
12. Avoid reaching overhead with heavy loads (use step stools, ladders, etc.).
13. Push rather than pull heavy objects. The exception to this rule is when on ramps, where you would pull from the higher level.
14. Slide or push objects, when possible, instead of lifting them.
15. Use carts and dollies to carry heavy loads. If possible, break up the load into several trips to avoid lifting heavy loads. Or have someone assist with the lifting of heavy objects.
16. Tilt containers or objects to avoid bending the wrist to pick up objects.

Note: Lifting and moving patients can be a particular challenge for health care professionals who work directly with patients. Many of the principles presented apply to these activities, but additional skills are also required that are beyond the scope of this book. The use of specialized lifting equipment may be available in these settings. Some hospitals have also developed lift teams that can be contacted for assistance in particularly problematic moves involving patients.

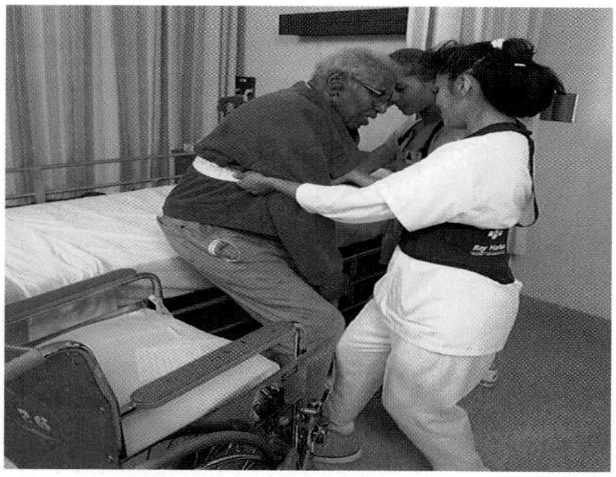

FIGURE 9–2 When lifting, maintain proper posture, position feet for wide base of support, and lift with the leg muscles. Also note that two health care professionals are working as a team for this difficult transfer.

Media Link

Learn more about how to properly move your body to prevent injury by viewing the Body Mechanics video on the Online Resources.

Back Belts

Back injuries account for nearly 20% of all injuries and illnesses in the workplace. This is estimated to cost the nation approximately 20 to 50 billion dollars per year.

In addition to applying body mechanics and learning how to lift properly, some facilities and health care professionals believe that back belts decrease lower back injuries. (See Figure 9–5.) Back belts may also be referred to as back supports or abdominal belts.

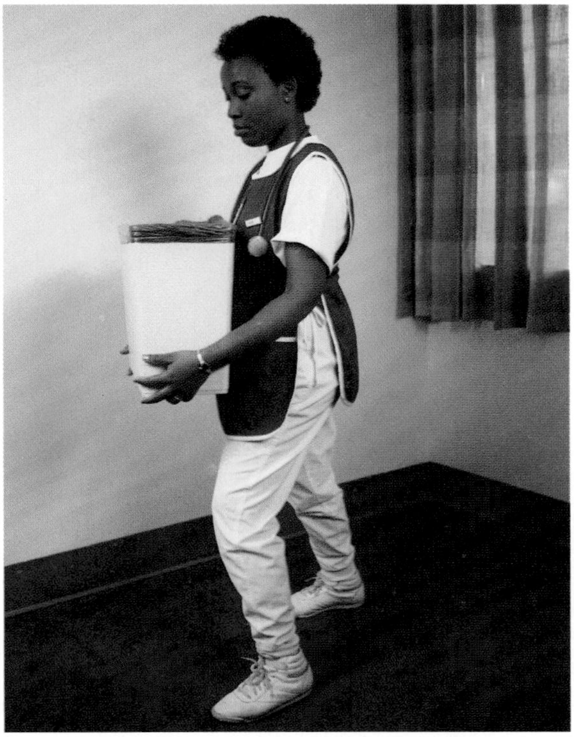

FIGURE 9–3 When lifting, maintain proper posture, position feet for wide base of support, and hold object close to the body at waist level using both hands.

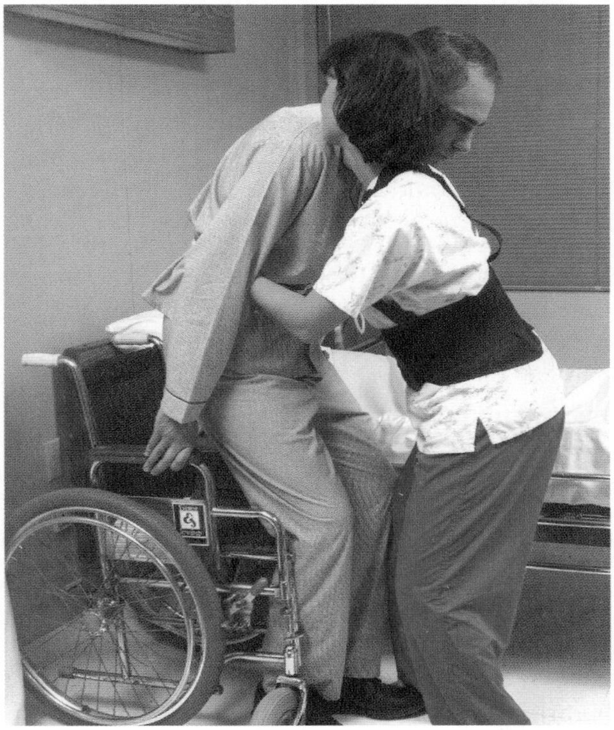

FIGURE 9–5 This health care worker is wearing a back belt as she helps transfer a patient from the bed to a wheelchair.

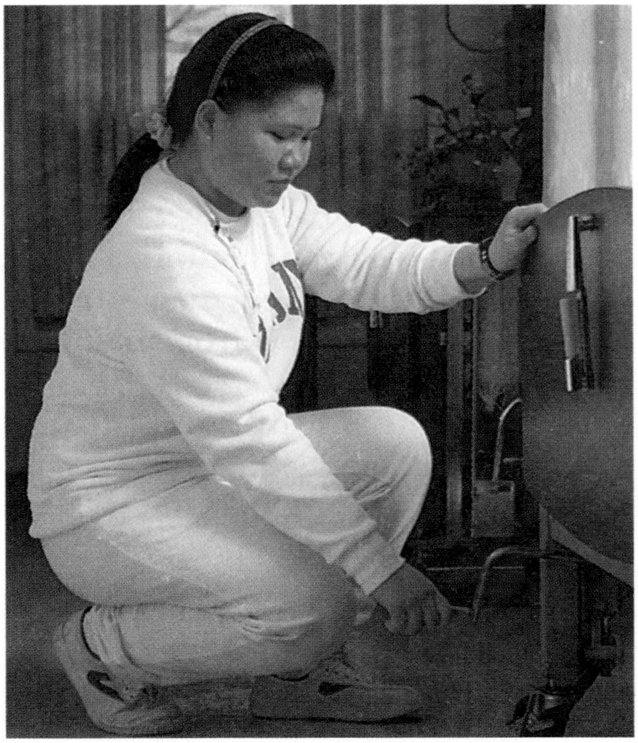

FIGURE 9–4 Maintain proper posture when bending from the hips and knees.

Back belt advocates state that they are helpful and that back belts increase intra-abdominal pressure, which creates support for the spine and back muscles when lifting. They also feel that the belts increase the flexibility of the stomach and back muscles by keeping them warm. Finally, it is argued that their presence serves as a reminder to workers to follow proper body mechanics.

Opponents to using back belts state that the belts increase the worker's blood and pelvic pressures, which can lead to cardiac problems. They also believe that the warmth and sweating created by wearing back belts can cause heat rashes, that improper fitting of belts can cause abdominal pain and injuries, and that they can give a false sense of security so that workers may attempt to lift heavier loads than their strength can safely handle. Finally, they suggest that, if used, back belts should be tightened only when lifting and left loose the rest of the time.

According to The National Institute for Occupational Safety and Health (NIOSH) there is inadequate scientific evidence to determine or deny the advantages of back belts. Go to cdc.gov/niosh/docs/94-127 to view a pamphlet detailing their findings.

The current theory is the most effective way to prevent back injury is to redesign the work environment and work tasks to reduce the hazards of lifting. Training in identifying lifting hazards and using safe lifting techniques and methods should improve program effectiveness.

Some facilities are incorporating other approaches into their ergonomic programs, such as lift teams and specialized equipment to decrease the possibility of back injuries.

COMPUTERS AND ERGONOMICS

Although ergonomics is not a new field, the advent of computers and expanding use of digital devices have increased awareness of the field because of the number of injuries being reported. In the past, keying of data was done by a small number of employees and the resulting RMIs were limited to relatively few workers. The prevalence of computers in offices, libraries, schools, and homes has resulted in a corresponding increase in injuries. Computers, along with smaller digital devices, are used not only at the workplace but also to play games, communicate with others, purchase items, and conduct research. Many users are now suffering from ailments that are the direct result of the repetitive motion of typing or using a mouse as a pointing device.

All computer users should take steps to protect themselves from potential RMIs. Health care professionals such as transcriptionists, insurance coders, information management technicians, admitting clerks, and others who work at computers each day should be especially careful about setting up workstations that fit their physical needs. Figure 9–6 illustrates proper positioning, and Box 9–4 includes tips for the safe use of the computer. Many facilities now provide computer stations that are mobile and adjustable. Many models provide the option to sit or stand while using the computer. The monitor angle is adjustable and its height along with the mouse and keyboard would ideally all be adjustable. Another advantageous feature would be locking wheels for easy portability plus stability. (See Figure 9–7.)

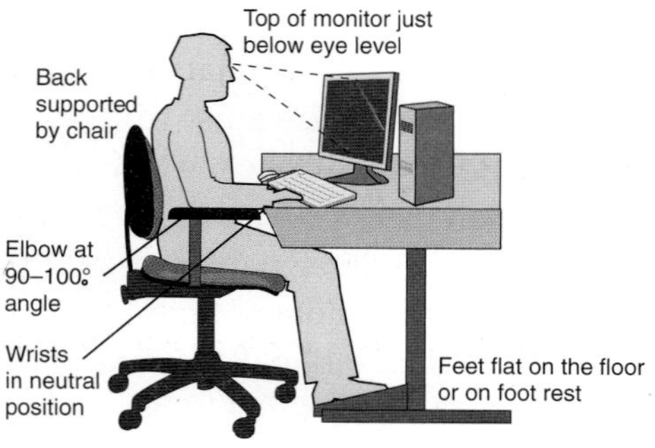

FIGURE 9–6 Proper positioning for seated use of the computer.

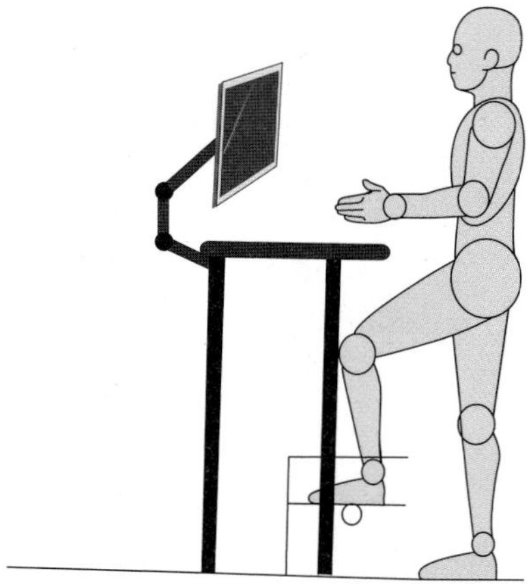

FIGURE 9–7 Proper upright standing posture includes a soft bend in the knees or alternating foot on the footplate of the cart, as demonstrated here.

Use of a Mouse as Pointing Device

The extensive use of the mouse as a pointing device when working with a computer has been shown to be a major contributor to RMIs. It is important that the mouse be within easy reach and that the user not stretch to use it. If a mouse is used on a keyboard tray, there needs to be enough room for the mouse so that it is positioned at the same level as the keyboard.

The chance of injury can be lowered by developing the ability to use the mouse with either hand and alternating hands throughout the day. Another preventive measure is to use the keyboard to give common commands. This involves simultaneously pressing the special function keys, such as "Ctrl" and "F1" and the lettered keys, or pressing the function keys alone. Examples include the following:

- Ctrl + s saves a document
- Ctrl + p prints a document
- Alt + F4 closes a program

Some keyboard commands are universal and apply to many software programs. Others are specific to programs such as Microsoft Office. Learning the commands for the programs used most often can speed input and help avoid computer injuries.

BOX 9–4

While Using the Computer:

1. Position the screen at arm's length to reduce eyestrain and head-forward posture.
2. Position the top of the monitor just below eye level directly in front of the body.
3. Place a document holder next to the screen rather than working from a document placed flat on the desk.
4. Place both feet flat on the floor or footrest to reduce back strain.
5. Keep your back in total contact with the back of the chair.
6. Position your abdomen close to the edge of the desk to prevent a forward-leaning posture.
7. Maintain your wrists in a neutral (straight) position when keying or using a pointing device.
8. Position the keyboard so your elbow is at the same height as the keyboard. Slant the keyboard as necessary to maintain your elbows at an angle of 90 to 100 degrees and a neutral wrist position.
9. Rest your eyes and reduce eyestrain by blinking your eyes rapidly, closing them, or focusing on another object away from the computer screen for 10 seconds every 15 minutes.
10. Stretch frequently (shrug shoulders, arch back, nod head, roll feet in circular motion). See Table 9–2 for computer exercises.
11. Use wrist rests during pauses to help maintain neutral position. They are not meant to be used during active keying.
12. Avoid resting wrists against hard surfaces and sharp edges.
13. Try using an ergonomically designed keyboard.

Table 9–2 Computer Exercises

Exercise	Description	Benefit
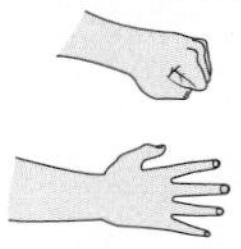	Make a fist, and then open your hands while spreading fingers apart.	Relaxes muscles of hands, wrists, and forearms
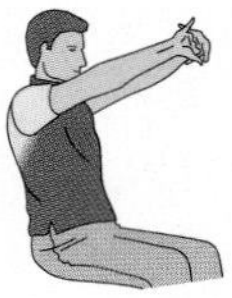	Interlace the fingers of both hands, then extend your arms at shoulder level, palms facing away from you.	Stretches the muscles of the arms, shoulders, and upper back
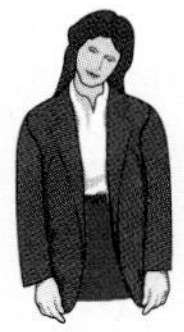	Slowly rotate your head by tilting it to one side, then roll it to a forward position, to the other side. Repeat.	Stretches the neck muscles and helps relieve tension
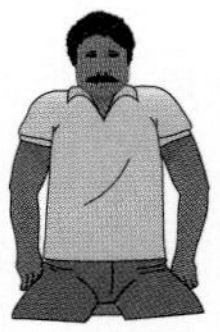	Shrug shoulders up toward the ears, then relax and let them return to their normal position.	Decreases tension in neck and shoulder muscles
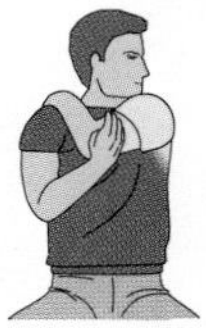	Place your left arm on your right shoulder and turn your head to the left. With your right arm, gently push your left arm for increased stretch. Repeat.	Stretches muscles of upper arm and upper back

Visual Problems

Visual discomfort is commonly reported as a result of computer work. Eyestrain and headaches are the most common problems. The eyes tire more quickly when looking at a computer screen than when reading printed materials. This is because of the different characteristics of the type. Printed material has dark, dense, consistent lines that are easy to focus on. Computer screens display images with a less consistent density; this results in the eyes having to work much harder to focus. This extra effort can result in eyestrain. See Box 9–5 for guidelines to prevent eyestrain.

People who wear bifocals have an additional challenge to overcome when working on the computer. The lower section of bifocals is used for reading and is adjusted to focus at a closer distance than the typical distance one sits from the computer. Bifocals are also angled downward for reading, so bifocal wearers will typically tilt their heads upward so they can view the screen at this angle. This moves the neck out of the neutral position and can lead to neck problems. One solution is to position the monitor lower than eye level. For the person who does a great deal of computer work, it is preferable to have the ophthalmologist prepare a set of bifocal lenses specifically designed for use at the computer.

BOX 9–5

To Prevent Eyestrain:

- Look away from the computer screen and focus on other objects in the environment at frequent intervals.
- Rest the eyes every 20 to 30 minutes.
- Adjust the contrast on the computer screen to a comfortable level.
- Keep the computer screen clean.
- Position the screen to avoid glare from surrounding lights and windows.
- Use a paper holder to prevent having to look down to see text.
- Use a glare screen on the monitor.

Thinking It Through

Gary Carlson is a nurse who works at an intermediate care facility. During the shift, he frequently needs to lift patients as he cares for or assists them during their activities of daily living. The facility has just implemented a new policy that all health care professionals must wear a back belt while lifting or moving patients. Gary attended the inservice on how to properly wear and use the back belt, but has several concerns. He has hypertension (high blood pressure) and fears that the back belt may elevate it further. He has also noticed that the increased perspiration from wearing the belt has caused an uncomfortable rash. He has decided to stop wearing the belt and hopes that his supervisor will not notice.

1. Are Gary's concerns valid?
2. Is Gary's solution to the problem appropriate?
3. Are there other solutions Gary could consider to resolve the problem?

WORKBOOK PRACTICE

Go to your workbook and complete the exercises for this chapter.

SUGGESTED LEARNING ACTIVITIES

1. If you have a computer area or office at your home, evaluate whether any changes to the workstation would improve the ergonomics.
2. Evaluate your work, academic, leisure-time, and household activities for areas that may cause overlap of repetitive movements. Did you identify any areas of concern? What can you do now to prevent future problems?
3. Observe health care professionals at work. What measures do they take to avoid workplace injuries?
4. Evaluate your compliance with the guidelines in this chapter. Do you have any "at risk" behaviors? What modifications can you make to decrease the risk of injury?

WEB ACTIVITIES

Ergoweb

www.ergoweb.com

Choose one of the news articles and write a report.

U.S. Department of Labor—Occupational Safety and Health Administration (OSHA)

www.osha.gov

Use the index to find ergonomics. Summarize the recommended elements that factor into implementing the ergonomic process to reduce the risk of musculoskeletal injuries.

Ergonomics

www.ergonomics.org

Record the three ergonomic principles that can significantly reduce risk of injury.

REVIEW QUESTIONS

1. What do the following terms mean?
   a. Body mechanics
   b. Ergonomics
   c. Repetitive motion injuries
2. What are the three most common RMIs, and why do they occur?
3. How can health care professionals protect themselves from injury when sitting, walking, standing, and lifting?
4. What are the characteristics of correct posture?
5. What guidelines should be followed to prevent injury when working at a computer?
6. Why is it important to do stretching exercises when spending extended time working at the computer? Describe exercises that stretch the neck, hands, arms, and upper back.
7. How can you decrease the risk of RMIs when using a mouse as a pointing device?
8. What is the cause of eyestrain when reading from a computer screen? What can you do to prevent this from occurring?

APPLICATION EXERCISES

1. What could Rene, in The Case of Broken Dreams at the beginning of this chapter, have done to decrease her likelihood of sustaining injuries?
2. John Jones, a health care student, has been saving for months to purchase a laptop computer to assist him with his classes. He plans to purchase a computer table and chair as soon as he saves the additional money. In the meantime, he will be using the computer on his lap or at the kitchen table.
   a. What possible injuries is John risking by not having an ergonomically sound setup?
   b. What criteria should he consider when purchasing a computer table and chair?
   c. What can he do in the meantime to adapt the kitchen to a safe working environment? Include RMI and eyestrain prevention. Describe in detail or prepare a sketch of your suggestions.

PROBLEM-SOLVING PRACTICE

Robert Sherman spends many hours at the computer. He loves to surf the web and play games and now he is also doing a great deal of word processing for his classroom projects. He has heard a lot of talk about carpal tunnel syndrome and wonders if he can prevent this from happening to him. Using the five-step problem-solving process, determine what Robert can do about prevention.

SUGGESTED READINGS AND RESOURCES

National Institute of Neurological Disorders and Stroke. www.ninds.nih.gov/

Occupational Safety and Health Administration. www.osha.gov/

This page intentionally left blank

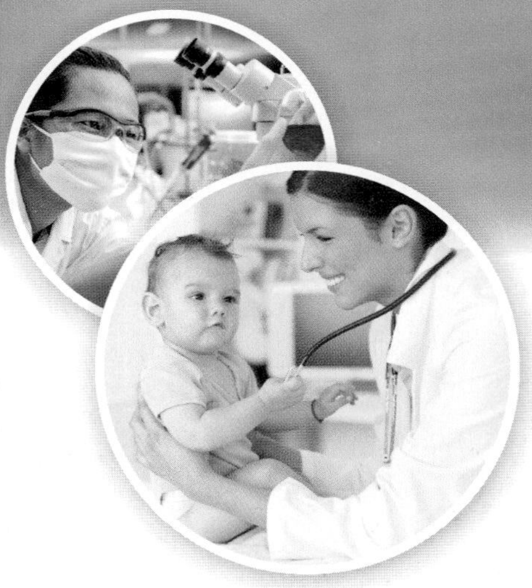

Chapter 10

Infection Control

OBJECTIVES

Studying and applying the material in this chapter will help you to:

- Understand and explain the importance of infection control practices in maintaining the safety of the health care professional, patients, and others.
- List the milestones that led to the development of germ theory and infection control.
- Identify the five types of microbes and give examples of infectious diseases caused by each type.
- Describe the chain of infection and list methods the health care professional can use to break it.
- Give examples of the body's defense mechanisms.
- Describe the CDC and OSHA and explain their roles in health care safety.
- Identify the preventive procedures included in the standard precautions.
- Identify situations when handwashing is indicated and demonstrate the technique.
- Identify the three types of transmission-based precautions and when they may be used.
- Describe neutropenic precautions and when they would be used.
- Explain the differences among antiseptics, disinfectants, and sterilization.
- Identify and describe the three major disease risks for health care professionals.
- Describe how pathogens become drug resistant and the impact this has on health care.
- Describe measures that will protect the health care professional and others from blood-borne pathogens.

KEY TERMS

aerobic
AIDS
anaerobic
antibiotic
antiseptics
asepsis (aseptic technique)
bacteria
bacteriocidal
bacteriostatic
Centers for Disease Control and Prevention (CDC)
chain of infection
communicable disease
contaminated
disinfectants
fungi (pl. of fungus)
germ theory
hepatitis B
HIV positive
host
immune response
infection control
infectious disease
medical asepsis (clean technique)

(continues)

KEY TERMS (continued)

- microbes
- microbiology
- microorganisms
- microscope
- neutropenic precautions
- normal flora
- nosocomial infection
- Occupational Safety and Health Administration (OSHA)
- opportunistic infection
- parasite
- pathogens
- protozoa
- rickettsia
- standard precautions
- sterile field
- sterilization
- surgical asepsis (sterile technique)
- transmission-based precautions
- tuberculosis (TB)
- viruses

The Case of the Traveling Microorganisms

Ralph Romero, a health care professional at a large metropolitan hospital, awakens in the middle of the night with coughing, sneezing, runny nose, and a temperature of 101°F. He is scheduled to work the next day and so takes medications to treat his symptoms and goes back to bed. He awakens still feeling ill and wishes he could stay home, but knows the hospital is always so busy on the weekends and decides to go despite being ill. He works his shift, being careful when he coughs or sneezes to turn his head away from the patient and use some handkerchiefs he brought from home when coughing, sneezing, or blowing his nose. He also makes sure that he washes his hands when entering each patient's room. In this chapter, health care professionals will learn their role in preventing the transmission of microorganisms while performing their duties.

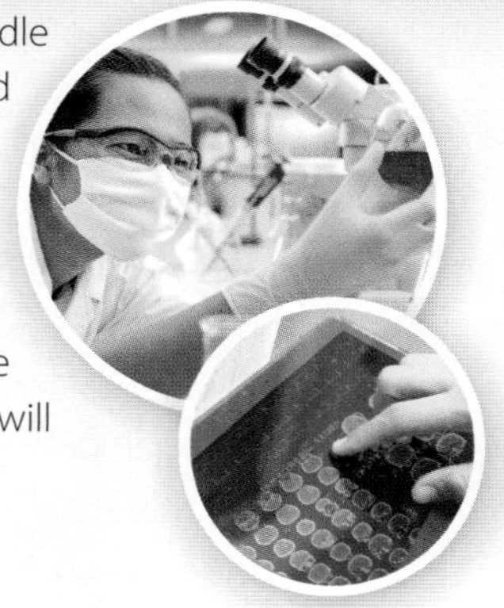

IMPORTANCE OF INFECTION CONTROL IN HEALTH CARE

Before entering a health care facility or having contact with a patient, it is essential to have a clear understanding of **infection control**. The main goal of infection control is to prevent the spread of infectious diseases. An **infectious disease** is any disease caused by the growth of **pathogens**, disease-causing microorganisms (germs), in the body.

It is essential that health care professionals maintain a safe environment by following specific policies and procedures designed to reduce the risk of transferring infectious diseases. Failure to prevent the spread of an infectious disease can cause unnecessary pain, suffering, and even death. Regulatory standards have been developed to prevent pathogens from being passed from patient to patient, staff to patient, patient to staff, or staff to staff. Improperly cleaned instruments and equipment are other means of transmitting pathogens. Strict adherence to proper procedures also prevents health care professionals and visitors to facilities from spreading pathogens to the community.

It is critical to identify any signs or symptoms of an infection as quickly as possible so an evaluation can be performed and treatment prescribed as indicated. An infection can be *generalized* (i.e., *systemic*, affecting the whole body), or *localized* (affecting one area of the body).

- Generalized (systemic) infections: Signs and symptoms commonly experienced are headaches, fever, fatigue, vomiting, diarrhea, and an increase in pulse and respiration.
- Localized infections: The area will be red, swollen, warm to the touch, and painful. There may also be drainage.

As infection control is central to all health care occupations, there is a great deal of material to cover on this subject. This chapter is organized by topic: microbiology, prevention through asepsis, infection control procedures, risks, and reporting procedures for accidental exposure.

MICROBIOLOGY

Microorganisms are very small, usually one-celled, living plants or animals. They exist everywhere in the environment but can only be seen with the aid of a **microscope** (an instrument fitted with a powerful magnifying lens). It is easy to forget their significance because their presence is not obvious. *But it is critical to remember that the actions of the health care professional can assist destructive microorganisms in their travel, allowing them to infect workers and others.*

The study of microorganisms is called **microbiology** and is derived from the Greek words *micros*, meaning small; *bios*, meaning life; and *logy*, meaning the study of. Although the microscope was invented in the 1600s by Anton van Leeuwenhoek, scientists did little more than simply observe microorganisms under the lens. No one questioned their origin or relation to other life forms. It was not until Louis Pasteur (a French biochemist and physicist) began to study the actions of specific microorganisms in the 1800s that the germ theory was developed. The **germ theory** states that specific microorganisms, called bacteria, are the cause of specific diseases in both humans and animals.

Important highlights in the history of infection control include the following:

- An article written in 1843 by Oliver Wendell Holmes stating that a *contagious disease* or **communicable disease** (a disease that may be transmitted either directly or indirectly from one individual to another) might be spread by the **contaminated** (presence of infectious material) hands of doctors and nurses.
- The observation by Ignaz Philipp Semmelweis, a Hungarian obstetrician, that mortality rates were higher when patients were attended by physicians or medical students who came directly from the morgue or autopsy room without first washing their hands.
- The development by Lord Joseph Lister in 1864 of *surgical aseptic technique* to prevent contamination of the wound and operative site.

Not all microorganisms are harmful. Many commonly reside in a particular environment on or in the body and are known as **normal flora**. The skin, vagina, and intestines are examples of areas that have normal flora.

Some microorganisms are even necessary to maintain normal function. For example, the bacterium *Escherichia coli* aids the digestive process in the colon. In this case *E. coli* is a nonpathogen. *E. coli* can also be a pathogen and create an infection when it invades an area of the body where it is not a part of the normal flora, such as the blood or urine.

Other microorganisms are part of the normal flora, but have no beneficial role. They normally do no harm unless the individual becomes susceptible to an infection due to an alteration in the normal physiological state of the body. This can occur through suppression of the **immune response**, which is a specific defense used by the body to fight infection and disease by producing antibodies (protective proteins that combat pathogens). Also, long-term **antibiotic** (medications capable of inhibiting the growth of or destroying microorganisms) therapy suppresses the normal flora and creates an imbalance that can decrease the body's ability to resist pathogens. When an infection occurs due to the weakened physiological state of the body, it is called an **opportunistic infection**. The ability of the body to resist infection is determined by age, presence of other disease, level of physical health, degree of mental stress, nutritional state, and certain medications.

Microorganisms are either **aerobic** (require oxygen to live) or **anaerobic** (do not require oxygen to live). Many microorganisms prefer a warm, moist, dark environment that provides a source of food. The human body meets these requirements and is thus an ideal environment within which microorganisms can flourish.

Some microorganisms derive nutrients for growth and reproduction from nonliving material and others from living organisms, or **hosts**. If this relationship is beneficial to the host, it is called *symbiosis*. If there is no effect on the host, it is called *neutralism*. But if damage is done to the host, the condition is *parasitic*. An organism that nourishes itself at the expense of other living things and causes them damage is called a **parasite**.

Fascinating Facts

Prior to the germ theory, it was believed that microorganisms spontaneously arose from decomposing nonliving matter. This theory was based on such observations as noting that maggots (fly larvae) were found in decaying meat and mice would appear when sweat laden shirts were stored with wheat in a dark area.

Types of Microbes

Microbes are pathogenic microorganisms. Plant and animal microbes are classified as bacteria, viruses, fungi, rickettsia, and protozoa.

Bacteria

Bacteria are one-celled organisms and can be either pathogenic or nonpathogenic. Many produce *toxins* (poisonous substances). Most bacteria require oxygen and grow best in moderate temperatures. When a group of bacteria grows in one place, it is called a *colony*. Bacteria are categorized according to their shapes: round, rod, and spiral. Each type causes certain diseases and conditions. (See Figure 10–1.)

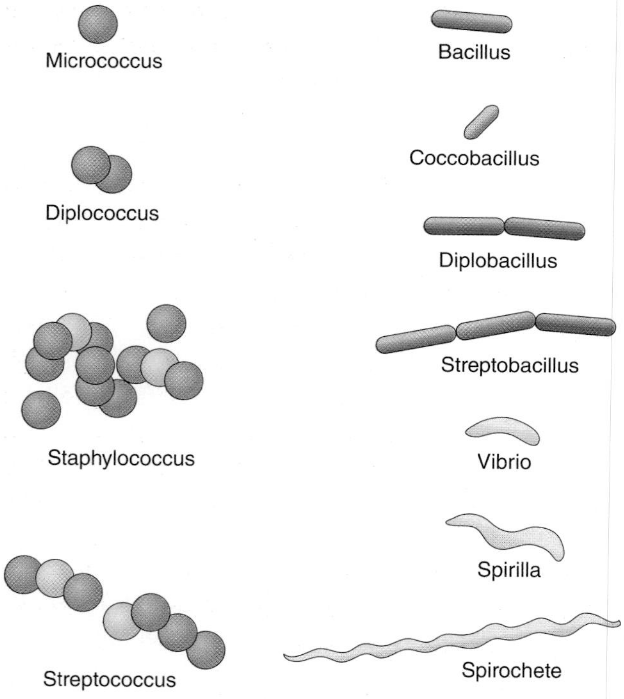

FIGURE 10–1 Bacterial cells vary in shape and arrangement.

Round- or *ovoid-shaped* bacteria are called *cocci*. Cocci can be further defined by a description of their appearance:

- Micrococci: Appear singly
- Diplococci: Appear in pairs
- Staphylococci: Appear as irregular clusters
- Streptococci: Form chains

Micrococci cause a variety of skin and wound infections. Diplococci cause gonorrhea, meningitis, and some types of pneumonia. Staphylococci are pus-producing and can cause other types of pneumonia, abscesses, boils, wound infections, and urinary tract infections. Streptococci can cause rheumatic fever and a severe sore throat referred to as strep throat.

Rod-shaped bacteria are called *bacilli*. Bacilli can also be further defined by description of their appearance:

- Bacilli: Appear singly
- Coccobacilli: Rods are somewhat oval
- Diplobacilli: Appear in pairs
- Streptobacilli: Attached end to end to form chain

Some common diseases caused by various bacilli are tuberculosis, tetanus, pertussis (whooping cough), botulism (severe form of food poisoning), diphtheria, and typhoid fever.

The third shape bacteria can take is *spiral*. Spiral-shaped bacteria can be further defined by their characteristics or appearance:

- Vibrios: Form curved rods
- Spirilla: Organism is rigid
- Spirochetes: Organism is flexible

Some common diseases caused by spiral-shaped bacteria include syphilis and cholera.

Although cocci are incapable of movement, some of the rod- and spiral-shaped bacteria have slender whip-like appendages called *flagella* (sing. flagellum) that give them the power of independent locomotion.

Diagnosing which bacteria may be causing an infection is essential for proper treatment. A laboratory method that is often used to identify the general category of a microorganism is called *Gram staining*. In this method, bacteria are stained with a substance called crystal violet. Bacteria react to staining differently, based on the makeup of their cell walls. This is why their reactions are clues to their identity. There are three categories of reactions:

1. Gram-positive: Retains the stain
2. Gram-negative: Loses the stain
3. Acid-fast: Retains the stain even when treated with acid

This information can be obtained rather quickly and helps determine the class of antibiotic to prescribe.

Another laboratory method usually performed at the same time is to grow the microorganism in various culture media (materials that promote the growth of microorganisms). It can take 24 to 72 hours for colonies to form, but the information obtained can result in the identification of the exact bacteria. Based on this more specific diagnosis, the choice of antibiotics can be reevaluated to determine if a more specific medication should be prescribed.

Fascinating Facts

It is estimated that each of us carries 10^{14} bacteria (100,000,000,000,000, or 100 trillion) in and on our bodies and that the total population of our planet excretes 10^{22} bacteria in feces every day (Thomas, 2013).

Almost all bacteria can be destroyed with antibiotics. However, several types of bacteria are resistant to antibiotics and are challenging to treat. They create a threat to the health of both patients and health care professionals. Resistant strains of bacteria are discussed later in this chapter.

Some bacteria have the ability to form spores. Spores are a thick capsule that the bacterium creates for self-protection. Spores are created when life-supporting conditions are not favorable and are referred to as the "resting stage." Spores are extremely difficult to kill and can lay dormant for months or even years. In this stage, bacteria are still alive but inactive and very resistant to heat, drying, and the action of disinfectants. When supportive conditions return, the bacteria become active again. Extremely high temperatures, such as that reached by steam, must be used for sterilization to ensure that all spores are killed.

Viruses

Viruses are the smallest of the microbes and cannot be seen under the traditional light microscope. A special piece of equipment called an electron microscope is necessary to identify them. (See Figure 10–2.)

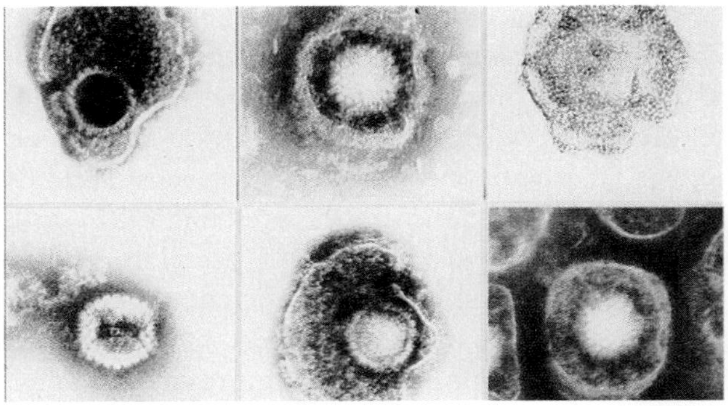

The Centers for Disease Control and Prevention, Dr. Erskine Palmer

FIGURE 10–2 Electron micrographs of herpes simplex viruses.

Viruses are not whole cells and depend on living cells to provide food, nutrients, and a means of reproduction. Because they can only live inside another living organism, they are referred to as *obligate intracellular parasites*.

More than 300 viruses have been identified by researchers. Some appear to be harmless, but others can cause infections that result in the common cold, influenza (flu), pneumonia, chickenpox, croup, hepatitis B, acquired immunodeficiency syndrome (AIDS), measles, mumps, herpes, warts, and polio.

Viral infections can be extremely difficult to treat because viruses multiply rapidly and are easily transmitted by blood and other body secretions. They are resistant to many disinfectants and are not killed by antibiotics, which kill bacteria.

Fungi

Fungi are a large group of organisms that are neither plant nor animal. They have unique characteristics that are not shared by other organisms and are thus placed in a Kingdom of their own. Two forms of fungi are potential pathogens: yeast and mold. Yeasts are one-celled and molds are multicelled organisms. Both are present everywhere. Fungi cannot produce their own nutrients, so they rely on *organic* (animal and vegetable forms of life) materials. Some use live and others use dead organic materials for nutrients. Fungi thrive in warm, moist, dark conditions.

Many yeasts and molds are nonpathogenic. In fact, penicillin, an important antibiotic, is produced from a mold. But as with other types of microorganisms, fungi can become pathogenic when the right conditions exist. When this happens they create an opportunistic infection. Fungal infections can range from merely annoying to life-threatening.

Some fungi cause chronic, recurrent infections. Superficial, or *cutaneous*, infections are infections of the skin or mucous membranes; these include fungi that cause ringworm, athlete's foot, and infections of the skin, hair follicles, and scalp. The most serious of the fungal infections are the systemic infections, such as *histoplasmosis* (a systemic respiratory disease). Infections that go beyond the cutaneous level are always difficult, if not impossible, to treat or cure. Treatment of systemic infections requires medications that are toxic to humans. Patients, therefore, must be closely monitored.

Fascinating Facts

A fungus is an organism that causes food spoilage. Who has not seen fuzzy or dark moldy spots on spoiled bread, fruits, and vegetables? And you are probably familiar with the characteristic "musty" smell of mold. But there are also commercial uses of fungi, such as the use of yeast in making wine from grapes and beer from malt, and creating the carbon dioxide necessary for dough to rise. Molds are also responsible for the flavor of Roquefort and Camembert cheeses.

Rickettsia

Rickettsia are much smaller than bacteria and have rod or spherical shapes. They stain as gram negative and do not move independently. Rickettsia must live inside the cell of another living organism and so are, like the viruses, referred to as obligate intracellular parasites.

Media Link

View the Infection Control animation on the Online Resources for an overview of microscopic organisms that cause diseases and the importance of handwashing in preventing the spread of infection.

Rickettsia cause several types of typhus and Rocky Mountain spotted fever. The microorganism is passed through the bite of fleas, lice, ticks, and mites. Historically, epidemic typhus has wiped out entire villages. Fortunately, typhus is rarely seen today.

Protozoa

Protozoa are the only microorganisms that are classified as animals. Consisting of one cell, they are plentiful in the environment and reside in and on the body. Like other microorganisms, they seek locations that provide nutrients, warmth, and moisture. This is why some of the 45,000 identified types of protozoa are constantly present in the intestines and on the skin and mucous membranes of the nose and throat.

Fascinating Facts

Here is a chilling fact that emphasizes the need to follow strict infection control procedures: Rickettsia get their name from the physician who first identified the causative agent of Rocky Mountain spotted fever, Dr. Howard T. Ricketts, an American pathologist. *He subsequently died from typhus, having been infected through his own research on the disease.*

Protozoa are also found in decayed materials, water contaminated with sewage waste, food washed in contaminated water or handled by unwashed hands, bird and animal feces, and insect bites. (See Figure 10–3.)

Some of the most common diseases caused by the pathogenic protozoa include the following:

- *Dysentery*, an intestinal infection resulting in abdominal pain, cramping, and diarrhea, is caused by *Giardia lamblia* and is commonly referred to as "traveler's diarrhea." It is the most common intestinal parasite in the United States. It is acquired through contaminated water or food and is diagnosed by examination of the feces.
- *Trichomoniasis* is a sexually transmitted genital infection.

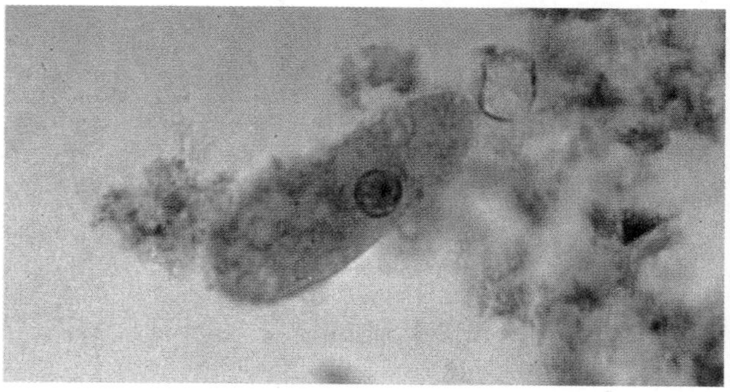

Electron micrographs courtesy of the Centers for Disease Control and Prevention, Atlanta, GA

FIGURE 10–3 Intestinal protozoan *Entamoeba coli.*

- *Toxoplasmosis* is of particular significance in pregnant women because it can pass to the unborn child and result in death, blindness, or mental retardation. It is found in the feces of birds and animals.
- *Pneumocystis pneumonia* is caused by a protozoan that is normally not pathogenic. But in patients with weakened immune systems, it is very serious and is a common cause of death among AIDS patients.
- *Malaria* is caused by a parasite that attacks the red blood cells and is characterized by periodic (every 48 to 72 hours) chills, fever, and sweats. The parasite is acquired through the bite of a specific kind of mosquito or through a blood transfusion.

Chain of Infection

The **chain of infection** is a useful model for explaining how infectious diseases occur and are transmitted. It consists of six elements that must be present for an infection to develop. (See Figure 10–4.)

1. Infectious agent: A pathogen must be present.
2. Reservoir host: The pathogen must have a place to live and grow. Examples of reservoir hosts are the human body, contaminated water or food, animals, insects, birds, and dead or decaying organic material. When humans or animals are capable of transmitting the pathogen but have no outward signs of the disease, they are referred to as *carriers*. Individuals who are carriers may not even be aware that they are spreading an infectious disease.
3. Portal of exit: The pathogen must be able to escape from the reservoir host where it has been growing. Examples of portals of exit are blood, urine, feces, breaks in the skin, wound drainage, and body secretions such as saliva, mucus, and reproductive fluids.

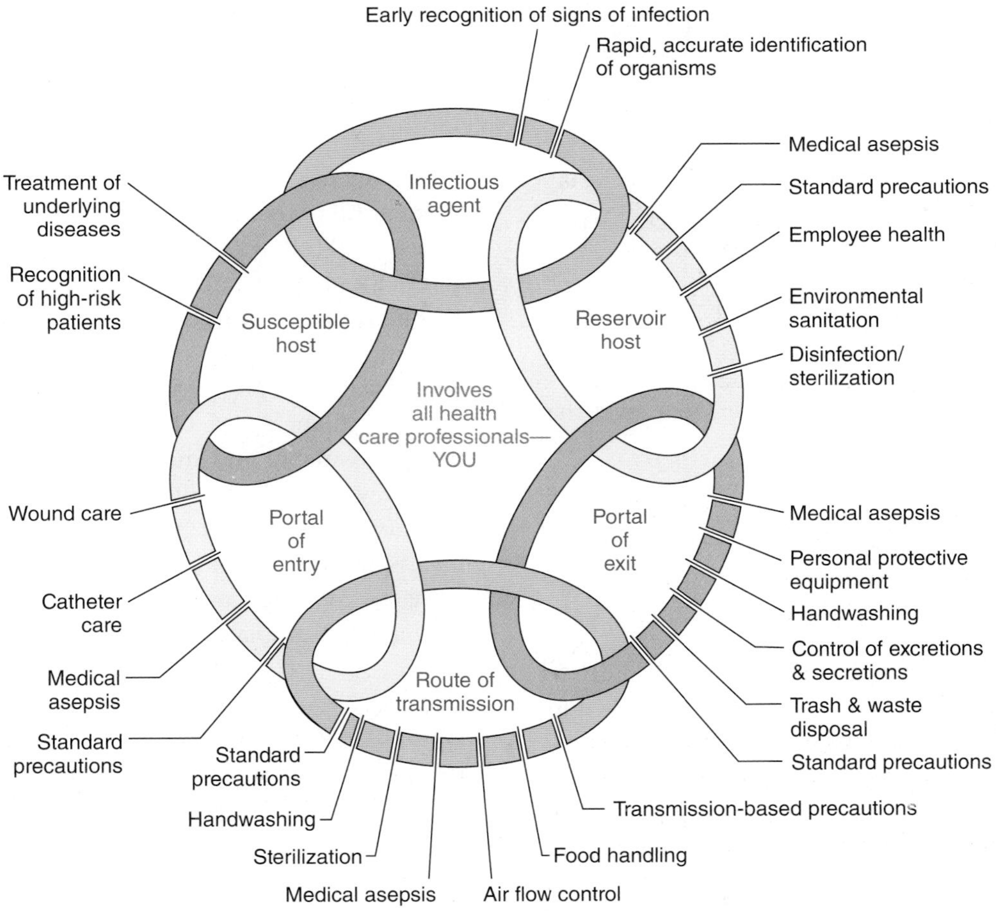

FIGURE 10–4 The chain of infection. Breaking at least one link stops the infectious disease. Examples of health care practices and procedures that impact the cycle are included.

4. Route of transmission: When the pathogen leaves the reservoir host through the portal of exit, it must have a way of being transmitted to a new host. Examples are air, food, insects, and direct contact with an infected person.
5. Portal of entry: The pathogen must have a way of entering the new host. Common ports of entry are the mouth, nostrils, and breaks in the skin.
6. Susceptible host: An individual who has a large number of pathogens invading the body or does not have adequate resistance to the invading pathogen will get the infectious disease.

Defense Mechanisms

One of the marvels of the body is the number of defense mechanisms present to resist infections. If the defense mechanisms are intact, along with a strong immune system, the individual can often resist the microorganism and not become ill. Examples of the body's natural defense mechanisms include the following:

- Cilia in the respiratory tract that catch and move pathogens out of the body
- Coughing and sneezing to propel pathogens outward
- Tears, which contain chemicals to kill bacteria
- Hydrochloric acid in the stomach, which destroys pathogens
- Mucous membranes of the respiratory, reproductive, and digestive systems, which serve to trap pathogens
- Rise in body temperature (fever) to a level that will kill microorganisms
- Production of additional leukocytes (white blood cells), which have the specific function of destroying pathogens

Scope of the Problem

It is important to realize that a health care facility by the very nature of its business, assisting patients with infections, has a higher concentration of microorganisms than is found in other environments. Combine this with patients who have lowered levels of resistance due to illness, and health care personnel who have frequent contact with body fluids, and there exists a potentially deadly situation.

The result is that infections are sometimes acquired through association with health care facilities. The term **nosocomial infection** (also referred to as health care–associated infection, or HAI) refers to an infection that occurs while a patient is receiving health care. Over the past 25 years, the rate of nosocomial infections per 1000 patient days has increased 36%. It is estimated that in U.S. hospitals alone, health care–associated (nosocomial) infections account for an estimated 1.7 million infections and 99,000 associated patient deaths each year (CDC Online). Of these infections:

- 32% are urinary tract infections
- 22% are surgical site infections
- 15% are pneumonia (lung infections)
- 14% are bloodstream infections
- 17% are other miscellaneous infections

The Centers for Disease Control and Prevention states that handwashing is the single most important procedure for preventing health care–acquired infections.

The fundamental ethic of health care is that a sick person must receive care. This premise carries an unstated consequence: an occupational risk to health care workers who respond to the needs of contagious patients. (See Table 10–1.)

When an employee contracts an infectious disease while at work, it is called an industrial illness. There are a number of diseases that the health care professional can be exposed to while caring for infected patients. All of them are preventable if the health care professional follows standard precautions (discussed later in the chapter) and other safety practices defined by the facility. Needlestick injuries are an important and continuing cause of exposure to serious and fatal diseases among health care professionals. Due to the high incidence of needlesticks, safer equipment is available and more devices are continually being developed by health care manufacturers, such as safety shields for syringes and needleless systems. It is essential that health care professionals learn and apply the means to avoid all types of risks encountered in the workplace.

Table 10–1 Occupational Deaths among U.S. Health Care Workers

Cause of Death	Number of Deaths per Year (3-year average)
Injury	77–93
Infection-related	80–260
Total	157–353

Source: CDC Online. www.cdc.gov

Regulatory Agencies

Two very important regulatory agencies have led the way in the battle against pathogens. They are responsible for developing the guidelines to safeguard health care professionals, their patients, and the public. Understanding the purpose of these agencies and learning the guidelines that pertain to specific occupations is an essential part of health care training.

The **Centers for Disease Control and Prevention (CDC)** is a government agency that is part of the U.S. Department of Health and Human Services. By studying the causes and distribution of diseases (*epidemiology*), the CDC is able to formulate safety guidelines to help prevent and control the spread of infectious diseases. Other major tasks include the licensing of clinical laboratories, maintenance of laboratory reference centers for microorganisms, and operation of extensive disease research programs.

The **Occupational Safety and Health Administration (OSHA)**, established in 1970, is a government agency that is under the Department of Labor. Its two main functions are to establish minimum health and safety standards for the workplace and to enforce those standards. OSHA is the "watchdog" of employee safety and has the authority to conduct onsite inspections to verify compliance with its standards. It is the agency that requires employers to have an exposure control plan and provide hepatitis B vaccines to employees with occupational exposure risk.

PREVENTION THROUGH ASEPSIS

The practice of **asepsis**, or **aseptic technique**, involves methods used to make the patient, the worker, and the environment as pathogen-free as possible. There are two types: medical and surgical.

1. **Medical asepsis**, or **clean technique**, includes procedures to decrease the number and spread of pathogens in the environment. Examples include handwashing, good personal hygiene, the cleaning of rooms between patient use, and disposal of gloves after contact with body fluids or contaminated objects.
2. **Surgical asepsis**, or **sterile technique**, includes procedures to completely eliminate the presence of pathogens from objects and areas. Examples of surgical asepsis are wearing sterile caps, gowns, masks, and gloves during surgery; sterilizing and using special techniques to handle instruments to be used with patients; maintaining sterile fields; changing dressings; and disposing of contaminated materials.

Breaking the Chain of Infection

The chain of infection demonstrates how infectious diseases occur and are spread. The most important concept to remember is *that breaking at least one link stops the infectious disease*. The practices and techniques that health care professionals use daily are designed to break the chain.

Recall that the chain of infection consists of six elements. These six elements are often summarized into the following three components:

1. Source of infecting microorganisms (elements 1 and 2—infectious agent and reservoir host—both involve the source of infection)
2. Means of transmission for the microorganism (elements 3, 4, and 5—portal of exit, route of transmission, and portal of entry—all affect transmission)
3. Susceptible host (element 6—susceptible host—is unchanged in this summarized format)

The best defenses, then, are to decrease the sources of microorganisms, prevent their transmission, and maximize the resistance of the host. Here are examples of how the health care professional can have an impact in each of these areas. (See Figure 10–4 for other examples.)

1. How can I decrease the source of microorganisms?
   - Perform proper handwashing.
   - Decontaminate surfaces and equipment (antiseptics, disinfectants, sterilization).
   - Avoid contact with patients and others when harboring infectious microorganisms; for example, the force of a sneeze can propel microorganisms for many feet (the spray travels in the shape of a cone, so as the distance increases from the nose, the spray widens).
2. How can I prevent the transmission of microorganisms?
   - Wear personal protective equipment (PPE) when indicated. PPE includes caps, gloves, gowns, masks, booties, and eye protection.
   - Follow isolation procedures when indicated. These are additional precautions used when working with patients who have highly contagious diseases.

3. How can I maximize the resistance of the host?
   - Provide good hygiene
   - Ensure proper nutrition and fluid intake
   - Decrease stressors that weaken the immune response

The first line of defense in medical asepsis and the most effective way to help prevent the spread of microorganisms is good handwashing technique. Many microorganisms are normal flora, always present on the body. For example, staphylococci occur naturally on the hands. But when transferred to a wound site, they can cause pus-producing infections.

Two types of normal flora are found on the hands. *Transient flora*, whether pathogenic or nonpathogenic, are picked up during our activities of daily living and are easily removed from the hands with frequent and thorough handwashing. *Resident flora* are present at all times, and considerable scrubbing is required to remove these deeply imbedded microbes. It is not possible to completely remove all the microorganisms from the hands, but the transient flora can be removed and the resident flora diminished with diligent handwashing. In individuals who do not maintain proper hygiene, it is possible that even the transient flora will become resident flora. This results in the person becoming a carrier of that particular organism.

Standard Precautions

It is impossible to know which pathogens a patient may carry, so specific procedures have been developed by the CDC. Known as **standard precautions**, it is essential that they be followed at all times and applied to every patient in the health care environment. (See Figure 10–5.)

Standard precautions must be followed to prevent contact with potentially infectious body fluids. Specifically, these fluids include the following:

- Blood
- All body fluids, secretions, and excretions except sweat, regardless of whether or not they contain visible blood
- Nonintact skin
- Mucous membranes
- Any unidentified body fluids

The following sections summarize the specific standard precautions needed by health care professionals.

Handwashing

Always perform proper handwashing technique as indicated to avoid transfer of microorganisms to you, your patients, others, or the environment. (See Figure 10–6.) Examples of appropriate times to do handwashing are as follows:

- When coming on duty
- When taking a break or leaving work
- Between patient contacts
- Before applying and immediately upon removing gloves
- Before and after touching your face in any way (manipulating contact lenses, applying lip balm, blowing your nose, coughing, sneezing)
- After contact with anything considered contaminated (picking up items from the floor, touching equipment or environmental surfaces that may be contaminated, handling soiled linens)
- Before touching any items considered clean, such as a patient's food or drink; before and after eating, drinking, or using the restroom

It is necessary to wash the hands between tasks and procedures on the same patient if there is the possibility of cross-contaminating different body sites. The hands must also be washed and the gloves changed before touching nonintact skin or mucous membranes and after touching nonintact skin, mucous membranes, blood, or any moist body fluid, secretions, or excretions.

Check the Infection Control Program policy in your facility to determine which type of soap to use. It may state to use plain (nonantimicrobial) soap for routine handwashing and an antimicrobial agent for specific circumstances. (See Figures 10–7 a–d and Procedure 10–1.)

Health care facilities will often have waterless handwashing foams, gels, or lotions available. The waterless hand-cleaning products contain alcohol as the antiseptic and a moisturizer to prevent drying of the skin. (See Figure 10–8.) A major advantage of this system is availability as they can be placed in multiple locations for easy access. The waterless system can be used between patients when hands are not visibly soiled and when there has been no contact with blood or body fluids. Enough product should be applied to all surfaces of the hands, fingers, nails, and wrists for it to take about 15 seconds of rubbing for the hands to feel dry. It is important to read the

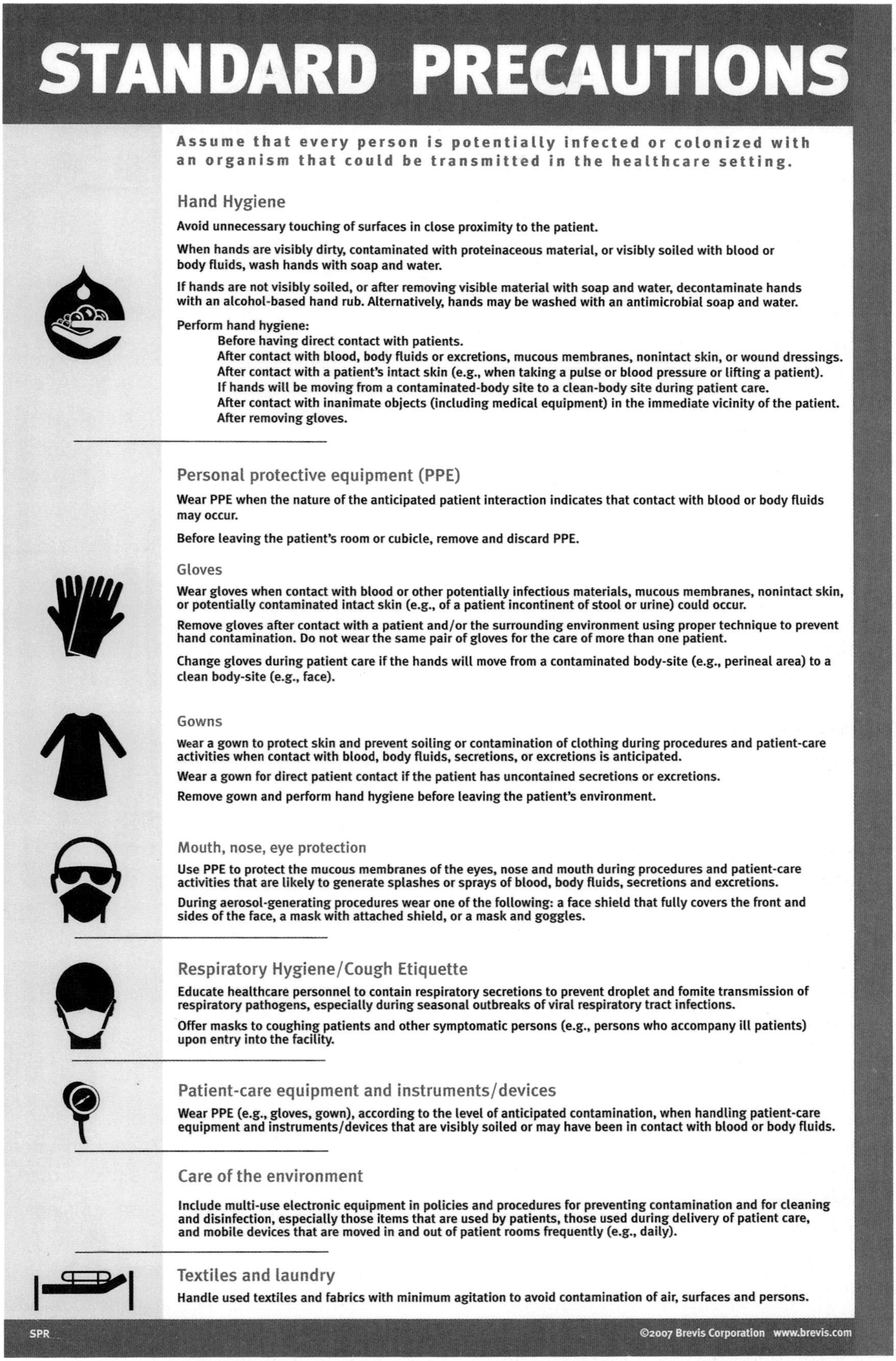
STANDARD PRECAUTIONS
Assume that every person is potentially infected or colonized with an organism that could be transmitted in the healthcare setting.
Hand Hygiene
Avoid unnecessary touching of surfaces in close proximity to the patient.
When hands are visibly dirty, contaminated with proteinaceous material, or visibly soiled with blood or body fluids, wash hands with soap and water.
If hands are not visibly soiled, or after removing visible material with soap and water, decontaminate hands with an alcohol-based hand rub. Alternatively, hands may be washed with an antimicrobial soap and water.
Perform hand hygiene:
Before having direct contact with patients.
After contact with blood, body fluids or excretions, mucous membranes, nonintact skin, or wound dressings.
After contact with a patient's intact skin (e.g., when taking a pulse or blood pressure or lifting a patient).
If hands will be moving from a contaminated-body site to a clean-body site during patient care.
After contact with inanimate objects (including medical equipment) in the immediate vicinity of the patient.
After removing gloves.
Personal protective equipment (PPE)
Wear PPE when the nature of the anticipated patient interaction indicates that contact with blood or body fluids may occur.
Before leaving the patient's room or cubicle, remove and discard PPE.
Gloves
Wear gloves when contact with blood or other potentially infectious materials, mucous membranes, nonintact skin, or potentially contaminated intact skin (e.g., of a patient incontinent of stool or urine) could occur.
Remove gloves after contact with a patient and/or the surrounding environment using proper technique to prevent hand contamination. Do not wear the same pair of gloves for the care of more than one patient.
Change gloves during patient care if the hands will move from a contaminated body-site (e.g., perineal area) to a clean body-site (e.g., face).
Gowns
Wear a gown to protect skin and prevent soiling or contamination of clothing during procedures and patient-care activities when contact with blood, body fluids, secretions, or excretions is anticipated.
Wear a gown for direct patient contact if the patient has uncontained secretions or excretions.
Remove gown and perform hand hygiene before leaving the patient's environment.
Mouth, nose, eye protection
Use PPE to protect the mucous membranes of the eyes, nose and mouth during procedures and patient-care activities that are likely to generate splashes or sprays of blood, body fluids, secretions and excretions.
During aerosol-generating procedures wear one of the following: a face shield that fully covers the front and sides of the face, a mask with attached shield, or a mask and goggles.
Respiratory Hygiene/Cough Etiquette
Educate healthcare personnel to contain respiratory secretions to prevent droplet and fomite transmission of respiratory pathogens, especially during seasonal outbreaks of viral respiratory tract infections.
Offer masks to coughing patients and other symptomatic persons (e.g., persons who accompany ill patients) upon entry into the facility.
Patient-care equipment and instruments/devices
Wear PPE (e.g., gloves, gown), according to the level of anticipated contamination, when handling patient-care equipment and instruments/devices that are visibly soiled or may have been in contact with blood or body fluids.
Care of the environment
Include multi-use electronic equipment in policies and procedures for preventing contamination and for cleaning and disinfection, especially those items that are used by patients, those used during delivery of patient care, and mobile devices that are moved in and out of patient rooms frequently (e.g., daily).
Textiles and laundry
Handle used textiles and fabrics with minimum agitation to avoid contamination of air, surfaces and persons.
SPR
©2007 Brevis Corporation www.brevis.com

FIGURE 10–5 Standard precautions.

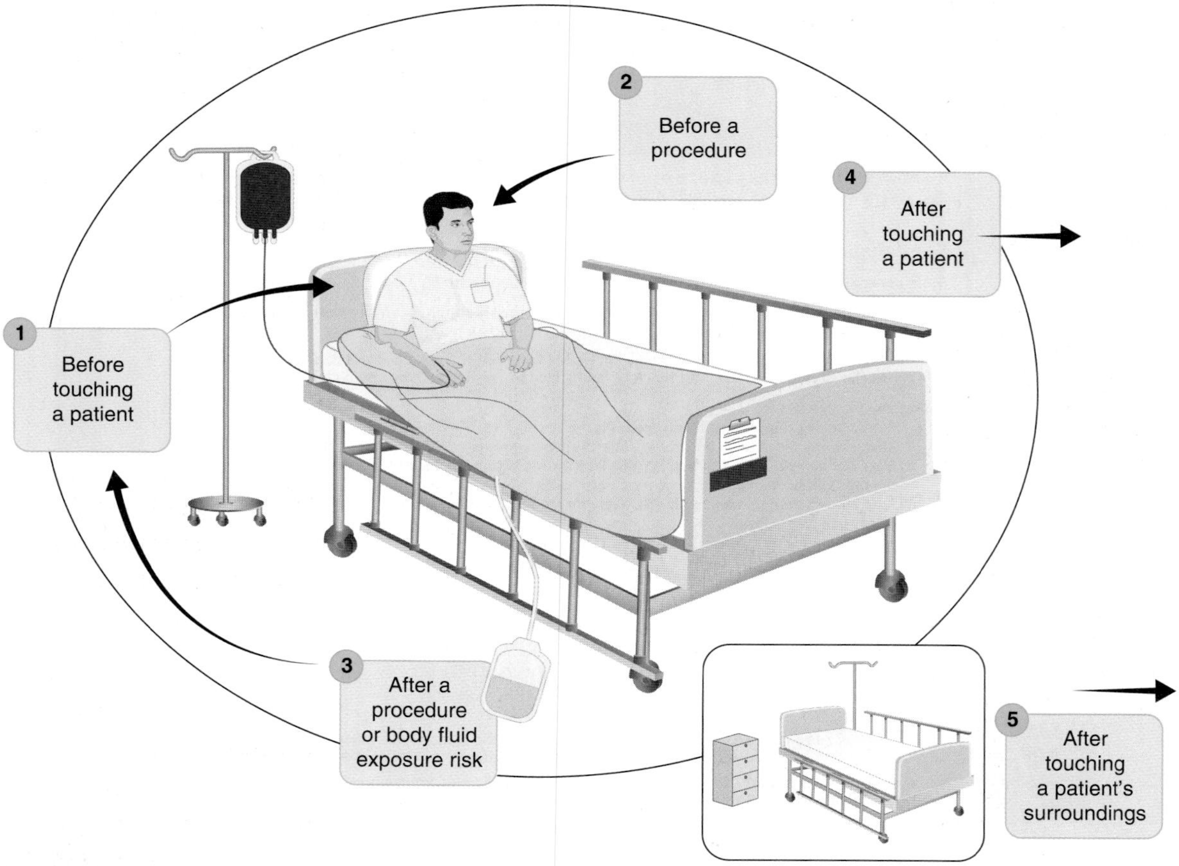

FIGURE 10–6 Clean hands are caring hands.

PROCEDURE 10–1

Handwashing

PROCEDURE	RATIONALE
1. Turn faucet on using a clean, dry paper towel. (See Figure 10–7a.)	Faucets are always considered contaminated.
2. Run warm water over hands and wrists.	Warm water helps remove superficial dirt and microorganisms.
3. Do not lean against the sink, and avoid splashing clothing with water.	The sink is always considered contaminated; water splashed from the sink is contaminated, and wet material easily conducts microorganisms.
4. Keep hands lower than arms during procedure, and keep fingertips pointing downward.	Prevents contaminated water from running up the arms and dripping on clothes.
5. Apply liquid soap to hands.	Bar soap can carry microorganisms.
6. Scrub palms in a circular motion while clasping hands together.	Creates lather, and the friction helps to remove microorganisms.

(continues)

PROCEDURE 10–1

Handwashing

(continued)

PROCEDURE	RATIONALE
7. Scrub wrists 1 to 2 inches above the hands by encircling one wrist with the other hand; then repeat for the other wrist.	Same as above.
8. Scrub the back of each hand with a circular motion by cupping one hand over the other. (See Figure 10–7b.)	Same as above.
9. Scrub between the fingers with a back and forth motion by interlacing fingers. (See Figure 10–7c.)	Same as above.
10. Scrub each individual finger and clean under the nails with a cuticle stick, a brush, or a fingernail on the other hand, or by rubbing it against the palm of the other hand.	Microorganisms can easily hide under the nails.
11. Scrub hands for at least 2 minutes.	Provides thorough cleaning of all surfaces.
12. Rinse each hand thoroughly with running water from the wrists down to the fingertips. (See Figure 10–7d.)	Soap residue can cause skin irritation.
13. Dry thoroughly with a disposable towel(s).	Moisture remaining on the skin can cause irritation; reusable towels can harbor microorganisms.

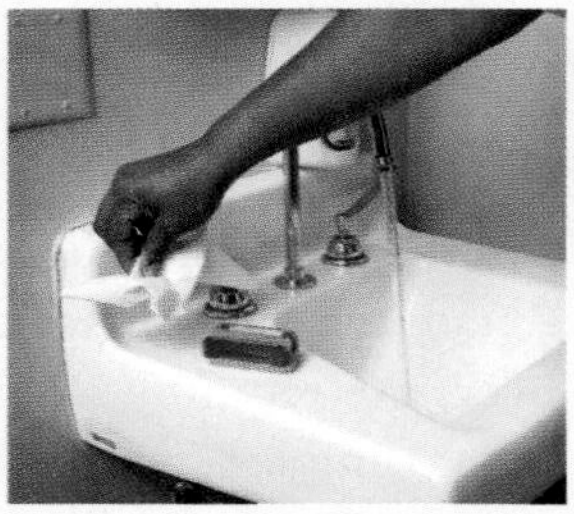

FIGURE 10–7a Use a clean, dry paper towel to turn the faucet on and off.

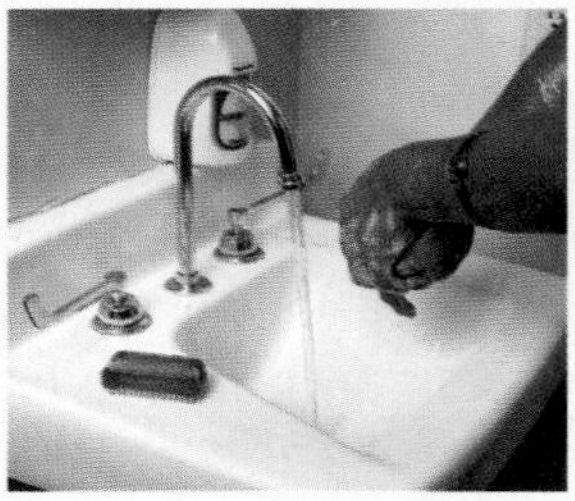

FIGURE 10–7b Keep the fingertips pointed downward. Scrub hands and wrists with a circular motion.

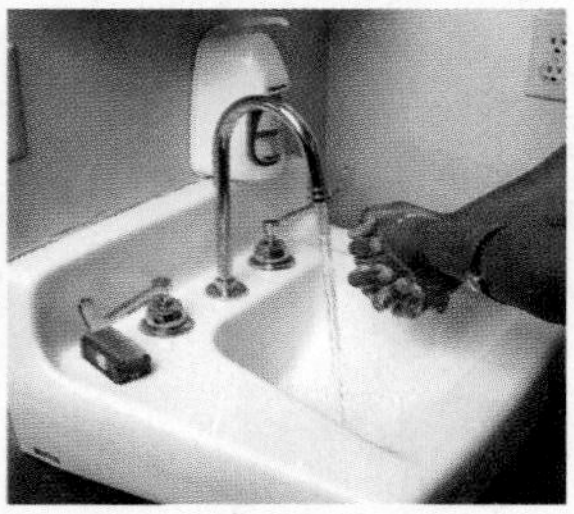

FIGURE 10–7c Scrub between fingers with back and forth motion by interlacing fingers.

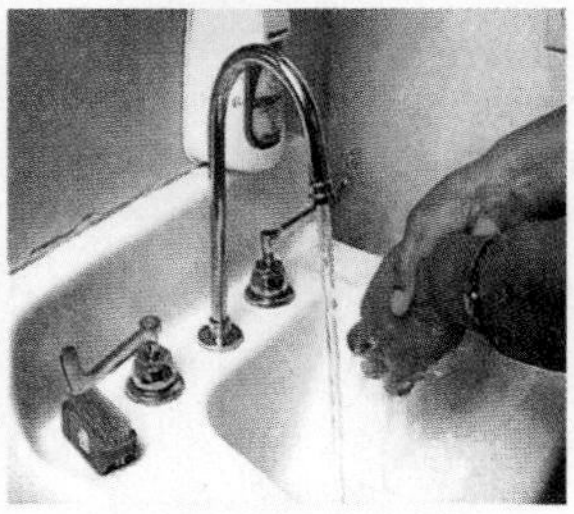

FIGURE 10–7d Rinse each hand thoroughly with running water from the wrists down to fingertips.

(continues)

PROCEDURE 10–1

Handwashing

(continued)

PROCEDURE	RATIONALE
14. Use another dry towel to turn off the faucet handle. (See Figure 10–7a.)	Prevents recontamination of hands from microorganisms on the faucet handles; a wet towel would allow microorganisms to travel from the faucet handle back to the hands.
15. Clean sink area using dry towels, being careful not to recontaminate hands by touching any surfaces.	Leaves the area ready for the next person; the faucets and sink are always considered contaminated; wet towels are considered contaminated.
16. Use lotion if desired.	Keeps hands soft and helps prevent chapping and cracking of hands, which are more susceptible to growth of microorganisms.

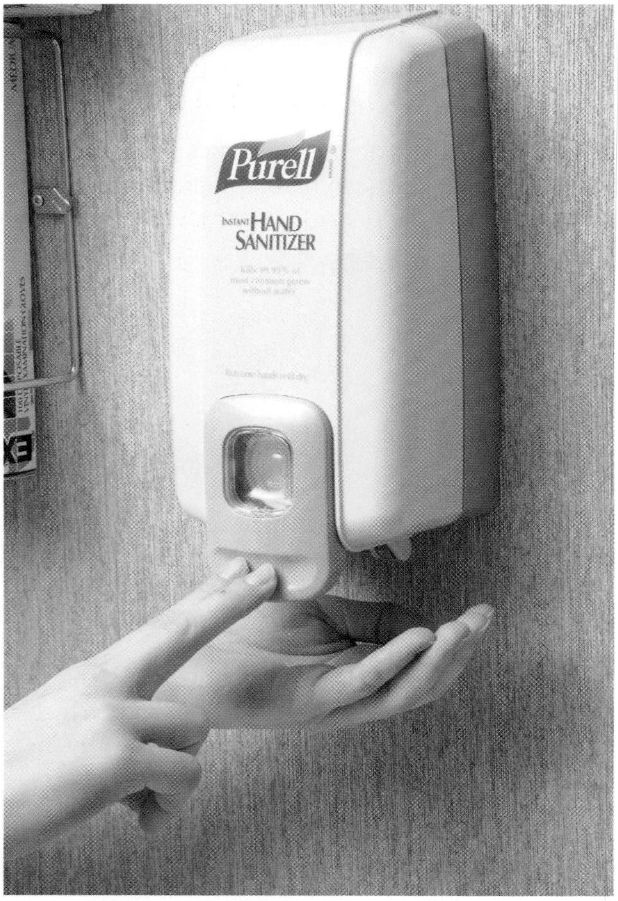

FIGURE 10–8 If your hands are not visibly dirty or contaminated with blood or body fluids, they can be cleaned with a waterless hand cleaner.

manufacturer's instructions before using any product and to be familiar with the written policies on hand hygiene for the health care facility.

Personal Protective Equipment

Personal protective equipment, commonly referred to as PPE, includes gloves, masks, protective eyewear, gowns, and caps. To be effective, these must be properly used in all situations that have the potential to infect the health care professional.

OSHA requires the use of PPE to reduce employee exposure to infectious hazards in the health care environment. Employers are required to determine what hazards exist and to implement a PPE program to address these hazards. This program should address the hazards present; the selection, maintenance, and use of PPE; the training of employees; and monitoring of the program to ensure its ongoing effectiveness.

Gloves

Wear clean, nonsterile gloves when you touch, or have the potential of coming in contact with, blood, body fluids, secretions, excretions, or contaminated items. Put on clean gloves just before touching mucous membranes and nonintact skin. Gloves should be changed between tasks and procedures on the same patient if there is contact with material that may contain a high concentration of microorganisms. Remove gloves promptly after use, before touching noncontaminated items and environmental surfaces, and before going to another patient. After gloves are removed, wash your hands immediately to avoid transferring of microorganisms to other patients or environments. See Figures 10–9 a–h and Procedure 10–2.

Mask, Eye Protection, Face Shield

Wear a mask and eye protection or a face shield to protect the mucous membranes of the eyes, nose, and mouth during procedures and patient care activities that are likely to generate splashes or sprays of blood, body fluids, secretions, or excretions. (See Figure 10–10.)

Gown

Wear a clean, nonsterile gown to protect the skin and to prevent soiling clothing during procedures and patient care activities that are likely to generate

PROCEDURE 10–2

Nonsterile Gloves (Applying Clean Gloves and Removing Contaminated Gloves)

PROCEDURE	RATIONALE
1. Use proper handwashing technique before applying gloves.	To remove microorganisms from hands.
2. Remove appropriate-sized clean gloves from the box and apply. Once the hands are washed, no specific technique is necessary for applying gloves, but touch only the gloves you will be using when removing them from the dispenser.	Gloves that are too small can split and expose skin, and gloves that are too large are difficult to work with and can expose skin by slipping down; do not contaminate the remaining gloves in the dispenser by touching them.
Removing contaminated gloves:	
3. Grasp the outside of one glove at the palm with the other gloved hand (see Figure 10–9a); pull the glove down (see Figure 10–9b) and turn it inside out while removing it. (See Figure 10–9c.)	At no time should the hands touch the outside of the contaminated gloves.
4. Hold the removed glove in the palm of the remaining gloved hand. (See Figures 10–9d and 10–9e.)	Same as above.

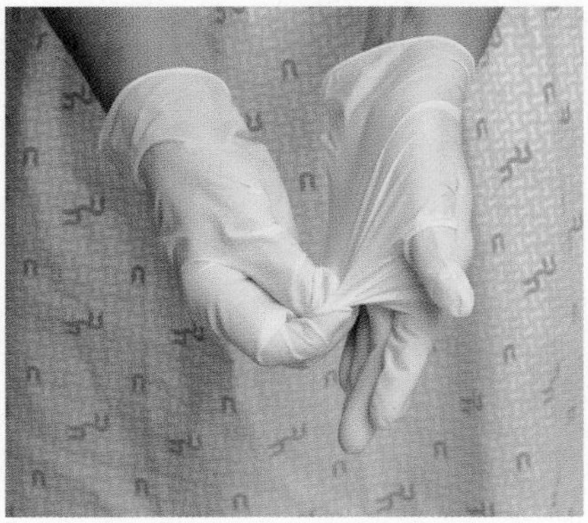

FIGURE 10–9a Grasp the outside of one glove at palm site with the other gloved hand.

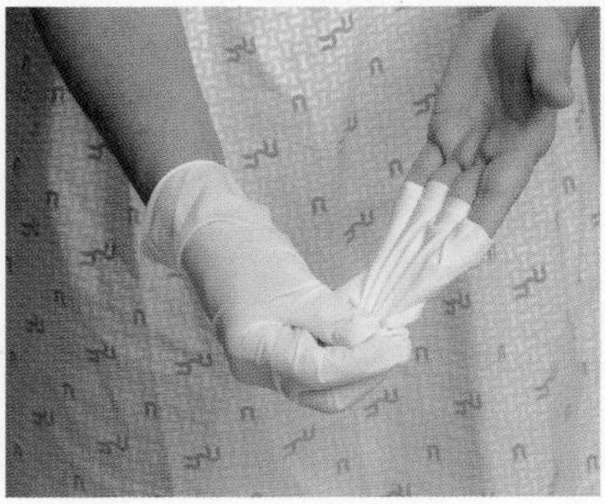

FIGURE 10–9b Begin removing the first glove.

(continues)

PROCEDURE 10–2

Nonsterile Gloves (Applying Clean Gloves and Removing Contaminated Gloves)

(continued)

PROCEDURE	RATIONALE
5. Take the ungloved hand and slide it under the cuff of the remaining glove (see Figure 10–9f) and push the glove off. (See Figure 10–9g.) The first glove is now inside the second glove that was removed. (See Figure 10–9h.)	Same as above.
6. Discard the gloves in an appropriate container according to facility policy.	Isolates the contaminated gloves from contact with other surfaces.
7. Wash hands immediately after removing gloves.	To remove microorganisms from hands.

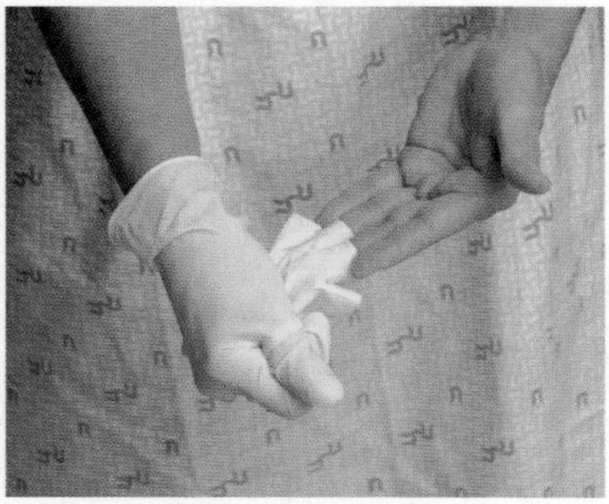

FIGURE 10–9c Turn the glove inside out while removing it. Take care not to touch bare skin with the contaminated glove.

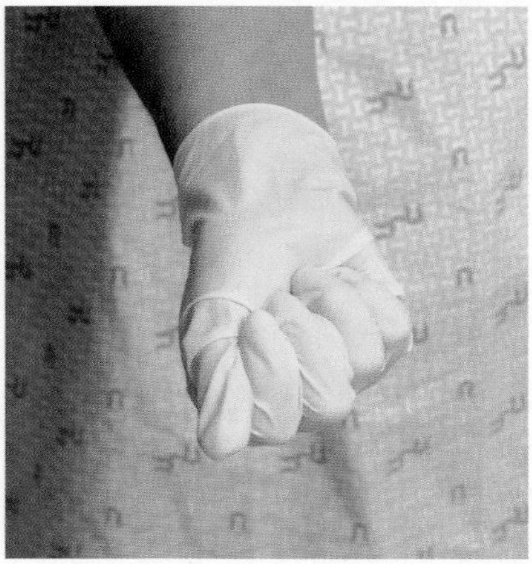

FIGURE 10–9e Contain the inverted glove completely in the gloved hand.

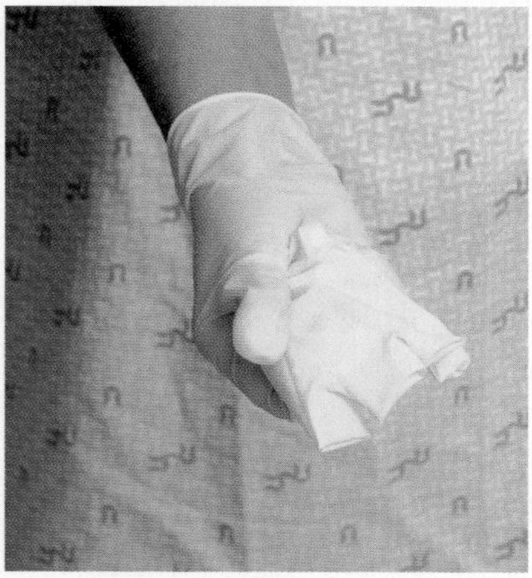

FIGURE 10–9d Inverted glove is completely removed into the contaminated glove.

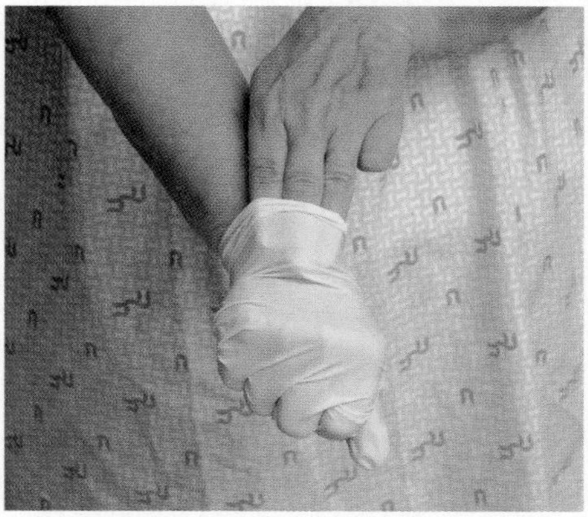

FIGURE 10–9f Take the ungloved hand and slide fingers under the cuff of the remaining contaminated glove.

(continues)

PROCEDURE 10–2

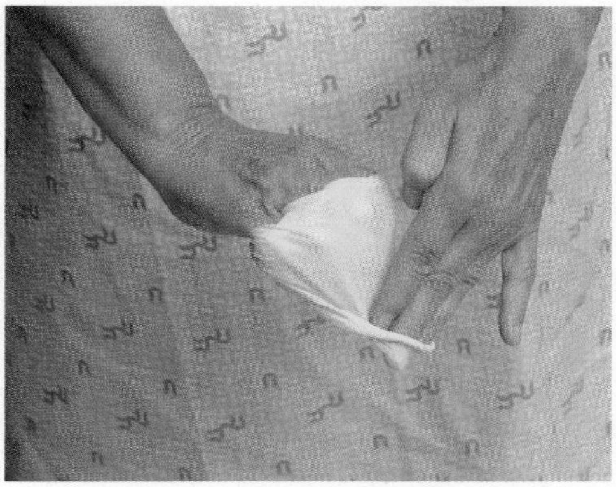

FIGURE 10–9g Push the glove off while inverting the second glove over the first.

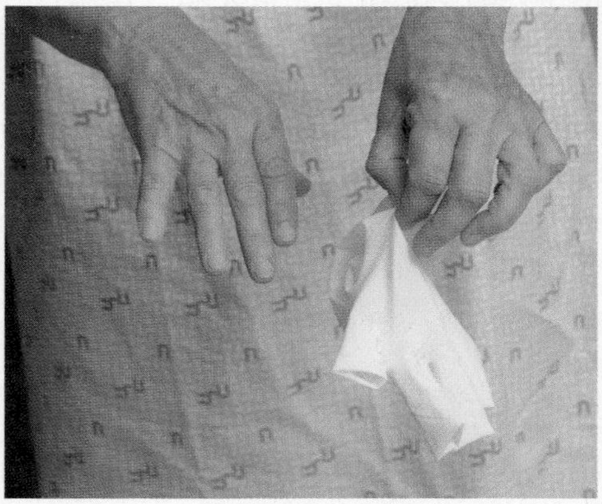

FIGURE 10–9h The first glove is now inside of the second glove that was removed. Dispose of gloves in appropriate container according to facility policy.

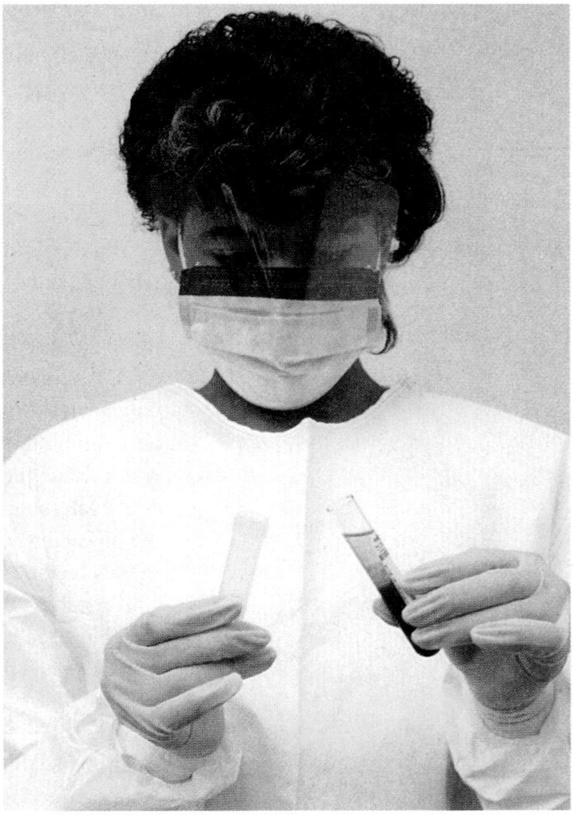

FIGURE 10–10 Gloves, mask, eye protection, and gown should be worn during procedures and patient-care activities that are likely to generate splashes or sprays of blood, body fluids, secretions, and excretions.

splashes or sprays of blood, body fluids, secretions, or excretions. Select a gown that is appropriate for the activity and amount of fluid likely to be encountered. Remove a soiled gown as promptly as possible and wash your hands to avoid transfer of microorganisms to other patients or environments.

Application of PPE

When working in contaminated areas, there are guidelines for applying and removing PPE. See Procedure 10–3, which includes the most commonly used equipment.

Patient-Care Equipment

Handle used patient care equipment that is soiled with blood, body fluids, secretions, and excretions in a manner that prevents skin and mucous membrane exposures, contamination of clothing, and transfer of microorganisms to other patients and environments. Ensure that reusable equipment is not used for the care of another patient until it has been cleaned and reprocessed appropriately. Be sure that single-use items are discarded properly.

Environmental Control

Procedures must be followed and consistently performed for the routine care, cleaning, and disinfection of environmental surfaces, beds, bed rails,

PROCEDURE 10–3
Applying and Removing PPE

PROCEDURE	RATIONALE
1. Use proper handwashing technique before applying PPE. (See Procedure 10–1.)	To remove microorganisms from hands.
2. Put on cap, mask, protective eyewear, and gown. No specific sequence of applying these items is required.	Complete coverage needed to protect against contamination.
3. To apply gown (See Figures 10–11 a–c): Put on the gown by placing your hands inside the shoulders. Slip your fingers inside the neckband to tie the gown at the neck. Overlap the back edges of the gown so your uniform is completely covered before tying the waist ties.	Be sure that the cap covers all the hair and ears, the mask fits snugly to the face (press metal clip on mask to fit snugly across bridge of nose), eyewear extends to protect the side of the face, and the gown completely covers the clothing.
4. Apply gloves last. Remove appropriate-sized clean gloves from the box and apply. Touch only the gloves you will be using when removing them from the dispenser.	Gloves that are too small can split and expose skin, and gloves that are too large are difficult to work with and can expose skin by slipping down; do not contaminate the remaining gloves in the dispenser by touching them.

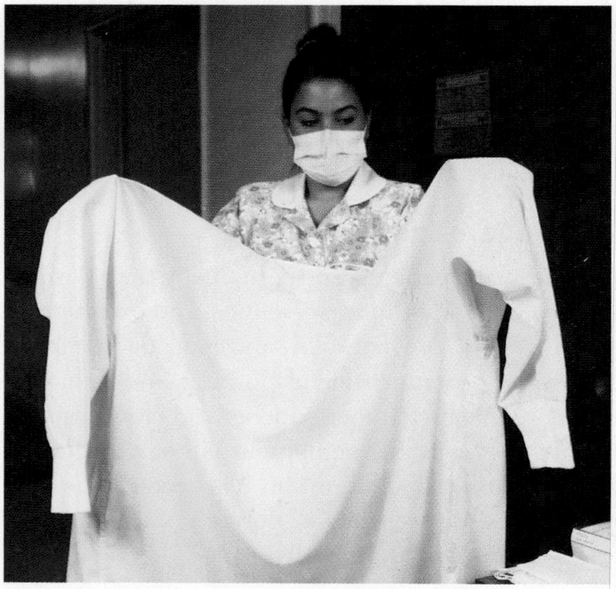

FIGURE 10–11a Put on the gown by placing your hands inside the shoulders.

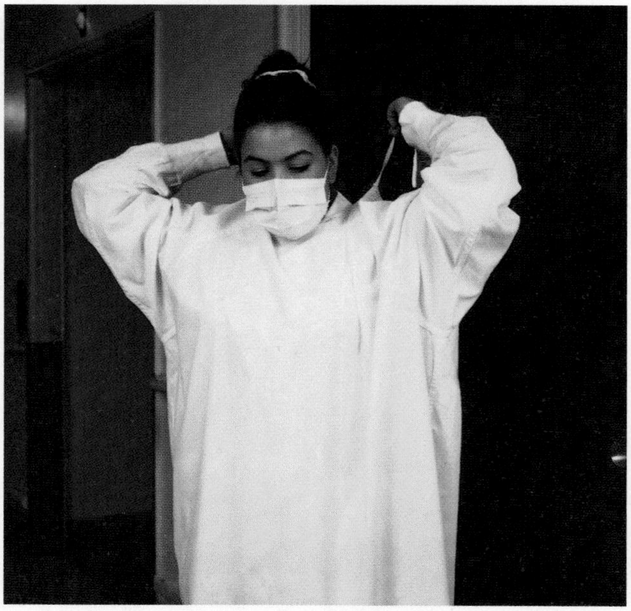

FIGURE 10–11b Slip your fingers inside the neckband to tie the gown at the neck.

(continues)

PROCEDURE 10–3
Applying and Removing PPE

(continued)

PROCEDURE	RATIONALE
5. Pull the cuffs over the sleeves of the gown to create a seal.	Creates seal against entrance of microorganisms.
Remove PPE prior to leaving the contaminated area, as follows:	
6. Untie the waist ties of the gown.	The waist ties of the gown are considered contaminated.
7. Remove contaminated gloves.	See Procedure 10–2.
8. Wash hands.	See Procedure 10–1.
9. Remove cap and protective eyewear gently.	Do gently to prevent dispersion of microorganisms.
To remove the gown (See Figures 10–12 a–c):	
Untie the neck tie of the gown and remove the gown.	The neck ties of the gown are considered clean.
To remove the gown, slip the fingers of one hand under the cuff of the opposite arm and pull the gown down until it covers the hand.	The outside of the gown is considered contaminated and should not be touched.
Using the gown-covered hand, grasp the outside of the gown on the opposite arm, and pull the gown down until it covers the hand.	The outside of the gown is considered contaminated and should not be touched.

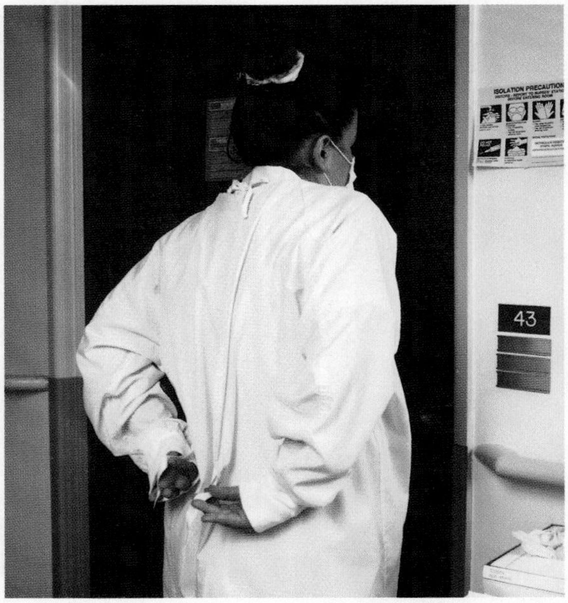

FIGURE 10–11c Overlap the back edges of the gown so your uniform is completely covered before tying the waist ties.

(continues)

PROCEDURE 10–3
Applying and Removing PPE

(continued)

PROCEDURE	RATIONALE
Both hands are now inside the gown and can be used to grasp the outside of the gown. Use your covered hands to grasp the gown at the shoulders and turn the gown inside out (contaminated side on the inside) as you remove it. Roll it up and place in appropriate container according to facility policy.	Keep gown in front of you and away from the body. Avoid excessive motion during procedure because motion causes the spread of organisms.
10. Remove the mask. Hold the mask by the strings to discard it.	The ties of the mask are considered clean. Do not touch any other part of the mask, as it is considered contaminated. The mask is always removed last if the contaminants are airborne.
11. Wash hands. (See Procedure 10–1.)	To remove microorganisms from hands.

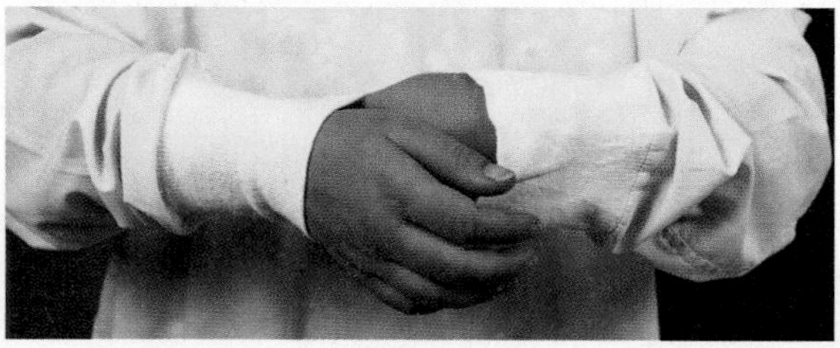

FIGURE 10–12a To remove the gown, slip the fingers of one hand under the cuff of the opposite arm and pull the gown down until it covers the hand.

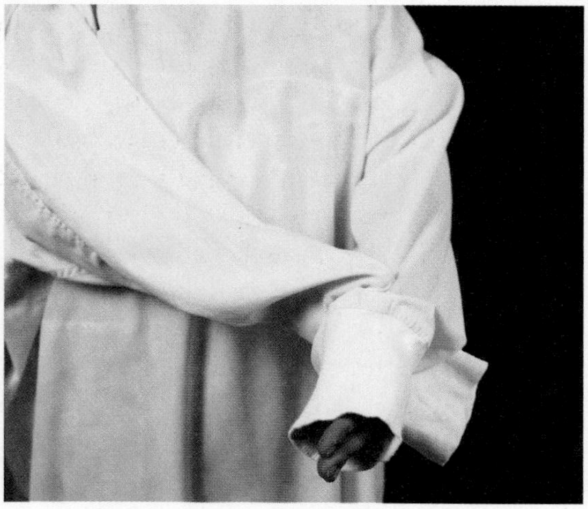

FIGURE 10–12b Using the gown-covered hand, grasp the outside of the gown on the opposite arm, and pull the gown down until it covers the hand.

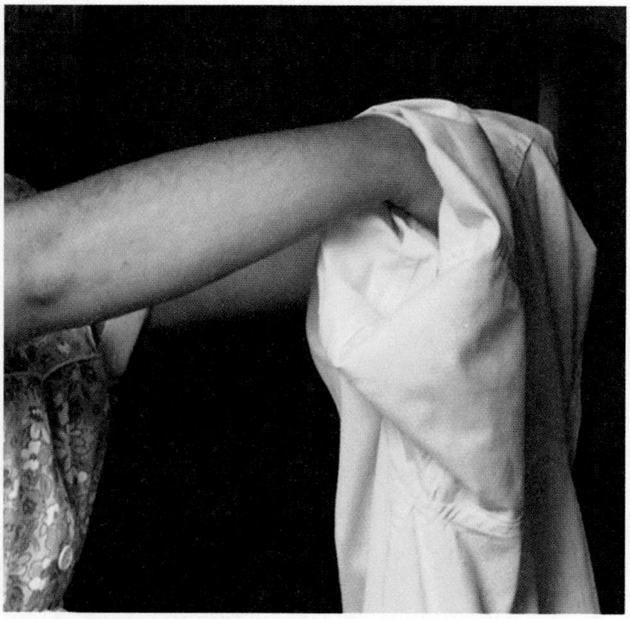

FIGURE 10–12c Both hands are now inside the gown and can be used to grasp the outside of the gown. Use your covered hands to grasp the gown at the shoulders and turn the gown inside out (contaminated side on the inside) as you remove it. Roll it up and place in appropriate container according to facility policy.

bedside equipment, and other frequently touched surfaces.

Linen

Handle, transport, and process used linen that is soiled with blood, body fluids, secretions, and excretions in a manner that prevents skin and mucous membrane exposures, contamination of your clothing, and transfer of microorganisms to other patients and environments.

Occupational Health and Blood-Borne Pathogens

Take care to prevent injuries when using needles, scalpels, and other sharp instruments or devices; when handling sharp instruments after procedures; when cleaning used instruments; and when disposing of used needles. Place used disposable syringes and needles, scalpel blades, and other sharp items in appropriate puncture-resistant containers. (See Figure 10–13.) These should be located as close as practical to the area in which the items are used. Place reusable syringes and needles in a puncture-resistant container for transport to the reprocessing area.

The following additional precautions must be followed when using needles:

- Never recap used needles. The health care professional needs to be familiar with the facility policies on how to handle contaminated needles because there may be an exception to this rule. Examples include using either a one-handed "scoop" technique or a mechanical device designed for holding the needle sheath.
- Do not remove used needles from disposable syringes by hand and do not bend, break, or otherwise manipulate used needles by hand.

Use mouthpieces, resuscitation bags, or other ventilation devices as an alternative to mouth-to-mouth resuscitation methods. Keep these devices available in areas where the need for resuscitation is predictable.

Patient Placement

Patients with infections who contaminate the environment or who do not—or cannot be expected to—assist in maintaining appropriate hygiene or environmental control should be placed in a private room. If a private room is not available, consult with infection control professionals regarding patient placement or other alternatives.

FIGURE 10–13 All needles and sharp objects should be discarded immediately in a puncture-resistant sharp container.

Transmission Precautions

Certain pathogens are especially dangerous because they are easily transmitted and have the potential of causing epidemics. The CDC recommends the use of **transmission-based precautions** with patients who are documented or suspected to be infected with these pathogens. There are three types of transmission-based precautions: airborne precautions, droplet precautions, and contact precautions. (See Table 10–2.) They may be combined for diseases that have multiple routes of transmission. *Either singularly or in combination, they are to be used in addition to standard precautions* (CDC Online). Some hospitals prefer to protect the patient's privacy and post a simple note stating that one must report to the nurse's station prior to entry into the room. (See Figure 10–17.)

Placing a patient on transmission precautions, however, often presents certain disadvantages to the hospital, patients, personnel, and visitors.

- It requires the patient to be in a private room unless it is shared with another patient with the same disease. The rationale for this is to confine the pathogen to the patient's unit.
- It may require specialized equipment and environmental modifications that add to the cost of hospitalization.

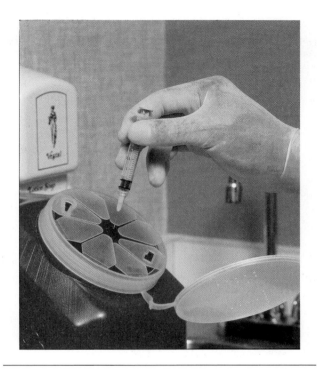

Table 10–2 Transmission-Based Precautions (Isolation Precautions)

Type of Precaution	Description	Examples
Airborne (Figure 10–14)	• Airborne droplets or dust particles containing the infectious agent remain suspended in the air for long periods • Can be dispersed widely by air currents within a room or over a long distance • Can be emitted during talking, sneezing, coughing, and whispering.	• *Mycobacterium tuberculosis* • Rubeola (measles) • Varicella (chickenpox)
Droplet (Figure 10–15)	• Propelled short distances through the air. • Deposited on the host's conjunctiva, nasal mucosa, or mouth • Can be emitted during talking, sneezing, or coughing, and during the performance of certain procedures such as suctioning and bronchoscopy	• Some forms of pneumonia, meningitis, and sepsis • Streptococcal pharyngitis • Mumps • Influenza • Rubella
Contact (Figure 10–16)	• Most important and frequent mode of transmission of nosocomial infections • Divided into two subgroups: direct-contact transmission and indirect-contact transmission • Direct-contact transmission occurs when touching the infectious patient's dry skin—for example, when performing patient care activities such as turning a patient or giving a bath; direct-contact transmission can also occur between two patients, with one serving as the source of the infectious microorganisms and the other as a susceptible host • Indirect-contact transmission occurs when a contaminated object is touched, such as coming in contact with instruments, needles, dressings, environmental surfaces, or patient care items	• Some gastrointestinal, respiratory, skin, and wound infections • Herpes simplex virus • Impetigo • Scabies

- It makes frequent visits by nurses, physicians, and other personnel inconvenient, and may make it more difficult for personnel to give prompt and frequent care that sometimes is required.
- Using a multipatient room for one patient uses valuable space that otherwise might accommodate several patients.
- Forced solitude deprives the patient of normal social relationships and may be psychologically harmful, especially to children and confused patients. As part of the health care team, you must do all you can to decrease these psychological stresses, not only for humanitarian reasons, but also because they compromise the immune system. So, even if it is inconvenient, check on the patient frequently. Remember you are isolating the pathogen, not the patient.

These disadvantages, however, must be weighed against the hospital's mission to prevent the spread of microorganisms that may cause an epidemic.

The proper disposal of hazardous waste (contaminated materials) is also essential to maintaining a safe environment. When a patient is in isolation, there will be specially marked hazardous waste containers for trash and for linen located in the room. The only way to remove the contaminated items from the room is

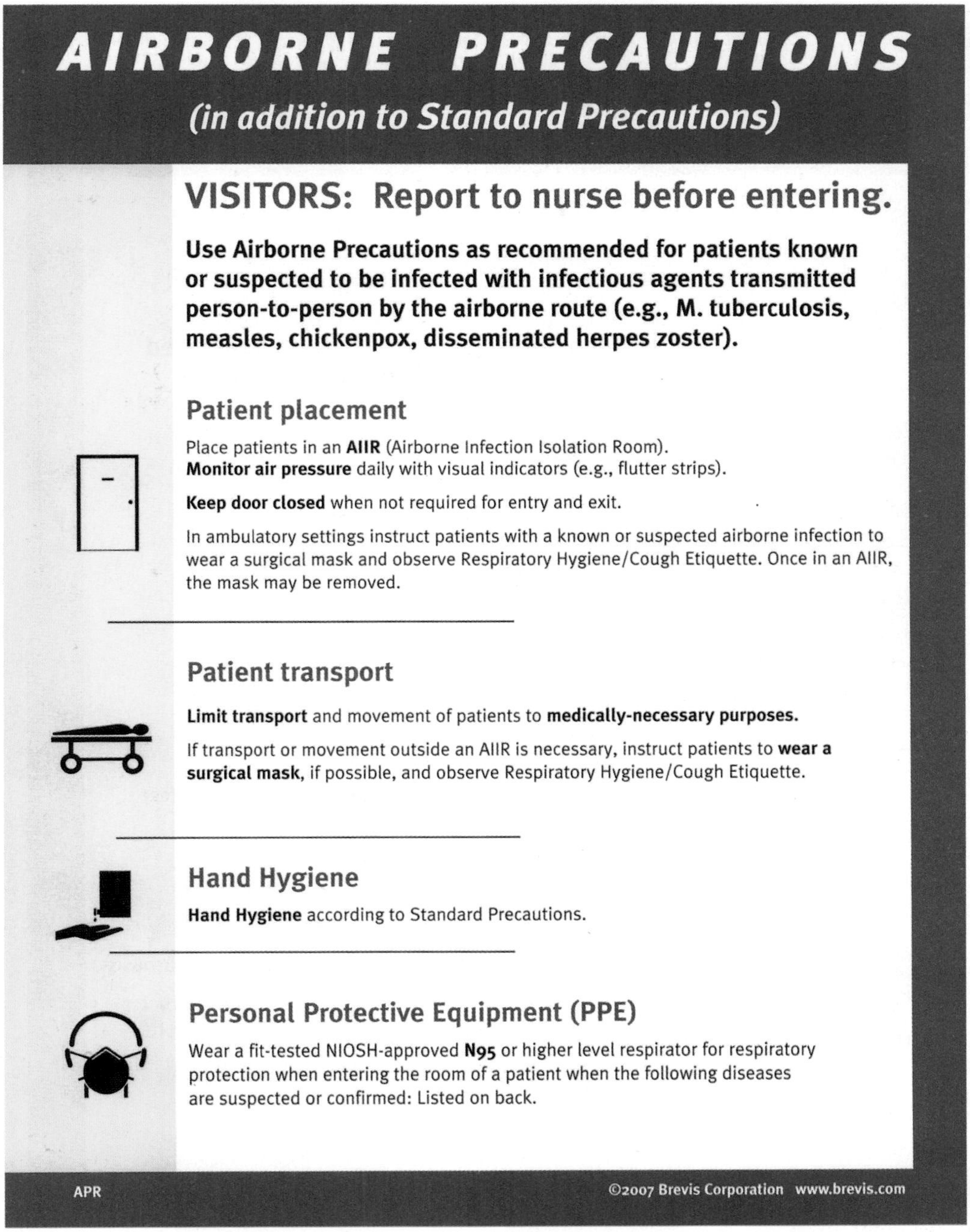
AIRBORNE PRECAUTIONS
(in addition to Standard Precautions)
VISITORS: Report to nurse before entering.
Use Airborne Precautions as recommended for patients known or suspected to be infected with infectious agents transmitted person-to-person by the airborne route (e.g., M. tuberculosis, measles, chickenpox, disseminated herpes zoster).
Patient placement
Place patients in an AIIR (Airborne Infection Isolation Room).
Monitor air pressure daily with visual indicators (e.g., flutter strips).
Keep door closed when not required for entry and exit.
In ambulatory settings instruct patients with a known or suspected airborne infection to wear a surgical mask and observe Respiratory Hygiene/Cough Etiquette. Once in an AIIR, the mask may be removed.
Patient transport
Limit transport and movement of patients to medically-necessary purposes.
If transport or movement outside an AIIR is necessary, instruct patients to wear a surgical mask, if possible, and observe Respiratory Hygiene/Cough Etiquette.
Hand Hygiene
Hand Hygiene according to Standard Precautions.
Personal Protective Equipment (PPE)
Wear a fit-tested NIOSH-approved N95 or higher level respirator for respiratory protection when entering the room of a patient when the following diseases are suspected or confirmed: Listed on back.
APR
©2007 Brevis Corporation www.brevis.com

FIGURE 10–14 Airborne precautions.

by using a *double-bagging* technique. Double-bagging involves taking the contaminated bag from the isolation room (the health care professional has appropriate PPE on) and slipping it into another bag held by a coworker outside the isolation room. Care is taken so that the coworker does not touch the contaminated bag, and the health care professional in the room does not touch the clean bag. The bags are labeled according to the facility policy with hazardous waste or linen markers to alert other personnel to the need for special handling.

Media Link

Learn more about transmission-based precautions by viewing the Pathogens video on the Online Resources.

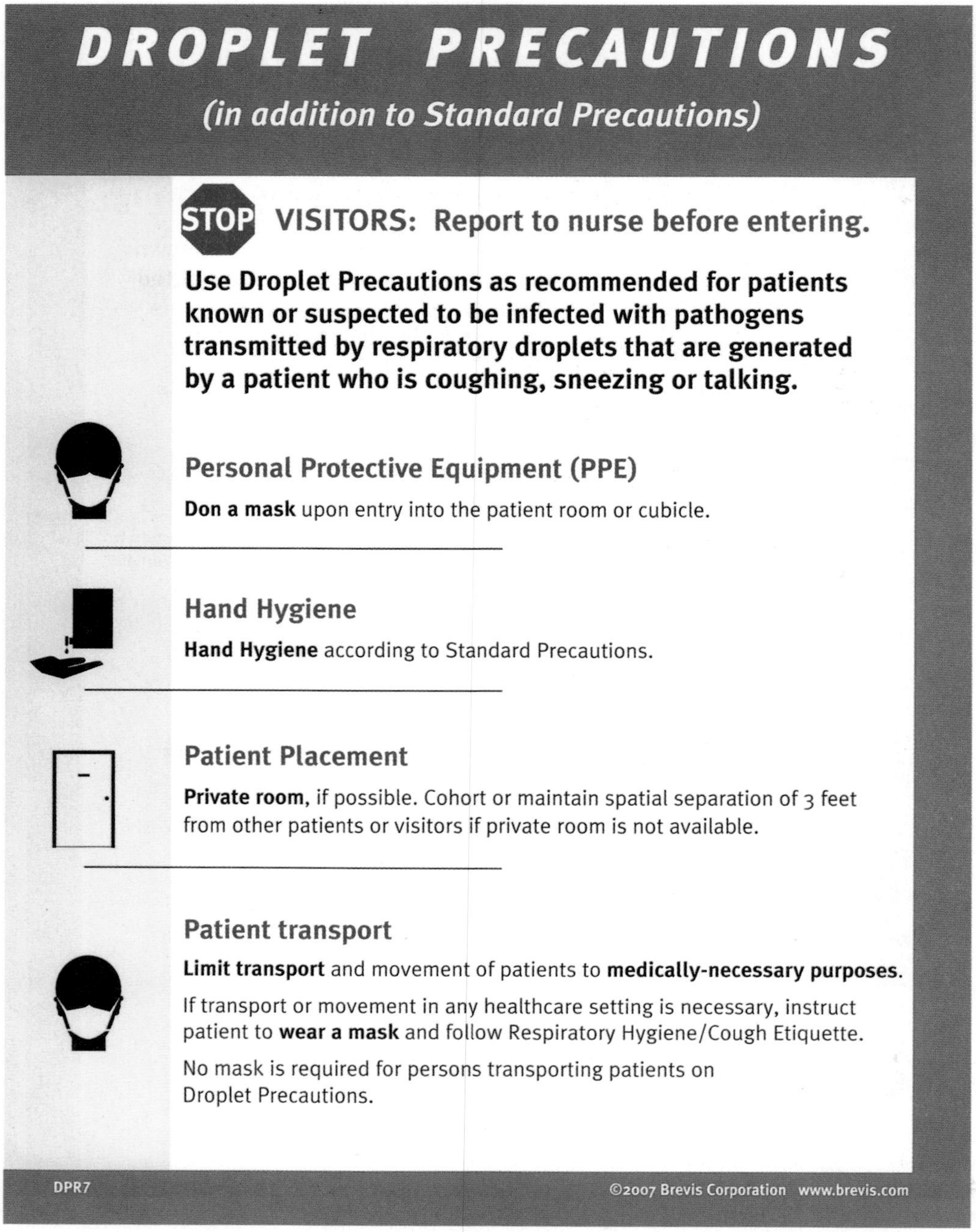
DROPLET PRECAUTIONS
(in addition to Standard Precautions)
STOP
VISITORS: Report to nurse before entering.
Use Droplet Precautions as recommended for patients known or suspected to be infected with pathogens transmitted by respiratory droplets that are generated by a patient who is coughing, sneezing or talking.
Personal Protective Equipment (PPE)
Don a mask upon entry into the patient room or cubicle.
Hand Hygiene
Hand Hygiene according to Standard Precautions.
Patient Placement
Private room, if possible. Cohort or maintain spatial separation of 3 feet from other patients or visitors if private room is not available.
Patient transport
Limit transport and movement of patients to medically-necessary purposes.
If transport or movement in any healthcare setting is necessary, instruct patient to wear a mask and follow Respiratory Hygiene/Cough Etiquette.
No mask is required for persons transporting patients on Droplet Precautions.
DPR7
©2007 Brevis Corporation www.brevis.com

FIGURE 10–15 Droplet precautions.

Neutropenic Precautions

Another type of precaution may be ordered for patients who are very susceptible to infections. The procedures followed are meant to protect the patient from infections brought in by people or other sources, rather than protecting the health care professional and visitors from patient infections. These precautions are called **neutropenic precautions**, or reverse isolation. This type of precaution will most commonly be seen with an oncology patient who has a repressed immune system secondary to the cancer treatment (i.e., chemotherapy, radiation). A sign similar to Figure 10–17 can be posted on the patient's door. The general guidelines, in addition to standard precautions, are as follows:

- The patient is placed in a private room.
- No one who has an infection should enter the room.

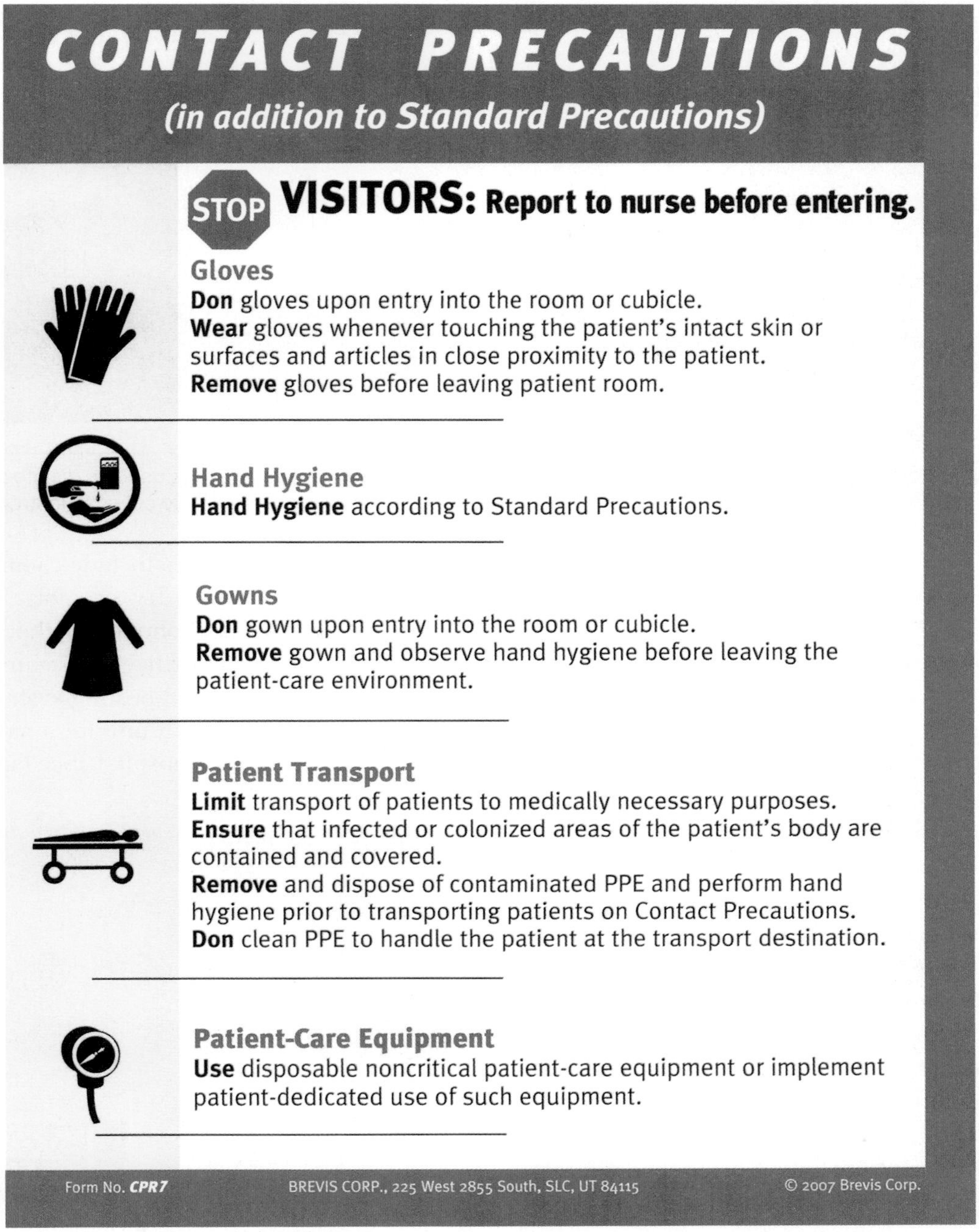
CONTACT PRECAUTIONS
(in addition to Standard Precautions)
STOP
VISITORS: Report to nurse before entering.
Gloves
Don gloves upon entry into the room or cubicle.
Wear gloves whenever touching the patient's intact skin or surfaces and articles in close proximity to the patient.
Remove gloves before leaving patient room.
Hand Hygiene
Hand Hygiene according to Standard Precautions.
Gowns
Don gown upon entry into the room or cubicle.
Remove gown and observe hand hygiene before leaving the patient-care environment.
Patient Transport
Limit transport of patients to medically necessary purposes.
Ensure that infected or colonized areas of the patient's body are contained and covered.
Remove and dispose of contaminated PPE and perform hand hygiene prior to transporting patients on Contact Precautions.
Don clean PPE to handle the patient at the transport destination.
Patient-Care Equipment
Use disposable noncritical patient-care equipment or implement patient-dedicated use of such equipment.
Form No. CPR7
BREVIS CORP., 225 West 2855 South, SLC, UT 84115
© 2007 Brevis Corp.

FIGURE 10–16 Contact precautions.

- No visitors who have infections or recent exposure to communicable diseases or vaccinations are allowed to enter the room.
- No unwashed fresh fruit or vegetables, raw eggs, or yogurt may be eaten.
- No flowers or plants are allowed in the room.
- Sources of stagnant water (e.g., denture cups, irrigating containers) should be avoided.

Antiseptics, Disinfectants, and Sterilization

A number of chemical agents and physical methods are used to inhibit the growth of or destroy microorganisms. If the method used only inhibits the growth of the microorganism, the action is described as **bacteriostatic**. If the method results in the microorganisms being killed, the action is **bacteriocidal** or

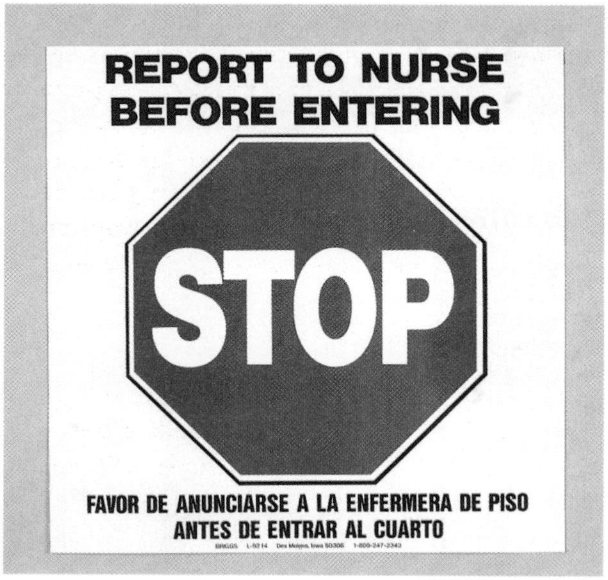

FIGURE 10–17 Report to nurse signage.

germicidal. The methods used can be broken into the following three categories:

- **Antiseptics:** Chemical agents that are antiseptics are only bacteriostatic. They are mild enough to be used on the skin. An example is cleaning with a 70% isopropyl alcohol wipe before giving an injection.
- **Disinfectants:** Agents or methods that destroy most bacteria and viruses. This method of cleaning is used for instruments that do not penetrate the skin and for cleaning the environment (e.g., floors, bathroom, equipment). *Chemical agents* are frequently used as disinfectants. Using a solution comparable to a 10% dilution of common household bleach in water for cleaning the environment (including blood spills) meets OSHA recommendations because it kills hepatitis B, human immunodeficiency virus (HIV), and tuberculosis organisms. Alcohol was mentioned earlier as an example of an antiseptic, but if instruments are soaked for 20 to 30 minutes, it acts as a disinfectant. (See Figure 10–18.) Carefully read and follow the manufacturer's directions when using chemical agents. *Physical disinfectant methods* include boiling instruments in water. This was once commonly used in home health settings, but with the availability of one-time-use equipment, it is rarely used today.
- **Sterilization**: Agents or methods that totally destroy all microorganisms, including viruses and spores. Examples include chemical agents, gas, radiation, and dry or moist heat under pressure. The most common method used is the autoclave, which sterilizes by steam that is created by a pressurized heating system. The size can vary from a small unit for a medical office to a large unit for a hospital. (See Figure 10–19.)

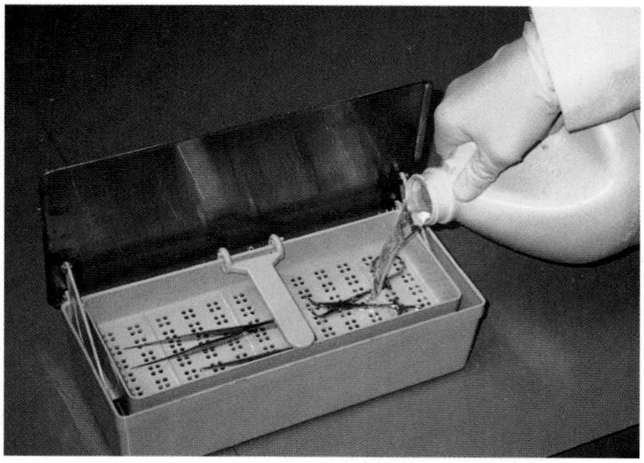

FIGURE 10–18 Chemical agent used as disinfectant. Pour in enough solution to completely cover all instruments.

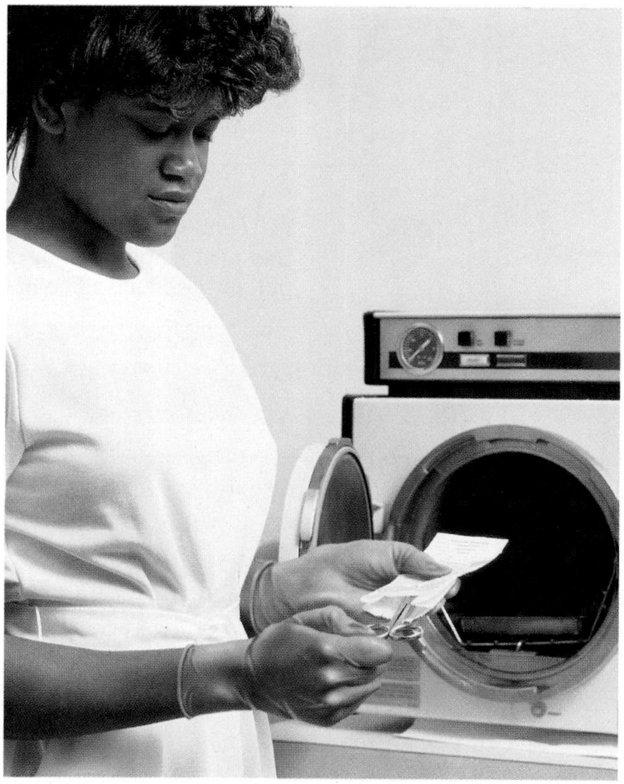

FIGURE 10–19 An autoclave is a pressurized heating system that sterilizes by steam.

Surgical Asepsis

Surgical asepsis (or sterile technique) is a group of principles and related procedures that eliminate the presence of pathogens from objects and areas. To correctly perform these procedures, it is necessary to understand the concept of a sterile field. A **sterile field** is an area that has been designated as free of microorganisms. An example is a sterile towel placed on a clean, dry surface. The towel now represents a sterile field. Many health care procedures, such as surgeries, require the use of sterile fields.

When working with a sterile field or sterile items, it is essential that contaminants not be brought into the field through actions such as touching it, allowing it to become wet, reaching across it, or talking directly over the surface. Sterilized items, such as instruments and surgical gloves, come in sealed packages that must be opened and handled properly to avoid contamination. It is also necessary for the health care professional to use sterile gloves, applying them in a way that prevents them from being contaminated. (See Procedure 10–4.) Always check for expiration dates on the package before using any sterilized items.

Media Link

Learn more about how to apply sterile gloves by viewing the Sterile Gloves and the Sterile Field video on the Online Resources.

PROCEDURE 10–4

Sterile Gloves (Applying Sterile Gloves and Removing Contaminated Gloves)

PROCEDURE	RATIONALE
1. Use proper handwashing technique (See Procedure 10–1.)	To remove microorganisms from hands.
2. Inspect glove package for tears or stains and do not use if present.	Tears and stains indicate the gloves are no longer sterile and must be discarded or used for nonsterile purposes.
3. Place package of gloves on a clean, dry, flat surface above waist level.	Using a contaminated surface can compromise the sterility of the sterile package.
To apply sterile gloves (See Figures 10–20 a–f):	
Open sterile gloves by pulling back on the tabs without touching the sterile inner border.	Extra caution must be taken to protect the sterility of the gloves.
The gloves should be opened with the cuffs toward you, the palms up, and the thumbs pointing outward. If the gloves are not positioned properly, turn the package around, being careful not to reach over the sterile area or touch the inner surface of the gloves.	Sterile gloves are packaged in this position for ease of application.
Pick up the first glove by grasping the glove on the top edge of the folded-down cuff. Do not drag or dangle the fingers over any nonsterile area.	Picking up the glove by grasping the inner cuff prevents the outer part of the glove from becoming contaminated. Strict adherence to the sterile principles is essential.
Maintain the grasp on the cuff, insert your other hand, and gently pull the glove on by the cuff.	Pull gently to avoid tearing the glove. If contamination occurs, discard the gloves and start again.

(continues)

PROCEDURE 10–4

Sterile Gloves (Applying Sterile Gloves and Removing Contaminated Gloves)

(continued)

PROCEDURE	RATIONALE
Slip the gloved fingers under the cuff of the second glove to lift it from the package and insert the other hand into the glove.	The outside of the second glove is sterile and may be touched only by another sterile surface.
Pull the glove on and adjust the glove into position, being careful not to touch the skin with the gloved hands.	Always be mindful of what is a sterile surface and what is contaminated.
Turn the cuffs up by manipulating only the sterile surface of the gloves (go under the folded cuffs, pull out slightly, and turn cuffs over and up).	Only sterile touches sterile.
Check the gloves for tears, holes, and imperfections.	If any flaws noted, discard and start again.
4. Once gloves are applied always hold the hands above the waist and away from the body with palms up.	Serves to increase awareness of sterile gloves and prevent inadvertently touching nonsterile areas.

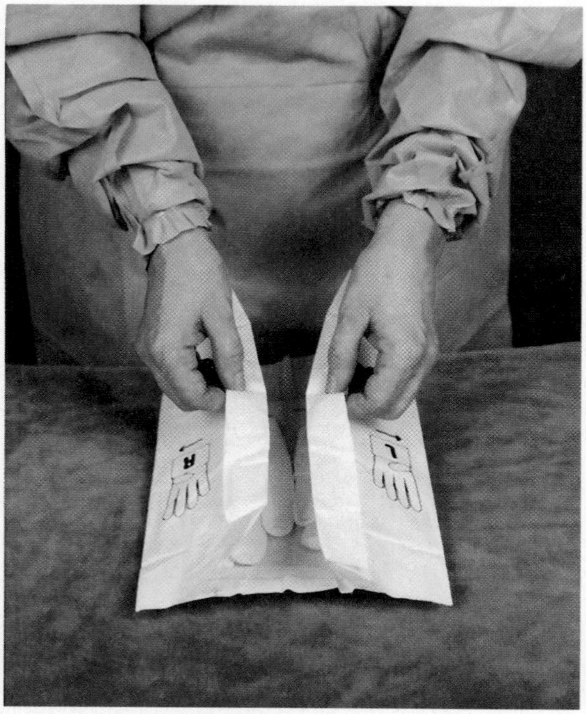

FIGURE 10–20a Open sterile gloves by pulling back on the tabs.

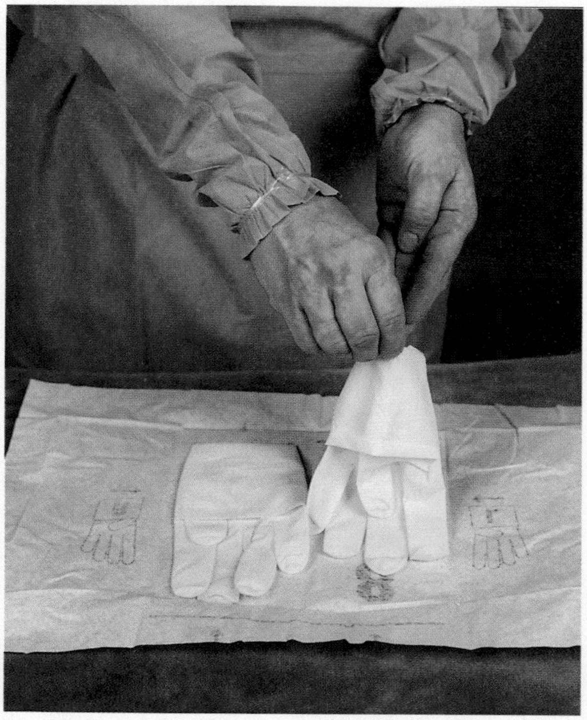

FIGURE 10–20b Pick up the first glove by grasping the glove on the top edge of the folded-down cuff.

(continues)

PROCEDURE 10–4

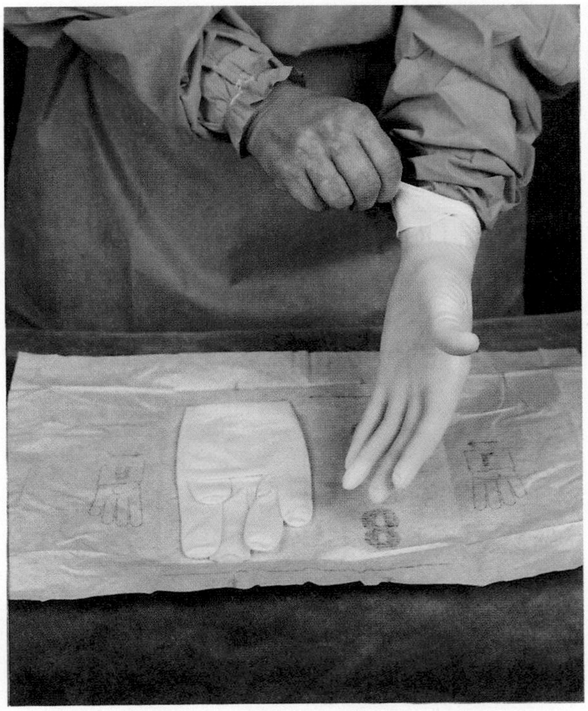

FIGURE 10–20c Maintain the grasp on the cuff, insert your other hand, and pull the glove on by the cuff.

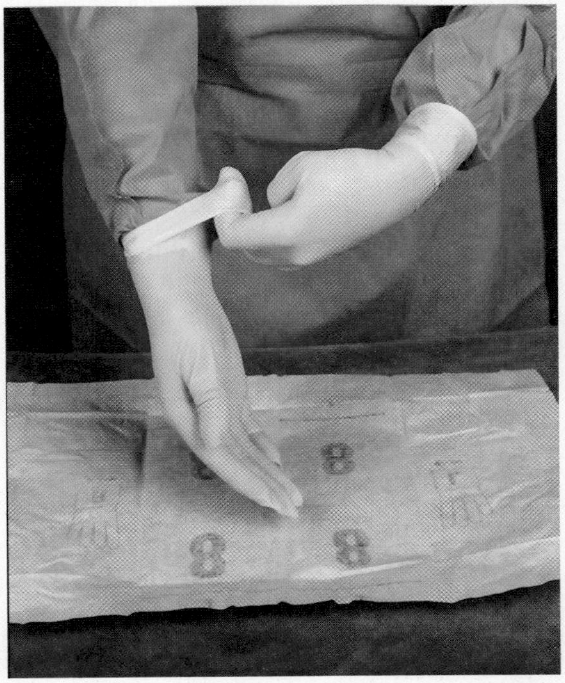

FIGURE 10–20e Pull the glove on and adjust the glove into position, being careful not to touch the skin with the gloved hands.

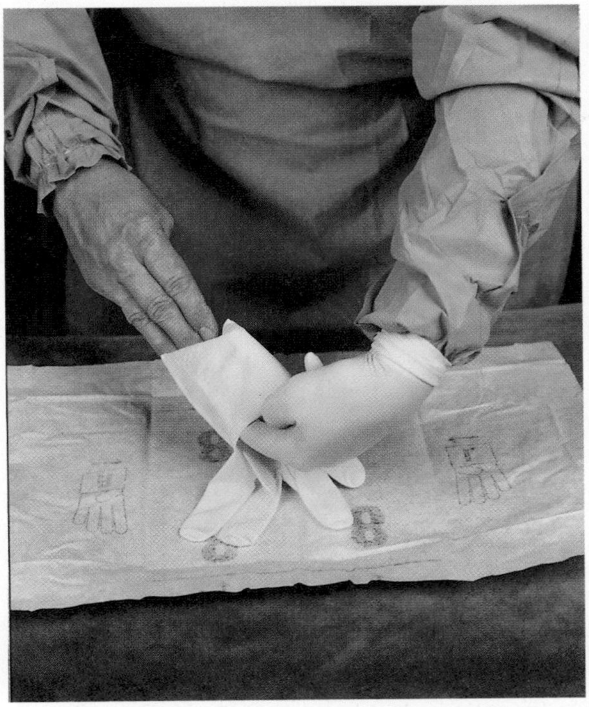

FIGURE 10–20d Slip the gloved fingers under the cuff of the second glove to lift it from the package and insert the other hand into the glove.

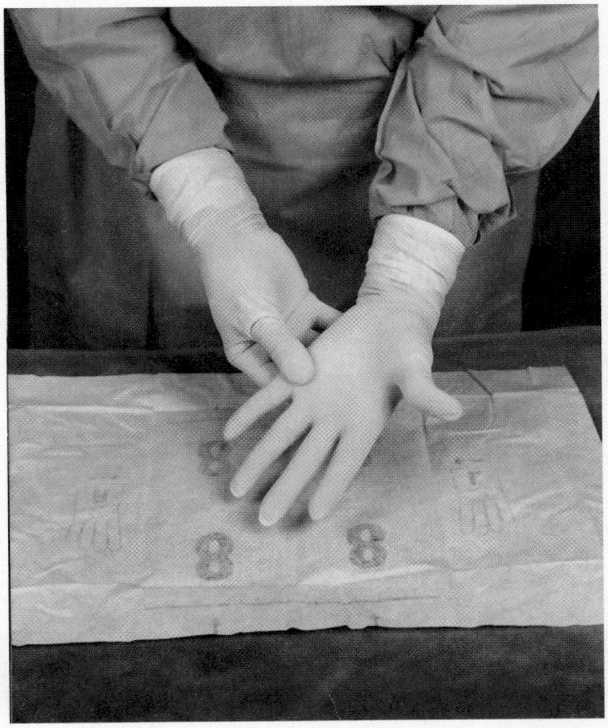

FIGURE 10–20f Check the gloves for tears, holes, and imperfections.

THE RISKS

Certain diseases pose special risks to the health care professional. These include two blood-borne pathogens, hepatitis B virus (HBV) and human immunodeficiency virus (HIV), and an airborne-transmitted disease, tuberculosis (TB). Also of great concern are two drug-resistant infections that create unique challenges.

The term *blood-borne* is used to identify pathogenic microbes that are spread through contact with blood. Blood, however, is not the only route by which they can be transmitted. Infections can also be transmitted through contact with nonintact skin, mucous membranes, secretions, excretions, or any moist body fluid except sweat.

Hepatitis B

Hepatitis B virus infection is the major infectious blood-borne occupational hazard for health care professionals. HBV can be spread via several routes:

- Parenteral: Blood transfusion, needle sharing by intravenous (IV) drug users, needlestick, or other sharp instrument
- Mucous membranes: Blood contamination of the eye or mouth
- Sexual contact
- Perinatal: From infected mother to newborn infant

(*Source:* OSHA Online)

When an individual becomes infected, the liver, in its attempt to destroy the hepatitis virus, causes an inflammation and subsequent destruction of liver cells. Symptoms range from very mild to severe jaundice (yellowing of the eyes and skin), dark urine, fatigue, loss of appetite, nausea, abdominal pain, and sometimes joint pain, rash, and fever.

Efforts for prevention in health care settings are focused on the administration of hepatitis B vaccine, use of PPE, prevention of puncture injuries, and disinfection and sterilization of equipment and surfaces. OSHA mandates that employers provide hepatitis B vaccine for all employees who have an occupational exposure risk. The hepatitis B vaccines are given in three doses over a six-month period. These vaccines, when given according to manufacturer's directions, induce protective antibody levels in 85% to 97% of healthy adults. If there is some doubt about a person's immunity, a blood test can be done to verify presence of the antibody (OSHA Online). An employee has the right to refuse the hepatitis B vaccine, but if declined, the employee must sign a form stating his or her refusal. This releases the facility from responsibility should the health care professional become infected.

Although hepatitis B is the most common hepatitis virus, there are other hepatitis viruses of which the health care professional must have knowledge. (See Table 10–3.) Note that hepatitis A (HAV) and hepatitis E (HEV) are transmitted by the fecal-oral route. Hepatitis B, hepatitis C (HCV), and hepatitis D (HDV) are transmitted by blood and body fluids.

> **Thinking It Through**
>
> Frank Gello is very excited about his new position as a surgical technologist at the local hospital, although he is somewhat intimidated by the person who is orienting him and is anxious to complete his training and work more independently. As they set up for the next surgery, his preceptor positions himself on the opposite side of the sterile field. As Frank opens the sterile instruments to place them on the sterile field, his preceptor talks him through the procedure and on several occasions he reaches across impatiently to move Frank's placement of the instruments. Frank also knows that he should check all of the packaging on the instruments for integrity to insure sterility has been maintained, but his preceptor abruptly states "I have already done that. Don't waste my time. Keep going as the surgeon is arriving in a few minutes."
>
> 1. Does this scenario refer to medical or surgical asepsis? What is the difference between medical and surgical asepsis?
> 2. Were any of the aseptic principles broken? If so, what are they?
> 3. Should Frank perform a double-check on the packaging to verify the integrity of the sterility of the instruments even if his preceptor states he has already performed that check?

Human Immunodeficiency Virus

HIV (human immunodeficiency virus) is the virus that causes AIDS (acquired immune deficiency syndrome). The virus destroys cells in the host that are

Table 10–3 Viral Hepatitis

Type	Infectious Agent	Route of Transmission	Prevention and Recommendations
A	Hepatitis A is an acute liver disease caused by the hepatitis A virus (HAV), lasting from a few weeks to several months. It does not lead to chronic infection.	Ingestion of fecal matter, even microscopic amounts; from close person-to-person contact; or ingestion of contaminated food or drinks. Once you have had HAV, you cannot get it again.	Hepatitis A vaccination is recommended for all children starting at age 1 year, travelers to certain countries, and others at risk, such as: • Men who have sex with men • Injecting and noninjecting drug users • Persons with clotting-factor disorders (e.g., hemophilia) • Persons with chronic liver disease Short-term protection is obtained when immune globulin is given within 2 weeks of contact with HAV. Always wash hands with soap and water after using the bathroom, changing a diaper, and before preparing and eating food.
B	Hepatitis B is a liver disease caused by the hepatitis B virus (HBV). It ranges in severity from a mild illness, lasting a few weeks (acute), to a serious long-term (chronic) illness that can lead to liver disease or cancer.	Contact with infectious blood, semen, and other body fluids from having sex with an infected person, sharing contaminated needles to inject drugs, or from an infected mother to her newborn.	Hepatitis B vaccination is recommended for all infants, older children, and adolescents who were not vaccinated previously, and adults at risk for HBV infection. Adults at risk include all health care professionals with an occupational risk.
	An infection occurs when blood or body fluids from an infected person enters the body of a person who is not immune.	Hepatitis B virus can remain active in dried blood for several days, so proper precautions must be followed when cleaning up dried blood.	Other recommendations: • If having sex with more than one steady partner, use latex condoms correctly and every time you have sex. If allergic to latex, use a condom made of polyurethane or other synthetic material. The efficacy of latex condoms in preventing infection with HBV is unknown, but proper use may reduce transmission. • If pregnant, get a blood test for hepatitis B; infants born to HBV-infected mothers should be given hepatitis B immune globulin (HBIG) and vaccine within 12 hours after birth.

(continues)

Table 10–3 Viral Hepatitis (continued)

Type	Infectious Agent	Route of Transmission	Prevention and Recommendations
			• Do not inject drugs; if you do, stop and get into a treatment program; if you cannot stop, never share drugs, needles, syringes, water, or "works"; and get vaccinated against HAV and HBV. • Do not share personal care items that might have blood on them (e.g., razors, toothbrushes). • Consider risks if you are thinking about getting a tattoo or body piercing. You might become infected if the tools have someone else's blood on them or if the artist or piercer does not follow good health practices. • If you have or had HBV, do not donate blood, organs, or tissue. • If you are a health care or public safety worker, get vaccinated against HBV and always follow routine standard precautions and safely handle needles and other sharps.
C	Hepatitis C is a liver disease caused by hepatitis C virus (HCV). HCV infection sometimes results in an acute illness, but most often becomes a chronic condition that can lead to cirrhosis of the liver and liver cancer.	Contact with the blood of an infected person, primarily through sharing contaminated needles to inject drugs.	There is no vaccine to prevent HCV. Several drugs can be taken, but they result in a cure in less than 50% of cases. • Do not inject drugs; if you do, stop and get into a treatment program; if you cannot stop, never share needles, syringes, water, or any personal care items and get vaccinated against HAV and HBV. • Do not share personal care items that might have blood on them (e.g., razors, toothbrushes).

(continues)

Table 10–3 Viral Hepatitis (continued)

Type	Infectious Agent	Route of Transmission	Prevention and Recommendations
			• If you are a health care or public safety worker, always follow routine barrier precautions and safely handle needles and other sharps; get vaccinated against HBV. • Consider risks if you are thinking about getting a tattoo or body piercing. You might become infected if the tools have someone else's blood on them or if the artist or piercer does not follow good health practices. • Can be spread by sex, but this is rare. If you are having sex with more than one steady sex partner, use latex condoms correctly and every time to prevent the spread of sexually transmitted diseases (if allergic to latex, use a condom made of polyurethane or other synthetic material); also get vaccinated against HBV. • If you are HCV positive, do not donate blood, organs, or tissue.
D	Hepatitis D is a serious liver disease caused by the hepatitis D virus (HDV), which relies on HBV to replicate. It is uncommon in the United States.	Contact with infectious blood, similar to the mechanisms by which HBV is spread.	There is no vaccine to prevent HDV. Recommendations are the same as for HCV.
E	Hepatitis E is a serious liver disease caused by the hepatitis E virus (HEV). It usually results in an acute infection and does not lead to a chronic infection. While rare in the United States, hepatitis E is common in many parts of the world. It is found in the stool (feces) of persons and animals with HEV.	Ingestion of fecal matter, even in microscopic amounts; outbreaks are usually associated with contaminated water supply in countries with poor sanitation. Transmission from person to person occurs less commonly than with HAV.	There is no vaccine to prevent HEV. • Always wash hands with soap and water after using the bathroom, changing a diaper, and before preparing and eating food. • Avoid drinking water (and beverages with ice) of unknown purity and avoid eating uncooked shellfish and uncooked fruits or vegetables that are not peeled or prepared by the traveler.

vital to the proper functioning of the immune system. Individuals infected with the virus are said to be **HIV positive**. This is not the same as having **AIDS**, which means that the immune system has become weakened as a result of the action of the virus. Some individuals carry the virus without becoming ill; most, however, eventually develop AIDS and die as the result of severe opportunistic infections. These are infections that individuals with normal immune systems rarely experience. The most common opportunistic infection and cause of death of persons with AIDS is *Pneumocystis carinii*.

Common signs and symptoms of AIDS include weakness, chronic fever, night sweats, swelling of the lymph nodes, weight loss, and diarrhea. There is no vaccine against AIDS and no known cure. The goal is to prolong life and manage the symptoms. New antiviral drugs have been and continue to be developed that have added many years to the life of someone with AIDS.

Carriers of HIV may not have symptoms or even detectable amounts of the virus in the blood during the first six months of infection. It is essential, therefore, that health care professionals understand how the virus is transmitted and follow standard precautions with *all* patients.

Infection with HIV may be identified through testing the blood for the presence of HIV antibodies. Most people infected with HIV have detectable antibodies within six months of infection, with the majority generating detectable antibodies between 6 and 12 weeks after exposure. Once individuals are HIV positive, they become lifelong carriers and can spread the virus to others.

HIV has been isolated from human blood, semen, breast milk, vaginal secretions, saliva, tears, urine, cerebrospinal fluid, and amniotic fluid; however, only blood, semen, vaginal secretions, and breast milk have been proven to transmit the virus. Common modes of transmission are sexual intercourse; using contaminated needles; blood exposure via parenteral, mucous membrane, or nonintact skin contact; transfusions; transplants; semen used for artificial insemination; and contact with perinatal fluids.

HIV is not transmitted by casual contact. No evidence exists that HIV is transmitted by shaking hands or talking; by sharing food, eating utensils, plates, drinking glasses, or towels; by sharing the same house or household facilities; or by "personal interactions expected of family members," including hugging and kissing on the cheek or lips. HIV is also not transmitted by mosquitoes or other animals (OSHA Online).

Fascinating Facts

More than 1.1 million people in the United States are living with HIV infection, and almost 1 in 6 (15.8%) are unaware of their infection. About 1 in 4 HIV infections are among youth ages 13 to 24. Most of them do not know they are infected, are not getting treated, and can unknowingly pass the virus on to others. (www.aids.gov).

The rate of infection from exposure is in relationship to the amount of infected material introduced into the body. For example, a person receiving a contaminated blood transfusion has a much greater chance of infection than a health care professional injured with a contaminated needle. In fact, only three to five health care professionals out of 1000 will become infected when injured with contaminated needles (OSHA Online). This is *not* to downplay the impact of acquiring such a devastating disease, but only to put the risk in perspective. Most health care professionals fear being infected by AIDS more than HBV, and yet the infection and death rates of HBV far exceed those of AIDS. (See Table 10–4.)

Tuberculosis

Tuberculosis (TB) is caused by *Mycobacterium tuberculosis*, an airborne pathogen. Working with tuberculosis patients require the use of special PPE, such as special masks fitted to the individual health care professional, to avoid inhaling the tiny droplets that carry the pathogen through the air. The TB bacteria are put into the air when a person with TB disease of the lungs or throat coughs, sneezes, speaks, or sings. People nearby may breathe in these bacteria and become infected.

TB is *not* spread by:

- Shaking someone's hand
- Sharing food or drink
- Touching bed linens or toilet seats

Table 10–4 HIV/AIDS

Route of Transmission	Major Symptoms	Treatment	Prevention
AIDS is caused by the blood-borne virus HIV and is transmitted by: • Vaginal, oral, and anal sex • Sharing needles to inject drugs, body piercing or tattooing • Contaminated blood products (rare) • Infected mother to newborn *Note*: It is *not* transmitted by shaking hands, social kisses, utensils, animals, hugging, swimming pools, toilet seats, food, insects, or coughing.	This disease mimics symptoms of many other infections, such as: • Flu-like illness • Swollen lymph nodes • Persistent fevers • Night sweats • Prolonged diarrhea • Unexplained weight loss • Purple bumps on skin or inside mouth and nose • Chronic fatigue • Recurrent respiratory infections *Note*: These symptoms are not specific for HIV and may have other causes. Most people with HIV have no symptoms at all for several years.	No preventative vaccine or cure is available. Early diagnosis and treatment can extend life for years. Keep immune system as strong as possible with medications and life style. Antiviral drugs slow cell processes and can extend life. Prompt treatment of AIDS-related illnesses decreases death due to complications. Medications are available for HIV-infected pregnant women to greatly reduce the chance of passing infection to newborn.	Prevention is similar to that for other blood-borne diseases: • Always use latex condoms/latex barriers during sex (if allergic to latex, use a condom made of polyurethane or other synthetic material). • Do not share needles for drugs, tattooing, or body piercings. • Limit number of sex partners. • Be tested and have potential partners tested for HIV; this can be done by providers, sexually transmitted disease (STD) clinics, and HIV counseling and testing sites. • Notify sex and needle-sharing partners immediately if HIV infected. A health care worker can prevent workplace exposure by following standard precautions and avoiding needlestick injuries.

- Sharing toothbrushes
- Kissing

Once considered to be nearly eliminated from the United States, cases of TB have increased and some bacteria have become resistant to drug therapy. This is because medications must be taken for at least six months. Failure by some patients to complete the full length of treatment has allowed certain strains of the bacterium to develop resistance to the drugs.

Although renewed efforts to control TB have resulted in a steady decrease in cases since 1992, it remains one of the most common infections in the world (one third of the world's population is infected with TB) and is the leading killer of people who are HIV infected. Globally, TB causes 1.3 million deaths annually (CDC Online).

The screening test for TB is a skin test. A positive test result does not necessarily indicate active disease, but does indicate that the person has had an exposure to the pathogen. A chest X-ray and other tests are done to determine if active disease is present. The signs and symptoms are lethargy, fever, night sweats, cough, weight loss, blood-tinged sputum, chest pain, and shortness of breath. TB primarily affects the lungs, but can affect other parts of the body, such as the kidney, spine, and brain. Patients hospitalized with suspected TB are placed in isolation for two to three weeks during which time antibiotic treatment is given.

Thinking It Through

Monica Stokes is a volunteer at a local extended care facility. Her duties include pushing a cart with books around to the patients' rooms to ask if they would like to borrow a library book. When she enters Mr. Haskin's room, the nurse asks her if she would please take the dirty linens and place them in the linen basket down the hall. She is new and unclear if this is one of her duties, but also desires to be helpful, and surely the nurse would not ask her if it were not appropriate. So she picks up the linens from the floor, carries them close to her, and places them in the linen basket. She notices some stains on her clothes, so she goes to the sink and rinses them off with cold water in the hope there will be no permanent stain. She then returns to her duties of distributing books to patients.

1. Was it appropriate for the nurse to ask the volunteer to assist with the linens?
2. Are all the links present in the chain of infection?
3. What breaks in standard precautions can you identify?

Not everyone infected with TB bacteria becomes sick. As a result, two TB-related conditions exist: latent TB infection and active TB disease. (See Table 10–5.)

- Latent TB infection: This condition is present when TB bacteria live in the body without making the person sick. In most people who breathe in TB bacteria and become infected, the body is able to fight the bacteria to stop them from growing. People with latent TB infection do not feel sick and do not have symptoms. The only sign of TB infection is a positive reaction to the tuberculin skin test. People with latent TB infection are not infectious and cannot spread TB bacteria to others. However, if TB bacteria become active in the body and multiply, the person will become sick with TB disease.
- TB disease: TB bacteria become active if the immune system cannot stop them from growing. Once the bacteria are active (multiplying in the body), the person will be sick with TB disease and can spread the disease to others. Some people develop TB disease soon after becoming infected (within weeks), before their immune system can fight the TB bacteria. Other

Table 10–5 Differences between Latent TB Infection and TB Disease

Person with Latent TB Infection	Person with TB Disease
Has no symptoms	Has symptoms that may include: • Bad cough that lasts 3 weeks or longer • Pain in the chest • Coughing up blood or sputum • Weakness or fatigue • Weight loss • No appetite • Chills • Fever • Sweating at night
Does not feel sick	Usually feels sick
Cannot spread TB bacteria to others	May spread TB bacteria to others
Usually has a skin test or blood test result indicating TB infection	Usually has a skin test or blood test result indicating TB infection
Has a normal chest X-ray and a negative sputum smear	May have an abnormal chest X-ray, or positive sputum smear or culture
Needs treatment for latent TB infection to prevent active TB disease	Needs treatment to treat active TB disease

Source: CDC Online. www.cdc.gov

people may become sick years later, when their immune system becomes weak for another reason. For persons whose immune systems are weak, especially those with HIV infection, the risk of developing TB disease is much higher than for persons with normal immune systems. (See Table 10–5.)

Fascinating Facts

Imagine ¼ teaspoon of HBV mixed into a 24,000-gallon swimming pool of water. Someone draws a ¼ teaspoon of that water into a syringe and injects you with it. Although the virus is diluted well, you will become HBV positive. Now imagine that 10 people are in a room. Someone takes ¼ teaspoon of HIV and mixes it into a quart of water. Then ¼ teaspoon of this solution is injected into each person. Only one person in the room will become HIV positive. Hepatitis B is thus a much greater threat to health care professionals than HIV (Acello, 2009).

Other Infectious Organisms

Other contagious diseases have received a lot of media coverage. Some of these are listed in Table 10–6. They have a global impact because organisms easily cross borders. So when an outbreak of a disease is first noted in another country, the United States immediately becomes involved to develop a plan of action. The CDC is actively involved in this process. The CDC works with partners throughout the nation and the world to monitor health, detect and investigate health problems, conduct research to enhance prevention, develop and advocate sound public health policies, implement prevention strategies, promote healthy behaviors, foster safe and healthful environments, and provide leadership and training (CDC Online).

Drug-Resistant Organisms

The development of drug-resistant organisms is a fairly recent occurrence. It is a result of antibiotic usage. Antibiotics and similar drugs, together called antimicrobial agents, have been used for the

Table 10–6 Other Contagious Diseases

Disease	Source	Major Symptoms	Prevention and Recommendations
Ebola virus	Body fluids of a person who is sick with or has died from Ebola; contaminated objects; infected animals (by contact with blood or fluids or infected meat).	Symptoms can occur 2–21 days after exposure and include fever, headache, diarrhea, vomiting, stomach pain, unexplained bleeding or bruising, and muscle pain.	Seek immediate medical testing if symptoms occur. Always follow standard precautions. Transmission precautions will be in effect for direct care.
Bird flu (H5N1 avian influenza)	Infected birds shed the virus in their saliva, nasal secretions, and feces; the virus was first isolated in 1961 in wild birds (terns) in South Africa and was thought to be limited to bird-to-bird contact. In 1997, the first documented case of bird-to-human transmission occurred. Because influenza viruses can mutate (change), it is possible that the virus could change so that it could infect humans and could be spread easily from person to person.	Symptoms range from typical influenza-like symptoms (e.g., fever, cough, sore throat, and muscle aches) to eye infections, pneumonia, acute respiratory distress, viral pneumonia, and other severe and life-threatening complications.	Prevention involves culling (killing) of sick and exposed birds; this includes both wild and domestic birds. Travelers to countries in Asia with documented outbreaks should avoid poultry farms, contact with animals in live food markets, and any surfaces that appear to be contaminated with feces from poultry or other animals.

Table 10–6 Other Contagious Diseases (continued)

Disease	Source	Major Symptoms	Prevention and Recommendations
Mad cow disease (bovine spongiform encephalopathy [BSE])	The exact cause of BSE is not known; it is thought to be caused by an infectious form of a type of protein, prions, normally found in animals. In cattle with BSE, these abnormal prions initially occur in the small intestines and tonsils and are found in central nervous tissues, such as the brain and spinal cord, and other tissues of infected animals experiencing later stages of the disease.	BSE causes the cow's brain cells to die, forming sponge-like holes in the brain. The cow behaves strangely and eventually dies. A disease similar to BSE called Creutzfeldt-Jacob Disease (CJD) is found in people. A variant form of CJD (vCJD) is believed to be caused by eating contaminated beef products from BSE-affected cattle.	BSE cannot be killed by cooking, freezing, or disinfectants. The U.S. Department of Agriculture (USDA) guidelines are as follows: • Prohibits imports of live ruminants or ruminant products (meat, feed, by-products) from Europe • Tests for BSE if any cattle showing abnormal behavior • Inspects all cattle used for food for signs of neurological diseases. Cattle with unidentified neurological disorders are rejected • Prohibits the use of mammalian proteins in making animal feed for ruminants FDA guidelines include the following: • The FDA has recommended that pharmaceutical companies should not use animal tissues from countries with BSE in making drug products (vaccines). • The FDA has asked blood centers to exclude potential blood donors who have spent five or more years in Europe from 1980 to present. In addition, the deferral criteria applies to persons who lived in the U.K. between 1980 and 1996. The CDC has issued guidelines to travelers in Europe: • Avoid beef and beef products altogether. • If eating meat, select beef or beef products that have less opportunity for contamination from nervous tissue (solid muscle cuts versus processed sausages or hamburgers). • Milk or milk products are not believed to pose any risk from the BSE agent.

(continues)

Table 10–6 Other Contagious Diseases (continued)

Disease	Source	Major Symptoms	Prevention and Recommendations
West Nile virus	This virus is transmitted by infected mosquitoes to humans and animals; an uninfected mosquito can become infected by biting an infected animal. There is no evidence of human-to-human or animal-to-human transmission.	Most people have mild or no symptoms at all; most common symptoms are similar to any other flu-like infection (fever, headache, rash, lymph gland swelling, and general muscular aches and pains). In severe cases, encephalitis (inflammation or swelling of the brain) can occur.	No specific treatment exists other than supportive care of symptoms; no vaccine is available. Prevention includes the following: • Protect oneself from mosquito bites by wearing long sleeves and long pants and applying insect repellent with DEET. • Eliminate breeding grounds near residences by ensuring there is no standing water. • Stay indoors at dawn, dusk, and early evening when mosquitoes are actively feeding.
Swine flu (H1N1 influenza)	H1N1 is a virus thought to spread mainly from person-to-person through coughing or sneezing of infected people. It may also be spread by touching infected objects and then touching your nose or mouth. It is a new virus of swine origin that first caused illness in Mexico and the United States in March and April 2009.	Common symptoms are high fever, cough, sore throat, runny or stuffy nose, body aches, headache, chills, fatigue, and sometimes diarrhea and vomiting.	Vaccine is available and recommended, especially for young children and those over 65 years of age or those who have certain health conditions that put them at greater risk. Everyday actions to stay healthy include: • Cover nose and mouth with a tissue when coughing or sneezing. Throw the tissue in the trash after use. • Wash hands often with soap and water, especially after coughing or sneezing. Alcohol-based hand cleaners are also effective. • Avoid touching eyes, nose, or mouth. Germs spread that way. Stay home if sick. The CDC recommends that people who are ill with swine flu stay home from work or school and limit contact with others to keep from infecting them.

Source: CDC Online. www.cdc.gov

past 70 years to treat patients who have infectious diseases. Since the 1940s, these drugs have greatly reduced illness and death from infectious diseases. However, these drugs have been used so widely and for so long that the infectious organisms the antibiotics are designed to kill have adapted to them, making the drugs less effective.

Each year in the United States, at least 2 million people become infected with bacteria that are resistant to antibiotics and at least 23,000 people die each year as a direct result of these infections. Many more people die from other conditions that were complicated by an antibiotic-resistant infection (CDC Online).

Another contributing factor is that antibiotics have routinely been overused by being prescribed for minor conditions. In addition, many patients fail to complete an entire course of antibiotic as prescribed. These two actions create conditions that encourage pathogens to become resistant to antibiotics. It is important to explain to patients why they must take all the medication prescribed for them, because they have a tendency stop taking the antibiotic when they feel better.

The CDC lists antibiotic-resistant microorganisms by threat level. The 2013 report has three at the urgent threat level, 11 at the serious threat level, and three at the concerning threat level. Two of these drug-resistant organisms commonly encountered in health care are *methicillin-resistant Staphylococcus aureus (MRSA)* and *vancomycin-resistant Enterococcus (VRE)*. Both are difficult to control and treat and can cause very serious infections. If there is a treatment available, it is usually very expensive and can have severe side effects, such as liver, kidney, and hearing damage. Because these infections occur most frequently in elderly patients who are more susceptible to the side effects and already have weakened resistance, they often result in death. (See Table 10–7.)

Another organism that the CDC states is an immediate public health threat requiring urgent and aggressive action is *Clostridium difficile*. Infections most often occur in people who have had both recent medical care and antibiotics. *C. difficile* causes life-threatening diarrhea. Although resistance to the antibiotics used to treat *C. difficile* is not yet a problem, the bacteria spread rapidly because they are naturally resistant to many drugs used to treat other infections. Deaths related to *C. difficile* increased 400% between 2000 and 2007, in part because a more resistant bacterial strain emerged. An estimated $1 billion in excess medical costs occur per year as a result of this infection.

Fascinating Facts

Persons exposed to TB may develop *latent* (inactive) TB infection. Almost 2 billion people (*one third of the world's population*) have latent TB infection, and about 10% of these infected individuals will develop active disease sometime during their lifetime. In an era marked by increased international travel and a global marketplace, no region of the world is immune from outside influences. International collaboration will be essential to eliminate TB (CDC Online).

The seriousness of these infections emphasizes the importance of always following standard precautions and any additional procedures developed by the health care facility to prevent their spread. Actions on the part of the health care professional can determine whether infections are kept under control or are spread among patients and other workers.

REPORTING ACCIDENTAL EXPOSURE

Any injury or accident that involves exposure to blood or body fluids should be washed immediately. After a thorough washing of the area, the next action is to report the incident to the supervisor. This must be followed by completion of a written incident or injury report according to facility or agency requirements. Prompt reporting allows for evaluation, appropriate treatment (if indicated), and follow up of any problems resulting from the exposure. Failure to report an incident can result in negative health consequences for the health care professional and others, as well as the need to take time off from work to recover.

OSHA regulations require every facility to have an exposure control plan. This plan has many components, including the predetermination of employee exposure risk to blood-borne pathogens, description of how employees at risk will be protected, and training and annual retraining and testing requirements for employees. Plans must also include policies and

Table 10–7 Drug-Resistant Infections

Infectious Agent	Source/Route of Transmission	Major Symptoms	Prevention and Recommendations
MRSA (methicillin-resistant *Staphylococcus aureus*) is most frequently (85%) seen in persons in healthcare facilities who have weakened immune systems. This is called HA-MRSA (health care-associated or acquired MRSA). MRSA infections occurring outside of the healthcare setting in otherwise healthy people is known as CA-MRSA (community-associated or acquired MRSA). *Note*: MRSA is a type of staph that is resistant to certain antibiotics, such as methicillin, oxacillin, penicillin, and amoxicillin.	*S. aureus* bacteria are commonly carried on the skin or in the nose of healthy people. Approximately 25% to 30% of the population is colonized (when bacteria are present, but not causing an infection) in the nose with staph bacteria and about 1% are colonized with MRSA.	HA-MRSA symptoms vary with location of infection (skin, surgical wound, bloodstream, urinary tract, pneumonia). CA-MRSA is usually manifested as skin infections, such as pimples and boils and can be red, swollen, painful, or have pus or other drainage.	To prevent HA-MRSA: • See guidelines for VRE below. To prevent CA-MRSA: • Keep hands clean by washing thoroughly with soap and water or using an alcohol-based hand sanitizer • Good general hygiene • Keep cuts and scrapes clean and covered with a bandage until healed • Avoid contact with other people's wounds or bandages • Avoid sharing personal items, such as towels or razors Diagnosis of MRSA is frequently done by culture, which can take 2–3 days. If available, Xpert MRSA is a test that provides results in about an hour.
VRE (vancomycin-resistant enterococci) *Note*: Vancomycin is an antibiotic that is often used to treat infections caused by enterococci. When enterococci become resistant to this drug, it is called VRE.	Enterococci are normally present in the human intestines, in the female genital tract, and are often found in the environment. VRE can also live here without causing disease (called colonization). However, sometimes it can cause infections of the urinary tract, the bloodstream, or of wounds. Transmitted from person to person by the hands of caregivers or after contact with contaminated surfaces.	Varies with the location of the infection	• Handwashing • Keeping surfaces clean • Wearing gloves • Standard precautions • Follow facility guidelines for contact precautions in caring for patients with VRE

Source: CDC Online. www.cdc.gov

procedures to be followed if exposure does occur. The policies and procedures should include the following:

- Actions to be taken immediately upon exposure, such as washing the exposed area immediately with warm water and soap, or, if the eye or mucous membranes are involved, rinsing with normal saline
- Time frames for reporting
- To whom the incident must be reported
- Form(s) to complete and information that must be included, such as how exposure occurred and the name of the patient
- Recommended procedure for evaluating the risk and outcome of the exposure. For example, a baseline blood test would be run on the health care professional and then repeated at specified intervals, the patient's blood would be drawn to determine HBV and HIV status, and postexposure treatment would begin if indicated. Blood draws and treatments require the consent of the involved individual
- Plan for counseling and information on safe practices to protect self and others

WORKBOOK PRACTICE

Go to your workbook and complete the exercises for this chapter.

SUGGESTED LEARNING ACTIVITIES

1. If you have access to a microscope, take samples from various areas, such as your skin or mucous membranes, stagnant pond water, or decaying food, and look for microorganisms.
2. Watch a medical program on television and evaluate the action for breaks in aseptic technique (medical and surgical).
3. Practice handwashing technique in your home environment.
4. Observe the handwashing techniques of others when out in the community.
5. Research additional sources and read about the lives and contributions made by Louis Pasteur, Oliver Wendell Holmes, and Lord Joseph Lister.
6. Practice donning and removing PPE using a robe as a gown, any type of gloves you may have, and a mask made with paper and a plastic strap.
7. Identify how your actions at work can affect the health and safety of your family.

WEB ACTIVITIES

Worldometers
www.worldometers.info

Go to this website and report on the total number of deaths due to communicable diseases this year.

Centers for Disease Control and Prevention (CDC)
www.cdc.gov

Do research on severe acute respiratory syndrome (SARS). Write a report on how it is transmitted, what symptoms are commonly seen, and how to prevent transmission.

Occupational Safety and Health Administration (OSHA)
www.osha.gov

Identify the role of OSHA in the workplace.

World Health Organization (WHO)
www.who.int

Identify a communicable disease and list the countries that are experiencing an outbreak.

REVIEW QUESTIONS

1. Why is it critical for health care professionals to apply infection control practices in the workplace?
2. What theories and discoveries led to microbiology as we know it today?
3. Name and describe the characteristics of each of the five types of infectious microbes. Include examples of diseases caused by each type.

4. What are the elements in the chain of infection, and how can the chain be broken?
5. What are three examples of defenses used by the body against infection?
6. What are the roles of the CDC and OSHA in protecting the public against infectious diseases?
7. What are the requirements of standard precautions?
8. What are medical and surgical aseptic techniques?
9. How do antiseptics, disinfectants, and sterilization differ?
10. What are the three types of transmission-based precautions?
11. Which three infectious diseases are major risks for health care professionals?
12. Name two drug-resistant organisms. What has caused the development of this resistance? What are the specific risks caused by these organisms?
13. What are the purpose and contents of an exposure control plan?

APPLICATION EXERCISES

1. What are the behaviors demonstrated by Mr. Romero in The Case of the Traveling Microorganisms that jeopardize both him and his patients?
2. Nurse Kristie Rudzinski oversleeps and has barely enough time to dress and get to work on time. She decides to wait until she gets to the hospital to change the adhesive bandage on the finger she cut while fixing dinner last night. When she arrives at work she hears a patient calling for help. No one else is there, so she immediately goes to the patient's room. On entering, Kristie discovers that the patient's IV has become disconnected and blood is running from the patient's vein onto the linens. Without delay she is at the bedside and solves the problem by reconnecting the tubing. The patient is very grateful for her prompt assistance. Kristie leaves the room very pleased that she was able to help, especially because this is a patient she has cared for many times. He is an elderly gentleman who is undergoing chemotherapy and has already had more than his share of problems.
   a. Evaluate the scenario to determine which elements in the chain of infection were present.
   b. What revisions to Kristie's actions would have to occur to follow the principles of medical and surgical asepsis?
   c. Which microorganisms would most likely be a threat to Kristie and to the patient?

PROBLEM-SOLVING PRACTICE

Gene Peterson works at Peaceful Retirement, a local skilled nursing facility, as a nursing assistant. He has always enjoyed working with the elderly population. He finds their wisdom, compassion, and humor very comforting. Prior to going to work, Gene has developed a routine of stopping to visit his grandfather and is just leaving for his visit when his mother calls to tell him his grandfather has been admitted to the hospital with tuberculosis. Gene is very concerned because he knew his grandfather had not been feeling well lately, but had no idea he was that ill. Using the five-step problem-solving process, determine what steps Gene should take next.

SUGGESTED READINGS AND RESOURCES

Centers for Disease Control and Prevention. www.cdc.gov

Kennamer, M. (2013). *Basic infection control for health care providers* (2nd ed.). Clifton Park, NY: Cengage Learning.

Occupational Safety and Health Administration (OSHA). www.osha.gov

World Health Organization. www.who.int

This page intentionally left blank

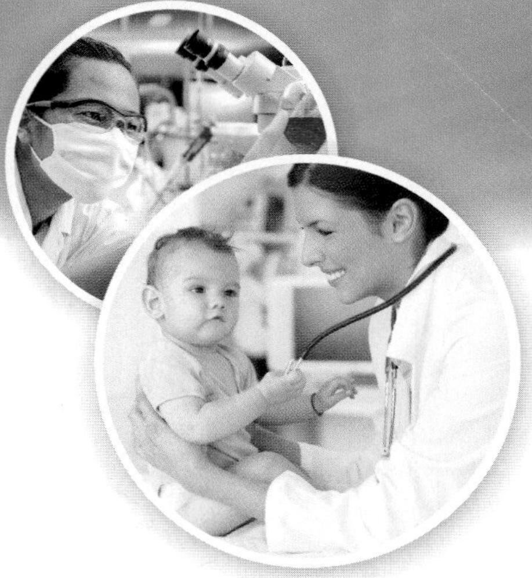

Chapter 11

Environmental Safety

OBJECTIVES

Studying and applying the material in this chapter will help you to:

- Understand and explain the importance of environmental safety in maintaining the safety of the health care professional, the patients, and others.
- Identify general safety guidelines that will help prevent injuries and accidents in health care facilities.
- Describe and give examples of how changes in the physical and mental health of a patient can increase the risk of injuries and accidents.
- Define what workplace violence is and discuss preventive measures.
- Describe and explain the purpose of an incident report.
- Identify the appropriate steps to take in the event of a fire.
- Identify the different classes of fire extinguishers and type of fire on which to use each.
- List ways to prevent electrical hazards.
- Discuss chemical, radiation, and infectious hazards and the role of the health care professional in their prevention.
- Describe the precautions necessary when oxygen is in use.
- Explain when an emergency preparedness plan would be implemented and define a triage system.

KEY TERMS

compatibility
emergency preparedness plan
environmental safety
flammable
incident report
inflammable
PASS
RACE
toxic
triage system

The Case of the Bomb Threat

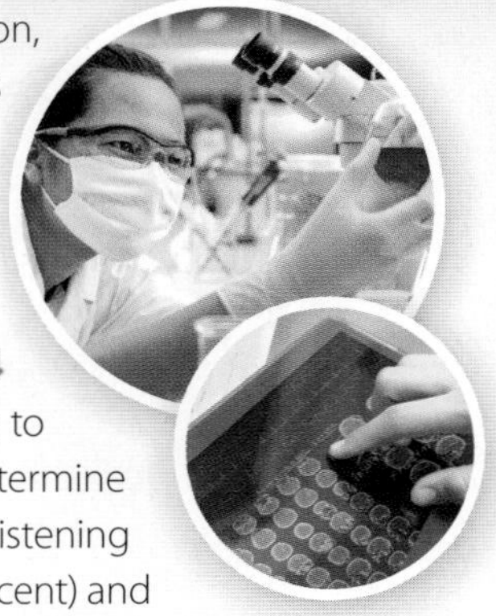

Johanna Welks is a clinical assistant at the community hospital. As she sits at the nursing station, she reflects on how lucky she is to have a job she loves and one that is located only a few blocks from where she lives. When the phone rings, she answers the phone in a cheerful, professional manner: "Hello, this is 4 West, Mrs. Welks speaking, how may I help you?" What she hears next sends chills down her body. The caller states, "Your hospital killed my little girl, and now I will get my revenge. I have placed a bomb in the hospital." Mrs. Welks feels on the verge of hysteria. She thinks of hanging up and leaving or starting to yell for everyone to evacuate the hospital immediately. But then her head clears, and she thinks about what would be the smartest thing to do in this situation. She tries to keep the caller on the telephone as long as possible in order to determine more specifically where the bomb is located and when it will explode. At the same time she is listening closely to the voice on the phone (to determine the sex, the age, and whether the caller has an accent) and also for any background noise (e.g., car horns, trains, bells, music). This chapter will address the many environmental hazards found in health care facilities and how to keep patients and workers safe. Also discussed are the nature of an emergency preparedness plan, when it is initiated, and the role of the health care professional when the plan is in effect.

IMPORTANCE OF ENVIRONMENTAL SAFETY IN HEALTH CARE

Environmental safety means identifying and correcting potential hazards that can cause accidents and injuries. See Table 11–1 for examples of some common health care hazards. The health care professional must understand and follow workplace safety policies and procedures that reduce hazards and prevent accidents, and know how to handle incidents correctly if they do occur.

The Occupational Safety and Health Administration (OSHA), in addition to the infection-control measures presented in Chapter 10, has many regulatory requirements that apply to other workplace safety issues. The exact policies and procedures may vary among health care facilities, but they must all meet the regulatory requirements of OSHA.

GENERAL SAFETY GUIDELINES

The best approach to safety is to focus on *prevention*. There are many ways that health care professionals can contribute to the prevention of common accidents and injuries that occur in the health care environment. Personal safety practices include ways to move safely within and dress for the workplace, work with patients, provide protection for oneself and others, and determine what, when, and how to report any accidents that do occur. The guidelines in this section present specific safety behaviors.

Moving Safely

Movement creates the potential for accidents such as falls. The following practices will limit such occurrences:

- Never run, even in an emergency. You can move swiftly without running if the situation warrants a fast pace.
- Stay to the right in hallways and be cautious when approaching intersections in order to prevent collisions. Pay attention to warning mirrors on corners.
- Remove any loose rugs from floors to prevent tripping or slipping.
- Open doors slowly to avoid injury to someone on the other side.
- Use handrails when climbing or descending stairs.
- Never run up or down the stairs.
- Never carry uncapped syringes or sharp instruments in hallways or between rooms.

Dressing for Safety

Work in health care requires specific types of clothing and grooming to ensure the safety of both workers and patients:

- Wear long hair tied back or up to prevent contact with contaminated material or the contamination of clean materials.

Table 11–1 Common Health Care Hazards

Type of Hazard	Description	Examples
Chemical	May have toxic effects through inhalation, absorption through the skin or mucous membranes, or ingestion. Some irritate the skin on contact	Chemotherapeutic agents, disinfectants, cleaning solutions, alcohol, anesthesia
Environmental	Unsafe conditions in the workplace	Slip, trip, and fall hazards; cramped working space, inefficient equipment, and inadequate equipment maintenance; fire and electrical hazards
Ergonomic (musculoskeletal)	Unsafe workplace design and lack of appropriate client- and material-handling tools and equipment contributing to increased risk of musculoskeletal disorders. Poor lighting, excessive vibration, and noise are also considered ergonomic hazards	Activities that require lifting heavy loads; twisting, bending, reaching, and holding body parts and other materials for long periods; standing for long periods; pushing, pulling, awkward postures, and repetitive motions; high detail work in dimly lighted area; noisy environment *Note:* Ergonomics is covered in Chapter 9.
Infectious (biological)	May cause infection through inhalation, direct contact with skin or mucosa, skin puncture, or through ingestion (eating or drinking)	Bacteria, viruses, fungi, and other living microorganisms *Note:* This topic is covered in Chapter 10.
Physical	Agents that can cause physical injury and tissue damage	Radiation, noise, explosive objects or substances (e.g., oxygen)
Psychosocial	Stressors in the workplace causing workplace anxiety and emotional fatigue	Providing constant emotional support, coping with emergency situations, inadequate staffing, lack of supervisor support, and frequent schedule changes; bioterrorism *Note:* Coping with stressors is covered in Chapter 12.
Workplace violence	Any physical assault or verbal abuse that is incurred during the course of performing one's duties at work	Being pushed, hit, or restrained; spoken to in a loud or demeaning manner, cursed at or berated; this type of hazard could also be listed under physical or psychosocial hazards depending on the nature of the violence

Source: Adapted from *Working Safely in Health Care: A Practical Guide*, by Deborah L. Fell-Carlson, 2008, Clifton Park, NY: Delmar Cengage Learning.

- Do not wear earrings that extend beyond the earlobe so that they cannot be grabbed or caught.
- Wear enclosed shoes with no more than a 1- to 1½-inch heel to prevent injury to the feet.
- Limit jewelry to a smooth wedding band.
- Keep fingernails short. The longer the nail, both natural and artificial, the more likely it is that bacteria reside under its free edge.

Working Safely with Patients

Patient safety is always a primary concern. Focusing on the task at hand and thinking through patient care activities are essential ways to promote safety.

- Do not perform any procedure on patients until you have received adequate training and do not alter the correct procedure (avoid shortcuts).

- Observe and note conditions in patients that might increase their risk of accident and injury. (See Table 11–2.)
- Be absolutely positive you have the correct patient. Always identify your patient by checking his or her wristband against the patient's record. In some health care settings, patients will not have a wristband (e.g., a physician's office). These patients can be identified by asking them to tell you their full name. Do not ask, "Are you Mr. Jones?" because many confused patients will reply affirmatively. Many facilities require two forms of identification, such as having them state their name and their birthdate.
- Always verify that the patient has given consent, because patients have the right to refuse any procedure or medication.
- Observe patients closely and report any changes immediately or assist them as needed. Do not leave patients unattended on treatment tables.

Table 11–2 Physical and Mental Changes That Increase the Risk of Injuries and Accidents

Physical or Mental	Change the Risk	Health Care Considerations
Changes in vision	Unable to see unsafe conditions and/or unable to judge distances	Identify yourself when approaching or entering the room. Provide unobstructed walkways. Place items needed by patients within their visual field. Explain the location of items orally.
Changes in hearing	Unable to hear warnings or approaching carts and equipment	Face the patient when speaking. Speak clearly, but do not yell. Notice when patients do not react to warning sounds.
Altered neurological function	Shaking or tremors can affect balance and increase the risk of falls; decreased sensation can prevent normal warning signals (e.g., can step on sharp object and not be aware of injury)	Pay increased attention to physical signs of injury. Give extra assistance, as needed. Do not leave patient alone on treatment table or under any conditions where falls might occur.
Changes in blood vessels	Dizziness when attempting to stand and increased risk of falls	Instruct patients to get up slowly. Assist patients as necessary.
Slowed reflexes (automatic reactions that cause us to pull away from danger)	Unable to move away quickly from danger (e.g., removing hand from hot surface or from under hot water, or unable to stop in time to avoid collision)	Provide patient and family with information about possible unsafe behaviors and ways to safeguard the home.
Changes in mental function	Confusion and forgetfulness can impair good judgment and decrease awareness of common dangers	Provide family with information about medications, home health resources, and safeguarding the home.
Weakness from illness or injury	More prone to falls	Observe patients carefully. Provide extra assistance. Instruct the family about extra precautions needed.
Taking medications	Side effects of some medications cause dizziness, visual disturbances, and other problems that increase the risk of injury	Instruct patient and family to report symptoms immediately. Monitor patients carefully when administering medications and do not leave them alone immediately afterward; watch for possible reactions.

- Leave the bed in a low position, side rails up (if needed), wheels locked, and place the call signal, telephone, and bed controls within the patient's reach.
- Keep the work area clean, dry, and organized for efficient use. Place all supplies and equipment in their proper storage location.

Protecting Yourself and Others

Health care environments contain many potential hazards. It is essential to apply safety practices that consider the well-being of others:

- Follow the standard precautions discussed in Chapter 10.
- Do not open more than one file cabinet drawer at a time to prevent tipping.
- Do not leave cabinet doors open because someone may hit his or her head or trip.
- Do not place food in a refrigerator that contains lab specimens or medications.
- Do not wear uniforms in nonwork settings.
- Keep floors clear by immediately picking up dropped objects. Use OSHA standards when cleaning up glass, spilled specimens, and liquids. Broken glass is best picked up with a brush or broom and dustpan (Figure 11–1) and placed in puncture-resistant wrap or container, prior to placing in a plastic bag. This will prevent cuts on the hands of anyone who handles the bag. When the spill involves bodily secretions or blood, follow standard precautions by using gloves and disposing of waste in special bags designated for biohazardous waste. (See Figure 11–2.)

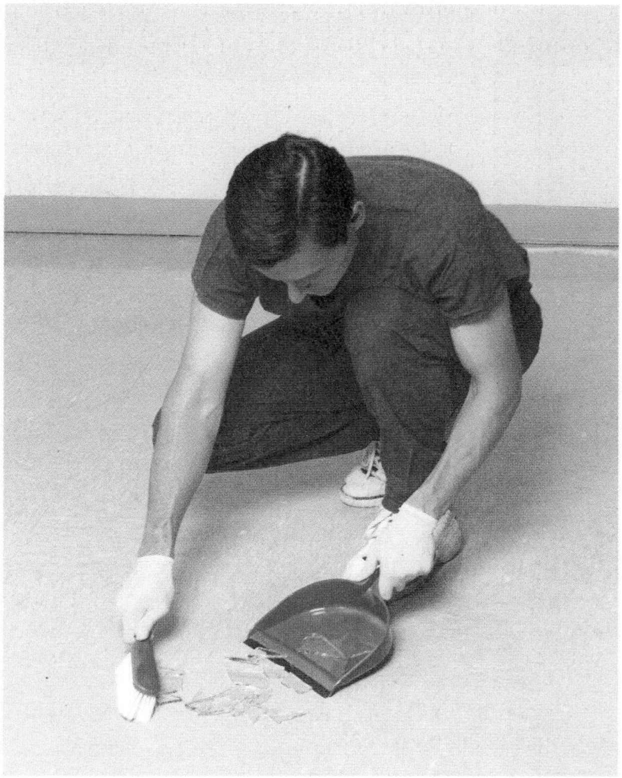

FIGURE 11–1 Sweep up broken glass. Wear gloves.

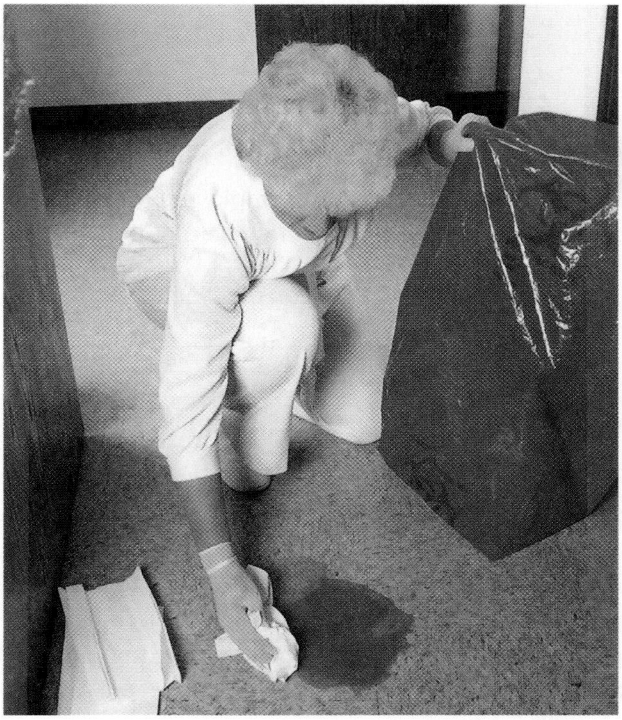

FIGURE 11–2 Clean up spills immediately. When bodily secretions or blood are involved, follow standard precautions.

Reporting for Safety

Properly reporting unsafe conditions and accidents provides a means of making corrections and preventing future problems.

- Report any unsafe conditions immediately, such as burned-out exit sign lights, equipment or flooring in need of repair, frayed electrical cords, and side rails or signal lights that do not work.
- Report any accidents or injuries immediately and complete an incident report. An **incident report** is a written document completed when any unexpected situation occurs that can cause

Thinking It Through

Peta Fry works as a respiratory therapist at a busy medical center. This particular day is busier than usual and it seems no matter how quickly Peta works, she cannot get her assignments done to keep on schedule. It is important for Peta to finish on time because she has a friend picking her up in front of the hospital right after work to go out for dinner. While working with Mrs. Homer, a bottle of water is accidentally tipped over because the patient did not see it due to her poor vision. Peta makes a mental note to call housekeeping when she finishes, so they can clean up the spill. When she finishes with Mrs. Homer, Peta realizes that she is going to be late and is afraid her friend will be upset. In an effort to save time, she decides not to change into the street clothes she brought with her to work and runs as quickly as she can to meet her friend.

1. Identify at least three behaviors of Peta that jeopardize environmental safety. What are the possible consequences of these unsafe behaviors?
2. What health care considerations could Peta have followed when working with the patient with impaired vision that may have prevented the bottle of water from spilling?

harm to a patient, an employee, or any other person. It contains only factual information, and most facilities have policies that specify not to include the report in the patient's chart or to refer to it in the documentation.

WORKPLACE VIOLENCE

Today health care professionals from many occupations perform a wide variety of duties. They are exposed to many safety and health hazards, including violence. The National Institute for Occupational Safety and Health (NIOSH) defines workplace violence as "violent acts (including physical assaults and threats of assaults) directed toward persons at work or on duty." In health care settings, the most common workplace violence is client aggression toward caregivers. In 2010, the Bureau of Labor Statistics (BLS) reported that health care and social assistance workers were the victims of approximately 11,370 assaults by persons, a greater than 13% increase over the number of such assaults reported in 2009. Almost 19% (i.e., 2130) of these assaults occurred in nursing and residential care facilities alone. Unfortunately, many more incidents probably go unreported.

Although anyone working in a health care environment may become a victim of violence, hospital nurses and nursing assistants who have the most direct contact with patients are at higher risk. Other personnel at increased risk of violence include emergency response personnel, hospital safety officers, and all health care providers.

Workplace violence ranges from offensive or threatening language to homicide. Examples of violence are demonstrated in the following actual case reports:

- An elderly patient verbally abused a nurse and pulled her hair when she prevented him from leaving the hospital to go home in the middle of the night.
- An agitated psychotic patient attacked a nurse, broke her arm, and scratched and bruised her.
- A disturbed family member whose father had died in surgery at the community hospital walked into the emergency department and fired a small-caliber handgun, killing a nurse and an emergency medical technician and wounding the emergency physician.

The circumstances of hospital violence differ from the circumstances of workplace violence in general. In other workplaces, such as convenience stores and taxicabs, violence most often relates to robbery. Violence in health care usually results from patients—and occasionally from their family members—who feel frustrated, vulnerable, and powerless.

The effects of violence go further than the actual injuries and psychological trauma. Violence may also have negative organizational outcomes, such as low worker morale, increased job stress, increased worker turnover, reduced trust of management and coworkers, and a hostile working environment.

Both the employer and the employee have a responsibility to decrease violent occurrences. Review Table 11–3 for some methods of preventing or decreasing violence.

Table 11–3 Workplace Violence Preventive Measures

Employer	Employee
Environmental designs: • Develop emergency signaling, alarms, and monitoring systems. • Install security devices such as metal detectors to prevent armed persons from entering. • Install other security devices, such as cameras and good lighting, in hallways. • Provide security escorts to the parking lots at night. • Design waiting areas to accommodate and assist visitors and patients who may have a delay in service. • Design the triage area and other public areas to minimize the risk of assault (provide staff restrooms and emergency exits, install enclosed nurses' stations, install deep service counters to increase distance from patients or bullet-resistant and shatterproof glass enclosures in reception areas, arrange furniture and other objects to minimize their use as weapons). Administrative controls: • Design staffing patterns to prevent personnel from working alone and to minimize patient waiting time. • Restrict the movement of the public in hospitals by card-controlled access. • Develop a system for alerting security personnel when violence is threatened. Behavior modification: • Provide all workers with training in recognizing and managing assaults, resolving conflicts, and maintaining hazard awareness.	Watch for signals that may be associated with impending violence: • Verbally expressed anger and frustration • Body language such as threatening gestures • Signs of drug or alcohol use • Presence of a weapon Maintain behavior that helps diffuse anger: • Present a calm, caring attitude. • Do not match the threats. • Do not give orders. • Acknowledge the person's feelings (e.g., "I know you are frustrated"). • Avoid any behavior that may be interpreted as aggressive (e.g., moving rapidly, getting too close, touching, or speaking loudly). Be alert: • Evaluate each situation for potential violence when you enter a room or begin to relate to a patient or visitor. • Be vigilant throughout the encounter. • Do not isolate yourself with a potentially violent person. • Always keep an open path for exiting—do not let the potentially violent person stand between you and the door. Take these steps if you cannot defuse the situation quickly: • Remove yourself from the situation. • Call Security for help. • Report any violent incidents to your management.

FIRE AND ELECTRICAL HAZARDS

Fires in health care facilities can result from a number of hazards, such as damaged equipment, overloaded circuits, defects in heating systems, spontaneous combustion, improper trash disposal, and smoking. It is important to familiarize yourself with the recommended policies and procedures for the health care facility in which you work. Once a fire starts, there is no time to read the policy and procedure manual, and valuable minutes are lost if you hesitate in acting promptly and correctly.

It is critical to stay calm during an emergency. A number of decisions must be made, and clear thinking is needed to properly assess the problem. If your safety is at risk, leave the area and sound the alarm. If the fire is small and contained and your safety and that of others are not at risk, determine which type of extinguisher is appropriate to use and proceed with the proper handling procedure. Remember that your safety and that of others come first.

Fires require three things to start: oxygen or air, an item that will burn to supply fuel (trash, linen, chemicals), and a source of heat (sparks, flames, matches). (See Figure 11–3.) To respond promptly and correctly to a fire, you must be knowledgeable in the following areas:

- The location of fire alarms and extinguishers
- How to use a fire extinguisher—carry the extinguisher upright. To help remember the proper sequence of operation, think **PASS**:
  1. **P**ull the pin.
  2. **A**im the nozzle at the *base* of the fire.

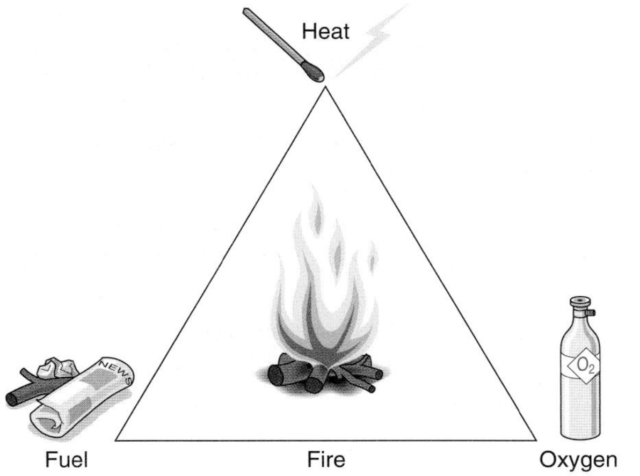

FIGURE 11–3 The fire triangle: elements needed for combustion (burning).

3. **S**queeze the handle.
4. **S**weep back and forth along the *base* of the fire. (See Figures 11–4 a–c.)

- How to respond to each type of fire—fire extinguishers vary for different types of fire. Using the wrong type of fire extinguisher can result in spreading a fire rather than putting it out. (See Table 11–4.)
- The emergency evacuation routes (See Figure 11–5.)

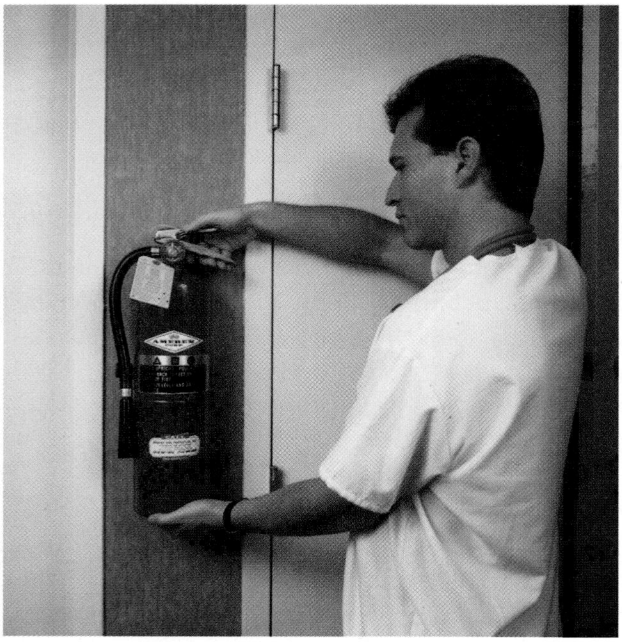

FIGURE 11–4a Verify that the fire extinguisher is the correct class to use.

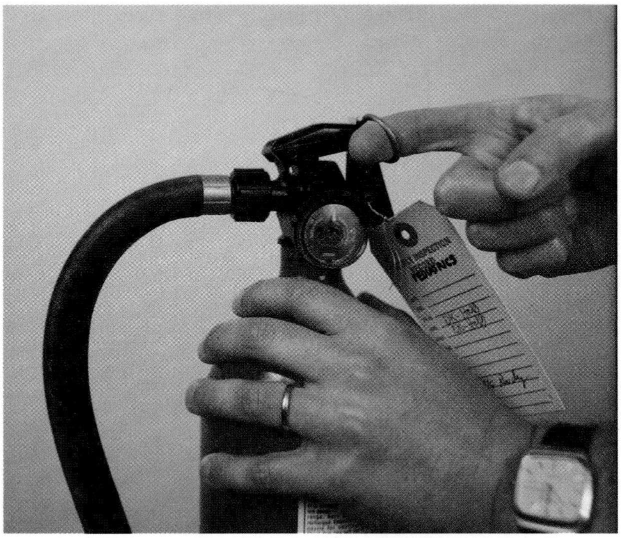

FIGURE 11–4b *Pull* the pin.

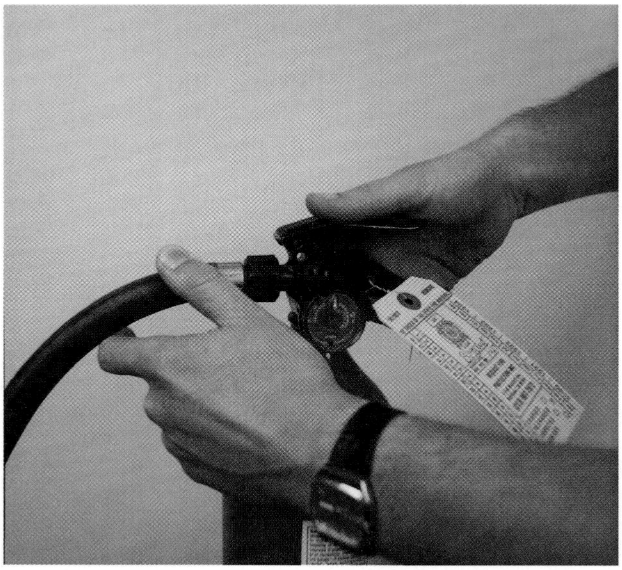

FIGURE 11–4c *Aim* the nozzle at the base of the fire and *squeeze* handle. *Sweep* back and forth along the base of the fire.

- What procedures to follow—although procedures may vary at individual facilities, there are generally accepted guidelines to use when a fire occurs. These are outlined in Table 11–5. To help you remember the proper sequence, think **RACE**:

1. **R**emove patients
2. **A**ctivate alarm
3. **C**ontain the fire
4. **E**xtinguish the fire or **E**vacuate the area (See Figure 11–6.)

Table 11–4 Types of Fires and How to Extinguish

Type of Fire	How to Extinguish	Cautions
Class A Most common type of fires (ordinary combustibles, e.g., paper, cloth, rubber, plastic, wood, trash, or mattress fires)	Use either water, a Class A fire extinguisher, or a Class ABC fire extinguisher. Class A extinguishers are water based and contain pressurized water or aqueous film-forming foam (AFFF). Class ABC extinguishers release a multipurpose dry chemical (monoammonium phosphate) that blankets the burning area and interrupts the chemical chain reaction.	Class A extinguishers—no special precautions; follow the proper sequence of operation (PASS) required with all extinguishers. Class ABC extinguishers—leave a white powdery residue irritating to skin and eyes. Do not stand too close to the fire. Take care when using extinguisher. Wash skin as soon as possible after extinguishing fire. The chemical is corrosive and will damage computers and electrical equipment.
Class B **Flammable** (easily set on fire; same as **inflammable**) and combustible liquids (e.g., gas, oil, paint, solvents, and cooking fat fires)	Use Class B, BC, or ABC fire extinguishers. Class B extinguishers release carbon dioxide (CO_2), which forms a cloud of dry ice or snow. The cloud displaces air and cuts off the fire's oxygen supply, thereby providing a smothering action.	Do not use water or a Class A fire extinguisher on a Class B fire because most burning liquids will float on top of the water, which spreads the fire further. Class B extinguishers—no special precautions; they are noncorrosive and do not damage computers and other electrical equipment, but are heavy and have a shorter discharge range. Class ABC extinguishers—see above.
Class C Electrical fires (e.g., electrical equipment, fuse boxes, wiring, and appliances)	Use Class C, BC, or ABC extinguisher. Same as Class B because carbon dioxide is used, which is nonconducting and provides a smothering action.	Do not use water or Class A extinguisher on this type of fire unless the electricity has been disconnected. Electrical fires are particularly hazardous because the possibility of electrocution is present. Class ABC extinguishers—see above.
Class D Burning metals (not typically seen in the health care environment)	Use Class D extinguisher or smother with dry sand. Class D extinguishers release a sodium chloride powder that when heated forms a crust. The crust excludes air and fire is smothered.	Do not use any of the other types of fire extinguishers on this type of fire.

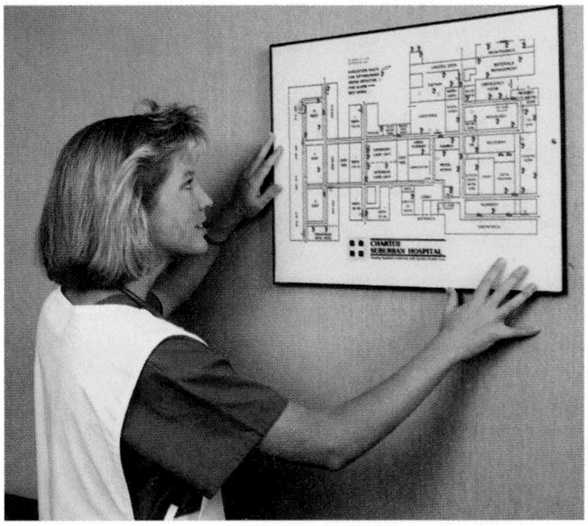

FIGURE 11–5 All personnel should be familiar with the emergency evacuation plan established by the facility in which they work.

- In case of a major fire, follow all instructions carefully. Your duties may include assisting patients into wheelchairs or onto stretchers. Advise ambulatory (able to walk) patients about evacuation routes.
- Many facilities have a policy that no personal electrical equipment can be brought into the hospital because the possibility that it may be defective is a fire risk. Larger facilities will have environmental safety personnel who verify the safety of facility equipment. Check the policy manual to determine if the environmental safety personnel will also check personal equipment. If so, they will attach a tag verifying the completion of the safety check.

Table 11–5 What to Do When You Discover a Fire: RACE

Guideline	Rationale
R	
Remove any patient who is in danger. Ambulatory patients can walk to safety; others may need wheelchairs or can be pushed in beds. Never use elevators during a fire; instead, carry nonambulatory patients in a linen sling, held at each end by a health care professional, while descending steps.	Places patient safety first. Fires can travel through elevator shafts, cables can be damaged, and elevators can get stalled between floors if power fails.
A	
Activate the fire alarm and notify the facility telephone operator/receptionist.	Pulling the fire alarm sends an alarm call to the fire station. The facility telephone operator(s) are often key to communication, and an exact location of the fire should be given to them
C	
Contain the fire by closing all windows and doors. Follow facility procedure for turning off oxygen and electrical equipment.	Decreases the amount of air available to the fire. Drafts (air currents) cause fire to spread more rapidly. Prevents explosions and further fueling of the fire
E	
Extinguish small fires with an extinguisher. Stand 6 to 10 feet from the nearest edge of the flame and aim at the base of the fire. For large fires, follow or start evacuation procedures.	Allows for immediate extinguishing of fire before it spreads farther. If fire is too large, do not attempt to put out; instead, use that time to initiate further evacuation procedures
Keep exits clear at all times.	Allows patients and workers to leave if necessary
Maintain an exit at all times—never let the fire get between you and the exit.	Prevents the health care professional and patients from being trapped in a confined area
If smoke is present, workers and patients should crawl or move close to the floor toward the exit.	Decreases inhalation of smoke because smoke rises. More oxygen is available closer to the floor. All fires give off toxic gases, which are in the smoke.
A damp towel or similar cloth may be used to cover the mouth and nose for breathing.	Decreases the temperature of inhaled air and filters soot particles from the air
Always check the temperature of a door before opening it. If a door is hot to the touch, do not open it.	Prevents burns caused by a sudden burst of flames escaping the room when the door is opened
If you are trapped in a room and the door is hot to the touch, stay in the room (lie on the floor for more oxygen and less smoke) and place wet towels or blankets under the door.	Wet towels decrease the smoke entering the room

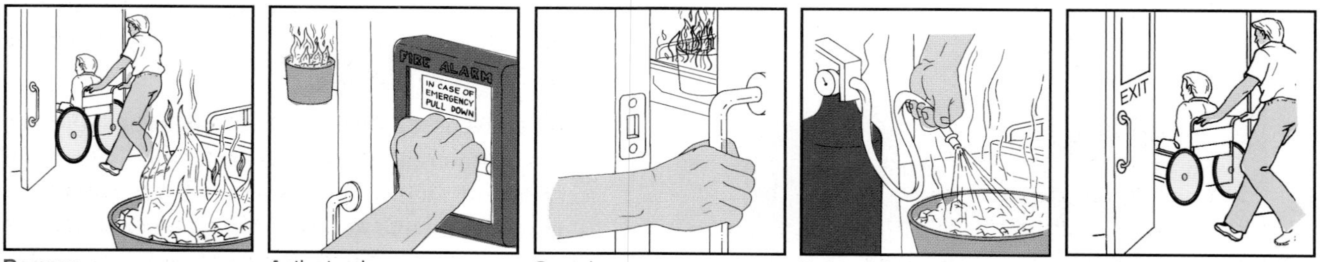

FIGURE 11–6 Remember the sequence of critical actions to follow in case of fire.

Most electrical hazards can be avoided by following a few general safety practices:

- Always be thoroughly familiar with any equipment before attempting to use it independently for the first time. Know and follow all safety precautions.
- Review and follow the manufacturer's operating instructions. The health care professional should not use shortcuts or experiment with unfamiliar equipment.
- If any damage to the equipment is noted, do not attempt to use it, but report it to the proper person for repair. If the health care professional is not trained in the repair of a particular piece of equipment, he or she should never attempt to repair it.
- Never use electrical cords that are not completely intact, use plugs that have been altered (i.e., have third prong removed), or use excessive force to insert a plug into an outlet.
- Never handle any electrical equipment around water because electrocution can occur (water conducts electrical currents). Holding electrical equipment with wet hands, standing in water, or removing equipment that has been accidentally dropped in water can be life threatening. Always dry hands, clean up any spilled water, and remove the power source.
- If someone is being shocked (electrically), do not touch the person or pull the plug from the wall because this places you at risk. Instead, turn the main source of power off immediately and be prepared to administer emergency care and call for help.

Media Link

Learn more about safety in the workplace by viewing the Fire Safety video on the Online Resources.

CHEMICAL HAZARDS

Hundreds of chemicals are used in health care, such as cleaning solutions, anesthesia, and drugs used for chemotherapy. Chemicals can often cause harm if swallowed, inhaled, or absorbed through the skin or mucous membranes. Some also create a fire hazard. Great care must be taken when working with or near these agents. As discussed in Chapter 10, OSHA requires all health care facilities to have an exposure control plan. In addition, material safety data sheets (MSDS) must be available to all employees. The MSDS includes the precautions to take when handling the chemical, safety instructions for use, requirements for clean-up and disposal, and first aid measures to take if exposure occurs. There are some general guidelines that apply whenever chemicals are handled:

- If the container is not properly labeled or if it cannot be read clearly, do not use it.
- Recheck labels at least three times. Read the label carefully when you first locate it, and then reread it after removing the solution and again before returning it to its proper location.
- Never mix any two chemicals together without first verifying **compatibility** (i.e., if they can be combined without unfavorable results).
- Avoid contact with the eyes and skin and do not inhale.
- Take precautions not to splash or spill solutions.
- Wear personal protective equipment (PPE) as indicated.
- Make sure chemicals are used only for their intended purpose.
- Store chemicals as directed on the labels. For example, does the chemical require room temperature storage or refrigeration? Can it be stored on the counter or does it require a dark environment? Never place chemicals in direct sunlight or close to heat.
- Do not pour **toxic** (poisonous), flammable, foul-smelling, or irritating chemicals down the drain. Instead place them in the specified container as per the policy and procedure manual.
- If you spill any solutions, clean up immediately according to established procedures and dispose of the debris properly.
- If a chemical does come in contact with the skin, rinse immediately under cool water for at least 5 minutes. Splashes in the eye should be rinsed for a minimum of 15 minutes, preferably with normal saline. Report any accidents immediately to the supervisor and seek medical assistance for evaluation and follow-up.

RADIATION HAZARDS

Health care professionals in areas where X-rays or radiation therapy are used must practice safety precautions to prevent exposure to radiation waves and particles. Excessive radiation exposure can put the employee at risk for developing tissue damage, contracting cancer, or becoming sterile (unable to have children) or may lead to infants being born with birth defects. Employees at risk for radiation exposure must wear safety monitoring film badges that record the amount of exposure. Safety guidelines have been developed that determine the maximum level of radiation exposure allowed per employee.

There are strict guidelines for the proper disposal of radiological waste. Radioactive waste must be placed in a special container and labeled as "radioactive." It should never be placed in the trash, incinerated, placed in a bag with other waste products, or put down a drain. Only a licensed removal facility can remove these wastes from the health care facility.

INFECTIOUS WASTE

Infectious waste is any item or product that has the potential to transmit disease. Infectious waste must be handled using standard and transmission-based precautions, placed in containers or bags labeled as to type of waste (e.g., linen, sharps, trash), decontaminated on site, or removed by a licensed removal facility for decontamination. It is the health care professional's responsibility to follow the facility's policies and procedures in the proper handling, containment, cleanup of spills, and disposal of infectious waste. Any direct contact with waste that puts the worker at risk of infection should be reported per facility policy.

OXYGEN HAZARDS

When a patient is unable to take in adequate oxygen on his or her own, the physician may order the administration of oxygen. The physician will order how much oxygen to give, what device to use for oxygen delivery (Figures 11–7a and 11–7b), and how long it is to be administered.

Special precautions are necessary when oxygen is in use:

- Most facilities have signs stating "Oxygen in Use" that are posted as specified in the facility policy.

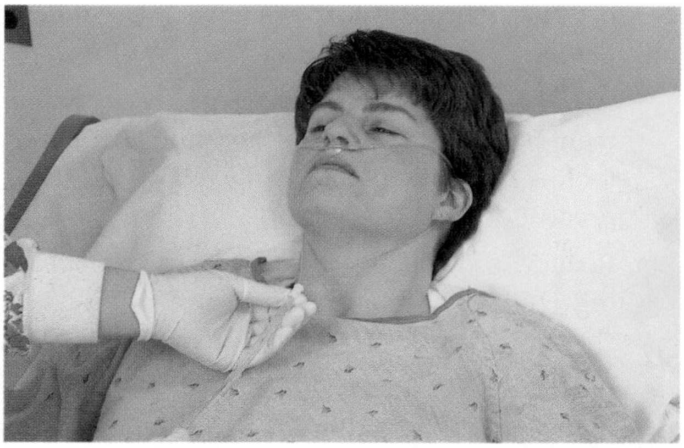

FIGURE 11–7a Oxygen being delivered by nasal cannula.

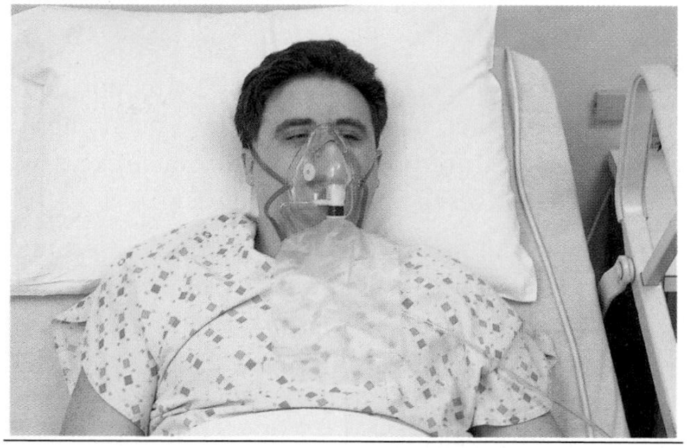

FIGURE 11–7b Oxygen being delivered by mask.

- Sparks may come from some electrical appliances, equipment, or toys. Before using any of these, always check with the supervisor. Examples include hair dryers, heating pads, space heaters, fans, radios, electric shavers, and hand-held computer games.
- Never use flammable liquids, such as alcohol, oils, adhesive tape remover, nail polish, or nail polish remover.
- An oxygen tank should be secured to prevent it from falling over. Do not place it in the sunlight or near heat. The stem-and-valve assembly on the tank is fragile and if mishandled the cylinder can become a missile as the pressurized gas is suddenly released.
- Smoking is not allowed when oxygen is in use, and smoking materials must be removed from the room. Fortunately, most facilities no longer allow smoking at any time, due to the health risk to the person and others. Always be alert

for those who disregard the rules. No lighted matches or open flames should be permitted in the area.

- Use cotton blankets, gowns, or clothing. Wool and synthetics are more apt to create static electricity.

BIOTERRORISM

Since the devastating attack on the United States that occurred on September 11, 2001, there has been a tremendous amount of discussion about and preparation for a bioterrorist attack. Bioterrorism is not new to our times. It extends back in history to the earliest of human records. In the 14th century, cadavers were catapulted into enemy camps to create an outbreak of plague or to create such a fear that the enemy would flee and thus be defeated. British forces were suspected of giving Native Americans blankets contaminated with smallpox that led to an epidemic. Over the years, there have been numerous examples of attempts to contaminate food sources and develop weapons for the purpose of dispensing biological organisms.

One of the functions of an emergency preparedness plan is the incorporation of a biological exposure readiness plan. The first step in this plan is to become aware of and report a suspected bioterrorism-related outbreak. If such an attack is suspected, the Federal Bureau of Investigation (FBI) would be immediately notified. But it may not be possible to wait for definitive evidence to determine if there is a biological threat, so the best approach would be to base the suspicion on epidemiological factors, such as a sudden and rapid increase of disease in a normally healthy population, large numbers of people with the same symptoms, or other atypical or unusual presenting factors.

There are numerous agents that could be used for bioterrorism-related diseases, but it is believed that the most likely biological weapon would be anthrax, smallpox, botulism, or plague. In the event of an outbreak, the appropriate type of transmission precautions would be in force. (Chapter 10 covers precautions.) Generally, agents of bioterrorism are not transmitted person to person, so the exposure can be contained by the proper precautions. (See Table 11–6.)

Fascinating Facts

Hospitals, dental offices, veterinary clinics, laboratories, nursing homes, medical offices, and other health care facilities generate more than 3 million tons of hazardous medical waste each year. Much of this waste is dangerous, especially when it is potentially toxic, radioactive, or infectious.

EMERGENCY CODE SYSTEM

Many health care facilities use a code system to communicate to the employees in the building when certain emergencies occur. Larger facilities with an overhead paging system will announce by using these codes along with a location (if appropriate). A code system is utilized to prevent patients and visitors from becoming overly concerned. Code Red (fire) and Code Blue (respiratory or cardiac failure) are known by many outside of health care, but many of the other codes will not be familiar. See Figure 11–8.

Table 11–6 Bioterrorism Agents

Disease	Transmitted Person to Person?	Type of Precaution Recommended
Anthrax, cutaneous	Possible	Standard
Anthrax, gastrointestinal	No	Standard
Anthrax, pulmonary	No	Standard
Botulism	No	Standard
Plague, bubonic	No	Standard
Plague, pneumonic	Yes	Droplet
Smallpox	Yes	Airborne/contact

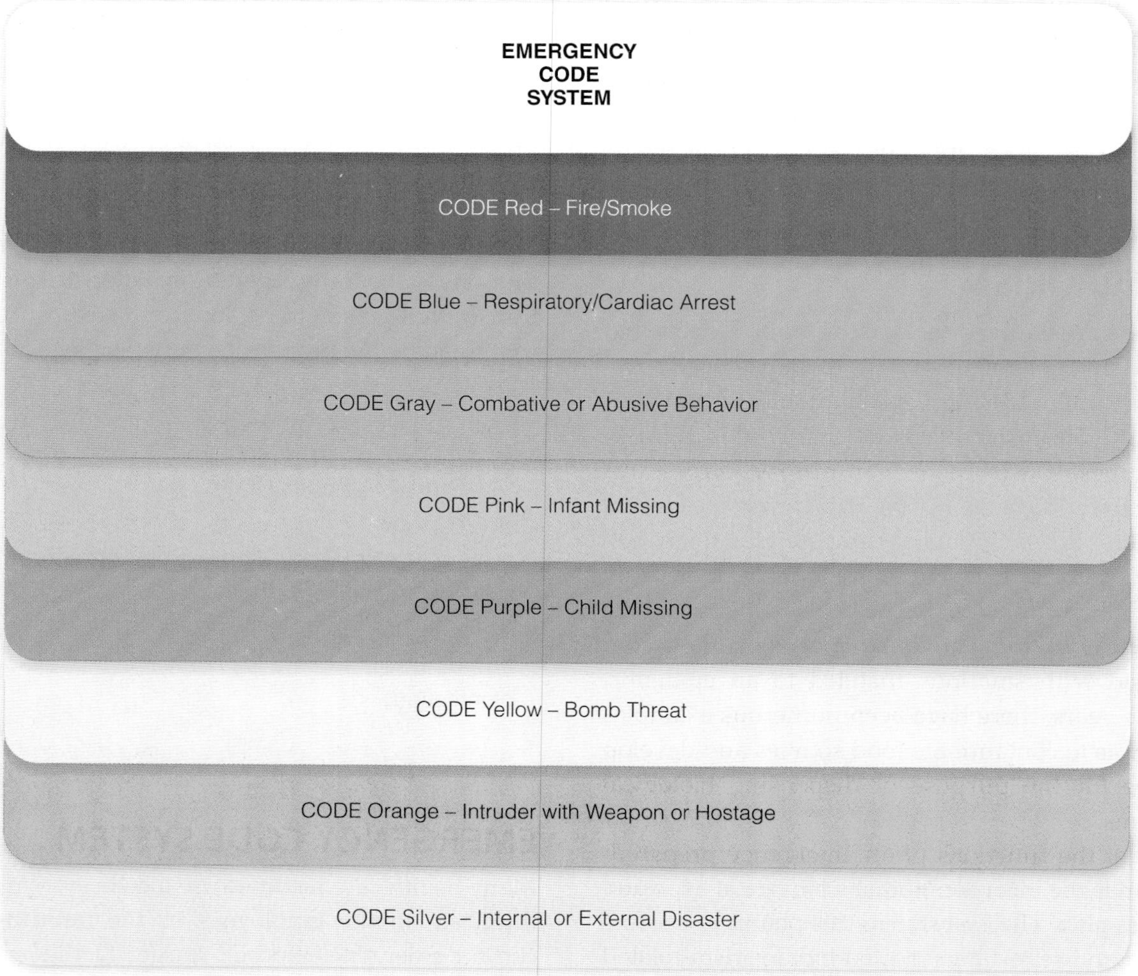

FIGURE 11–8 Example of an emergency code system. Each page color matches the code name. When the employee opens to any of the colored pages, they will find the criteria to follow upon hearing the code announcement.

EMERGENCY PREPAREDNESS PLAN

Federal law requires every health care agency to have an emergency preparedness plan and to practice twice each year. Each health care professional should know his or her place in the plan. OSHA requires health care facilities to have an **emergency preparedness plan** for handling large numbers of patients in the event of a catastrophe, such as an earthquake, a flood, a tornado, a hurricane, or a bombing. It is the responsibility of health care professionals to be familiar with the requirements and understand their roles. Procedures will vary based on the type of facility, but some examples of what may be included are as follows:

- Whether you should report to work
- How to protect yourself and your patients
- Your specific duties
- How to get communications and updates

Whatever your role, always remain calm. This will help you think clearly, as well as provide needed stability to those who are confused, injured, and frightened. This is a critical time for the health care team to work efficiently and cooperatively.

The following general guidelines are to be followed when an emergency preparedness plan is in effect:

- Stay calm. There will be a great deal of chaos and confusion in a severe emergency, but panic can escalate the fear and related difficulties. Everyone involved will benefit from an approach by the health care professional that communicates control of the situation, competence, and compassion.

- Know who is in charge and report your availability.
- Report to the person in charge at regular intervals for further directions or changes in assignments.
- If unsure about what to do in a particular situation, ask someone in authority.
- Communicate clearly and be cooperative.
- Use telephones only for official business, not for personal calls.

Triage

An effectively managed emergency response rests on an established **triage system**. *Triage* is a French word that means "to select." Specially trained personnel follow established triage guidelines to assess patients' conditions and determine where they should be sent and what treatment they should receive.

Triage systems are not just for major natural emergencies but are also used in the emergency department when multiple patients need medical care, for example, when a bus accident with multiple passengers or a passenger train that derails sends multiple victims to the emergency department. When there are multiple victims, the available services are overstrained, so the triage personnel must determine who to treat first, what lab or diagnostic tests receive priority, what procedures to perform immediately, and who to send to surgery. They continually reassess patients who are waiting for services to determine if their condition has changed and if their priority needs to be updated.

A less obvious triage system is in place at all times in the emergency department. For example, there may be a patient waiting to be seen for an earache or another who fell off a bike and may have a possible broken collarbone. Then a third patient arrives with complaints of chest pain and may be having a heart attack. The patient with the potential heart attack will be seen first, because his or her need is more urgent and lack of immediate care could lead to death.

WORKBOOK PRACTICE

Go to your workbook and complete the exercises for this chapter.

SUGGESTED LEARNING ACTIVITIES

1. Visit your local fire station and ask for information about common fire hazards, prevention, use of fire extinguishers, and availability of training sessions for the public.
2. When you enter a health care facility, look for the fire alarms and evacuation route plan (usually posted on a wall).
3. Look around your own home and when you are out in public. What potential hazards can you identify?
4. If someone in your family required oxygen to be administered at home, would anything need to be changed to make the situation safe?

WEB ACTIVITIES

National Institute for Occupational Safety and Health (NIOSH)

www.cdc.gov/niosh

Choose one of the workplace safety items and write a one-page report.

National Safety Council

www.nsc.org

Review the "News" and identify something you did not know about safety.

REVIEW QUESTIONS

1. What are the general safety guidelines to prevent injuries and accidents in the health care workplace?
2. What are the different hazards commonly encountered in a health care environment?
3. What are the physical and mental impairments that make patients more prone to injuries and accidents?
4. What is an incident report, and when should it be completed?
5. What do RACE and PASS mean?

6. What types of portable fire extinguishers are available? How would you decide which one to use? What are the precautions for their use?
7. What are the guidelines for preventing electrical hazards?
8. What precautions must be taken when oxygen is being administered, and why?
9. What is an emergency preparedness plan, and what is the health care professional's role?
10. What is the meaning of *triage*?

APPLICATION EXERCISES

1. Refer to The Case of the Bomb Threat at the beginning of the chapter and answer these questions:
   a. What would have been the possible consequences if Mrs. Welks had acted on her initial response to flee or yell out for an evacuation?
   b. How could the outcome of this situation be affected by obtaining more information about the location of the bomb and what time it was set to explode?
   c. Why do you think she was trying to listen so carefully to the voice and background noise?
   d. What should Mrs. Welks do when the telephone call is terminated?
   e. Should an emergency preparedness plan be initiated?
2. While at work, Jack Thompson, a health care professional, smells smoke and goes to investigate. He discovers the trash can in the restroom has smoke billowing from it, and he runs to get a fire extinguisher. The fire extinguisher is not where he thought it was, and by the time he returns to the restroom, there is smoke coming out from under the door. Jack opens the door, pulls the pin out of the extinguisher, moves as close as he can to the flames, and aims directly down into the trash can. He then hears someone coughing in one of the bathroom stalls and discovers a patient slumped on the floor. Jack pulls the patient out of the bathroom, but in the process, some of the white powdery residue from the fire extinguisher gets on the patient's skin. Jack is pleased with his actions and thinks to himself, "This patient might have died if I hadn't smelled the smoke and put the fire out."
   a. Evaluate the scenario to determine if Jack followed the recommended procedure. Did he follow RACE and PASS?
   b. What revisions to Jack's actions would have to occur to ensure safety for himself, patients, and coworkers?
   c. Can you determine from the information given, which class of fire extinguisher was used? Was it the correct extinguisher for a trash fire?
   d. Is it of concern that the patient has some of the white powdery residue on his skin?

PROBLEM-SOLVING PRACTICE

After reading the section on workplace violence, Maria Foust finds herself very upset about pursuing a career in health care. She has wanted to work in health care for as long as she can recall. She was raised in a community that was very violent and has finally been able to remove herself from that situation. Now the thought of working in a violent workplace is bringing back a lot of bad memories. Using the five-step problem-solving process, determine what Maria can do about her career choice concerns.

SUGGESTED READINGS AND RESOURCES

American Association of Poison Control Centers. www.aapcc.org

Klinoff, R. (2011). *Introduction to fire protection* (4th ed.). Clifton Park, NY: Delmar Cengage Learning.

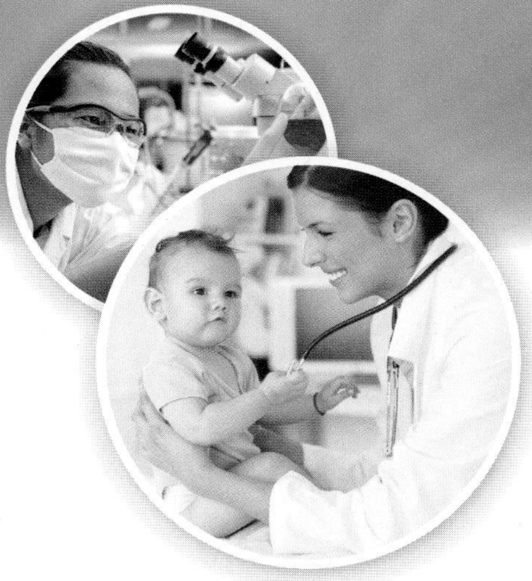

Unit 5

Behaviors for Success

This page intentionally left blank

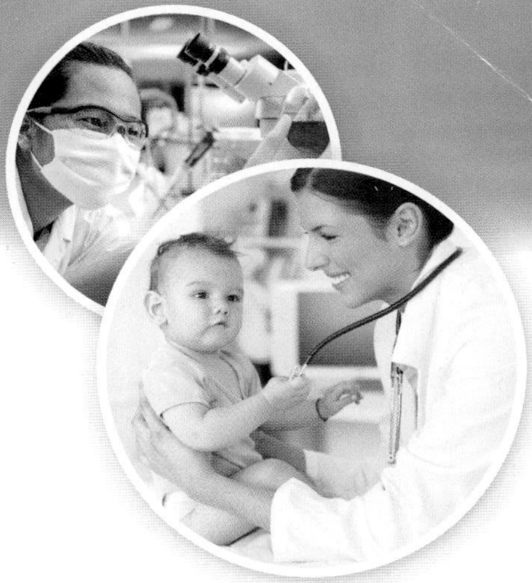

Chapter 12

Lifestyle Management

OBJECTIVES

Studying and applying the material in this chapter will help you to:

- Explain why it is important for health care professionals to practice a healthy lifestyle.
- List six techniques for developing positive habits.
- List the essential nutrients and the function of each.
- Describe how each of the following contributes to healthy living: diet, physical activity, sleep, and preventive measures.
- Define stress and list several common causes.
- Describe five ways of effectively dealing with stress.
- Explain the major health risks encountered by the health care professional.
- List the causes and symptoms of and preventive measures for burnout.
- Explain how health care professionals can help patients develop good health habits.

KEY TERMS

aerobic exercise
amino acids
anorexia nervosa
assertiveness
attitude
binge eating
body mass index (BMI)
bulimia
burnout
calories
carbohydrates
cholesterol
Choose My Plate
controlled substance
diet
fats
fiber
free radicals
legumes
meditation
metabolism
minerals

KEY TERMS (continued)

nutrients
nutrition
obese
organic
organic food
osteoporosis
overweight
prioritize
processed foods
proteins
relaxation
stress
stressors
trans fat
type 2 diabetes
vitamins

The Case of the Cardiac Unit Nurse

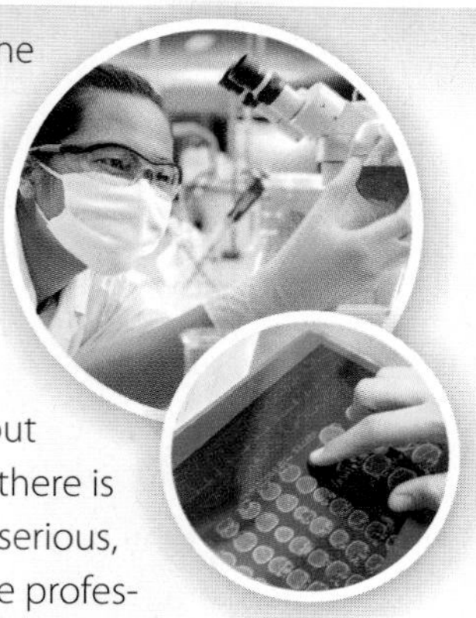

Gracie Chin is a nurse working in the cardiac care unit at a large metropolitan hospital. Many of the patients in the unit are recovering from open heart surgery and require continual monitoring and attention. Gracie works three 12-hour shifts each week, and her duties require that she be on her feet during most of that time. She checks each patient frequently and performs such tasks as turning and bathing patients, adjusting the levels of their beds, placing patients on and removing them from bedpans, repositioning and maintaining equipment, and reaching to change intravenous fluid bags or to adjust monitoring devices that are located above bed level. In addition to the physical requirements of her job, Gracie must remain mentally alert throughout her shift. Her work requires keen observation skills and good judgment because in patient care, there is no room for error. She must also deal with the stress of working with patients who suffer from serious, often fatal conditions. In this chapter you will learn about personal habits that enable health care professionals like Gracie to maintain the physical and mental fitness necessary to promote their own and their patients' welfare.

IMPORTANCE OF A HEALTHY LIFESTYLE

The human body consists of systems that are extremely complex and delicately balanced. Cared for properly, the average body is capable of repairing itself and giving many years of service.

Our state of wellness is largely under our own control. Although the causes of many conditions are still unknown, the top four causes of death in the United States today—heart disease, cancer, chronic lower respiratory diseases, and stroke—are often influenced by personal habits. Unlike previous generations who did not understand the causes of and ways to prevent disease, we have the knowledge and power to make healthy choices. To a great extent, individuals today can choose what to eat, how to deal with stress, and how much to exercise each day. Opportunities to raise our level of wellness lie within us, but *each person must accept the responsibility to take advantage of these opportunities.*

Practicing good health habits is especially important for the health care professional. The health professions require adequate physical energy and the ability to handle stress, two results of healthy living practices. Health care professionals owe it to themselves and to their patients, employers, and families to take care of themselves. In doing so, they can increase their effectiveness and ability to make professional contributions.

In addition, today's health care professional has an important responsibility to serve as a role model for patients. Patient education is a growing part of the health care professional's duties, because patients are assuming more responsibility for their own health. People tend to learn more from example than from words and advice. The wellness behavior demonstrated by the health care professional can have a positive effect on others.

Habits and Health

Maximizing health often requires a change in habits, and this is not always easy. As you read this chapter, you may decide that there are lifestyle habits you would like to change. Perhaps to improve time management skills, develop an exercise program, or change eating habits. Being *willing* to change current behavior is the first step. Here are some additional tips for eliminating old habits and developing new ones:

1. Recognize that making changes may not be easy at first. Accepting this fact will help prevent you from becoming discouraged in the beginning.
2. Be patient with yourself. Changes do not occur overnight.
3. Set reasonable goals. Do not try to make so many changes at once that you feel defeated from the start.
4. Focus on the positive. Think about the long-term benefits you will enjoy.
5. Track your progress. Make a chart, write a journal or diary, or create some other personal recording system.
6. Plan rewards for your achievements.

Some habits, such as smoking, involve the use of addictive substances. These habits are particularly difficult to change. Many people have found that seeking professional assistance or participating in self-help groups are the most effective ways of dealing with addictive behaviors.

The purpose of attaining good health is more than hoping to prevent disease and extend the length of life. It includes improving the *quality* of living throughout the entire life span. It means waking up refreshed with the energy and well-being necessary to enjoy each day. The following sections of this chapter contain general guidelines and suggestions for achieving maximum wellness. What is appropriate for each individual will vary. Identify your strengths and weaknesses, and develop a plan that works for you.

DIET AND NUTRITION

Eating right is one of the cornerstones of good health. What we eat determines, to a great extent, our risk for heart disease, stroke, cancer, and diabetes. Not only does eating a healthy diet help prevent disease, it provides us with the energy and feeling of well-being to live an active, productive life. The importance of diet has been recognized since ancient times. More than 1600 years ago, Hippocrates said, "Let food be your medicine and medicine be your food."

To many people, the word "diet" means an eating plan designed to help them lose weight. However, the more general meaning of **diet** is the kinds of food a person or people habitually eat. For example, we might say that a typical Japanese diet contains more fish than the diet of most Americans. The word diet is also used to describe various types of eating plans, such as a vegan diet or low-salt diet.

Nutrition means the process of obtaining food necessary for health and growth. **Nutrients** are the various substances the body uses to grow and function properly. There are six classes of nutrients and each is essential to good health:

1. **Proteins**: food substances containing **amino acids**, which are necessary for both building and maintaining the structural components of the body. Common sources are meat, fish, eggs, **legumes** (plants with seed pods), nuts, seeds, and grains.
2. **Carbohydrates**: food substances composed of units of sugars that provide the body with immediate energy. Common sources are fruits, breads, cereals, and pasta.
3. **Fats**: food substances consisting of fatty acids that provide the most concentrated forms of energy for the body. In addition to oils and butter, fats are found in meat, fish, nuts, eggs, and certain plants such as olives and avocados.
4. **Vitamins**: **organic** (related to or derived from living organisms) substances found in foods that are essential, in very small quantities, for growth, health, and life.
5. **Minerals**: inorganic (not derived from living matter) substances that must be supplied to the body, in very small quantities, in order for it to function properly. (See Table 12–1 for examples of key vitamins and minerals.)
6. Water: essential for life. Water makes up 55% to 80% of human body weight, depending on age.

In addition to the nutrients listed above, fiber is an important component of the diet. **Fiber** is food content that cannot be fully digested. Its principal benefits are maintaining a healthy bowel and normalizing bowel movements (preventing constipation). Fiber is found in fruits, vegetables, whole grains, and legumes.

The body requires energy from foods to function. The potential energy a food can provide the body is measured in **calories**. A gram of carbohydrates has

Table 12–1 Key Vitamins and Minerals that Contribute to Good Health

Nutrient	Essential for	Examples of Food Sources
Vitamin A	• Growth • Prevention of infection • Good vision and healthy skin	Liver, fish oils, eggs, dark green vegetables
Thiamin (Vitamin B_1)	• Production of energy from carbohydrates	Whole or enriched grain products, pork, organ meats
Riboflavin (Vitamin B_2)	• **Metabolism** of nutrients into energy	Dairy products, organ meats, enriched and fortified grains
Niacin (Vitamin B_3)	• Metabolism of nutrients into energy	Poultry, fish, beef, legumes, enriched or fortified grains
Vitamin B_6	• Manufacture of amino acids and red blood cells	Fortified cereals, sweet potatoes, chicken and beef liver
Vitamin B_{12}	• Production of red blood cells • Maintenance of central nervous system	Beef, dairy products, shellfish
Vitamin C	• Healing of wounds • Healthy bones and gums	Fruits and vegetables (especially citrus fruits and cabbage)
Vitamin D	• Absorption of calcium • Formation and maintenance of bones and teeth	Vitamin D–fortified milk and cereals, cod liver oil *Note*: The skin produces vitamin D when it is exposed to sunlight.
Vitamin E	• Normal function of muscles • Defense of cells against **free radicals**	Vegetable oils, wheat germs, nuts, seeds, leafy greens
Vitamin K	• Blood clotting	Eggs, cereal, leafy greens
Calcium	• Building and maintenance of bones • Maintain muscle and nerve function	Dairy products, leafy greens
Folate	• DNA synthesis in making protein	Fortified cereals, enriched grains, leafy greens, legumes, asparagus
Iron	• Transport of oxygen in red blood cells to body cells	Meats, eggs, dark leafy vegetables
Magnesium	• Energy production • Nerve function	Legumes, nuts, whole grains, green vegetables
Phosphorus	• Growth and repair of supporting tissue • Bone and teeth formation	Milk, meat, poultry, fish, eggs, legumes, nuts
Potassium	• Nerve function • Muscle contraction (including heart muscle)	Fruits, vegetables, meat, poultry, fish, milk
Zinc	• Reproduction of cells • Tissue growth and repair	Meat, eggs, seafood, whole grains

4 calories, a gram of protein has 4 calories, and a gram of fat has 9 calories. Our bodies "burn" calories and either use them for immediate energy needs or store them as body fat. This is why many weight-loss diets are based on reducing the number of calories taken in and increasing the amount of physical exercise to use up calories that have been stored as body fat.

Many Americans include a large number of **processed foods** in their diet. These are defined as foods that are packaged in boxes, cans, or bags. Examples include canned soups, chips, cookies, and microwave meals. One component of many processed foods that you want to *avoid* rather than include in your diet is trans fat. A **trans fat** results when hydrogen is added to vegetable oil, which is then identified on food labels as "partially hydrogenated oil." The problem with trans fats is that they raise the level of low-density lipoprotein (LDL) cholesterol ("bad cholesterol") while decreasing high-density lipoprotein (HDL) cholesterol ("good cholesterol"). **Cholesterol** is a fatty substance that can clog the arteries. Many food makers have decreased or eliminated trans fats from their processed cookies, crackers, and other foods.

Another component of processed foods is sodium, often in large amounts. While a certain amount of sodium is necessary for the body to function properly, excessive amounts contribute to high blood pressure. Some processed foods contain more sodium in one serving than the recommended amount for one day. The Institute of Medicine (IOM) recommends 1500 mg of sodium per day as the *adequate intake level* for most Americans and advises everyone to limit sodium intake to less than 2300 mg per day, which is identified as the *tolerable upper limit* (Centers for Disease Control and Prevention [CDC], February 2011).

Types of Diets

Many types of diets are currently advocated for reaching and maintaining optimal health. The most important factors in choosing a diet are to make sure you include a variety of foods that provide all the nutrients listed in the previous section, and that you choose a diet you can make part of your daily life.

The U.S. Department of Agriculture (USDA) has developed dietary guidelines, which are updated every few years, to help Americans eat for wellness. The guidelines describe a healthy diet as follows:

- Emphasizes fruits, vegetables, whole grains, and fat-free or low-fat milk and milk products
- Includes lean meats, poultry, fish, beans, eggs, and nuts
- Is low in saturated fats, trans fats, cholesterol, and added sugars (U.S. Department of Agriculture, 2014)

A visual icon, known as **Choose My Plate**, was created by the USDA to help individuals apply the dietary guidelines and make healthy food choices. (See Figure 12–1.) The "plate" is divided into four sections of different sizes to show the recommended proportions of five food groups:

1. Vegetables
2. Grains
3. Protein
4. Fruits
5. Dairy

The USDA's website, www.choosemyplate.gov, helps individuals determine the proportion of food from each group they should eat each day. The USDA emphasizes seeking variety and balance in foods, as well as engaging in adequate physical exercise.

Low-fat and reduced-salt diets are advocated as ways to prevent conditions such as heart disease and certain types of cancer. This is because excess fat can accumulate in the arteries, a condition that increases risk for heart attacks (myocardial infarction). High

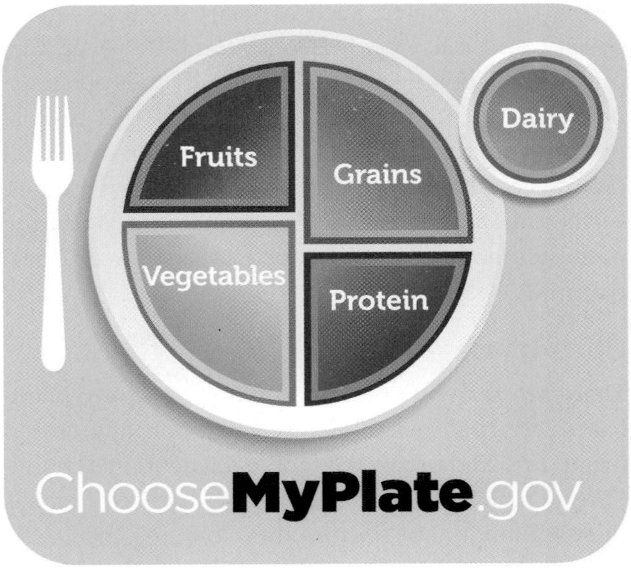

Courtesy of the U.S. Department of Agriculture.

FIGURE 12–1 Choose My Plate was developed by the USDA to encourage Americans to make healthy food choices.

amounts of salt can increase blood pressure to higher than recommended levels, a condition that can cause the blood vessels to weaken or clog.

Vegetarian Diets

Vegetarian diets consist mainly of plant-based foods, such as vegetables, fruits, whole grains, beans, nuts, and seeds. There are at least four types of vegetarian diets:

1. Vegan: Includes only plant-based foods. People who follow this diet do not eat any foods produced by animals such as milk, cheese, and eggs. The meaning of the term *vegan* has expanded beyond food choices and frequently relates to a philosophy that promotes animal rights. Vegans do not use or wear any animal products. When referring to dietary practices, the term *plant-based diet* is a more accurate descriptor than vegan.
2. Lacto-vegetarian: Includes milk and milk products along with plant-based foods.
3. Lacto-ovo vegetarian: Includes eggs, milk, and milk products along with plant-based foods.
4. Flexitarian (semi-vegetarian): A mostly plant-based diet, but may occasionally include small amounts of meat, poultry, or fish.

A growing number of scientific studies show that plant-based diets are healthier than meat-based diets. Vegetarian diets may prevent many of the chronic diseases and conditions that have become epidemic in the United States, such as heart disease, cancer, obesity, and diabetes. It is important, however, that plant-based diets be well-planned to include adequate nutrients. A common misconception is that animal products are the only source of protein, but this is not true. Recall that protein is also provided by legumes, seeds, nuts, and grains. A variety of vegetarian eating pyramids have been developed to assist with meal planning.

Other Diets

There are many diets that, while not entirely plant-based, are healthier than a diet that is heavy on red meats, fats, and processed foods. As mentioned previously, a major problem with many processed foods is the high amount of sodium they contain. The DASH diet, endorsed by the National Heart, Lung, and Blood Institute, is designed to lower blood pressure by reducing fats and sodium (National Heart, Lung, and Blood Institute, June 2014).

The Mediterranean diet, recommended for heart health by organizations such as the Mayo Clinic, incorporates the cooking and eating styles of countries such as Italy and Greece:

- Generous amounts of fruits and vegetables
- Substitution of olive and canola oils for saturated fats, such as butter
- Herbs and spices instead of salt seasoning
- Small portions of nuts
- Very little red meat
- Fish or shellfish at least twice a week (Mayo Clinic, June 2013)

Current research has identified specific foods that are especially beneficial for health, including the prevention of certain types of diseases. See Box 12–1 for examples of foods that are believed to promote heart health, in part because of their cholesterol-lowering properties. At the same time, news about "healthy foods" can be misleading. For example, there have been reports about olive oil promoting heart health. This has led many people to add olive oil to their diets. However, olive oil is a high-calorie fat. To obtain any potential health benefits, olive oil should be limited to small amounts and substituted for, not added to, other fats in the diet.

Food Labels

Food labels, intended to help individuals make good choices, are often confusing and incomplete. For example, low-fat milk labeled as 1% milkfat actually obtains 18% of its calories from fat. This figure is not given on the label: it can only be obtained by dividing the number of calories provided by fat (20) by the number of calories in an 8-ounce serving (110).

BOX 12–1

Examples of Heart-Healthy Foods

- Oatmeal
- Soy
- Salmon
- Spinach
- Walnuts

Source: Academy of Nutrition and Dietetics. Top Foods for a Healthy Heart, *http://www.eatright.org/resource/health/wellness/preventing-illness/top-foods-for-a-healthy-heart www.eatright.org/Public/content*

Another example is the use of the word "natural" to imply healthy. A popular "natural granola" cereal lists sugar as the second ingredient. One-half cup contains 210 calories, a relatively high number for that amount of cereal. The "all-natural" combination of oats, almonds, brown sugar, and honey results in something more like cookies than a healthy breakfast food.

Organic Foods

Organic foods are growing in popularity. The term organic, when applied to foods refers to the way they are grown and processed. Table 12–2 lists the major differences between organic and conventional farming methods. The USDA has established an organic certification program that includes standards in order for foods to be designated as organic:

- "100% organic": Completely organic
- "Organic": At least 95% organic
- "Made with organic ingredients": Contains at least 70% organic ingredients

Other terms that apply to foods include "all-natural," "free range," and "hormone-free," but these are not the same as organic. They can also be misleading. For example, the term *free range* implies that animals are allowed unlimited movement during their lifetime. However, they may have limited space and be allowed their freedom for only a few hours each day. And all-natural products may have natural ingredients, but they can also have a high sugar content that removes them from a healthy food list.

Studies comparing the nutritional value of traditionally grown foods with organic foods have led to conflicting results: Some researchers have shown that organic produce is far superior in nutritional value while others have found no significant difference for most food products. People who are concerned about chemical residues on food may prefer to eat organically grown products. (It should be noted that all fruits and vegetables, regardless of whether organic or not, should be thoroughly washed before eating.) In addition, people who are concerned about chemicals in the environment may be interested in organic foods. The major disadvantage of organic foods is that they are more expensive to grow than conventional foods and therefore cost more to purchase.

Improving Eating Habits

Improving eating habits sometimes requires individuals to make significant adjustments because the typical American diet contains many processed foods that are high in calories and sodium (salt) and low in nutritive value and fiber. To add to the problem, many people eat on the run and depend on fast-food suppliers—or worse, vending machines—for at least one of their daily meals. The following suggestions may be helpful when attempting to adopt a healthier diet:

- Eat moderate amounts. Go for flavor, not quantity.
- Look for nutritional value. Find foods you enjoy that contain essential nutrients. (See Figure 12–2.)

Table 12–2 Conventional versus Organic Farming Methods

Conventional Farming	Organic Farming
Use chemical fertilizers	Use natural fertilizers such as compost and manure
Spray insecticides	Use insects and birds that eat pests Disrupt mating of pests. Set traps
Use chemical weed killers	Rotate crops Hand weed Apply mulch
Give animals antibiotics and other medications, and growth hormones Food and Drug Administration (FDA) regulations allow rendered animal by-products and waste to be added to the feed	Give animals organic feed Provide animals with access to the outdoors to prevent spreading disease Use various preventive measures to help prevent disease

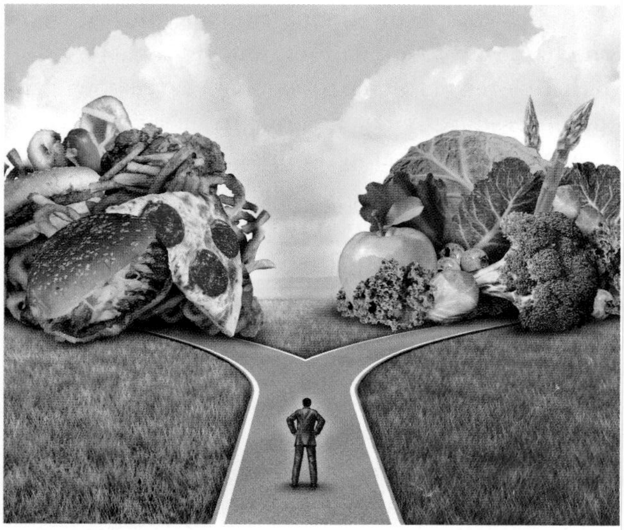

© Lightspring/Shutterstock.com.

FIGURE 12–2 Strive to make healthy food choices for most of your meals.

- Avoid excessive amounts of salt, fat, and sugar. Everyone enjoys a chocolate bar, popcorn, or a bag of chips from time to time, but these should not be eaten every day or substituted for meals.
- Eat adequate amounts of fiber. Not only does it contribute to a feeling of fullness, it also helps maintain colon health by forcing the muscles to work to remove the fiber from the body.
- Prepare your own sack lunch and dinner. Find foods that carry well, such as fruits, raw vegetables, nuts, seeds, cheeses, and peanut butter. (*Note:* Although the last four foods listed are high in calories, eaten *in moderation*, they are good sources of protein.)
- Eat slowly and enjoy each bite. You may find that you are satisfied sooner and do not need to eat as much.
- Drink sufficient water. The average adult body consists of 55% to 65% (up to 80% for elderly persons) water and depends on it to bathe cells and tissues, remove waste, and dissolve substances necessary for normal body function.
- Plan meals and snacks to include recommended amounts of vitamins and minerals.

Maintaining a Normal Weight

Along with good nutrition, maintaining a healthy weight has repeatedly been proven to contribute to wellness and the prevention of disease. However, it is estimated that at least 69% of adults in the United States are overweight (above a weight considered normal) or seriously overweight (with too much body fat), with 35% of adults age 20 and older obese (CDC, May 2014). This number may actually be higher because official statistical reports lag by several years and the trend is toward growing numbers of overweight individuals. Of particular concern is the increasing number of children and adolescents who are overweight, as shown by the following percentages for the years 2005 and 2006:

- Ages 2 to 5 years: 12%
- Ages 6 to 11 years: 18%
- Ages 12 to 18 years: 18.4% (CDC, May 2014)

Young people who are overweight tend to have weight problems as adults.

Body Mass Index

Height–weight charts were used for many years to determine if a person was overweight, but the **body mass index (BMI)** is increasingly being used. BMI measures the relationship of weight to height using a mathematical formula. (See Box 12–2.) A BMI of 25.0 to 29.9 is defined as **overweight**. A BMI of 30.0 or higher is considered **obese**.

Overweight and Obesity

The increasing numbers of overweight and obese Americans is being called by some the public health challenge of our time. Thousands of deaths and billions of health care dollars are the direct result of

BOX 12–2

Calculating Body Mass Index

1. Multiply weight in pounds by 703.
2. Divide the result by height in inches.
3. Divide the result from step 2 by height in inches.

Example: Calculate the BMI for a man who is 5 feet, 10 inches tall and weighs 236 pounds.

Step 1	236 × 703 = 165,908
Step 2	5'10" = 70 inches
	165,908 ÷ 70 = 2370
Step 3	2370 ÷ 70 = 33.86

BMI = 33.86

obesity, making it one of the leading causes of preventable deaths in the United States. This is because excess body weight contributes to a number of uncomfortable conditions and serious diseases, such as the following:

- High blood pressure
- Elevated levels of fats in the blood, including cholesterol
- Type 2 diabetes
- Heart disease
- Stroke
- Gallbladder disease
- Osteoarthritis
- Sleep apnea (condition in which a person stops breathing while sleeping)
- Respiratory problems
- Cancers (endometrial, breast, prostate, and colon)
- Depression

Researchers are investigating why the percentage of overweight and obese Americans continues to grow even as we learn more about the health benefits of maintaining a healthy weight. It is believed there are a number of reasons why Americans continue to gain weight:

- Increase in the total amount of food consumed
- Availability of inexpensive, calorie-dense foods
- Increased consumption of high-calorie and high-fat foods
- Heavy use of the automobile as a means of transportation
- Increased number of hours watching television, using the computer, and playing video games
- Lack of active recreational exercise
- Increases in technology and decreases in tasks that require manual labor

Recall that calories provide the body with energy. When more calories are taken in than are needed by the body to function, the unused energy is stored as fat. Thus, an increase in calories with a corresponding decrease in physical activity results in weight gain. (See Figure 12–3.)

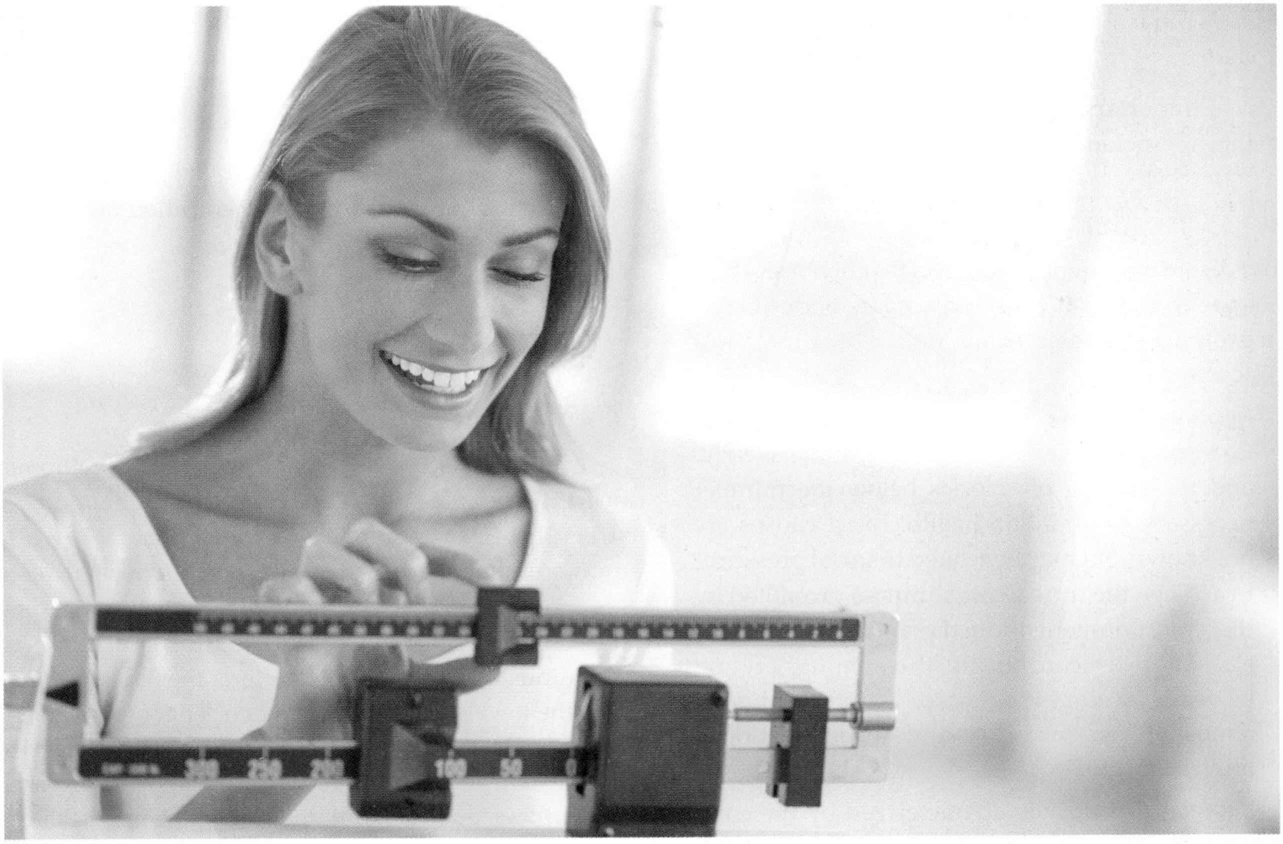

FIGURE 12–3 Maintaining a healthy weight requires balancing energy intake and output: burning all the calories contained in the food eaten.

Another contributing factor to weight gain is that decreased activity results in a loss of muscle mass, which in turn leads to a decreased number of calories needed to maintain the body's weight. This is because muscle tissue uses more energy to support itself than fat tissue does. Therefore, lack of exercise contributes to increased weight in two ways: by lowering the number of calories burned throughout the day and by reducing the body's caloric requirements.

Stress, anxiety, and boredom are sometimes causes of overeating. If you believe this to be true for you, try the stress-reducing techniques discussed later in this chapter. Eliminating the causes of overeating may not only resolve a weight problem but can improve other areas of life as well.

Dozens of diets and methods have been proposed for losing weight. Many of the most popular diets contradict each other, and it can be difficult to sort fact from fiction. Most nutrition experts believe that excess calories cause excess body weight. Any diet that provides fewer calories than are burned is likely to result in weight loss. Weight-loss diets that emphasize one type of food over another or eliminate a whole category of foods that provide essential nutrients can result in a shortage of one or more essential nutrients. Therefore, when planning a weight-loss diet, it is important to make sure that all necessary nutrients are included.

Eating Disorders

Eating disorders, often caused by a fear of obesity and the desire to conform to an unrealistic body image, are a growing problem. Following are the three most common conditions:

1. **Anorexia nervosa**: The distorted belief that one is overweight, even when severely underweight, and the cutting of calories below the number necessary to maintain health. Exact causes are not known, but may be related to social pressures to achieve the unrealistic slimness promoted by the entertainment industry and fashion models. Anorexia can be life threatening, ending in death by starvation. Medical intervention is almost always necessary, and hospitalization is often required.
2. **Bulimia**: A condition characterized by the compulsive eating of huge quantities of food, followed by self-induced vomiting and/or the use of large amounts of laxatives. These actions may be accompanied by feelings of guilt and the fear of being "found out." Stomach acids in vomit may cause the erosion of tooth enamel, development of dental cavities, and eating away of the esophagus.
3. **Binge eating**: The compulsive consumption of large quantities of food, beyond that needed to satisfy hunger. This uncontrolled eating is sometimes used as an escape from boredom, as a means to handle anger, and for other reasons related to handling emotional issues.

Medical assistance, counseling, and support groups offer help with eating disorders.

PHYSICAL ACTIVITY

Like good nutrition, physical activity has been found to have a significant influence on health. It has even been said that if exercise could be put in a tablet form, it would be considered a wonder drug. Exercise has benefits for every body system and can help prevent and treat many illnesses. The many benefits of physical activity include the following:

- Promotes feelings of well-being through the body's production of endorphins, substances that naturally raise the pain threshold and produce sedative effects
- Relieves stress and improves mental outlook
- Improves memory and concentration
- Improves the quality of sleep
- Helps with weight control
- Increases energy level
- Helps prevent lower back pain
- Reduces symptoms of arthritis

Exercise also reduces the risk of developing heart disease. The heart is a muscle and therefore is strengthened by regular exercise that forces it to work by increasing the heartbeat beyond its normal resting rate, within a target range. For a healthy person, the maximum desired heart rate during exercise is 220 minus his or her age. Therefore, the older the person, the lower the target heart rate. This type of exercise, known as **aerobic exercise**, increases the heart's strength. In addition to helping prevent heart disease, the number one cause of death in the United States, physical activity decreases the incidence of type 2 diabetes, **osteoporosis**, and certain types of cancer, including breast and colon.

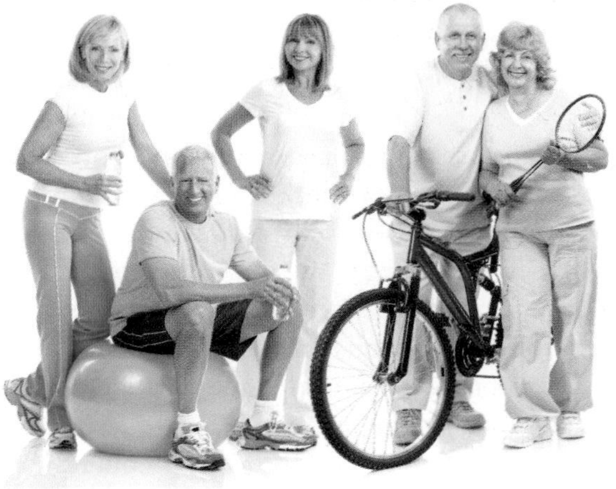

FIGURE 12–4 Physical exercise is a key component of good health. Find something you enjoy doing.

It is recommended that adults exercise for at least 30 minutes on five or more days a week. Children and teens need 60 minutes a day. This time may be broken into segments of 10 or 15 minutes and still provide health benefits. In addition to periods of planned exercise, physical activity can be incorporated into daily life. A few alterations can result in a built-in exercise program that does not take too much time in an already busy life. Here are a few ideas:

- Whenever possible, leave the car at home. Walk to the store, library, church, and so on. When using the car, park at the far end of the mall or grocery store parking lot.
- Use the stairs instead of elevators.
- Wash the car instead of going to the car wash.
- Do jobs yourself that require physical effort, such as mowing the lawn and washing windows.
- Find a sport or activity you enjoy, such as swimming or dancing. Or shoot baskets with the kids and walk around the neighborhood with a friend. Substitute activity for a few hours of television each week. (See Figure 12–4.)

SLEEP

An adequate amount of sleep is necessary because it is during sleep that the body recuperates from the day's activities. Body functions slow down and body temperature drops. It is believed that during the last few hours of sleep before awakening, the time when most dreams occur, mental recuperation takes place. Studies have shown that during sleep the brain is preparing itself for learning and taking in new information (Washington University School of Medicine, 2009). This is why it is especially important that students and others who are engaged in learning activities make it a point to get enough sleep. "Enough" varies among individuals but is generally believed to be six to nine hours for adults.

Sleep provides the energy necessary to function efficiently throughout the day and deal with stress. Getting enough sleep is a good investment because it can increase productivity. Busy students may appreciate the benefits but are wondering just how to get the recommended amount of sleep when trying to balance the responsibilities of school, work, family, and personal activities. This is a common problem. Here are some suggestions for increasing the length and quality of sleep:

- Avoid caffeine—found in coffee, tea, cola drinks, and chocolate—late in the day if it keeps you awake.
- Try to avoid stressful activities or communications just before going to bed.
- Keep a "worry log" to write down things to think about at a set "worry time." Keep the "appointment" and use the time to focus on finding solutions. Knowing that it is possible to get back to worries later can help clear the mind at bedtime.
- Use the time management techniques described later in this chapter to increase personal efficiency and increase the time available for sleep.
- Engage in some form of exercise each day, but avoid very vigorous exercise just before going to bed.
- Develop a routine for getting ready for bed and try to use it every day. This will signal the body to become sleepy.
- Keep the bed for sleeping. Do not do homework and other chores there or the body may program itself to become alert when getting into bed.

PREVENTIVE MEASURES

Many health problems can be avoided by practicing preventive measures. These include the following:

- Regular visits to physician or health care practitioner for routine checkups. (See Figure 12–5.)

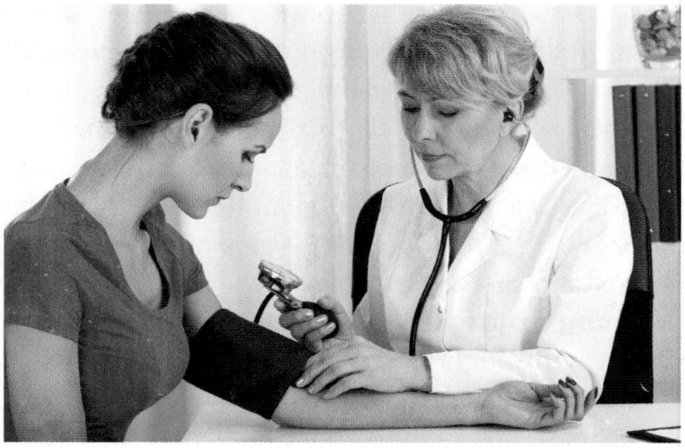

FIGURE 12–5 Regular checkups and screening tests are important for maintaining good health.

- Periodic screening for risks associated with your gender and age group.
- Regular visits to the dentist and the practice of proper dental hygiene, including regular flossing. Most gum disease, which can cause the loss of teeth, can be avoided. Untreated tooth decay and abscesses can result in serious infections in other parts of the body, including the heart.
- Treatment of illnesses in their early stages. Positive outcomes are more likely with early treatment.
- Immunizations. Many health care employers offer hepatitis B vaccinations for all employees whose work requires them to be exposed to body substances. An annual vaccination against influenza is also highly recommended. Although this illness may seem like "just the flu," it causes tens of thousands of death each year. (CDC, July 2014.)

STRESS IN MODERN LIFE

Stress refers to the body's reactions when it responds to danger, either real or imagined. In seeking a state of readiness for action, the body undergoes a series of physical changes that include the following:

- Increased heart rate
- Increased rate of breathing
- Elevated blood pressure
- Raised blood sugar level
- Dilated blood vessels in the muscles to give them the immediate use of sugar
- Dilated pupils of eyes (Harvard Medical School, 2011.)

These reactions, characteristic of the "fight or flight" response explained in Chapter 7, serve individuals well when they must protect themselves, run from a scene, or perform an emergency procedure under pressure. (See Table 7–3.) But the body cannot distinguish between physical danger and fears and worries experienced in the mind or the emotional strain resulting from negative circumstances. For example, worries about losing a job or handling financial problems create the same reaction as being in danger of physical attack. When psychological pressures are continuous or occur frequently, the body can literally wear itself out making preparations to face danger. Responses originally meant to be helpful become sources of harm.

Research studies in recent years have looked for a correlation between stress and various illnesses. Although the evidence is not conclusive, some researchers and physicians believe that the experience of chronic psychological and emotional stress weakens the body's immune system. This reduces the

Thinking It Through

Mikel Korsov is a recent graduate of a licensed practical nurse program. He has been hired to work in the pediatric ward at Samuelson Hospital. Mikel loves working with children and has a real talent for calming their fears and helping them cope with necessary procedures and medications. He finds, however, that he is physically exhausted at the end of each day. He has little energy left to do much more than drag himself home, eat whatever is available or quick to prepare, and then watch television until bedtime. Mikel weighs about 60 pounds more than the weight suggested for his height and does not participate in much physical exercise beyond that required on the job.

1. What might be the long-term consequences of Mikel's current habits? Consider this from both personal and professional viewpoints.
2. Discuss the possible impact of his health habits on the attitudes of his patients regarding their own health.
3. Suggest five things he can do that can help increase his energy level.

body's ability to defend itself against disease. Stress is also believed by many health professionals to contribute to high blood pressure, heart disease, cancer, and other diseases. In addition to possibly increasing the risk of serious health problems, excessive stress interferes with personal effectiveness, productivity, relationships, and the enjoyment of life.

External and Internal Stressors

Modern life presents many **stressors** (causes of stress). External stressors are those outside one's immediate control. Examples include the fast pace of life, the high cost of living, crowded cities and freeways, and demanding patients. We have limited control over external stressors, although changes can be made in how we perceive and deal with them. (See the section on attitude in this chapter.)

Internal stressors are self-generated and within the individual's control. Examples include a negative attitude, unrealistic goals, poor time management skills, and lack of problem-solving ability. Internal stressors can be controlled by acquiring additional skills, making changes in personal habits, and adjusting one's mental outlook.

Dealing with Stress

There will always be stressors in life. The future may bring achievements and satisfaction, but there is no perfect job or ideal set of conditions that are stress-free. And some degree of stress is actually healthy because it provides the motivation for action. Health care work, by its very nature, can be stressful because workers must be able to do the following:

- Interact with people who are ill or injured
- Remain calm in difficult situations
- Remain constantly attentive
- Apply thinking skills
- Perform tasks accurately
- Work under time constraints
- Respond to changing needs of patients and the facility

Dealing effectively with stress starts with identifying the major stressors in life. Are they internal or external? Which are within your control? Are you adding to your own stress level with ineffective personal habits? Which stressors are outside your control and require adaptive and coping techniques?

Marcos, a respiratory therapy student, is a perfectionist when it comes to his homework assignments. He goes over each one several times, reworking them until he feels satisfied that they are "just right." As a result, Marcos frequently turns in assignments late and never feels caught up. The need for perfection is causing Marcos stress and may be a serious problem when he becomes employed. Workplace tasks, although needing to be performed correctly, must also be completed in a timely way. In this example, knowing when work is satisfactory can alleviate unnecessary stress.

Setting Priorities

Stress can be created by the inability to prioritize. To **prioritize** means to rank tasks that need to be done in order of importance. Adult learners often experience conflicts between their many responsibilities. School and work are priorities and, at times, choices must be made in order to reduce stress. Ellen, a mother of three, agreed to serve on a parents' committee at her children's school. After enrolling in a dental hygiene program, she found that she did not have the time for both the committee meetings and responsibilities and studying for her classes. She completed the tasks she had already committed to do, then met with the chairperson to explain her situation and resign from the committee.

Examining your values and determining which current activities will result in long-term benefits can help you decide what is most important to you. Where can you make compromises now in exchange for future benefits? The time and effort you invest in your studies, for example, will determine your future employment success. And time spent with children is essential to their healthy development. (See Figure 12–6.) The ability to prioritize will continue to be an important skill both on the job and as you balance professional, family, and personal responsibilities.

Time Management

Poor time management is a major cause of stress. Fortunately, it is possible to have more control over time than we may realize. Although it is impossible to increase the number of hours in a day, the ones that are available can be used more effectively. Improving the use of time can reduce stress, improve personal performance, and increase feelings of personal power.

Start by doing an honest review of your daily habits. It will help to keep a record for a week, listing

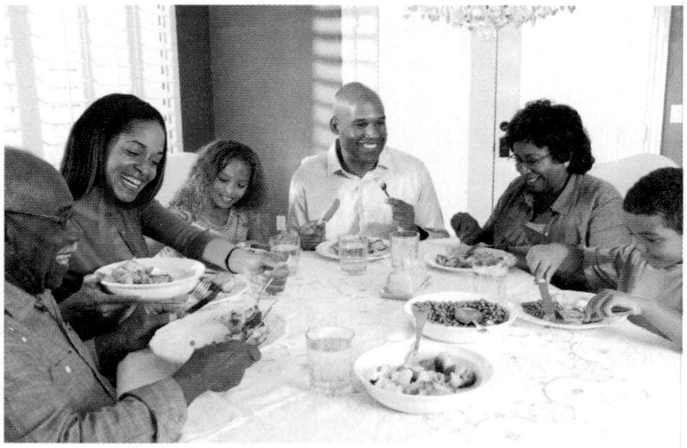

FIGURE 12–6 Spending time with family and friends supports emotional and physical health and should be a priority.

the amount of time spent on each activity. Are there hours when time is simply "killed" instead of being used effectively or enjoyed? Television, the telephone, and the Internet can eat up hours. They may not provide enjoyment in proportion to the time spent. Are there others? Is there adequate time built in for resting and thinking, or is everything too rushed? Are there actions you can take to prevent a future crisis that can be very time-consuming? Try prioritizing activities as a means to identify those that bring the most benefits or enjoyment for the time invested.

Procrastination is a stress producer for many people. This is illustrated by Mohammed, a health information management student. He has assignments that are due throughout the semester. Last semester he was in a continual state of panic and last-minute rushes to complete them. Unexpected delays and interruptions created a sense of emergency. Feelings of desperation mounted and made it difficult to concentrate. Mohammed thought about why he procrastinated and realized that he was afraid to start projects because they seemed overwhelming. He developed the following plan:

1. Break large projects into smaller steps that are more manageable.
2. Set completion dates for each step, starting with the project deadline and moving backward on the calendar.
3. Schedule time to work each day or every other day in order to feel a sense of accomplishment and keep the project moving. (It is important to work even when not in the mood for it.)
4. Seek appropriate help and gather information as needed.
5. Focus on the feelings of accomplishment and control being experienced.

Many time-management techniques can be incorporated into a busy daily schedule:

- Keep a calendar of assignments, tests, field trips, appointments, birthdays, and other "must-remember" activities.
- Write a daily to-do list in the order of most to least important tasks. At the end of each day, cross off completed tasks and carry over undone tasks for the next day.
- When possible, do the hardest things first.
- Keep other lists to help stay organized: shopping, freezer contents, children's chores.
- Organize errands so that several can be accomplished in one trip.
- Keep things in their place so that time is not wasted looking for them.
- At work, know the priorities of your supervisor or department.

Time management is a critical work skill. With emphasis on cost containment and efficiency, health care professionals are expected to use time well and accomplish required duties within prescribed time periods. Learning to manage time will contribute to workplace success. See Chapter 26 for more ideas about time management on the job.

Relaxation Techniques

Relaxation, as used here, refers to releasing tension in the muscles. This reduces stress, both physical and emotional, by improving blood circulation and allowing the release of blood lactate, a substance that some studies have shown to be associated with anxiety. Using relaxation techniques also produces the sensation of being rested. With practice, it is possible to quickly identify and release muscle tension when it begins to occur.

There are several methods for doing muscle relaxation exercises. Although it is outside the scope of this book to provide extensive information, instructions for one popular method can be found in Box 12–3.

Meditation

When individuals are awake, the mind is continually engaged in thinking. **Meditation** is a process

BOX 12–3

Muscle Relaxation Technique

1. Choose a time and place where you can arrange not to be interrupted.
2. Sit in a comfortable position with the spine straight and feet flat on the floor.
3. Starting at the toes, tighten the muscles of each section of the body, experience the feeling of tension, and then relax. Move up as follows:
   a. Toes (flex)
   b. Legs
   c. Hips and abdomen
   d. Chest and upper back
   e. Hands (make a fist) and arms
   f. Shoulders (lift toward ears)
   g. Face, head, and neck (be sure to relax the jaw afterward)
   h. Eyebrows (raise and lower, pull together and release)
4. Tighten the entire body at once, hold as long as possible, then relax as much as possible. (Important note: This step is not recommended for people with hypertension [high blood pressure].)
5. Repeat to yourself: "I am relaxed."
6. Sit for several minutes and experience the lack of tension. If you become aware of any areas of tension, tighten and then release the muscles in that area.

Source: Adapted from Understanding Human Behavior: A Guide for Health Care Providers *(7th ed.), by M. E. Milliken & A. Honeycutt, 2004, Clifton Park, NY: Delmar Cengage Learning.*

for quieting the mind by clearing it of thoughts. It slows the rate of brain waves experienced during normal activity. The regular practice of meditation has been shown to bring about physiological changes that result in both psychological and physiological well-being. An increasing number of health care professionals are recommending meditation as a therapeutic technique because some research suggests that it may help manage the symptoms of the following:

- Anxiety disorders
- Asthma
- Cancer

Thinking It Through

Janice Nelson, dental assistant for Dr. Grady, is worried about the conversation she had with Dr. Grady this afternoon. He spoke with her privately and expressed concern about her time management practices. He pointed out that Janice had arrived late for work three times in the last two weeks, had left early one day due to child-care problems, and had several times failed to complete assigned work tasks in the designated time. Dr. Grady explained that in a small practice with only a few employees, Janice was having a significant impact on work flow in the office. He warned her that she must improve if she was to continue working there.

1. Discuss the possible impact of Janice's actions on patients, coworkers, and Dr. Grady.
2. Suggest ways that Janice can improve her personal organization and time management.

- Depression
- Heart disease
- High blood pressure
- Sleep apnea (Mayo Clinic, November 2014)

The positive, long-term effects that can be achieved through daily meditation, when it is practiced over an extended period, include the following:

- Changes in perception of self, others, and life events
- A freeing of emotions, especially suppressed emotions
- Greater compassion
- Increased capacity for self-love and love for others
- Improved ability to cope with life situations (Milliken & Honeycutt, 2004)

You may have had the experience of finding the solution to a problem when you stopped focusing on it and just "let the mind go." Meditators report similar experiences occurring after completing a meditation session.

There are a number of meditation methods. See Box 12–4 for an example.

The meditation procedure may sound incredibly simple, but it has been proven over the centuries to be effective. Like many practices that result in improved

BOX 12-4

A Meditation Method

1. Choose a time and place where you can arrange not to be interrupted.
2. Set a timer. Twenty minutes is best, 10 is the minimum.
3. Sit in a comfortable position in a chair or on the floor. Straighten the spine and place the hands on the thighs.
4. Take a few deep breaths and let your body relax.
5. While breathing naturally, start counting each time you exhale. When you reach four (four breaths), start over.
6. Focus on the counting, not on the breaths.
7. If thoughts enter your mind, let them go by, refocusing on the counting.

Source: Adapted from Understanding Human Behavior: A Guide for Health Care Providers *(7th ed.), by M. E. Milliken & A. Honeycutt, 2004, Clifton Park, NY: Delmar Cengage Learning.*

health and stress relief, it is free and fairly easy to learn. It does take practice, however, and must be done regularly over time. This requires the willingness to set aside 20 minutes each day or every other day.

Attitude

The close relationship between the mind and body is increasingly being recognized. Our quality of life is dependent to a great degree on whether our thoughts are generally positive or negative. **Attitude** refers to how a situation is viewed mentally. Every situation in life can be viewed in many different ways. For example, problems can be viewed as dreaded difficulties or as challenges that keep life interesting.

Fascinating Facts

Many sources state that 10 to 20 minutes of meditation are equivalent to a 2-hour nap.

Health care professionals face many situations that can be approached either positively or negatively. Let's look at an example:

Mr. Chang is an 86-year-old resident in an extended care facility. He spent most of his life in Hong Kong, moving to the United States when he was in his 60s. His wife died two years ago, and his children live in other parts of the country. He rarely has visitors. Mr. Chang is difficult to understand because of his accent, complains a lot about being in the care facility, and is considered generally unpleasant to be around.

Two staff members have contrasting experiences with Mr. Chang:

1. Anne dreads having to enter Mr. Chang's room each morning. He complains and grumbles as she gets him up and dressed. Anne hurries through her tasks and limits her conversation to necessary instructions.
2. Charles works the evening shift and looks forward to working with Mr. Chang. Charles did some research on Chinese culture and learned that for Mr. Chang, living in a care facility away from family is different from how life would have been in Hong Kong, where senior family members are highly respected and cared for at home. Charles asks Mr. Chang questions and listens carefully. As a result, he has learned a lot about life in another culture and has learned to appreciate the importance of family ties. He has shared stories about his family with Mr. Chang and offered the elderly resident friendship and relief from loneliness.

When faced with difficult situations, look for ways to turn them into learning experiences or deal with them in ways that create the least amount of stress. Ask yourself:

- Do I fully understand the situation?
- Is my behavior contributing to the problem?

Thinking It Through

Mary Payongayong is stressed out from her job as a radiology technician in a mid-city orthopedic clinic. Her work load has increased as the result of staff reductions, and her current supervisor is demanding. Mary finds it difficult to communicate with him and feels that he is unresponsive to the needs of the staff.

1. What might Mary do to improve her situation at work?
2. What might she do to relieve her stress?

- If so, what can I do differently?
- Are there any positive possibilities, such as those that Charles found, that I have overlooked?

Some situations, in spite of the health care professional's best efforts, do not turn out to be as positive as the example with Charles and Mr. Chang. The best approach in these cases is to perform work in a professional manner, keep emotions under control, and avoid mentally dwelling on the negative aspects of the situation. Engaging in physical exercise, meditation, and other health-promoting activities can help reduce or relieve external stressors over which we have no control.

MINIMIZING HEALTH RISKS

Being aware of commonly encountered health risks enables health care professionals to take preventive measures. These actions provide benefits for workers themselves, as well as for the patients they serve. Armed with knowledge about health risks, workers are better equipped to educate patients about ways to achieve maximum wellness.

Smoking

Most people are familiar with the risks associated with cigarette smoking. It has been linked to many serious health conditions and is estimated to have contributed to approximately 438,000 or one in five deaths annually (CDC, February 2014). The major causes of these deaths are diseases related to smoking, such as cancer and respiratory and vascular diseases. Added to this are the 42,000 deaths each year linked to secondhand smoke (CDC, February 2014).

Unfortunately, understanding the dangers does not necessarily make it easy to stop smoking. Nicotine is a physically addictive substance. Although the long-term benefits of quitting are many, the discomfort of withdrawing from the use of tobacco discourages many people who would like to quit. There are methods that some individuals find helpful:

- Groups that meet regularly and offer a structured program that involves quitting gradually. Leaders are usually ex-smokers who offer encouragement. Buddy systems are often organized to provide support between meetings.
- Classes and support groups offered by health care facilities
- Hypnosis
- Methods that allow the gradual withdrawal from nicotine through the use of skin patches and/or gum
- Medications that reduce the need for nicotine

Withdrawal symptoms vary among individuals. They may include anxiety, inability to concentrate, headaches, irritability, and strong cravings for a cigarette. (These are an indication of just how strong the effect of nicotine is on the body!) Knowing what to expect and keeping in mind that the symptoms *will disappear* may offer encouragement to stay with the quitting process. Most ex-smokers agree that the temporary discomfort is worth it for them to feel better now and to decrease the risks of illness and premature death.

Substance Abuse

Substance abuse is a growing problem that increases the risk of stress, disease, and injury, accounting for tens of thousands of deaths annual. Paradoxically, it is to *escape* from stress that many individuals turn to alcohol and drugs. However, these habits are likely to create problems and become *additional* sources of stress. Drinking excessive amounts of alcohol in an effort to "relax" after work is an example. At best, alcohol offers only temporary relief. At worst, it can result in poor job performance and dismissal, in addition to health problems, such as liver damage and increased risk of accidents. The Centers for Disease Control and Prevention reports that approximately 88,000 deaths annually in the United States are attributable to excessive alcohol use (CDC, August 2014).

Fascinating Facts

In 2012, health care providers wrote 259 million prescriptions for painkillers. This was enough for every American adult to have a bottle of pills.

Source: Centers for Disease Control and Prevention. (Last updated October 17, 2014). Prescription drug overdose in the United States–Fact Sheet. *Retrieved November 13, 2014 from the World Wide Web: http://www.cc.gov/homeandrecreationalsafety/overdose/facts.html.*

The abuse of drugs, especially prescription drugs that are **controlled substances** (have potential for addiction), has become a serious public health problem. Prescription and over-the-counter overdoses now result in 9 out of 10 poisoning deaths, killing an average of 114 people every day. The vast majority of these overdoses are unintentional (CDC, October 2014). This problem extends to an increasing number of health care professionals. Information available on the subject estimates that between 10% and 15% of health care professionals are addicted to drugs or alcohol (Nebraska Department of Health and Human Services, 2011).

There are a number of reasons for drug use among health care professionals:

- Easy access to controlled substance medications
- Stressful job conditions
- Self-medication
- Perceived ability to improve work performance and alertness (U.S. Department of Justice, n.d.)

Another contributing factor is that some health care professionals are able to call in unauthorized prescriptions for themselves to pharmacies because they know the vocabulary and procedures for ordering.

The dangers of drug abuse, whether with illegal substances or prescription drugs, cannot be overemphasized. Patient care is compromised when health care professionals perform under the influence of either drugs or alcohol because they can cause the following:

- Faulty judgment
- Blackouts
- Memory loss
- Inability to adequately perform tasks requiring physical coordination
- Illegible written documentation

Improper drug use can result in negative physical effects on the health care professional, along with the problems caused by the need to use larger amounts of the substance as the degree of physical tolerance rises. Stealing prescription drugs from a facility is a crime. In addition, patient care can be seriously compromised if health care providers consume the drugs needed by the patients. Even in cases not involving theft, the use of any type of drug or alcohol on the job can result in severe consequences. The fortunate employee may be required to enter a rehabilitation program. The less fortunate one faces imprisonment and a lifetime ban from working in certain health care occupations. Health care students should be aware that a conviction for using illegal drugs can permanently disqualify them from licensure in certain occupations.

There are many effective programs for treating substance abuse, including ones designed especially for health care professionals. The counseling office at most schools is a good source of information about community services. Anyone who believes that he or she may have a problem with drugs or alcohol should seek help immediately.

Occupational Hazards

Health care professionals encounter various risks on the job: exposure to infectious disease, to chemicals, and to potentially dangerous equipment. Most risks can be minimized by using proper safety precautions and following facility rules. Occupational safety is discussed throughout this text:

- Avoiding injury through the use of proper body mechanics: Chapter 9
- Protecting oneself against infection and bloodborne pathogens: Chapter 10
- Practicing environmental safety: Chapter 11
- Using the computer safely: Chapter 9

Fascinating Facts

The National Highway Traffic Safety Administration reports that in 2013, 10,076 or almost 30 people a day, died in alcohol-related traffic accidents. This represents 31% of all traffic fatalities.

Source: CDC, Impaired Driving–Get the Facts. *http://www.cdc.gov/motorvehiclesafety/impaired_driving/impaired-drv_factsheet.html*

At each facility where you are employed, carefully read all the safety manuals and instruction books that apply to your work. Never hesitate to ask questions about anything you do not understand. Your safety, and that of patients and coworkers, depends on your knowledge and use of safe practices.

Safe Sex

Sexual practices have become a necessary topic of discussion due to the global spread of the human immunodeficiency virus (HIV). Although the number of new cases has remained stable at 50,000 per year, there are 1,144,500 individuals living with HIV (CDC, December 2013). And although not fatal, genital herpes has reached epidemic proportions in the

United States. According to the CDC, one person in six is infected with the virus that causes genital herpes. The number may actually be much higher because many people do not experience symptoms.

There are a number of other sexually transmitted diseases (STDs) that health care professionals should be aware of. Some of the most common include:

- Human papillomavirus (HPV)
- Chlamydia
- Gonorrhea
- Syphilis
- Trichomoniasis

The only 100% effective means of preventing STDs is abstinence from sexual activity. For individuals who choose to be sexually active, basic precautions can minimize the risk of contracting STDs:

- Discuss risk factors with your potential partner before beginning a sexual relationship. Ask if he or she is aware of having an STD. Herpes is problematic because symptoms can be so mild that many people do not know they are infected.
- With any new partner, mutually agree to be tested for HIV. (*Note:* This is only effective if it has been at least six months since the last sexual contact. It can take that long for the virus to become detectable.)
- Use condoms.
- Get regular screening because some diseases have no signs or symptoms.
- See a physician immediately if symptoms of any STD are experienced. These include sores in the genital area, unusual odors, discharges, and itching.

Burnout

Burnout is a form of physical and emotional exhaustion that can be caused by a variety of personal and environmental stressors experienced over an extended period. Burnout occurs in all professions, but health care professionals can be particularly susceptible due to the nature of their work. Examples of stressors that can lead to burnout include the following:

- Long hours working under difficult conditions
- Lack of adequate rest
- Inability to deal effectively with frustrating situations
- Inadequate emotional support
- No time for recreational activities
- Emotional involvement with patients who are suffering from terminal diseases
- Poor diet and insufficient exercise

The symptoms of burnout vary among individuals. Commonly noted changes in behavior include the following:

- Negative feelings about work
- Feelings of not being appreciated
- Increased absences due to minor illnesses
- Physical symptoms such as fatigue, gastrointestinal disorders, and headaches
- Irritability
- Making errors and taking longer than previously required to complete tasks

  (*Source:* Adapted from *Understanding Human Behavior: A Guide for Health Care Providers* (7th ed.), by M. E. Milliken & A. Honeycutt, 2004, Clifton Park, NY: Delmar Cengage Learning.)

Health care professionals should be on the alert for signs of burnout. The daily practice of good health habits and regular use of stress-prevention techniques are good ways to prevent its occurrence. Developing good **assertiveness** (expressing feelings freely in a nonthreatening manner) and communication skills (see Chapters 15 and 16) can help resolve workplace issues that might otherwise result in burnout.

Working cooperatively in high-risk situations can help everyone deal with a difficult workload. The nurses in a neonatal unit at a northern California hospital found the stress of caring for heroin-addicted newborns who cried constantly for days at a time to be overwhelming. They agreed to share their assignments so that no one had more than two consecutive shifts working with these babies (P. Bird, personal communication, June 1999). The Cleveland Clinic, rated as one of the best hospitals in the world, has initiated a Code Lavender response team to assist health care professionals in need of emotional support after experiencing troubling or exhaustive times, such as when experiencing the death of a patient (Gregoire, 2013).

HELPING PATIENTS DEVELOP HEALTHY LIFESTYLES

In addition to serving as role models, many health care professionals are required to provide patient education. All the health-promoting techniques described in this chapter can be applied to patients. You may also be expected to give specialized instructions, like the dental hygienist who teaches proper flossing and brushing techniques. Including information about healthy lifestyles is an excellent form of preventive care. Some dental patients, for example, can also benefit from learning the nutritional guidelines that improve dental and general health.

Physical therapy assistants teach exercises as part of their daily work. But other health care professionals, such as medical assistants, also have opportunities to explain the benefits of exercise. The fact is that almost every health care professional has opportunities to share information that will help patients develop healthier lifestyles.

(*Note:* Be sure that your supervisor is aware of and has approved any information and materials you share with patients.)

WORKBOOK PRACTICE

Go to your workbook and complete the exercises for this chapter.

SUGGESTED LEARNING ACTIVITIES

1. Find articles from credible sources about the benefits of proper nutrition and exercise. What does current research report about best practices?
2. Start a scrapbook of articles and information from journals and the Internet about healthy habits.
3. Read packaged food labels. What are the major components of your favorites? Are you surprised by what you discover?
4. Try eating new foods that are high in nutritional value.
5. Start a collection of recipes for healthy dishes.
6. Develop a personal exercise program. Set a reasonable goal, such as three times a week for 20 minutes. Record your progress.
7. Look for examples of stressors in your environment. Which are internal and which are external?
8. Try the relaxation or meditation exercises for two weeks. Do you notice any benefits?

WEB ACTIVITIES

United States Department of Agriculture
www.choosemyplate.gov

Explore this website to learn more about nutrition and healthy eating. List 10 facts you did not know before researching the site. Then write a short report about how you can apply what you learned to your daily eating habits.

National Library of Medicine–Medline Plus
http://medlineplus.gov

Click on "Health Topics," then on "Health and Wellness" and "Fitness and Exercise." Follow the links until you find an article or news report of interest to read and summarize.

Healthy Living
www.mayoclinic.com

Click on the "Patient Care & Info" tab, then on "Healthy Living." Choose a topic of interest and use what you learn to prepare a short pamphlet with healthy lifestyle suggestions for health care professionals.

REVIEW QUESTIONS

1. Why is it important for health care professionals to practice good health habits?
2. How can old habits be changed or new habits be formed?
3. What are the six classes of nutrients and the purpose of each?
4. What are the major components of the USDA's dietary guidelines?
5. What does the USDA's Choose My Plate icon communicate?
6. Describe how organic foods are grown differently from conventionally grown foods.

7. List five recommendations for improving one's daily eating habits.
8. Describe the three major eating disorders.
9. Give six examples of health problems caused by overweight and obesity.
10. What are five benefits of physical exercise?
11. What are the possible negative consequences of getting an inadequate amount of sleep?
12. Describe the following health risks and what can be done to prevent or minimize them:
    a. Smoking
    b. Substance abuse
    c. Occupational hazards
    d. Sexually transmitted diseases
13. What are some methods the health care professional can use to deal with stress?
14. What are the major health risks faced by health care professionals today?
15. List the symptoms of burnout and suggested preventive measures.

APPLICATION EXERCISES

1. Refer to The Case of the Cardiac Unit Nurse at the beginning of this chapter. Describe the lifestyle habits, based on what you learned in this chapter, that enable Gracie Chin to stay fit for her job as a cardiac nurse.
2. Jorge Chavez is a surgical technologist at a busy ambulatory surgical center. His full-time job requires that he spend many hours on his feet, that he stay mentally alert, and that he quickly and correctly respond to surgeons' requests. Jorge must balance his job with a busy family life. He and his wife have two small children whom he cares for while his wife attends college two evenings a week. Using the information in this chapter, develop a plan that will help Jorge stay healthy, avoid burnout, and remain an effective member of the health care team.

PROBLEM-SOLVING PRACTICE

Sandra is enrolled in a physical therapist assistant program and looking forward to getting her first job. Her father died recently and her elderly mother is making many demands on Sandra's time and energy. She calls Sandra at least once a day to ask questions, complain about how lonely she feels, or ask her daughter to run errands for her.

How can Sandra use the five-step problem-solving process to find ways to help her mother and, at the same time, ensure that she graduates and maintains a job?

SUGGESTED READINGS AND RESOURCES

Academy of Nutrition and Dietetics. www.eatright.org

Alcoholics Anonymous. www.alcoholics-anonymous.org

American Heart Association. www.heart.org

American Sexual Health Association. www.ashastd.org

Drug Abuse Information and Treatment Referral Line. 1-800-662-HELP (4357)

Mayo Clinic. www.mayoclinic.com

MedlinePlus. http://medlineplus.gov

Milliken, M. E., & Honeycutt, A. (2012). *Understanding human behavior: A guide for health care providers* (8th ed.). Clifton Park, NY: Delmar Cengage Learning.

Mind Tools (Extensive information on stress management). www.mindtools.com

My Plate www.choosemyplate.gov

National Council on Alcoholism and Drug Dependence. www.ncadd.org

National Eating Disorders Organization. www.nationaleatingdisorders.org

National Institute on Alcohol Abuse and Alcoholism. www.niaaa.nih.gov

Smoke Free. smokefree.gov

Substance Abuse and Mental Health Services Administration. http://www.samhsa.gov

U.S. Department of Agriculture, Center for Nutrition Policy and Promotion. www.usda.gov/cnpp

U.S. Department of Health and Human Services (HIV/AIDS information). http://aids.gov

This page intentionally left blank

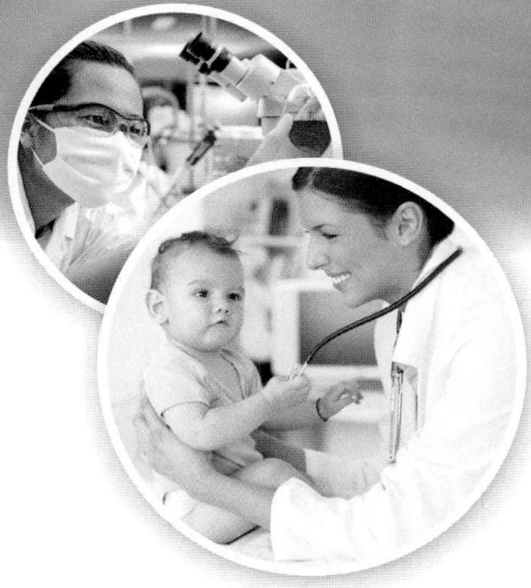

Chapter 13

Professionalism

OBJECTIVES

Studying and applying the material in this chapter will help you to:

- Explain the meaning of professionalism for individuals who work in health care.
- Describe each of the following components of professionalism:
  - Attitude
  - Behaviors
  - Health care skills
  - Appearance
- Explain the meaning of "professional distance."
- Explain how health care professionals can effectively handle difficult situations.
- Describe how to accept criticism professionally.
- Explain how professional organizations help individuals who work in health care increase their level of professionalism.
- Identify the characteristics of a health care leader.

KEY TERMS

continuing education
leadership
professional distance
professionalism

The Case of the Lost Opportunity

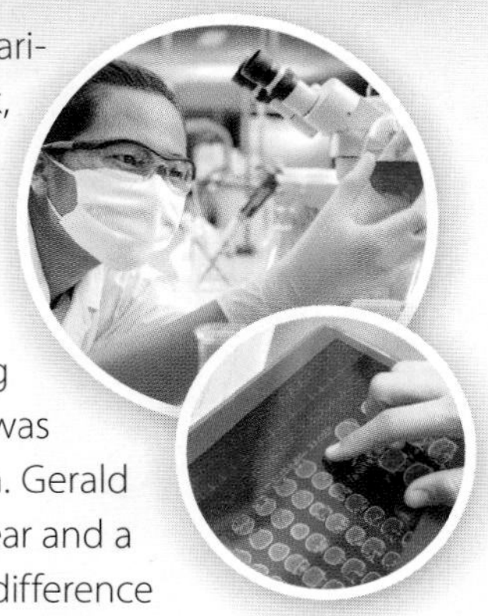

Gerald Lenz has worked as an ultrasound technician for just over three years. He performs a variety of duties at a large imaging center. Gerald does what is necessary to complete his work, but believes that his job consists of using his technical skills. He performs them adequately, but makes no effort to "go out of his way" for either his coworkers or patients. Although he is never rude, it is clear to patients that working with them is simply a job Gerald performs in exchange for a salary. Gerald never volunteers to work on extra projects, never contributes new ideas at staff meetings, and never participates in special activities offered outside working hours. Ultrasound technicians are in short supply in Gerald's city, so he remains employed. He was recently passed over for a promotion because his supervisor believed he lacks professionalism. Gerald was disappointed and could not understand why someone who had worked there for just a year and a half got the position instead of him. In this chapter you will learn about behaviors that make the difference between just getting by on the job and making a positive, professional contribution.

THE MEANING OF PROFESSIONALISM

Professionalism is an essential quality for everyone who works in health care. We often hear someone described as being "very professional" or "acting professionally." Professionalism is difficult to define because it consists of many characteristics and behaviors. Individuals in all health care occupations display professionalism by dedicating themselves to doing their best on the job and providing and maintaining high-quality service. "Caring competence" is one way to express the meaning of **professionalism** in health care.

The confidence patients have in the care they receive is influenced by each individual they have contact with in the health care system. Health care professionals represent the facilities in which they work. Their actions are a reflection of all the services and people who work there.

Professional Attitude

Attitude, discussed in Chapter 12, refers to the way a person thinks and feels about someone or something. Individuals working in health care who have professional attitudes approach work as positively and enthusiastically as possible. They think in terms of what they can give rather than what they can get. Patient welfare is the primary focus of the employee with a professional attitude, and studies have shown that the attitude of the health care professional has a significant effect on patients. This is true whether the task is preparing accurate billing statements or providing direct patient care.

A professional attitude in health care work can be expressed in many ways:

- Be committed to your work. Believe in the value of what you are doing and your ability to do it.
- Keep in mind your impact on patient care and services. Aim to contribute positively to the well-being of patients and their perception of the facility.
- Use an objective approach to situations. This means considering the facts rather than responding emotionally. For example, if a patient you have assisted is rude, think about possible causes. The rudeness may be a reaction to fear or pain and have nothing to do with you personally.
- View problems as opportunities for positive action. Problems are part of everyday life, and learning to deal with them effectively is essential for achieving work success and satisfaction. (Review the five-step problem-solving process described in Chapter 1.)
- Develop and practice self-discipline. Knowing you can depend on yourself to accomplish what needs to be done results in both competence and self-confidence.

Fascinating Facts

When employees in two large-scale studies were asked, "What makes you feel successful at work?" more than half the respondents answered, "Doing a good job."

Professional Behaviors

A professional attitude provides the foundation for developing professional behaviors, and these behaviors are what demonstrate "caring competence." The actions of health care professionals directly influence the level of patient satisfaction. Poor outcomes as well as malpractice lawsuits increase when patients are dissatisfied with the service they receive. Patients are health care consumers, and good service increases consumer loyalty. (See Chapter 23.)

The following behaviors are important expressions of professional conduct:

- Be dependable. Follow through on assignments, meet deadlines, and be on the job and on time as scheduled.
- Perform all duties as assigned and needed. "It's not my job" is rarely heard in today's facilities because employees who say it are not employed for long. (An exception is if a health care professional is asked to do a task that he or she is not trained or legally allowed to perform.) Willingness to always do one's best is the sign of a true professional.
- Be flexible. Health care work is continually changing. Willingness to adapt to these changes is essential.
- Accept differences. Today's patient population is increasingly diverse. (See Chapter 15 for information on cultural diversity.)
- Be aware of how your actions affect others. Treat everyone with courtesy and consideration.
- Practice good communication skills. (See Chapters 15 and 16.)
- Put personal problems aside during work time. Do not discuss them with coworkers or patients. And *never* complain about your work, supervisor, or the facility while you are in the workplace. Patients who hear such complaints may lose confidence in the care they are receiving. Complaining can also negatively affect the morale of coworkers. Keep your conversations focused on creating positive relationships and solving problems rather creating them. (See Figure 13–1.)
- Be well organized and plan your work. For example, gather all equipment and supplies before beginning a procedure so the patient does not have to wait.

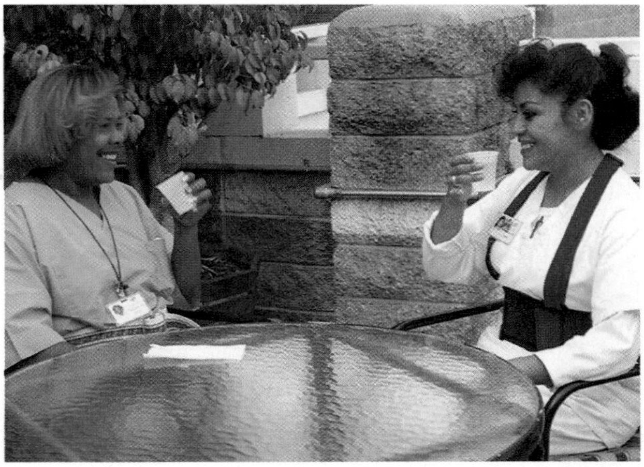

FIGURE 13–1 Keep conversation positive. Avoid complaining about the workplace with coworkers. Instead, focus on how you and your coworkers can make helpful contributions.

- Behave ethically at all times and set high personal standards. (See Chapter 3.)
- Conduct yourself calmly. This is especially important in emergencies and upsetting situations, when it is necessary to think clearly. Remaining calm also helps patients, who look to health care professionals for reassurance.
- Serve as a role model for good health. As a health care professional, you have an opportunity to encourage good health habits in others. (See Chapter 12.)
- Set professional goals and aim for continual improvement.

Fascinating Facts

According to Stephen Covey, author of best-selling books on personal effectiveness, the average person spends 80% of his or her time interacting with others. For most people, then, the majority of their waking hours is spent interacting or communicating with other people—or dealing with the poor results of that interaction.

Professional Health Care Skills

Achieving and maintaining a high level of skill is a critical component of professionalism. Tasks must be performed correctly and carefully. Pay attention and think about what you are doing at all times. Nothing can be taken for granted or become routine. Approach each patient as an individual who deserves your best efforts. Here are additional suggestions for developing your skill level:

- Develop an in-depth understanding of your work. Learn as much as possible about the theories that support your skills. This will increase the level of your performance and provide a foundation for good decision making and problem solving.
- Observe and listen carefully. Question situations that do not seem right given the circumstances.
- Consult the employee manual at your workplace or ask questions if you are unsure about a policy or procedure.
- Perform all work as neatly and accurately as possible.
- Dedicate time to acquiring new knowledge and skills. (See Chapter 14.)

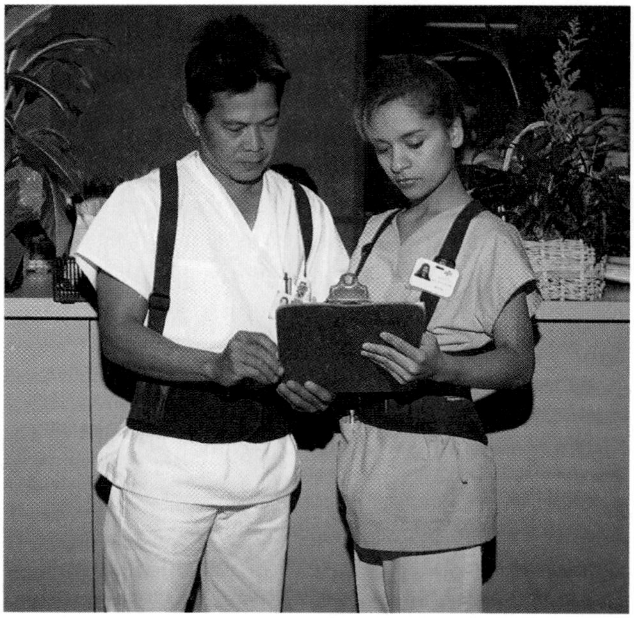

FIGURE 13–2 What positive messages are communicated by the appearance of these health care professionals? What effect do you think they have on patients?

Professional Appearance

The appearance of those who work in health care occupations is an outward sign of their level of professionalism. It strongly influences the way they are perceived by patients and coworkers. A professional appearance communicates the message, "I take my job and myself seriously. I have self-respect and want patients to have confidence in my abilities."

Professional appearance in health care settings is generally conservative. Some popular fashion trends, such as tattoos and body piercing, were at one time associated with antisocial groups. This is why some patients find them offensive and even frightening. As more people have tattoos and piercings, they are becoming accepted by increasing numbers of employers. However, because extremes in appearance can undermine patients' confidence in the care they receive, it is still best to maintain a fairly conservative appearance. This may or may not include wearing a uniform. It is a sign of respect for patients to consider their feelings when planning your appearance. (See Figures 13–2 and 13–3.) Maintaining a professional appearance includes the following:

- Practice personal cleanliness. This includes the hair, hands and fingernails, clothing, and shoes.

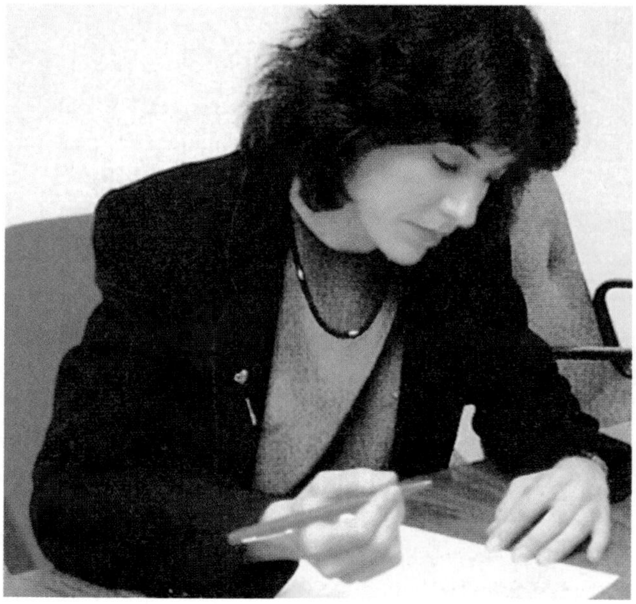

FIGURE 13–3 When the job requires regular clothing, it should be neat and conservative.

- Avoid long and/or painted fingernails. Color on nails can hide dirt that harbors bacteria.
- Use a deodorant or antiperspirant daily.

- Pay attention to dental hygiene. Flossing and regular dental care help prevent bad breath.
- Avoid the use of perfumes and strong-smelling hair sprays and other personal products. Some people are allergic to fragrances. Many others find them offensive, especially when they are ill. Some fragrances can even trigger asthmatic attacks.
- Avoid extreme styles in dress and grooming, such as unnaturally colored hair and green nail polish. When possible, wear clothing that covers tattoos.
- Consider personal safety and that of others. Avoid wearing anything that can be grabbed or caught, such as dangling earrings and untied long hair. Wear closed-toed shoes to protect your feet from injury.

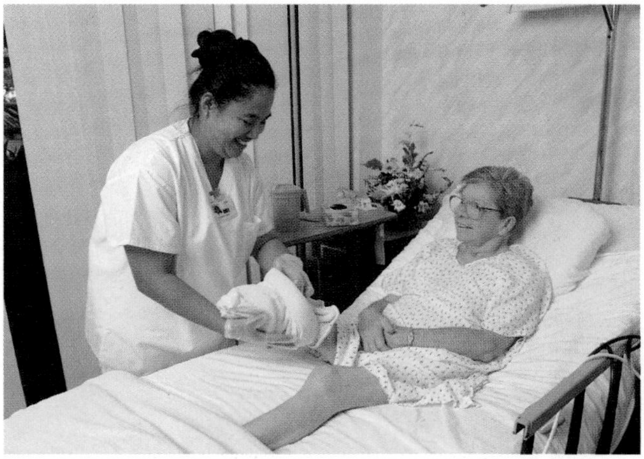

FIGURE 13–4 Professional distance requires focusing on the health care needs of the patient while expressing caring concern.

Professional Distance

Professional distance refers to a healthy balance in the health professional–patient relationship. It means demonstrating a caring attitude toward patients without the goal of becoming their friend. Although it is appropriate to seek personal satisfaction from work, it is inappropriate to personally depend on the friendship and approval of patients. Working to please, rather than serve appropriately, can be counterproductive. Keep your focus on the patients' health goals and what must be done to achieve them. At the same time, it is appropriate to demonstrate a caring attitude toward patients. (See Figure 13–4.)

Handling Difficult Situations Professionally

Health care professionals sometimes deal with challenging and stressful situations. It is natural to react emotionally when faced with an emergency, the death of a child, or an angry patient. Such a response, however, can interfere with your effectiveness. An objective, although not unfeeling, response is necessary for the health care professional to perform professionally and constructively.

Being professional requires that you know yourself well and make an effort to understand the basis of your reactions to workplace problems. Learning to recognize the causes of a behavior can help you change it, if necessary. For example, Keith has always had a quick temper. He finds it difficult to be patient and becomes easily irritated by incidents involving disorder, delays, and disorganization. His work as a pharmacy technician in a busy hospital does not always go smoothly, and Keith's impatience is negatively affecting his relationships with coworkers. When he takes time to analyze his behavior and sees that it follows a lifelong pattern, he realizes that he must learn to make adjustments and adapt to workplace conditions.

The problem-solving model described in Chapter 1 provides a constructive way to deal with difficult situations. Reviewing and gathering information, as described in the model, helps to separate fact from emotion. Facts provide a basis on which to identify potentially effective resolutions to problems and to make sound decisions.

Professional Acceptance of Criticism

Criticism and correction can be valuable learning resources. These opportunities to learn are often lost because it is hard for people to admit that they might be wrong. It is common to react defensively in these situations and miss the message. Responding gracefully to criticism is a sign of professionalism and self-confidence. Health care professionals who feel secure about themselves are comfortable with suggestions about their work and conduct. They are able to evaluate the information and decide if it applies to them. Being willing to recognize and work

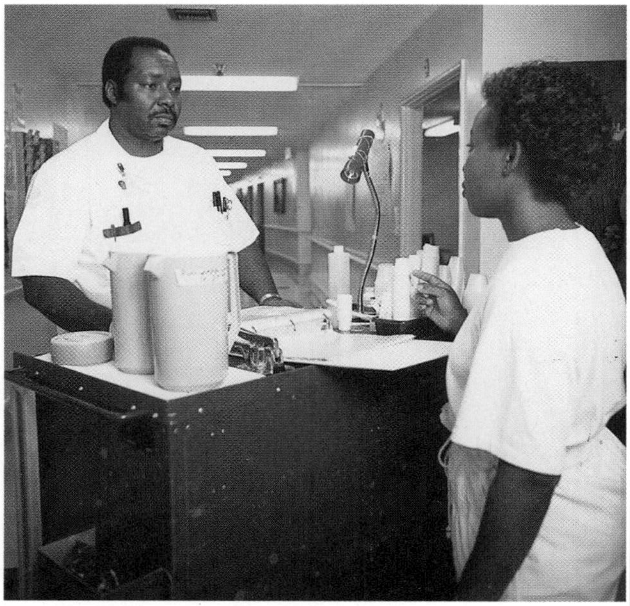

FIGURE 13–5 Accepting criticism gracefully is the sign of a professional who is willing to see it as a learning opportunity.

on imperfections is a sign of emotional maturity and professionalism. (See Figure 13–5.) Chapter 23 contains more information about giving and receiving criticism.

Thinking It Through

An important part of Torst Borgen's work as a physical therapy assistant is working with postoperative patients in their homes. His job is to help them regain strength and range of motion. Exercises prescribed by the supervising physical therapist are often uncomfortable and Torst must encourage as well as instruct patients to perform them. Torst lives alone and enjoys the social aspects of working with patients. He wants them to like him. This sometimes makes it difficult for him to insist that they engage in necessary exercises that are painful.

1. How might Torst's need to be friends with patients interfere with their full recovery?
2. What changes are needed in his view of his role as a physical therapy assistant?
3. What actions in his personal life can he take to achieve the professional distance necessary to best assist patients in their recovery?

Thinking It Through

Certified nursing assistant Barbara Sterndorf has difficulty working independently in her job at Pinehurst Care Home, an extended care facility. Barbara was raised by parents who were quite critical, and she lacks self-confidence. She is afraid of making mistakes and only does exactly what she is directed to do by her supervisor, Carla Thomas. In spite of her self-doubts, Barbara always performs high-quality work and is well liked by the residents. Carla believes her to be well trained and among the most competent CNAs on the staff and tells her this during Barbara's performance evaluation.

1. What might Barbara do to increase her self-confidence at work?
2. How might her self-image and work habits hold her back from advancing in her career?

PROFESSIONAL ORGANIZATIONS

Participating actively in a professional organization can contribute positively to professional development. Most health care occupations have an organization whose purposes include the following:

- Promoting the profession
- Ensuring quality patient care by making certain that professionals have the necessary knowledge and skill sets
- Sponsoring **continuing education** (learning experiences beyond those needed to earn the initial certificate or degree to work in an occupation). Some organizations, such as the American Association for Respiratory Care, offer leadership courses to help their members advance in their professions.
- Encouraging networking among members
- Supporting legislation on behalf of the profession and health care in general

Serving on committees, volunteering to help with projects, and running for office are excellent ways to become involved. There are many advantages for health care professionals who participate at any level:

- Learning to work in a group to achieve common goals
- Meeting established professionals who can offer career advice and serve as positive role models

- Keeping current in the field
- Developing management skills
- Receiving the support and encouragement of colleagues

See Appendix 1 for a list of health care professional organizations.

PROFESSIONAL LEADERSHIP

Leadership involves encouraging people to work together and do their best to achieve common goals. Leaders combine visions of excellence with the ability to inspire others. They promote positive changes that benefit their professions and the people they serve. A leader may or may not be a supervisor. It is possible to set an example of excellence and encourage others without having a position of authority.

Characteristics of effective leaders in health care include the following:

- A high level of competence in their profession
- Commitment to providing high-quality service
- Willingness to recognize and support the work of others
- Dedication to meeting high standards
- Belief that necessary changes and improvements can be accomplished
- Willingness to serve as an example and complete the tasks necessary to achieve the goals of the group
- Ability to communicate effectively

Media Link

To test your mastery of this material, go to the Online Resources to play interactive games and complete the quiz for this chapter.

WORKBOOK PRACTICE

Go to your workbook and complete the exercises for this chapter.

SUGGESTED LEARNING ACTIVITIES

1. Find examples of people you think exhibit professional characteristics. Explain why you chose them.
2. Rate your own level of professionalism in each of the following categories:
   - Attitude
   - Conduct
   - Appearance
   - Health care skills

Based on your ratings, create a plan to develop and/or improve your professionalism.

3. Interview a health care supervisor about his or her definition of professionalism.
4. Using the material in this chapter as a guide, create your own description of professionalism in your occupational area.

WEB ACTIVITIES

National Consortium for Health Science Education
www.healthscienceconsortium.org

On the left of the screen in the Navigation box, click on "Healthcare Standards." In the body of the linked page, click on "National Healthcare Foundation Standards and Accountability Criteria." Review the 11 standards. Choose one and discuss how the criteria relate to health care professionalism.

Professional Organizations

Explore the website of the professional organization(s) for careers of interest. (See Appendix 1 for a list of professional organizations and their contact information.) Does the organization contain a definition of professionalism for its members? What opportunities does it provide for members to develop professionally?

REVIEW QUESTIONS

1. What is meant by professionalism in health care?
2. Give five examples of how professionalism is exhibited in each of the following areas:
   - Attitude
   - Behaviors
   - Skills
   - Appearance
3. Explain the meaning of "professional distance."

4. How can learners prepare themselves to handle difficult situations they may encounter in the workplace?
5. What is meant by accepting criticism professionally?
6. What are the benefits of participating in a professional organization?
7. What are seven characteristics of a leader?

APPLICATION EXERCISES

1. What changes does Gerald Lenz, described in The Case of the Lost Opportunity at the beginning of the chapter, need to make in order to increase his level of professionalism as an ultrasound technician?
2. Karin is a dental receptionist for Dr. Sims. She arrives at the office on Monday morning to face the beginning of "one of those days." A long-time patient who has suffered all weekend with a toothache is waiting at the door. The dental hygienist is ill and will not be in, leaving seven patients without appointments. When notified that they will have to reschedule, two patients are very unhappy and express their irritation to Karin. Later in the morning, the office computer freezes up, and the scheduling and billing programs cannot be accessed. In the afternoon, an elderly patient returns to the office after his appointment to say that his car won't start. He asks for help to get it started or to find other transportation home. Discuss how Karin can handle each situation professionally. Include professional attitude as well as actions.

PROBLEM-SOLVING PRACTICE

Max is a licensed practical nurse who has been working in the oncology (cancer) unit of a local hospital for just over a year. He is finding it more and more difficult to remain objective and not become emotionally involved with the patients and their families. It is beginning to disrupt his sleep and he is worried that his feelings might negatively affect his ability to provide the help his patients need. How can Max use the five-step problem-solving process to help maintain a healthy professional distance?

SUGGESTED READINGS AND RESOURCES

Makely, S. (2013). *Professionalism in health care: A primer for career success* (4th ed.). Upper Saddle River, NJ: Prentice Hall.

Mind Tools. www.mindtools.com (Click on "Leadership Skills.") http://ispub.com/IJANP/10/1/10734

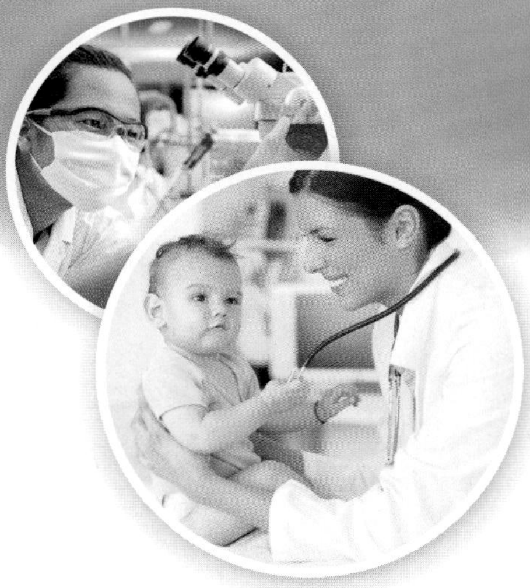

Chapter 14

Lifelong Learning

OBJECTIVES

Studying and applying the material in this chapter will help you to:

- Understand and explain the importance of lifelong learning for the health care professional.
- List the reasons for participating in continuing education opportunities.
- Describe ways you can earn continuing education units.
- List ways to incorporate self-directed learning into your daily life.
- Create a personal plan for self-directed learning.

KEY TERMS

continuing education units (CEUs)
continuing professional education (CPE)
demographics
lifelong learning
self-directed learning

The Case of Lifetime Success

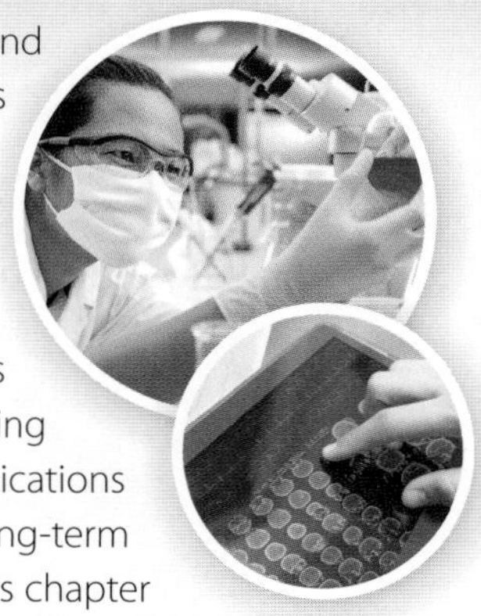

Mabel Bennett has worked in medical records for many years—so many that she likes to joke and tell people that records were handwritten with feather pens when she started. Mabel enjoys tasks that involve detail and order. She has always received satisfaction from the challenge of maintaining complete and accurate records and has risen to the position of medical records manager at a large suburban rehabilitation hospital. Over the years, Mabel has seen many changes in her field. Her first position was keeping paper records for a country doctor at a time when no one had even thought about desktop computers. Through the years, Mabel has pursued every available opportunity to learn more about her field and has enjoyed her learning experiences. She was one of the first in her profession to realize the potential of computer applications in medical records and became an expert user of computer technology. Mabel credits her long-term career success to her interest in learning all she can and working with the future in mind. In this chapter you will learn ways in which successful health care professionals like Mabel acquire the knowledge they need to stay current and advance in their fields.

IMPORTANCE OF LIFELONG LEARNING

Lifelong learning refers to all purposeful learning activities, both formal and informal, that take place throughout our lives. Today, lifelong learning is more important than ever, because the world is changing faster than at any other time in history. Until the mid-20th century, people could expect to live in much the same way as their parents and grandparents had. Current advancements in technology now produce significant changes during a single lifetime. For example, people who today are in their seventies grew up without television. Those in their fifties began their professional lives without personal computers, handheld calculators, cellular phones, and many other products that are now considered necessities in the workplace.

Today, most people take change for granted and incorporate it into their lifestyles. They are no longer surprised by the constant stream of new products available, or the speed of the changes in these products that require them to be updated even before they are worn out by use. What new health care professionals may find surprising is *how much learning will be required after graduation* in order to keep up with the many changes that affect the way jobs are performed. For example, many people in the workforce today learned to use a personal computer *after* they had completed their formal education and were already employed. They had to take the time to read manuals, attend workshops, watch videos, or use tutorials to learn to use what has now become an essential tool in most workplaces. And the need to learn in the area of computers alone will continue to grow as new applications and updated versions of software and hardware are developed. (See Chapter 18.)

Keeping Up with Changes in Health Care

Changes in the delivery of health care are taking place continually. Knowledge quickly becomes outdated, and within a few years of entering the health care field, an individual who fails to keep up with current information will become incompetent. Your graduation, then, marks the end of formal training and the beginning of lifelong learning.

In addition to technology, the social and **demographic** changes and trends discussed in Chapter 2 require that health care professionals acquire new knowledge and skills. See Table 14–1 for examples of changes and the corresponding learning requirements for health care professionals. Standard precautions, explained in Chapter 10, are now common knowledge in the workplace. And yet they are actually a recent development, created in 1987 in response to the spread of the human immunodeficiency virus (HIV) and hepatitis B. Health care professionals who work in certain positions must be trained and tested on various standards, including undergoing annual reviews. Health information professionals must continue to update their knowledge of contract management, patient eligibility, and billing procedures. And the shift in patient demographics has meant that a

Table 14–1 Changes That Affect Health Care

Changes	Corresponding Learning Needs of Health Care Professionals
People living longer	Developmental stages and needs of older adults Patient care skills for long-term care Care of patients with chronic conditions
Increasing numbers of patients diagnosed with Alzheimer's disease and other forms of dementia	Care of dementia patients
Hospital stays that are much shorter than in the past	Home health patient practices and techniques Patient education delivery techniques
Increased ethnic and cultural diversity of U.S. population	Diverse customs and health habits Languages other than English
Growing patient interest in complementary health care practices, such as acupuncture and holistic medicine	Knowledge of complementary and alternative medicine Understanding of how the use of complementary and alternative health care practices is affecting Western medical practices
Increase in third-party payers	Coding and billing practices Contract administration, obtaining preauthorizations for treatment, and permission for referral to specialists
Emphasis on wellness and patients' responsibility for their own health	Prevention practices to ward off diseases and disorders Patient education on wellness and prevention techniques
Increased computerization	Computer applications in health care: administration, diagnostics, treatment, and education Computer operation skills and knowledge of software programs
Increased use of electronic health records, along with the use of more specific diagnostic and treatment codes	Knowledge of electronic health records and new codes
Spread of hepatitis viruses, return of communicable diseases, such as measles, and threat of viruses due to globalization	Use of standard precautions Symptoms, treatment, and prevention of specific diseases
Increase in drug-resistant bacteria	Ability to educate patients about proper use of antibiotics, including when they are not necessary
Expansion of roles for health care professionals	Increased skill base Flexibility and willingness to perform a variety of tasks
Increased specialization and use of teams to provide patient care	Teamwork skills Intraprofessional and interprofessional communication skills
Development of increasingly sophisticated equipment	Operation of equipment and interpretation of results
New information about how the human body functions	New discoveries that affect the professional's occupational area
New diagnostic procedures and treatments	Information and skills that apply to the professional's occupational area
Implementation of the Patient Protection and Affordable Care Act	Education of new patients in how to use the health care system

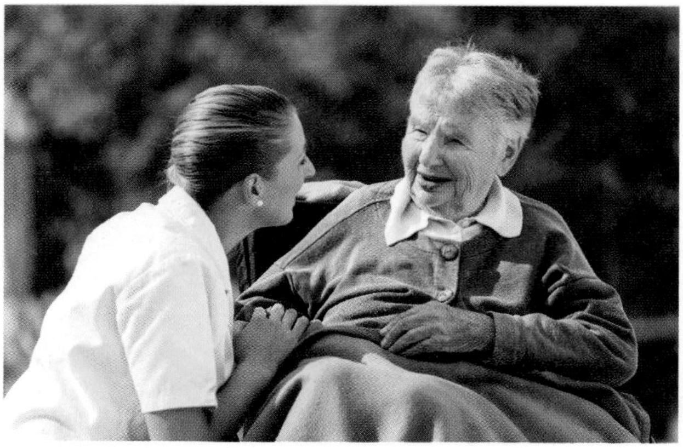

FIGURE 14–1 Health care professionals must continue to learn about the needs of older patients in order to provide appropriate care for this growing segment of the population.

large percentage of those who provide direct patient care will spend much of their time working with older adults. (See Figure 14–1.)

Many health care occupations have expanded their scope of practice in an effort to increase the efficiency of patient care delivery. Professionals who previously performed a limited set of tasks are now being cross-trained and becoming multi skilled. Examples of additional duties some facilities are assigning to medical assistants include the following: serving as health coaches and navigators, visiting homes of patients to perform risk assessments, working as pharmacy technicians, and performing the duties of a limited license radiological technician. (Note that some of these duties require additional formal training.)

CONTINUING EDUCATION UNITS

Continuing education units (CEUs) are the credits granted for certain types of learning that take place after the completion of formal education. This type of education is also referred to as **continuing professional education (CPE)**. Most forms of professional approval, such as licensure, certification, and registration, require that a specific number of CEUs be earned in order to be renewed. Health care professionals should find out the requirements for their occupations well in advance of licensure and certification renewal dates to allow adequate time to meet them. Most professional organizations and licensing boards have sites on the Internet that explain their continuing education requirements.

The amount of time, as well as the activities involved, vary for earning CEUs. Some credits are granted for assignments completed or tests passed; others require class or workshop attendance. Many schools and organizations offer classes and activities that award CEUs. However, the organizations that grant licenses, certifications, and registrations decide which CEUs they will accept. Not all courses and activities are accepted by all organizations. Before engaging in any activity for the purpose of earning CEUs, be sure that it has been approved by the necessary professional or regulatory organization.

If you participate in workshops or other activities, be *sure* to sign in. Also, ask for a certificate verifying attendance or completion of work. These will be needed as proof that units were earned. Keep certificates in a safe place. Some approval agencies require that they be kept for at least four years. Inquire whether your professional organization maintains a tracking system for CEUs earned by members. Some make a practice of sending out regular "statements" of units earned. These may be kept online and available for you to review. This is a good way for health care professionals to avoid getting caught short at renewal time.

Ways to Earn CEUs

There are many ways to earn CEUs. Health care professional organizations offer a variety of convenient ways to help their members stay current in their field. They can provide you with information about how many CEUs are needed, which subject areas they must be in, and how they can be earned. In addition to traditional classes and workshops, there are other ways to obtain CEUs:

- Special sessions and workshops offered at annual meetings, conferences, and conventions sponsored by professional health care organizations; may require taking a quiz, completing an assignment, or demonstrating in some other way that you have met the objectives

  Example CEUs can be earned at the national convention of the American Physical Therapy Association.

- Home study materials published in professional journals

  Example Members can read designated articles published in *CMA Today* (published by the

American Association of Medical Assistants [AAMA]) and earn units by passing online quizzes about the articles' content. The AAMA articles are available both in the print form of the journal and online.

- Online study courses sponsored by professional organizations

  Examples The American Association for Respiratory Care has online courses, some of them free, in various formats, including live webcasts; the National Association for Practical Nurse Education and Service offers a variety of courses online at its Online Learning Center.

- Home study courses offered by approved educational providers

  Examples Tech Lectures (www.techlectures.com) is a company that offers a series of printed lectures and exams that enable pharmacy technicians to earn CEUs that are accepted by the Pharmacy Technician Certification Board and the Institute for the Certification of Pharmacy Technicians. Speedy CEUs offers courses for nurses that are approved by the California Board of Registered Nurses and accepted by all states except Delaware.

- Distance education courses offered by colleges and universities—many courses are now available over the Internet; a growing number of institutions provide for-credit classes that include interaction with the instructor and other students

  Example University of Phoenix, based in Phoenix, Arizona, was one of the first to develop and offer distance education courses for credit. Its Web address is www.phoenix.edu. Today, dozens of colleges and universities offer online courses.

Fascinating Facts

Evidence of the vast amount of medical and health information available: The U.S. Library of Medicine indexes articles from 5400 of the world's leading biomedical journals. To make this information searchable for readers, there are 27,149 descriptors (subject headings) related to the articles.

Source: U.S National Library of Medicine Fact Sheet: Medical Subject Headings (MeSH®). http://www.nlm.nih.gov/pubs/factsheets/mesh.html.

Thinking It Through

Jan Summers loves her work as an occupational therapy assistant. One of the reasons that Jan wanted to be an occupational therapy assistant was because she likes to interact with other people. Her outgoing personality helps her develop good relationships with patients, and her cheerful disposition makes her a popular assistant. Jan looks forward to the annual occupational therapy conferences, held in different cities around the country. They provide opportunities to see friends she has made in the profession and catch up on all the news. What Jan does not enjoy is attending the informational meetings and workshops. She finds them "boring." She has talked some of her friends into signing her name on the attendance rosters and, so far, has not been caught. In this way she manages to accumulate the credits needed to renew her certification to practice.

1. Even if Jan is not caught, what are the possible future consequences of her failure to attend the meetings and workshops?
2. Is Jan maintaining professional ethical standards? Why or why not?
3. What is the possible impact on her patients?
4. What is the possible impact on her future career?

Not all providers of learning opportunities are high quality, and not all courses are beneficial simply because they grant CEUs. Consider the following criteria for choosing courses and materials that offer maximum value for the time and money invested:

- Recommendations from your professional and/or certification organization
- Skill and knowledge requirements of your current job
- Future career goals
- Credibility and reputation of the educational provider
- Areas of personal and professional weakness that need improvement
- Personal and professional interests

SELF-DIRECTED LEARNING

Knowing how to learn is essential to updating your knowledge and acquiring new skills throughout your career. Learning is not limited to formal classroom

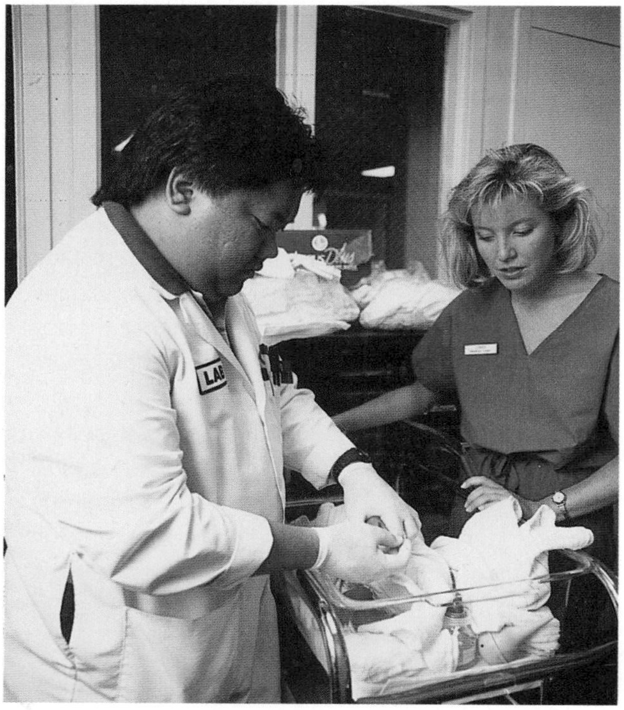

FIGURE 14–2 Health care professionals can learn a lot by observing others at work.

settings or experiences for the purpose of earning CEUs. **Self-directed learning** refers to all activities that you plan and participate in to increase your knowledge and skills. There are many ways to incorporate learning into your daily life:

- Observe others: Watch how successful, experienced professionals perform their duties. (See Figure 14–2.)
- Ask questions: Learn from the expertise of others. Most people are happy to share what they know. Be sure to choose an appropriate time to ask questions. For example, do not ask questions about patients in their presence or when the other professional is very busy and cannot stop to talk.
- Read books and journal articles: Plan a regular time to keep up on publications related to your occupational area. Most professional organizations publish a newsletter or journal. In addition, there are hundreds of specialized journals that cover medical and health care topics. A list of medical journals, including links to articles accessible at no charge, is available at www.biomedcentral.com. Many large health care facilities have libraries for employees. Some have libraries open to patients and the public. Many universities and colleges allow the public to use their libraries. Some offer checkout privileges for an annual fee. Libraries have become highly computerized. Do not hesitate to ask the librarian for assistance if you have trouble locating materials.
- Study in a small group: Organize a study group with other employees at work. Or, if you belonged to a study group at school, consider encouraging the members to meet regularly after you graduate. You can learn by sharing workplace experiences and working on selected topics to keep current in your field. (See Figure 14–3.) Important note: Remember that sharing personal or identifiable information about your patients is a breach of confidentiality.
- Study with a partner or mentor: You may prefer to work with just one other person who can support your learning efforts.
- Attend professional conferences and meetings: These often include lectures, workshops, and discussions of current topics.
- Watch online presentations, such as those on youtube.com, DVDs, and educational television programs; many DVDs are available for checkout at public libraries. Learning channels, public television stations, and those managed by local

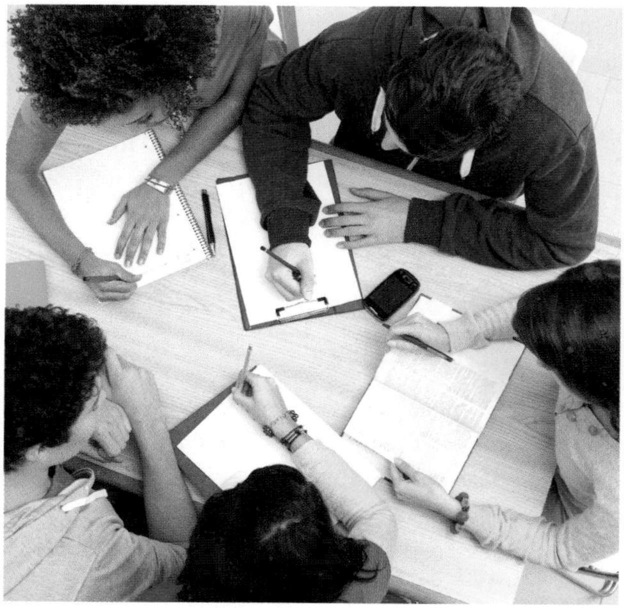

FIGURE 14–3 Studying in a small group allows the exchange of ideas and can be a productive way to learn.

universities often feature programs of interest to the health care professional. There are also cable channels devoted exclusively to medical issues.

- Explore the Internet: Information is available on all kinds of topics and in a variety of formats, including webcasts and videos.

Here are a few reliable health care websites to get you started:

- Centers for Disease Control and Prevention
  www.cdc.gov
- Mayo Clinic
  www.mayoclinic.com
- National Center for Health Statistics
  www.cdc.gov/nchs
- National Library of Medicine
  www.medlineplus.gov
- National Institute of Mental Health
  www.nimh.nih.gov
- National Institutes of Health
  http://health.nih.gov
- Web MD
  www.webmd.com

See Chapter 18 for tips on evaluating Internet sources.

Planning your own study activities allows you to take advantage of your preferred styles of learning, discussed in Chapter 1. Look for ways to make learning enjoyable and incorporate them into your daily life. Think of the world as a giant classroom that offers endless opportunities for learning. Keeping up with changes and adding to your knowledge and skill base should be part of your work routine. You will have the satisfaction of knowing that you are staying current and competent.

In addition to developing health care skills, you can advance your career by improving nontechnical skills. Oral and written communication, interpersonal relations, computer applications, and time management are examples of important skills that will help you get ahead.

WORKBOOK PRACTICE

Go to your workbook and complete the exercises for this chapter.

SUGGESTED LEARNING ACTIVITIES

1. Develop the habit of scanning popular magazines, such as *Bloomberg Businessweek*, and your local newspaper for health-related articles.
2. Visit your local public or university library. Review periodicals and books on health care. Are there helpful resources in your subject area? Many journals can now be accessed on the Internet.
3. Request a continuing education catalog from a local college or university. What types of courses are offered? Do you see any that might help you develop your personal or professional skills?
4. Choose a health topic you find interesting and conduct an Internet search. Record your findings and develop a webliography (a list of sites with name, Web address, and brief description of contents) of useful sites.
5. Explore the websites mentioned in this chapter.

WEB ACTIVITIES

National Library of Medicine—Medline Plus
www.medlineplus.gov

Choose three news articles listed under "Health News" to read and summarize.

National Library of Medicine—Medline
www.medline.gov

Click on "Videos & Cool Tools," then choose a topic of interest. View the slide show and write a list of facts you learned about the topic.

Innovation—Pharmaceutical Research and Manufacturers of America
www.innovation.org

Choose a topic to explore. Write a report describing what you learn about the role of pharmaceutical products in health care today.

Professional Organizations

Explore the website of the professional organization(s) for your career. (See Appendix 1.) What information does it contain about CEUs? Are there minimum requirements for your certification/licensure/registration (if applicable for your career)? What are various ways you can earn CEUs?

REVIEW QUESTIONS

1. Why is it essential for health care professionals to participate in lifelong learning activities?
2. What are five recent technological and demographic changes that require experienced health care professionals to acquire new knowledge and skills?
3. What is a continuing education unit?
4. Who determines which CEUs are accepted by professional and regulatory organizations?
5. What are five methods of earning CEUs?
6. What are eight ways to continue learning after graduation?

APPLICATION EXERCISES

1. Describe the methods for keeping up to date that Mabel Bennett, described in The Case of Lifetime Success, may have used throughout her career.
2. Debbie Yano is a practical (licensed) vocational nurse working for Dr. Cerutti in a single-physician office in a small town. Dr. Cerutti is a general practitioner and, because of the limited number of health care facilities in the area, many long-time patients rely on this caring physician for the majority of their health care needs. Debbie enjoys the variety of experiences encountered in her work with Dr. Cerutti: patients of all ages with all types of health issues. An important professional goal is to keep her skills up-to-date and to continue to acquire new ones. Learning opportunities are limited by her busy work schedule and family responsibilities and by living in a small town. Develop a comprehensive, long-term plan for Debbie to achieve her goal.

PROBLEM-SOLVING PRACTICE

Laura is pleased to have passed her exam and earned her certification as an occupational therapy assistant. How can she use the five-step problem-solving process to be sure she both stays up to date in her field and maintains her certification?

SUGGESTED READINGS AND RESOURCES

Agency for Healthcare Research and Quality. www.ahrq.gov

Mayo Clinic. www.mayoclinic.com

Medline Plus. www.nlm.nih.gov/medlineplus

National Center for Complementary and Alternative Medicine. http://nccam.nih.gov

National Center for Health Statistics. www.cdc.gov/nchs

National Institute of Mental Health. www.nimh.nih.gov

National Institutes of Health. http://health.nih.gov

National Library of Medicine. www.medlineplus.gov

World Health News (Harvard School of Public Health). http://worldhealthnews.harvard.edu

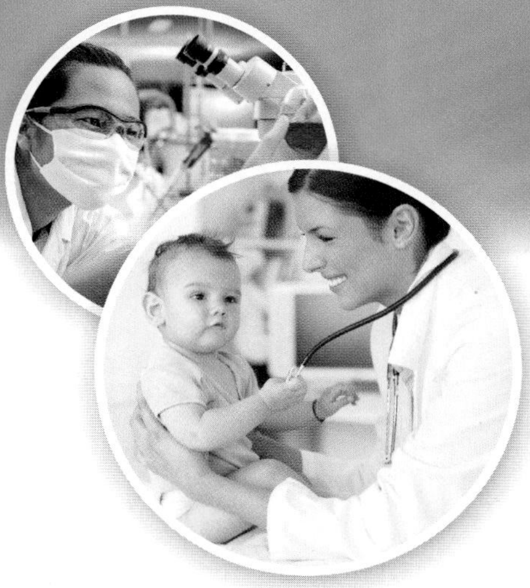

Unit 6

Communication in the Health Care Setting

This page intentionally left blank

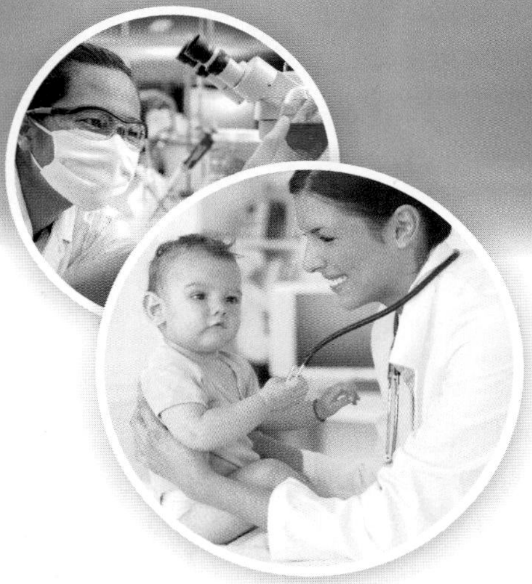

Chapter 15

The Patient as an Individual

OBJECTIVES

Studying and applying the material in this chapter will help you to:

- Explain the meaning of the philosophy of individual worth and how it applies to work in health care.
- Define *culture* and describe how it influences all aspects of human beliefs and behavior.
- Give examples of how different cultural groups approach issues of health.
- Describe how to determine the effect of cultural influences on the needs of patients.
- List the five levels of Maslow's hierarchy of needs and give an example of each.
- Recognize common defense mechanisms encountered in health care situations.
- Explain how the health care professional can help patients deal with the experience of loss.

KEY TERMS

culture
defense mechanism
dominant culture
Maslow's hierarchy of needs
personal space
philosophy of individual worth
physiological needs
prejudice
self-actualization
self-esteem

The Case of the Polite Patient

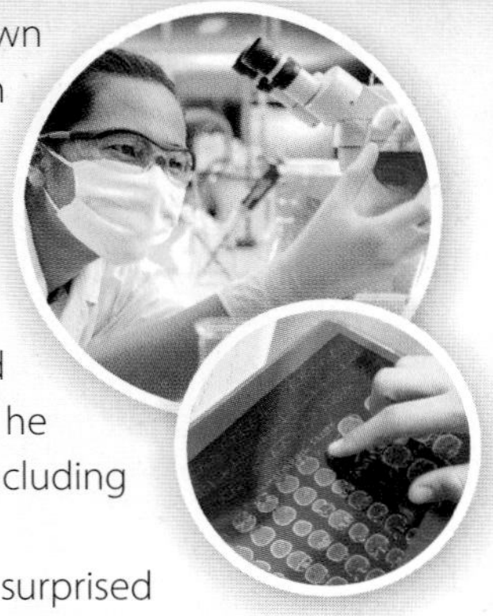

Shortly after graduation from a medical assistant program, Carley Ford moves from her small town to a large city 50 miles away. She has always wanted to experience city life and is excited when she is hired to work in a large downtown clinic. During her first week at the clinic, she meets with Mr. Alvarez, who was recently diagnosed with diabetes. His physician, Dr. Washington, believes that if Mr. Alvarez follows a diabetic diet and a regular plan of exercise, he may avoid having to take insulin injections. Carley spends about 10 minutes carefully explaining the eating plan recommended by Dr. Washington. She speaks slowly and clearly because she has noted that Mr. Alvarez does not speak English fluently. From time to time Carley asks Mr. Alvarez if he understands, and he nods to indicate that he does. She gives him a set of written instructions, including an eating plan, advising him to follow it carefully.

When Mr. Alvarez arrives for his follow-up appointment six months later, Dr. Washington is surprised that his condition has worsened. When he questions Mr. Alvarez—in Spanish—he learns that the elderly widower did not understand much of what Carley had explained to him. The written instructions were not helpful because Mr. Alvarez reads very little Spanish and no English at all. He has not cooked for himself since his wife died. Mr. Alvarez did not say anything to Carley about not understanding because "she was so nice and took her time" so he "didn't want to hurt her feelings." He also did not want to inconvenience the neighbors and family members who supply his meals by asking them to cook in a different way than they do for their families. This chapter discusses how to learn about individual patients in order to best help them meet their health care needs.

PATIENTS AS INDIVIDUALS

The well-being of patients depends on more than the technical competence of health care professionals. It is also very much affected by the attitude and concern expressed by everyone who works with them in the health care setting. Each patient is a complex individual who represents a combination of cultural influences, personal experiences, and basic human needs. Working effectively with patients, as well as with coworkers, requires understanding and appreciating the differences that make each person unique. The wide variety of people who make up the population of the United States today has been compared with a garden filled with flowers of every color and shape. Although each one is different, they all contribute to the overall beauty of the garden. The lesson for health care professionals is that working with a variety of patients can enrich their experience of giving service to fellow human beings. (See Figure 15–1.)

Philosophy of Individual Worth

The **philosophy of individual worth** is based on the belief that every human being, "regardless of personal circumstances or personal qualities, has worth and is entitled to respect as a human being" (Milliken & Honeycutt, 2004, p. 25). Health care professionals have the obligation to strive to give the same level of care to every patient, regardless of race, cultural background, economic status, behavior, physical condition, or sexual orientation. This is not always easy because patients can be rude, demanding, and uncooperative, behavior that is not uncommon when people are in pain, frightened, or anxious. Health care professionals have many tasks to accomplish in a limited amount of time. It is natural to resent people who

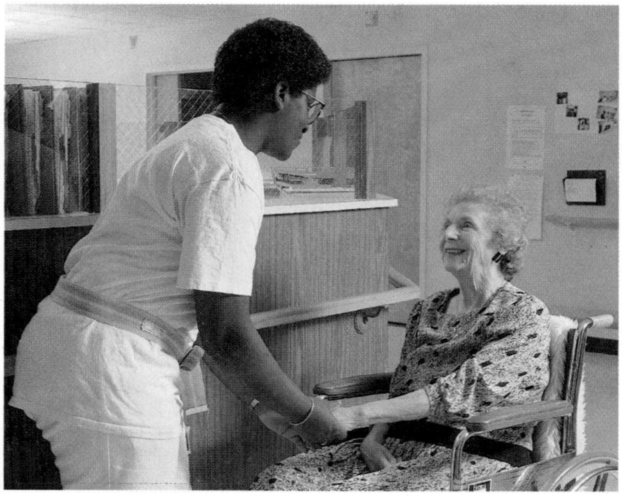

FIGURE 15–1 Every patient is worthy of your full attention and respect.

are unpleasant and make life more difficult. But it is at precisely these times that the philosophy of individual worth should serve as a reminder and motivator for health care professionals to do their best for every patient. Providing equal care to all, even under demanding circumstances, demonstrates the highest level of professionalism. Florence Nightingale, the founder of modern nursing, stated, "Souls deserve to be cared for" (Portillo, in Steefel, 2000). Caring for them effectively requires making sincere efforts to understand and accept them as they are.

Dealing with Prejudice

Prejudice, as used here, means having negative feelings about a person because he or she belongs to a specific cultural or racial group. It means assigning certain characteristics to an individual, often negative, based on assumptions about a group. Prejudice also refers to making unfavorable judgments about individuals because of characteristics such as obesity, poverty, and sexual preference. Prejudice prevents people from being considered as unique individuals.

Almost everyone has prejudices of some type. They are not always easy to recognize in ourselves because they become incorporated into our belief systems. They are taken for granted and become part of one's reality. It can be difficult to understand and accept that there are other acceptable ways of viewing the world. Health care professionals should make an effort to recognize their own prejudices by examining honestly how they regard others.

At the same time, it is not necessary to agree with all the beliefs and actions of others. In fact, some behaviors may be harmful to the health of the individual, and it is the duty of health care professionals to encourage positive changes. In order to do this, however, they must understand their patients' beliefs and motivations. And this understanding can only come by listening carefully and resisting the temptation to judge what is heard. When hearing information believed to be "incorrect," a common reaction is to stop listening. This prevents gathering the very information needed to begin to understand other people's points of view and the reasons for their beliefs.

THE MEANING OF CULTURE

The term **culture** refers to a wide range of factors that include values, shared beliefs and attitudes, social organization, family and personal relationships, language, everyday activities, religious practices, and concepts of time and space. Every individual is influenced, to a great extent, by his or her cultural background. Belief systems and customs are developed over time to help people make sense of their world. Accepted customs provide guidelines for behavior and actions so that daily life can proceed without constant decision making. They give life predictability and stability and provide the means for people to live together in relative harmony.

> **Fascinating Facts**
>
> Perhaps the greatest example of the application of the philosophy of individual worth was demonstrated by the life of Mother Teresa, who dedicated her life to working with, in her words, "the poorest of the poor." From 1948 until her death in 1997, Mother Teresa worked in Calcutta, India, caring for desperately poor people who were ill, abandoned, and dying. She founded the House for the Dying in 1952 to provide a place for people to die in peace and dignity. Over the years she created other sites that offered medical care and shelter to the needy all over the world. Mother Teresa put into action her belief that *every* human being is worthy of respect and loving care.

Culture gives direction to all aspects of life and provides a set of lenses through which the world is seen and interpreted. It is natural to take our own beliefs and way of life for granted. This is a common source of miscommunication because behaviors that are considered positive in one culture may be a sign of disrespect in another. For example, most people in the United States consider direct eye contact to be a sign of honesty and sincerity. In some cultures, however, it is a sign of boldness and disrespect. We often pat children on the head as a sign of affection. But in certain Asian cultures, the head is considered to be the location of the soul and touching it is a grave offense. It is important for health care professionals to recognize that everyone sees the world and interprets behavior in different ways.

Individuals and Culture

The United States is home to an increasingly diverse number of people from a variety of cultural backgrounds. Significant portions of the population are

Table 15–1 California Population Groups

Group	Percentage
White persons, not Hispanic	39%
African American	6.6%
Persons of Hispanic or Latino origin	38.4%
Asian person	14.1%
Foreign born	27.1%
Language other than English spoken at home	43.5%

Source: U.S. Census Bureau, http://quickfacts.census.gov/ qfd/states/06000.html

made up of people once considered to be members of "minority groups." Table 15–1 contains statistics that demonstrate the percentages of ethnic groups that made up the population of California in 2013. (See Figure 15–2.)

Immigrants come to the United States for a variety of reasons. Many who have arrived over the past 40 years have fled wars and unstable political conditions in their own countries. These immigrants are the most likely to live in close-knit communities. Older members tend to retain their native language and many customs.

There also exist other subcultures whose members, although born in the United States, have not fully integrated. The Chinese community in San Francisco is an example of a group that has retained the language and customs of the original culture over many generations. This does not mean that most members of ethnic groups, including recent immigrants and those who choose to retain traditional beliefs and customs, fail to learn the customs necessary to be successful in the United States. Many customs are quickly learned and integrated into daily life. Some behaviors retained from the culture of origin, however, are based on deeply held beliefs about what is important in life. Making the required changes to life in the United States may involve adopting new behaviors that are considered inappropriate in the original culture. Attitudes are much more difficult to recognize and change when they are based on important values.

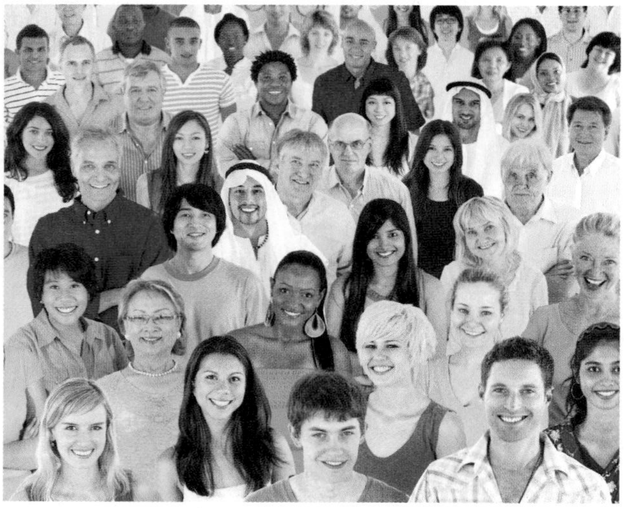

FIGURE 15–2 America's population is made up of dozens of ethnic groups.

Health care professionals must recognize that differences among people are sometimes based on cultural background. At the same time, they must take care to identify which cultural characteristics each individual patient or coworker has chosen to identify with and integrate into his or her lifestyle. Making assumptions about individuals based on the group to which they are believed to "belong" is disrespectful because it *takes away from their worth as individuals.* Assumptions also lead to mistakes in communication and misunderstandings. It is essential that health care professionals learn to observe, ask meaningful questions, and listen carefully to the responses. Using these skills, described later in this chapter, they can better meet the needs of all patients.

There is value in learning about the beliefs and practices of the cultural groups that health care professionals might encounter in their work. Gathering cultural information enables them to do the following:

- Realize and appreciate that there are many valid approaches to life. There is never an "only way" or even a "best way"
- Enrich and improve their own lives by increasing their knowledge of other cultures and discovering new ideas they might want to incorporate
- Avoid making the assumption that everything health care professionals do and say will be understood and appreciated
- Understand that certain beliefs *might* be held and certain customs *might* be practiced because of an individual's background
- Be sensitive to the possible needs of individuals who *appear* to be from specific cultural backgrounds and avoid taking actions that might

be offensive until more information can be obtained

- Ask appropriate and useful questions

When learning about different cultural groups, it is important to recognize that many common cultural groupings are actually composed of many subgroups that differ in customs and beliefs. For example, Asian Americans come from a wide variety of countries, including China, Japan, the Philippines, Korea, Laos, Cambodia, and Vietnam. Each of these countries has its own history, language, and customs. Spanish-speaking peoples, collectively called *Hispanics*, come from dozens of different countries and represent a variety of races and cultures.

Dominant Culture

The term **dominant culture**, as used here, refers to what are generally considered to be the foundational beliefs and ideal behavior of a society or country. These beliefs are generally considered to be necessary in order to be successful. This text, for instance, contains examples of attitudes that belong to the dominant culture of the United States:

- The importance of "being on time" and "using one's time effectively": Not all cultures believe that time is something to be controlled—or even that it *can* be controlled. Nor is punctuality an important concern. In some cultures, the belief is that everything will happen in its "own time" with or without the intervention of humans.
- The need to work efficiently: Interactions with people, even if a medical appointment or work assignment takes longer as a result, are given high priority by some cultures. If a health care professional moves quickly, even though competently, through a procedure and fails to inquire about the patient's family and engage in personal conversation, this may be viewed as indicating a lack of interest in and respect for the patient.
- The need to shake hands firmly when meeting new people: Recommended and even rehearsed for important occasions such as job interviews, this behavior is not universally practiced. In some cultures, only men are expected to shake hands and the handshake should be light, not firm. In others, handshakes are not common among persons of either sex. Other forms of greeting, such as a bow, may be used.

Personal Space and Personal Contact

Health care professionals who have close interactions with patients and coworkers daily, should understand customs regarding personal space and personal contact. **Personal space** refers to the distance at which people feel most comfortable when carrying on a conversation. In the dominant culture of the United States, a distance of about 18 inches is considered appropriate for people who know each other very well, such as family members and close friends. Two feet is considered appropriate for acquaintances and friends. In other cultures, such as some Middle Eastern societies, people stand very close together when talking. It is appropriate that each speaker feels the breath of the other. People from some of the Asian cultures, on the other hand, tend to maintain more distance when engaged in conversation.

Thinking It Through

Many nurses from the Philippines emigrate to work in the United States. Their educational training is similar and they can speak English. One thing that surprises them when they start work here is that part of their job is to provide personal care to patients. In the Philippines, it is family members who feed and help with hygiene tasks. One nurse reported that in the Filipino hospital where she worked, she had never seen a patient alone.

1. How do you think this might shape Filipino nurses' impressions of typical families in the United States?
2. How would you explain to them why in this country, personal care is typically performed by the nursing staff, such as nursing assistants?

In one U.S. health care facility, a Filipino nurse was reported to spend a lot of time on her phone during her shift. It was assumed that she was talking with her family and friends. It turned out that she was speaking with Filipino nurses in other parts of the hospital who considered her an expert and were calling her for advice.

1. Why do you think the nurses were calling a colleague in a different department, rather than asking for help from their supervisors or the other nurses on their shift?

Source of examples: Vestal, V., and Kautz, D. D. (2009). International perspectives: Responding to the similarities and differences between Filipino and American nurses. *Journal of Nursing Administration, 39*, 8–10. DOI: 10.1097/NNA.0b013e31818fe726.

The issue of touch is also relevant in health care. Many medical procedures involve parts of the body considered private by all cultural groups. It is important to be aware that the degree to which any type of physical contact is tolerated varies. For example, some cultures consider the examination of a female by a male physician to be unacceptable.

Harmless touching in one culture may be improper in another. As previously mentioned, patting a child on the head can cause extreme distress for some members of Asian cultures, including Vietnamese, because they believe that the spirits of their ancestors reside there. People who believe in reincarnation (rebirth of the soul in another body) may consider the issue of touch to be important even after death. The Hmongs, a group from Asia who immigrated to the United States as a result of the Vietnam War, fear that autopsies will cause the deceased to be born mutilated in the next life (Lee & Pfeifer, 2009/2010).

The most important point to understand is that generally there are no "correct" customs. Exceptions—that is, "incorrect customs"—would be those that are harmful or dangerous to oneself or others. The most important consideration for health care professionals is to establish an environment that is comfortable and reassuring for patients and that promotes their welfare. See Table 15–2 for information about major groups of American subcultures.

Table 15–2 Major Cultural Subgroups of the United States

African Americans		
Communication	**Time Orientation**	**Space**
May use African-American English	Present over future	Close personal space
May use slang, such as "bad" meaning "good" and other unique expressions	Flexible	Touching hair of another is sometimes offensive
Head-nodding does not necessarily mean agreement		
Nonverbal communication very important		
Direct eye contact often viewed as very rude		
Family	**Religion**	**Implications for Health Care**
Large, extended networks	Baptist (nearly 50%)	Do not label Black English as incorrect
Kinships formed with non-blood relatives	Often very religious	Clarify meaning of patient's words
Families often headed by female	Church is important in community	Clarify meaning of nonverbal communication
Unity and cooperation very important	Clergy highly respected	Be flexible with time
		Understand presence of extended family
Asian Americans		
Communication	**Time Orientation**	**Space**
Silence is valued	Present	Avoid physical closeness
Criticism, disagreement, and the word "no" are avoided		Usually do not touch others during conversation
Up-turned palm considered rude		Casual touch unacceptable with members of opposite sex
Direct eye contact considered rude		Head considered sacred, unacceptable to touch the head of another person

(continued)

Table 15–2 Major Cultural Subgroups of the United States (continued)

Asian Americans		
Family	**Religion**	**Implications for Health Care**
Structured and hierarchical	Buddism	Avoid excessive touch
Welfare of family valued above individual	Taoism	Touch head only when necessary and explain why
Ancestors are respected	Islam	Limit eye contact
Sharing, tradition, and loyalty very important	Christianity	Avoid gesturing with your hands
		Avoid confrontation and appearance of conflict

European Americans		
Communication	**Time Orientation**	**Space**
Eye contact is indication of interest and sincerity	Future over present	Northern European:
	Punctuality important	Close physical contact
		Handshakes for formal greetings
		Southern European:
		May hug, touch casually when conversing
Family	**Religion**	**Implications for Health Care**
Nuclear family—parents and children—is the basic unit	Christianity	Respect personal space
	Judaism	Use direct eye contact
		Respect patient's time

Hispanic Americans		
Communication	**Time Orientation**	**Space**
Many speak both English and Spanish	Present	Close personal space
Direct confrontation is disrespectful	Flexible concept of time	Comfortable hugging and touching, even kissing
Expression of negative feelings is impolite	Arriving after agreed upon hour not considered rude	
Gestures and facial expressions may be dramatic		
Avoidance of eye contact indicates respect and attentiveness		
Politeness very important		
Privacy and modesty important		
Family	**Religion**	**Implications for Health Care**
Family is primary unit of society	Catholicism	Priest may attend to needs of the very ill
Extended family important		Protect privacy and modesty
Godparents remain close		Avoid rigid scheduling
Family needs more important than those of individual		Ease into serious conversation

(continued)

Table 15–2 Major Cultural Subgroups of the United States (continued)

Native Americans		
Communication	**Time Orientation**	**Space**
May speak tribal languages as well as English Silence indicates respect for the speaker Proper to speak in low tone of voice Body language important part of communication Eye contact is sign of disrespect	Present	Personal space very important Will lightly touch hand of other person during greetings Touching a dead body is prohibited
Family	**Religion**	**Implications for Health Care**
Extended family is the basic unit Family is very important Grandparents may be family leaders and elders are honored Children taught to respect traditions	Sacred myths and legends provide spiritual guidance Religion and healing practices are united	Be aware of the importance of family input and need to be with patient Do not interpret lack of eye contact negatively Clarify messages

Important Note: This table contains generalities about ethnic groups. Health care professionals should *not* assume that members of these groups will necessarily demonstrate these behaviors or hold these beliefs.

HEALTH CARE BELIEFS

Health care beliefs and practices vary widely among cultural groups. Traditional Western medicine, defined here as that which is practiced by most physicians in the United States, focuses on the physical aspects of the body and employs scientific methods of diagnosis and treatment. The effect of the mind on the body is not generally considered to be of great importance, except in the case of holistic practitioners, discussed in Chapter 2. An exception for traditional practitioners is stress, which is becoming recognized as having an impact on health. Illness is generally attributed to factors that can be measured and explained, such as infection, environmental conditions, and physical changes in the body's structure. Treatment methods, such as medications, must be proven to be both effective and safe through carefully controlled clinical trials. There is emphasis on formal training and official verification of the competence of health care practitioners through licensing and certification.

Traditional Western medicine is beginning to acknowledge the possible effects of the mind on the functions and health of the body. Some cultures have always believed that there is a strong connection. Traditional beliefs of many Native Americans, for example, emphasize the relationship among the mind, body, and spirit. Illness may result when the harmony among these three human components is disrupted.

Thinking It Through

Kelly O'Connor handles the billing for Dr. Sinclair's busy orthopedic practice. Patients are sent to Kelly to give her information about their insurance coverage, make payment arrangements, and pay their portion of office calls. One day she is collecting a payment from an elderly patient who came to Dr. Sinclair for treatment of arthritis. He had moved to the United States from a small island in the South Pacific a few years ago. The patient is visibly upset. Kelly asks if Mr. Juarez is all right. He says, "Everything here is so rush-rush. The doctor has no time."

1. How can Kelly appropriately respond to the patient?
2. Are there questions she might ask him to learn more about his feelings?
3. How should she follow up?
4. Should she share this encounter with anyone else in the office? Why?

Religious Beliefs and Health

Religious and spiritual beliefs influence the health practices of many cultural groups and individuals. For example, the traditional healers in some Native American communities have religious status. Known as medicine men or women, they receive a calling similar to that experienced by spiritual leaders in other cultures. They serve as the mouthpiece of the spirits they believe exist throughout the universe. They use diagnostic and healing methods that have been employed for centuries. These include the widespread use of herbs and special healing ceremonies. A number of ethnic groups living in the United States retain their beliefs in the skills of these healers. At the same time, modern medical science is often combined with traditional methods.

Faith healing is practiced by some Christians. They believe they can be cured from illness and disabilities through prayer and strong religious faith. In fact, the National Institutes of Health reports that more than 60% of Americans use prayer to assist their healing from injury and illness. Some Christians believe that certain members of the clergy have the power to assist with healing. Christian Scientists believe that illness and health are controlled by God and that the patient's mind, not medical treatment, is the means to recovery.

Islam is a religion that is predominant in many parts of the world, including North Africa, the Middle East, and Indonesia. Many Muslims believe that what happens in life, including illness, is due to the "will of Allah" (God's will). Illness, then, can be avoided by religious means. These include the use of prayers, reciting verses from the Koran (the sacred text of Islam), and wearing charms.

Some cultures believe in the effects of evil spirits and the "evil eye," a stare from someone believed to have the power to cause harm. Some Caribbean peoples, for example, wear charms and carry special objects, such as engraved stones, to ward off evil spirits. This is not unlike athletes who have lucky objects, such as a special pair of shoes, that they believe they need to perform well. Some Latin American peoples have special customs to avoid encountering the evil eye. They are especially protective of young children.

The Catholic religion plays a major role in the life of many people and is the predominant religion in Spanish-speaking countries. Illness is considered by some Catholics to be a form of punishment for sins. Prayers are believed to be helpful, especially when they call upon specific saints for help and are accompanied by the purchasing and lighting of votive candles.

Harmony and Health

The concept of harmony as necessary for good health is common to many cultures. The balance of mind, body, and spirit, part of Native American culture, is also part of the belief system of some African Americans. The phrase "mind-body connection" is being heard more often in the United States as people are discovering the benefits of a more holistic approach to medicine. (See the section in Chapter 2 on Complementary, Alternative, and Integrative Health.)

The Chinese civilization is thousands of years old and has developed many time-honored health care practices. Chinese medicine is based in part on the belief that the body has two energy forces, known as *yin* and *yang*. Illness occurs when these forces are out of balance. Diseases and treatments are classified by their relationship to these forces. Activities and treatments believed to promote the integration of the mind and body and enhance the flow of the life force (*qi*) are widely practiced. An example is *t'ai chi*, an ancient form of martial arts, in which slow, relaxed movements are carried out while focusing the mind. T'ai chi is now becoming a popular method in the United States for promoting relaxation, balance, flexibility, and healthy joints.

Traditional beliefs among some Hispanic groups include the theory that the body is controlled by four basic body fluids, known as *humors*. These humors are classified as follows: hot and wet, hot and dry, cold and wet, and cold and dry. Illness results when the humors are out of balance. Disorders and corresponding treatments are organized according to the hot–cold principle. It is believed that cold illnesses should be treated with hot remedies and hot illnesses with cold ones. For example, a headache is classified as a cold condition. Appropriate hot foods include cereals, eggs, beef, and spicy foods; appropriate medical remedies include aspirin, cinnamon, and garlic. See Box 15–1 for more examples.

In addition to beliefs about hot and cold remedies, members of some cultural groups, such as the Chinese, prescribe specific foods as treatments for various conditions.

BOX 15–1

Hot and Cold Conditions and Treatments

Hot Conditions	Cold Conditions
Constipation	Cancer
Fever	Colds
Infections	Headache
Sore throat	Pneumonia
Ulcers	Tuberculosis
Cold Food Remedies	**Hot Food Remedies**
Dairy products	Cereals
Milk	Eggs
Lima beans	Beef
Vegetables	Oils
Honey	Spicy foods
Chicken	Wine
Raisins	
Cold Medical Remedies	**Hot Medical Remedies**
Bicarbonate of soda	Aspirin
Milk of magnesia	Cinnamon
Orange flower water	Cod liver oil
Sage	Garlic
	Penicillin

Fascinating Facts

There are 62 schools in the United States accredited by the National Association for Acupuncture and Oriental Medicine. These schools offer certificates through doctoral degrees.

Herbs and Plant Medicines

Plants and herbs have been used for thousands of years to treat various ailments. Asian cultures have developed thousands of herbal remedies that are widely used today. There has been growing interest in the use of medicinal herbs in the United States by many people who believe that, because they are natural, they have fewer dangerous side effects than pharmaceutical drugs. It is important that health care professionals be aware that "natural" treatments are not necessarily safe. Many plants and herbs *can* have harmful side effects. Also, some herbs interact negatively with traditional prescribed medications. Herbal remedies and food supplements are not regulated by the government as are pharmaceutical products.

Some older members of African-American communities are recognized for their ability to provide effective home remedies, including the preparation of medications from herbs and roots. As with other cultural groups, popular remedies may be handed down from one generation to the next.

See Boxes 15–2 through 15–5 for examples of culturally influenced approaches to health.

BOX 15–2

Definitions of Health

- Absence of disease
- Balance of body energy (yin and yang)
- Balance of hot/cold and wet/dry forces in the body
- Harmony with nature
- Integration of body, mind, and spirit

BOX 15–3

Sources of Good Health

- Nutritious food, rest, and practice of good hygiene
- Gift from ancestors
- Good self-care practices, such as exercise and not smoking
- Reward from God
- Will of God
- Good luck

BOX 15–4

Causes of Illness

- Blockage or imbalance of body energy
- Disharmony between self and environment
- Disharmony caused by demons or spirits
- Punishment for sins
- Receiving the evil eye or a bad fright
- Scientifically explained phenomena, such as microbes
- Supernatural forces
- Violation of taboo (prohibited activity)
- Will of God

BOX 15–5

Methods of Treatment

Acupressure

Acupuncture

Consultation with traditional healers

Exercise and changes in eating habits

Fasting (giving up eating all or certain foods for a specific period of time)

Herbs

Meditation

Pharmaceutical drugs

Prayer

Restoration of balance of energy or other bodily forces

Restoration of mind–body–spirit harmony

Rituals and ceremonies

Roots from plants

Surgery

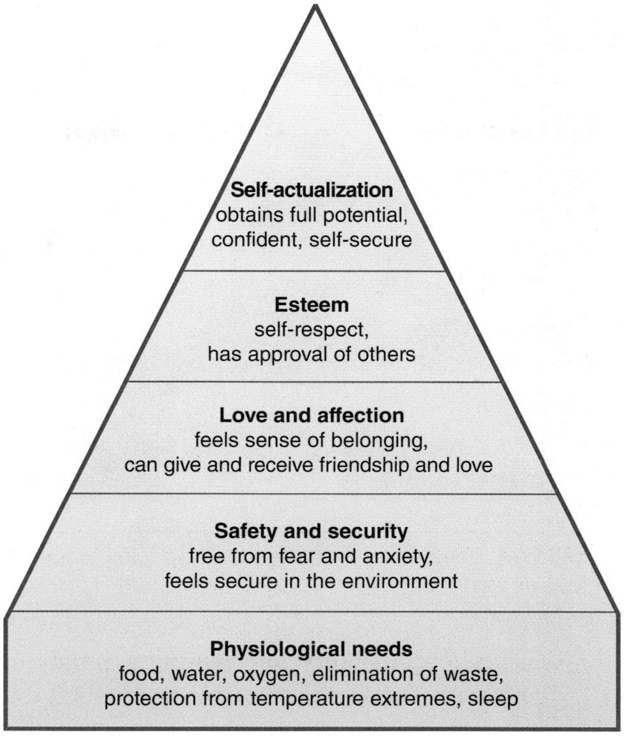

FIGURE 15–3 Maslow's hierarchy of needs.

MASLOW'S HIERARCHY OF HUMAN NEEDS

Cultural backgrounds form the frameworks for the physical, psychological, and spiritual development of human beings. Within these frameworks, however, each individual develops a unique combination of characteristics and behaviors.

There are many approaches to describing and explaining the complexities of human behavior. One useful approach for the health care professional is based on understanding basic human needs. A model that has helped health care professionals to better understand their patients was developed by American psychologist Abraham Maslow. According to Maslow, human behavior is motivated by each individual's efforts to fulfill certain requirements for complete physical, mental, and emotional well-being. He originally developed five categories of human needs, which he then ranked in order of importance for human fulfillment. As he continued to study human behavior, he added three more categories of needs: knowledge, beauty, and transcendence (the need to help others achieve self-actualization). Figure 15–3 contains a triangle that shows the relationship of the original five groups. This is known as **Maslow's hierarchy of needs** (a hierarchy being an arrangement in order of rank or grade) and is the version shown in most references to Maslow's work.

- Level 1: **Physiological needs**, which must be satisfied in order to maintain life. These include necessities such as oxygen, water, and food.
- Level 2: Need for physical and psychological security such as living free from the fear of physical harm.
- Level 3: Need for maintaining satisfying relationships with other people, in the form of love and affection. This need is met by enjoying friendships and attaining intimacy with another. (See Figure 15–4.)
- Level 4: Need for **self-esteem**, the opinion that an individual has of himself or herself. People with high self-esteem are comfortable with themselves and usually able to cope satisfactorily with stress. Being accepted into peer groups has an important influence on self-esteem.
- Level 5: **Self-actualization**, which Maslow defined as the achievement of one's greatest potential. The individual who reaches this level experiences a sense of personal control and

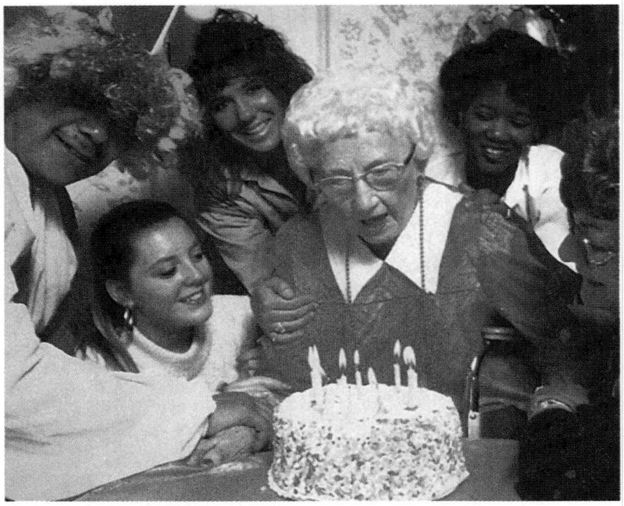

FIGURE 15–4 Celebrating with friends helps fulfill the need for love and affection.

accepts responsibility for creating a satisfying life. Another characteristic of individuals at this level is their willingness to help others.

Individuals change and develop over time. They do not remain at one level until every need at that level is met. In fact, some great works are achieved by people who live in extreme poverty or in difficult condition, such as prison camps. Life is a dynamic process that involves movement up and down the hierarchy in response to events and experiences in an ongoing effort to satisfy various needs.

An individual's behavior at any given time to meet the needs described by Maslow are determined by his or her personality, the current situation, and the opportunities available. For example, securing food for survival can be achieved in several ways: earning money, farming, trading, begging, or stealing. The method selected will be influenced by such factors as parental training, educational level, economic status, job availability, physical condition, level of self-esteem, and moral beliefs.

Fascinating Facts

Many people throughout history have achieved their greatest potential, labeled by Maslow as self-actualization, in spite of personal difficulties that may have prevented them from fulfilling lower needs on the hierarchy.

Helen Keller: Graduated from college and became an author, political activist, and lecturer in spite of being deaf and blind.

Franklin D. Roosevelt: Served four terms as president of the United States although severely disabled as a result of polio.

Ludwig van Beethoven: Wrote some of the world's most beautiful music after losing his hearing.

Stephen Hawking: Considered one of the most brilliant minds of the 20th century, he became a theoretical physicist and cosmologist despite early-onset amyotrophic lateral sclerosis (ALS), diagnosed when he was 21 years old.

PATIENT NEEDS

Illness and injury alter the nature of human needs and the means available to satisfy them. When patients enter the health care world as a result of illness or injury, they may have to develop new strategies for adjusting and coping. Health care professionals must understand how the need to meet basic needs affects patient behavior and recovery. They should also recognize the significant role they play in helping patients meet these challenges.

We will use the example of a patient named Carlos to illustrate the application of Maslow's hierarchy of needs throughout the recovery process. Carlos is a 29-year-old welder. His wife cares for their two children and maintains their home. Carlos is involved in a motorcycle accident in which he suffers a spinal cord injury that results in paraplegia, paralysis from the waist down. His injuries will make it impossible for him to ever walk again.

Carlos's needs are significantly changed as a result of the accident. His progress through the long recovery process begins with the most basic physiological need, which is to survive the physical trauma of the accident. If Carlos meets his needs at each level, his chances of moving up the hierarchy and achieving self-actualization are increased. His progress will not necessarily be smooth and steady and may not take place in an orderly way. Maslow's hierarchy of needs, like other models developed to explain human behavior, serves only as a guide to help us understand others.

Physiological Needs

Carlos's survival depends on whether his physiological needs can be met to deal with his injuries. This requirement is carried out by emergency room staff members who provide immediate medical care. He is now dependent on others to meet his physical needs. The emphasis at this time is providing the medical care necessary to save his life. His needs, like those of other patients in similar situations, include the following:

- Reassurance
- Knowledge that he is receiving competent care
- Information about where he is and what has happened

After receiving the basic care necessary to save his life, Carlos will remain dependent on the health facility for some time to attend to his physical needs. These include the food and shelter that he used to provide for himself and others.

Safety and Security Needs

Being confined to a health care facility can threaten a patient's feelings of safety and security. Carlos feels uncomfortable in this strange environment, separated from the familiar surroundings of his home and the presence of family members. The feeling of security is increased for patients when they know the following:

- The names of the staff providing their care
- How to contact staff when they need assistance
- The routine for their care, including when to expect meals, personal care, and treatments
- Pain or discomfort they are likely to experience
- Availability of pain medication

Carlos faces a future full of unknowns, and this is causing him considerable anxiety. He often expresses concern about how he will be able to pay for his medical expenses and continue to support his family. Do not try to trivialize his worries, even if well intentioned. Saying, "Now, you shouldn't worry about that—just concentrate on getting well," does not show respect for Carlos nor does it help him find solutions for his problems.

As Carlos learns to trust the members of the health care team, his feelings of security will increase. Team members can encourage the development of trust by demonstrating acceptance of and respect for the patient. They can accomplish this by listening attentively, withholding judgment, and providing answers to questions. Questions from patients that the health care professional is not qualified to answer should be referred promptly to his or her supervisor.

Love and Affection Needs

Paraplegia brings a set of serious challenges, and one of the most difficult areas is how it affects the need for friendship, love, and affection. Before the accident, Carlos's social life centered on active pursuits with his friends. He knows that he will no longer join in on Saturday soccer games and that his days of riding motorcycles are over. Many of the guys have visited him in the hospital, but he wonders how long they will keep spending time with someone who is confined to a wheelchair. Worse yet are his fears about how his wife is adjusting to having a disabled husband. Does she still love him? Will they be able to have sex?

All aspects of Carlos's previous social life seem altered, and the future looks very lonely. He is experiencing intense frustration and fear, and these emotions lead to occasional angry verbal attacks on the health care professionals who provide his care. Understanding the motivation for this behavior, a reaction to threats against the fulfillment of his basic needs, helps the health care team realize that Carlos's outbursts are not meant to be personal attacks, but are the result of his frustration. Although it is a natural response to avoid prolonged contact and communication with an angry patient, it is often at this time that human contact is most needed. If Carlos fears rejection and loneliness, avoidance will only reinforce his belief that he is unlikable and unlovable.

Ways to help patients meet their need for love and affection include the following:

- Expressing sincere interest in them and their well-being
- Behaving in a compassionate way when they exhibit difficult behavior
- Listening attentively
- Touching them on the hand or shoulder as a form of greeting or reassurance
- Allowing them to express themselves even if the topic is difficult or unpleasant
- Helping family and friends feel welcome and comfortable during visits
- Encouraging family and friends to come and celebrate holidays or special events with patients

The health care professional can also alert the supervisor or other appropriate members of the health care team about Carlos's current behavior and possible needs. For example, occupational therapists help patients like Carlos rebuild their lives and achieve the highest level of activity possible, including sexual function. (Remember, however, that legal considerations of confidentiality restrict any discussions about patients to *only* those health care practitioners who work with them.)

Self-Esteem Needs

The feelings that individuals have about themselves at a given time and their opinions of their value as people are known as self-esteem. Self-esteem can fluctuate, and whether it is high or low depends on the person's experiences and perceptions at the moment. Injuries and illnesses that disfigure and cause loss of function often result in a decrease in self-esteem that can last for extended periods. Most people place importance on what others think of them and base their self-esteem, to a great extent, on the opinions of others. Before the accident, Carlos defined himself in terms of his roles as husband, father, son, friend, and worker. In other words, he based his personal value on *what* rather than *who* he was. His relationships with others and his role in the community were sources of self-esteem. He took pride in his skills as a welder and was confident of his ability to provide for his family.

In the weeks following the accident, Carlos's self-esteem has plummeted. Maslow's hierarchy can help explain why. Carlos has lost control over his ability to meet the needs that make up the first three groups of the hierarchy. Let's look at each one. In caring for his physical needs, he will learn to perform many tasks for himself when he enters rehabilitation. For now, however, he must depend on others to take care of these requirements. Regarding security, he has not yet determined how he will provide for his own financial security or that of his family. Finally, he still has doubts about how he will be treated by friends and family during his long rehabilitation and future life as a paraplegic.

Health care professionals can help reinforce Carlos's self-esteem by sending the message that "You are worth my time. Your disability does not detract from your value as a person." Ways to express this idea to patients include the following:

- Taking the time to listen
- Showing interest by referring back to something the patient said in the past or remembering an occasion or event that is important to the patient
- Allowing patients the opportunity to express their needs
- Asking for and respecting their preferences
- Protecting their privacy
- Treating them with respect and dignity
- Asking for their approval before giving care
- Asking for patients' opinions of what works best for them *if* there are options

Self-Actualization Needs

Although the means available for Carlos to reach his highest potential have been altered by his accident, it is still possible for him to achieve self-actualization. Some people who have suffered serious health problems see their circumstances as an opportunity to make positive life changes. They even find that their quality of life improves, because they realize the value of each day and more fully appreciate what they have. Common life changes include the following:

- Finding work that is more meaningful
- Making time for things they have always wanted to do, such as painting or working with children
- Sharing their recovery experiences with others who are experiencing similar injuries or illnesses
- Becoming involved in health care fund-raising activities to pay for research into and treatment of their condition

Actor Christopher Reeve, star of the Superman movies, was paralyzed from the neck down when he was thrown from his horse in 1995. He returned to films as a director and worked vigorously to promote research focused on developing new treatments for spinal cord injuries until his death in 2004. He remains an example of responding in a self-actualized manner to a catastrophic event. Another example is popular television and movie actor Michael J. Fox, who was diagnosed at age 30 with early-onset Parkinson's disease. In addition to continuing his acting career (including a sit-com about a newsman who is diagnosed with Parkinson's), he works to raise public awareness of the disease and funds for research to find a cure.

Many factors will influence to what extent Carlos attempts to achieve self-actualization. The way he is treated as an individual in the various health facilities during his recovery is important. Health care professionals must realize how their interactions with patients can affect the patients' ability to move up the hierarchy and meet their needs at the highest level possible.

Maslow's hierarchy of needs serves as a useful model for understanding the behavior of all patients, not just those like Carlos who are suffering from very serious conditions. For example, one's sense of security can be threatened by visits to the dentist and physician for annual exams. And the self-esteem of an overweight patient can be undermined during a procedure that requires disrobing. It is important that health care professionals keep in mind that what is routine to them can be threatening to their patients. Being sensitive to the needs of patients is a prerequisite for establishing good communication.

DEFENSE MECHANISMS

The need to maintain one's self-esteem at an acceptable level is a driving force in shaping human behavior. **Defense mechanisms** are a special category of responses to perceived threats to self-esteem. They help provide relief from the mental discomfort and anxiety caused by internal conflict and are usually performed unconsciously (Milliken & Honeycutt, 2004). For example, a student may believe that his inability to arrive on time to class is due to sleep patterns inherited from his father, when in reality it is due to his habit of partying late at night. In this case, he is using rationalization to justify his behavior. Although defense mechanisms provide temporary relief, they do not resolve the underlying, anxiety-producing problems that need to be addressed. For example, Mrs. Azordegan discovers a small lump in her left breast. She is afraid that it might be cancer and refuses to take any action. She puts off calling her physician or telling anyone in the family about the lump. Her *denial* is a defense mechanism whose purpose is to avoid facing a potentially unpleasant truth. By the time she seeks medical attention, she learns that she does have cancer and that delaying treatment has allowed it to metastasize (spread to other parts of the body). The use of a defense mechanism has worsened the very problem that Mrs. Azordegan feared most and hoped to avoid. Even if the lump had not been cancerous, Mrs. Azordegan would have experienced prolonged and unnecessary stress caused by the delayed diagnosis. In either case, ignoring the situation only caused additional problems.

Defense mechanisms are commonly used at times of stress and anxiety, such as those experienced during illness or injury. Table 15–3 describes some of the defense mechanisms that health care professionals may encounter when working with patients. Recognizing defense mechanisms can help health care professionals understand patient behavior and reduce the amount of threat experienced by patients. Examples of ways the health care professional can do this include the following:

- Demonstrating acceptance
- Showing sincere interest in patients' well-being
- Providing education and instructions to increase patients' control over their own health issues (see Figure 15–5)
- Allowing them to discuss what is really bothering them, if they wish to do so
- Respecting their need to use defense mechanisms, which may be needed to get through a very difficult situation

DEALING WITH LOSS

Having to deal with loss can significantly influence patient behavior. Suffering an illness or injury or even undergoing the normal aging process can result in many types of loss. These include loss of independence, a body part or function, control over one's life, appearance and self-image, privacy, financial security, familiar surroundings, and significant other. The patient who must remain in a health care facility for a long time is likely to suffer multiple losses. Even the removal of a tooth in the dentist's office represents a loss. It can be traumatic for the middle-aged patient who experiences this as the beginning of the dreaded aging process and only the first of future physical problems and losses. Any health care encounter can represent loss of control for patients.

Just as the methods used to fulfill basic needs vary among individuals, so will their reactions to loss.

Table 15–3 Examples of Common Defense Mechanisms

Defense Mechanism	Definition	Example
Acting out	Expressing feelings difficult to communicate by performing an extreme behavior	Husband kicking the wall when angry over wife's criticism of him
Compensation	Attempting to meet a need by substituting something that does not actually satisfy the need	Recently divorced woman overeating to deal with loneliness
Control	Trying to exert excessive control over others to make up for a loss of control elsewhere	Hospitalized patient insisting on being given an exact time schedule for care
Denial	Pretending that something is not true, especially something unpleasant	Business executive refusing to acknowledge testing positive for human immunodeficiency virus (HIV)
Displacement	Transferring feelings that one has about one person to a different person	Nurse becoming angry with her children after working with a demanding patient
Malingering	Pretending to be ill when one is not	Student faking symptoms to avoid taking a test at school
Projection	Failing to see one's own weaknesses or problems while seeing them in others	Overweight mother criticizing her overweight daughter's poor eating habits
Rationalization	Explaining behavior by using a socially acceptable reason	Graduate nurse delaying taking a licensing exam because she is "too busy" when in reality she is afraid she will fail
Regression	Behaving in ways that are more appropriate for a younger person	A 10-year-old boy returning to thumb-sucking after being hospitalized
Repression	Keeping unpleasant thoughts or memories in the subconscious and out of awareness	Young woman lacking conscious memory of having been sexually assaulted as a child
Withdrawal	Refusing to communicate with others or participate in social activities	Teenage boy refusing to take calls from friends or attending social activities after being diagnosed with leukemia

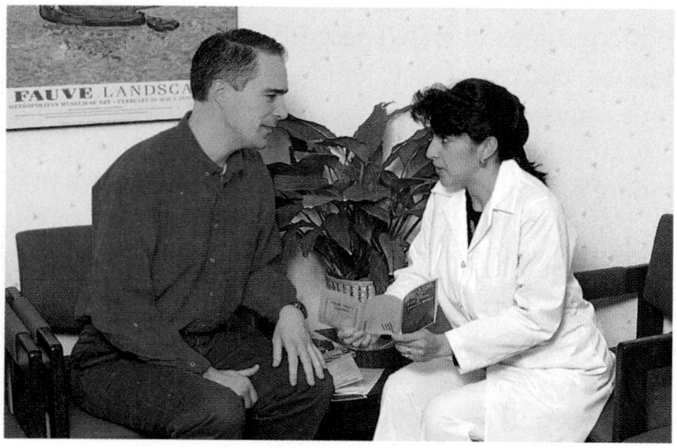

FIGURE 15–5 Educating patients about self-care techniques can reduce anxiety by increasing their control over personal health issues.

Some common examples of ways of dealing with loss include the following:

- Seeking support from family and friends
- Finding comfort in religion
- Drawing on self-esteem
- Employing problem-solving techniques
- Using defense mechanisms
- Becoming angry
- Experiencing depression

Health care professionals can help patients deal with loss by realizing its significance to patients, understanding their reactions to loss and their need to grieve, and being willing to talk with patients who

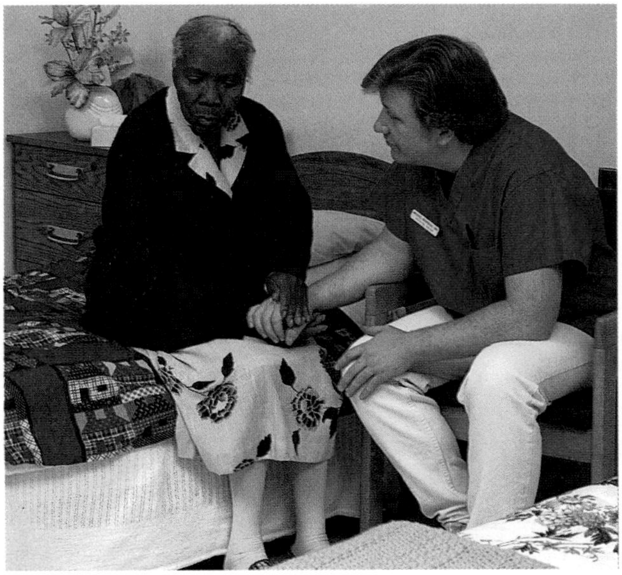

FIGURE 15–6 Listening and expressing concern can help patients deal with loss.

wish to discuss their loss. This gives patients the opportunity to share their feelings, if they wish to do so, and to explore ways to grieve and deal with their loss. (See Figure 15–6.) Death and dying is discussed in Chapter 8.

DETERMINING INDIVIDUAL NEEDS

The effectiveness of the health care professional's interactions and communication with patients depends largely on understanding and respecting individual differences. Although it is not suggested that the practice of modern health care be compromised to accommodate all the traditional beliefs of patients, knowing something about the content and basis of these beliefs can help provide a foundation on which to build effective helping relationships. Being sensitive to the variety of perceptions that patients bring to the health care setting enables health care professionals to better meet patient needs. There are a number of ways to learn about patients as individuals:

1. Observe the patient's behavior and ways of interacting with others.
    - Eye contact
    - Degree of formality in conversation and body movements
    - Outward signs of possible emotions such as nervousness, fear, or suspicion
    - Presence of family members
    - Interactions with family members
    - Reaction to touch and close personal contact
2. Determine whether language barriers are present.
    - Ask patient in what language he or she is most comfortable communicating
    - Ask about language preferences for written information and instructions
    - Ask if patient needs an interpreter when discussing health care information and treatments
3. Ask questions to determine individual preferences.
    a. Health beliefs and practices
        - What do you do to help you stay healthy?
        - What do you usually do when you are sick or not feeling well?
        - Who do you go to first when seeking help with health problems?
        - Who in your family is primarily responsible for making health care decisions for members of the family?
        - Who will help you at home if you need assistance with health problems?
        - In coping with this illness/injury, what are your expectations of the health care team and of yourself?
        - What do you think will be the most important factor in your recovery?
        - Are you aware of any medical procedures or practices that contradict your spiritual beliefs?

    b. Communication styles
        - What are the ways you show respect and disrespect?
        - Do you have preferences or restrictions related to touching, personal space, making eye contact, or social behaviors that you would like to tell me?

    c. General
        - Is there anything you would like to tell me that might help us understand your needs?
4. Listen carefully to the patient's responses.
5. Explain what you are doing and why when performing procedures or asking questions that

may be difficult for the individual based on what you have learned.

(*Source*: Adapted from *Health Assessment and Physical Examination,* (4th ed.), by M. E. Z. Estes, 2009, Clifton Park, NY: Delmar Cengage Learning.)

In addition to being aware of cultural and individual differences, understanding human motivation and the need to preserve self-esteem will help you communicate effectively and provide appropriate care. The next chapter presents communication techniques such as listening, observing body language, and creating clear messages.

WORKBOOK PRACTICE

Go to your workbook and complete the exercises for this chapter.

SUGGESTED LEARNING ACTIVITIES

1. Brainstorm ideas on how you can apply the philosophy of individual worth, described in this chapter, in your personal and future work life.
2. Learn more about the various cultural groups in your area. Attend local cultural events, such as diversity fairs and informational workshops.
3. Research two cultural groups that are different from your own. Choose five aspects to compare and contrast between the two groups and with your own.
4. Use illustrations from magazines to create a poster that represents the cultural groups represented in the United States today.
5. Observe the behavior of people around you. Identify attempts to meet the needs described by Maslow. Now observe your own behavior in terms of Maslow's hierarchy of needs.
6. Start a journal of your own behavior in which you observe and note your attempts to meet the needs described by Maslow.
7. Watch for examples of possible defense mechanisms used by people around you: friends, family members, and classmates. Why do you think these mechanisms were employed?
8. Think about your own behaviors and reactions to events in your life. Are you using any defense mechanisms?

WEB ACTIVITIES

American Medical Association Foundation
www.youtube.com/watch?v=cGtTZ_vxjyA

Health literacy video. Although created for physicians, this video has excellent information about communicating with the many patients who have difficulty understanding the information they receive from their health care providers. After watching the video, write a summary that describes why patients have trouble understanding health information and suggestions for health care professionals to improve their communication with patients.

University of Washington
https://ethnomed.org

Explore the various subject areas covered in this website. Then choose three articles to read or videos to watch. What did you learn about the effects of culture on health care? What can health care providers do to help patients from other cultures?

Psych Central
http://psychcentral.com

1. Enter "defense mechanisms" in the search box. Write a brief description of the mechanisms that are not included in this chapter.
2. Choose a mental health condition to read about and report on possible ways it can affect physical health. What should health care professionals understand about the condition to work effectively with patients who might have the condition?

Simply Psychology
www.simplypsychology.org

Click on "Perspectives" to learn about different approaches to psychology and human behavior. Choose a perspective that interests you and explain why. How can having a basic understanding of psychology help you work more effectively with patients?

REVIEW QUESTIONS

1. Explain the philosophy of individual worth and how it relates to work in health care.
2. What is the definition of *culture*?
3. Give examples of contrasting traditional beliefs and behaviors among the major American ethnic groups.
4. Give three examples of different cultural approaches to health care for each of the following categories:
   - Definition of health
   - Sources of good health
   - Causes of illness
   - Methods of treatment
5. What are the five levels of needs described by Maslow?
6. Give an example to demonstrate the meaning of each level of need.
7. What are the common defense mechanisms encountered in health care situations?
8. What are three ways the health care professional can help patients deal with the experience of loss?
9. What are four ways that the health care professional can determine the individual needs of a patient?
10. Give five examples of questions to ask to discover a patient's needs.

APPLICATION EXERCISES

1. Refer back to The Case of the Polite Patient at the beginning of the chapter. What assumptions did Carley make? How could she have learned more about Mr. Alvarez? Once she learned about his situation, what could she have done to better help him understand and carry out the diet and exercise program prescribed by Dr. Washington?
2. You are working as a medical assistant in the private medical office of an oncologist (cancer specialist). Mrs. Ramirez, an elderly woman who lived in Guatemala until she was 56, comes to the office accompanied by her granddaughter. Mrs. Ramirez speaks very little English, but her granddaughter is bilingual. This visit was at the granddaughter's insistence after her grandmother admitted finding a small lump in her breast. Mrs. Ramirez is very anxious about the visit. Describe how you would work with this patient, including a review of cultural factors and individual needs.

PROBLEM-SOLVING PRACTICE

Katelin works as a nurse in a public school. Many of the children with whom she works are from homes with parents who are immigrants from a variety of countries. Katelin often finds herself unable to communicate with these parents. How might she apply the problem-solving process to improve her ability to work with families from different cultural backgrounds?

SUGGESTED READINGS AND RESOURCES

Cultural diversity in health care. Links to articles by University of California Los Angeles professor Geri-Ann Galanti. www.ggalanti.com

Dienemann, J. (Ed.). (1997). *Cultural diversity in nursing: Issues, strategies, and outcomes.* Washington, DC: American Academy of Nursing.

Diller, J. (1999). *Cultural diversity: A primer for the human services.* Pacific Grove, CA: Brooks/Cole.

Milliken, M. E., & Honeycutt, A. (2012). *Understanding human behavior* (8th ed.). Clifton Park, NY: Delmar Cengage Learning.

Munoz, C., & Luckmann, J. (2005). *Transcultural communication in nursing* (2nd ed.). Clifton Park, NY: Delmar Cengage Learning.

Neff, N. *Folk medicine in Hispanics in the southwestern United States.* www.rice.edu/projects/HispanicHealth/Courses/mod7/mod7.html

Purtilo, R., & Haddad, A. (2012). *Health professional and patient interaction* (8th ed.). St. Louis: Elsevier.

U.S. Census Bureau. www.census.gov

Van Servellen, G. (1997). *Communication skills for the health care professional: Concepts and techniques.* Gaithersburg, MD: Aspen.

This page intentionally left blank

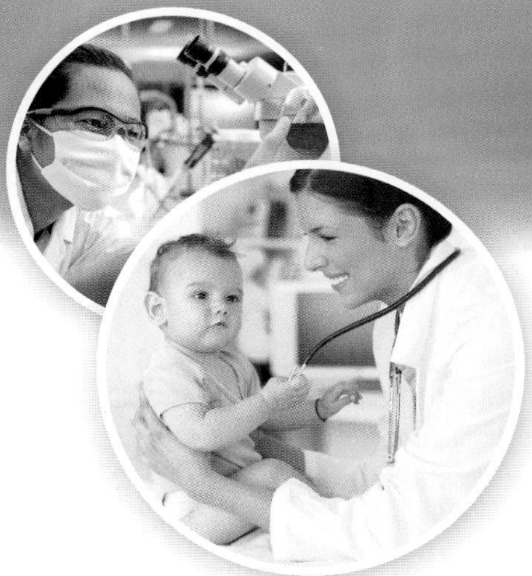

Chapter 16

The Communication Process

OBJECTIVES

Studying and applying the material in this chapter will help you to:

- Explain the importance of effective communication in health care.
- Describe the relationship between effective communication and patient well-being.
- List and describe the six steps of the communication process.
- Define and explain the use of the four types of questions.
- Explain the meaning of nonverbal communication and give examples of three types.
- Explain the meaning of *active listening*.
- Define *empathy* and explain its application in health care.
- Explain the meaning of *feedback* and how it is used in communication.
- Recognize common barriers that can prevent effective communication.
- List the techniques to use when communicating with patients who have special needs.
- Demonstrate professional telephone techniques and explain why it is important to apply them in the health care facility.
- Describe the elements that make up effective patient education.
- List strategies for preparing and giving presentations to groups.
- List three ways to handle situations that involve gossip.

KEY TERMS

active listening
asking questions
barriers
clinical depression
closed-ended questions
communication
empathy
feedback
leading questions
learning objectives
nonverbal communication
open-ended questions
pantomime
paraphrasing
probing questions
receiver
reflecting
requesting examples
sender
sympathy
therapeutic communication

The Case of the Coder Who Lacked Confidence

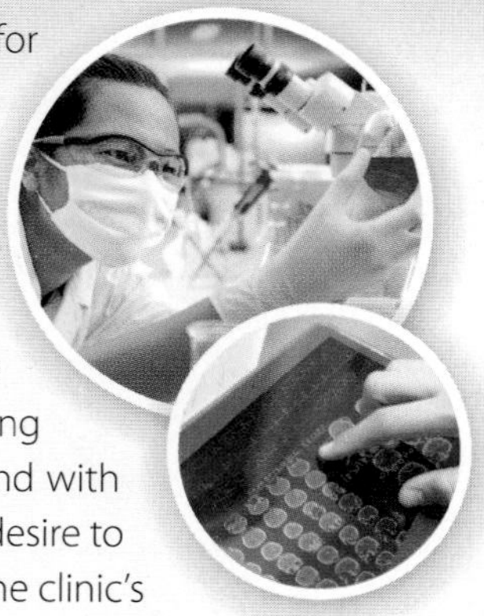

Jenny McAbee has worked as a medical insurance coder and biller for Appleton Medical Clinic for three years. She enjoys working with detailed information and performing tasks on the computer. Her coding is accurate and very few claims she submits to insurance companies are denied. Jenny chose this career partly because she is shy and enjoys working by herself. Dr. Morton, the director of the clinic, has noted that many patients are confused about their insurance coverage, which payments are their responsibility, how to fill out and submit the proper paperwork, and other insurance details. He believes it would be helpful if Jenny could spend less time on paperwork and more time interacting with patients, answering their questions, and explaining their insurance plans. Therefore, he provides her with an assistant so she will have time to spend with the clinic's patients. Although Jenny has a thorough understanding of medical insurance and a desire to help the clinic's patients, she does not feel confident about her communication skills. Many of the clinic's patients have hearing impairments. Others speak very little English. She wonders how she can best help them. This chapter covers the communication process and techniques for becoming an effective communicator.

IMPORTANCE OF COMMUNICATION IN HEALTH CARE

Communication is a process in which messages are exchanged between a sender and a receiver. The **sender**, also referred to as the speaker, is the person who creates and delivers a message. The **receiver**, also called the listener, is the person to whom the sender directs the message. Communication is successful when the receiver interprets the sender's message as it was intended. Throughout a communication encounter, the sender and receiver exchange roles. Messages can be exchanged in at least four ways:

1. Orally
2. Nonverbally (discussed in this chapter)
3. In written form (see Chapter 17)
4. Electronically (see Chapter 18)

In order to function effectively, modern health care systems rely on the efficient and accurate delivery of large amounts of information. Diagnoses and treatments are often based on a variety of data that must be shared among many health care providers. There are vast networks of primary care providers, specialists, therapists, testing centers, medical facilities, and insurance companies that work together to provide and coordinate patient care. It is critical that all information be both accurate and delivered in a timely way.

Several of the health care trends discussed in Chapter 2 have increased the need for communication excellence:

- Increase in the number of large health care systems: Effective delivery of patient care depends on the coordination of information among various facilities and staff members. Chances of miscommunication increase as systems become larger and more complex.
- Increasingly complex coverage of health care costs: Costs covered by private insurance, Medicare, Medicaid, and other insurance plans can be difficult to identify and understand. Patients need clear communication to determine which treatments and drugs they qualify for.
- Significant decrease in the length of time patients spend in hospitals and other health care facilities: Patients are now more responsible for their own follow-up care and need clear instructions to correctly carry out necessary self-care procedures.
- Shift in major causes of death from infectious diseases to cancer, heart disease, chronic obstructive pulmonary disease (COPD), and stroke: There has been an increase in chronic illness because people are living longer. An important part of the health care professional's responsibilities is providing patient education about factors that promote wellness. Effective communication is necessary to provide good education.

The ability to communicate well can be as important to the professional success of the health care professional as the phlebotomist's ability to safely draw blood and the respiratory therapist's command of ventilation therapy. The well-being of patients depends on more than technical competence. For example, if a nurse is instructing a patient about how to change the dressing on a wound, the patient's understanding of these instructions is critical for successfully carrying out self-care practices at home. Studies have shown that health and treatment outcomes are significantly influenced by the quality of communication between patients and health care providers.

Communication and Patient Well-Being

The ability of health care professionals to communicate effectively is influenced by their attitude. The first step in achieving communication excellence is to develop respect for and an understanding of individual patients and their needs, as discussed in Chapter 15. Effective communication skills involve more than applying a set of techniques. They must be based on sincere compassion and concern for patients and their welfare. (See Figure 16–1.)

The health care world can be intimidating for patients. They may be anxious about receiving negative test results and learning that they have serious medical conditions. Or they may be fearful about experiencing pain and discomfort during necessary treatments. Still others are worried about losing control over portions of their lives as a result of their physical conditions. These concerns, combined with the physical stress caused by illness or injury, can negatively affect patient recovery. Health care professionals can help relieve patient stress by showing compassion, providing appropriate information, and answering questions. *Good communication has been shown to increase the speed of patient recovery.*

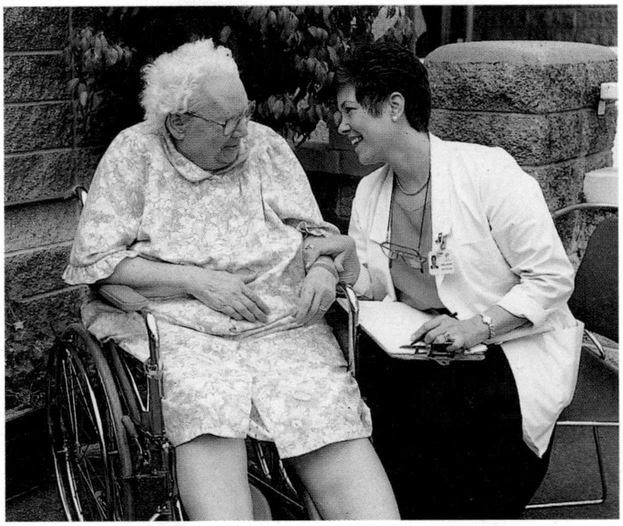

FIGURE 16–1 Good communication skills, combined with sincere caring about others, are essential for effective patient care.

Loneliness and depression are commonly experienced by patients during their stay in health care facilities. This is especially common among older patients in facilities such as nursing homes. Health care professionals may be their principal contact with the outside world. Being willing to talk and, even more important, to *listen* to patients can lift their spirits. One of the most important goals in health care communication is to help others to feel good about themselves (Collins, 1983).

Situations do not have to involve a direct threat to health to be stressful experiences for patients. As discussed in Chapter 15, any health care encounter can represent a loss for the patient and be a source of anxiety. Well-chosen words and a willingness to listen can help relieve anxiety. Patients' satisfaction is determined, to a great extent, by the quality of their communication with health care staff.

Patient care delivery is dependent on communication among members of the health care team, as well as on health care professional–patient interactions. The quality of care can be negatively affected when poor interpersonal and interprofessional relations exist among members of the team. As a future member of this team, it is your responsibility to make every effort to ensure that patient care is never compromised by a lack of attention to communication skills. Poor communication can lead to fatal consequences.

THE COMMUNICATION PROCESS

It is commonly believed that communication consists of simply talking and listening, activities that most people have been doing all their lives. We carry on dozens of conversations daily with family members, friends, classmates, and coworkers. Effective communication in health care, often referred to as **therapeutic communication**, is specifically aimed at meeting the needs of patients. It involves the application of a highly developed set of skills, and acquiring these skills takes effort, concentration, and practice.

In this text, communication is organized into a six-step process. This process provides a structured approach for studying and learning the variety of skills that make up effective communication. Individuals who have practiced and mastered good communication skills go through these steps quickly and automatically. Like other health care skills, communication cannot be taken for granted or performed in a routine manner. Each communication encounter presents its own set of circumstances and demands the health care professional's full attention. In other words, communication requires the application of the thinking skills presented in Chapter 1.

The Six Steps of the Communication Process

1. Set communication goals: Determine what is to be accomplished. This requires considering patient needs, current circumstances, and the duties assigned to the health care professional.
2. Create the message: Select and organize appropriate content based on the communication goals.
3. Deliver the message: Choose the delivery method best suited for ensuring that the receiver will understand the intent of the message.
4. Listen to the response: Employ listening and observational techniques to determine whether the message was received as intended.
5. Offer feedback and seek clarification: Rephrase what is heard or ask questions to check your understanding of the response.
6. Evaluate the encounter and revise the message: Determine whether the goal was met. If not, why not? What other options are available? What should be the next step?

Step One: Set Communication Goals

The first step in the communication process is for the sender to determine the goal. What is to be accomplished? Much of everyday communication is spontaneous and superficial and requires little or no planning. This includes everyday greetings ("Hi, how are you?"), which are said automatically and from which little real information is usually expected. Interactions in health care settings are more purposeful and contribute to providing appropriate patient care. They require skill. Suppose a nurse has a goal of learning about the current health status of a patient. Instead of asking the patient "How are you?" which usually results in a programmed response of "Fine," she needs to ask more specific questions. These will be based on communication goals. Examples of specific questions include the following:

- On a scale of 1 to 10, what is your pain level?
- Do you have any questions about your care?
- Are you feeling nervous about the procedure?

Communication goals come in many forms. The following examples are typical goals in health care situations:

- Gather as much objective and subjective information as possible from a patient.
- Instruct individuals on postsurgical home care procedures so family members will understand and follow them correctly.
- Inform a patient about the benefits of the treatment procedure you are administering.
- Report patient care information to a coworker who is taking over the care of the patient.

In addition to goals that are specific to the situation, there are three more that should be included in every patient interaction:

1. Demonstrate sincere concern for the patient's welfare.
   - Have a warm smile.
   - Use a gentle manner.
   - Do not act hurried.
   - Listen carefully.
2. Establish trust.
   - Establish eye contact as culturally appropriate.
   - Explain why a procedure, treatment, or test is necessary.
   - Explain in advance everything you are going to do.
   - Follow through with anything you say you will do (return in five minutes, call patient at home to check on progress, and so on).
3. Enhance the patient's self-esteem.
   - Involve the patient in decision making whenever possible.
   - Clarify the patient's communication if you're unsure of meaning.
   - Address the patient properly and respectfully.
   - Provide for privacy.
   - Ask the patient for input on how he or she wants things done, when appropriate.

These goals are based on the philosophy of individual worth, discussed in Chapter 15. It may seem unrealistic to try to achieve these goals in the brief time the health care professional spends with patients. There are other tasks to accomplish, such as taking a blood sample or performing a breathing treatment. Good communication, however, depends more on quality than quantity. A warm smile and informative reassurance are not time-consuming and can be included in any encounter. Patients today receive much of their care from strangers who are in a hurry. It is for this very reason that an effort should be made to personalize interactions and treat patients as individuals.

Collect Information

An important part of goal setting is to collect and review information that might affect communication. This includes the cultural and behavioral factors discussed in Chapter 15 as well as circumstances specific to the situation. The following factors should be considered:

- Patient's level of understanding
  - Is the patient very young?
  - Does the patient speak English?
  - If so, is English the second language?
  - Does the patient have a learning disability that affects his or her ability to understand?
  - Does the patient appear to be confused or disoriented?
  - What is the patient's ability to retain information? Is there short-term memory loss?
  - What is the appropriate terminology to use?
- Emotional factors
  - Does the patient's behavior indicate fear or anxiety?
  - Are there signs that the patient is using a defense mechanism? (See Chapter 15.)
  - Is the patient ready to accept the information that is to be offered?
- Physical factors
  - Is the patient in pain?
  - Is the patient on medication that causes drowsiness or affects the ability to concentrate?
  - Does the patient have a hearing, visual, or speech impairment that affects the communication process?
- Urgency of the communication
  - Must the communication take place now?
  - Is this the appropriate setting for the communication?
  - What are the consequences if it does not take place? Or if it is unsuccessful?

Learning to make these determinations quickly is an important health care skill that is developed over time. One technique for new health care professionals is to use mental checklists to help them prepare for communication encounters.

Step Two: Create the Message

Creating an appropriate message requires the selection of content and language that is based on the answers to the questions listed earlier. (Creating a message is also called "encoding.") Health care communication usually takes place at a deeper level than everyday conversation and must be clear and accurate. It may involve sharing very personal information, such as a patient's fears. Health care professionals must learn to carefully observe and listen for clues.

Information must be presented in a manner that the receiver understands. For example, although the use of medical terminology helps ensure accuracy in communications with other health care professionals, it can confuse and intimidate patients. Even everyday language may have to be simplified into common terms for some patients, depending on their age and language skills. For example, "number two" might be substituted for "bowel movement." At the same time, take care not to talk down to patients. (See Figure 16–2.)

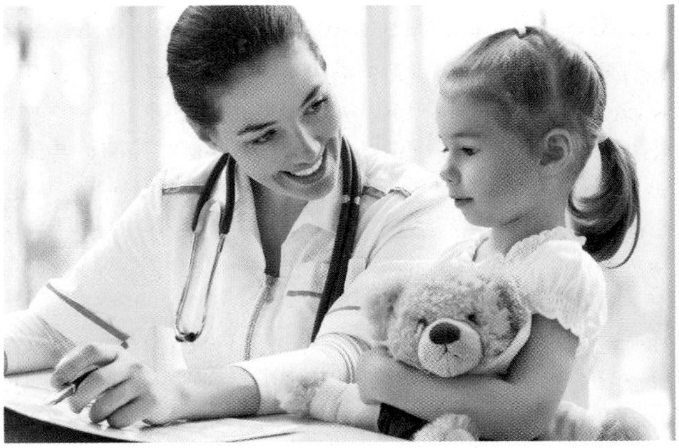

FIGURE 16–2 Your communication must be adjusted to the age and other characteristics of the receiver.

In general, it is best to use language that is not limited to specific ages or cultural groups. Similar to clothing, the language appropriate for professional settings may differ from that used in social situations. The overuse of filler words such as "you know" and "like" should also be avoided. They can be irritating to the receiver and distract from the message. Television news announcers are good models for standard American speech.

Organize long messages so they are easy for the receiver to follow. Here are some examples of organizational strategies:

- Explain what you plan to do and what the patient should expect to hear, feel, and so on.
- Rank information in order of importance.
- List a sequence of steps for the patient to follow.
- State facts and follow each with an explanation.
- Present an overview of a procedure before detailing the individual steps.
- Give instructions along with a description of possible consequences if they are not followed.
- Break information into sections, if possible, so the patient can grasp each part or set of facts before moving on to the next.
- Ask clarifying questions or have the patient demonstrate understanding, by the patient explaining the information or performing the task or exercise being taught, before going on to the next level.

Asking Questions

Some messages may be phrased as questions. There are several types of questions as well as a variety of ways to maximize their effectiveness.

1. **Closed-ended questions** can be answered with a single word or a response of "yes" or "no." This type of question is used to gather factual information. For example, the health care professional may ask closed-ended questions when obtaining background information about a patient. Closed-ended questions are not recommended when checking for understanding. Many patients will answer "Yes" to the question "Do you understand?" even if they do not. They are afraid of appearing stupid or do not want to "bother you" by having the information repeated.
2. **Open-ended questions** cannot be answered with a simple "yes" or "no." They require a more complete response and are used to encourage patients to provide more detailed information or explanations. These questions can be used to learn about the patient's symptoms, to encourage the sharing of feelings and opinions, or to check understanding of the message.
3. **Probing questions** are requests for additional information or clarification. For example, they can be used to lead patients to more fully discuss their symptoms. If a patient states, "My stomach hurts," appropriate probing questions would inquire about the exact location and type of pain, when it first occurred, and at what time it is experienced. It is important not to confuse the purposeful use of probing questions with digging for unnecessary personal details, which patients may find offensive.
4. **Leading questions** are those in which all or part of the answer is included in the wording of the question. Leading questions should be avoided when they encourage the receiver to give the answer believed to be correct or what the health care professional wants to hear. This is most likely to happen when a patient is concerned about appearing to be stupid or does not understand the question. Leading questions can be useful when used with patients who have difficulty speaking or who do not understand English well enough to phrase a complete answer. In these situations, take extra care to check for understanding to ensure that the patient is not simply agreeing with you. See Table 16–1 for examples of each type of question.

After asking a question, it is important to pause and give the receiver sufficient time to respond. Some people need more time than others to formulate answers. Do not interrupt or finish sentences for the receiver. If it is obvious that the intended receiver does not understand the question or is unable to reply, reword the question and provide another opportunity for a response. The state of each patient and his or her ability to answer questions must be considered. For example, Mrs. Feinstein is an elderly patient who has difficulty remembering. Hospitalized for severe back pain, she cannot accurately respond to questions about how she is feeling today compared to yesterday. A more effective way to get the needed information is to ask her to rate her pain level on a scale of 0 to 10, with 0 being no pain and 10 being the highest level

Table 16–1 Common Types of Questions

Question Type	Examples
Closed-ended	What is your date of birth? Are you taking any medications?
Open-ended	How did you fall? Why do you think you are feeling sad?
Probing	You said that you've been experiencing pain in your chest. Where, exactly, in your chest do you feel the pain? When is it the most severe? Can you tell me more about when you get these headaches?
Leading	Would you describe the pain as sharp, dull, throbbing, or aching? Do you feel more nauseated in the morning, afternoon, evening, or during the night?

she can imagine. (See Chapter 20 for more information about assessing pain.)

Using Humor

Messages need not always be serious. The careful use of humor can offer temporary escape from the difficult situations faced by patients and their families. It can help relieve tension and promote the open discussion of sensitive issues. Humor, however, should *never* be at the expense of anyone, even in that person's absence.

Patients will sometimes joke about their condition as a cover-up for fear or embarrassment, but the health care professional should never initiate this type of humor. Listen carefully in these situations, because these jokes may indicate the patient's need for help in dealing with a difficult condition. It is appropriate to let patients know that if they wish, they can discuss fears they have or request information they need.

> **Thinking It Through**
>
> Robin Winters is starting her career as a dental hygienist for Dr. Castro at an urban dental clinic. Robin has noted that many of the patients appear to have poor dental care habits: Their teeth have accumulations of plaque and a high number of caries (cavities), and the patients suffer from gingivitis (inflammation of the gums). When she asks patients if they take care of their teeth at home, most respond, "Yes."
>
> 1. How can Robin use questions more effectively to learn about her patient's dental care habits?
> 2. Give examples of questions that she might ask.

Step Three: Deliver the Message

It is important to first determine to whom the message should be delivered. This is not always obvious. For example, if the patient is a child or elderly person, should communication be directed to the patient or to a family member? Patients who are able to understand any or all of the message should be addressed directly. Detailed information or instructions can also be given to a family member later. For example, a medical assistant who greets 87-year-old Mrs. Hernandez by asking her daughter, "How is your mother doing today?" is failing to show respect for the patient. This can undermine the self-esteem of older patients, who are often faced with the biases of a youth-oriented society. Using titles, such as Mrs., Ms., and Mr., demonstrates respect for patients. It is also generally inappropriate to address older persons as "dearie" or "hon." Although this may be considered a sign of affection, it is offensive to some patients. A common guideline for health care professionals is to address patients older than themselves more formally than those who are the same age or younger. If in doubt, it is best to ask patients how they wish to be addressed.

Some cultural groups designate a family member, often the oldest or a male, to make decisions on behalf of the patient. Although it is important for the health care professional to understand the dynamics of the patient's family, this does not suggest that the laws governing confidentiality can be broken in order to accommodate cultural preferences. Well-meaning family members and friends, the patient's insurance company, and others who may appear to have a valid right to know *cannot* be given information unless the patient has signed a release. It is essential to recognize which messages have a restricted audience and exactly who that audience is.

Advance directives and a health care power of attorney, discussed in Chapter 3, serve as the links between health care professionals and patients who have lost their ability to communicate. It is essential to know what medical treatments patients desire to be performed and who may receive information and speak on their behalf.

It is believed that many patients who cannot speak or respond can hear and experience touch. Under these circumstances, health care professionals can provide comfort by maintaining communication. They should speak reassuringly and consider making appropriate physical contact, such as touching the patient's hand or shoulder when speaking.

Nonverbal Communication

The manner in which a message is delivered can either reinforce or change the intended meaning. It can communicate more than the words that make up the content. For example, an otherwise friendly remark, stated in a sarcastic voice, distorts the intended message. The words "that's a nice thing to say" can be delivered in a way that indicates the sender's pleasure. The same words, delivered in a mocking tone with stress on the word "that's," convey the opposite meaning. It sends the message that what was said was hurtful.

Nonverbal communication includes tone of voice, body language, gestures, facial expressions, touch, and physical appearance. Up to 70% of the meaning of messages is expressed nonverbally. Nonverbal communication is usually the most accurate expression of what the sender truly feels and believes. This is because it comes from within and is conveyed without the awareness of the sender. It takes place subconsciously.

Health care professionals must be aware of the nonverbal communication of both themselves and others. The nonverbal communication of patients should always be observed. For example, if a patient reports feeling "fine" but appears very tense and nervous, the verbal and nonverbal messages do not match. In such cases, the health care professional needs to observe carefully, ask questions, and provide opportunities for the patient to share what is really being experienced.

The appearance of the health professional is a form of nonverbal communication. It can influence the patient's confidence in the worker's competence, which in turn can affect how messages are perceived. (See Chapter 13 for a discussion of professional appearance.)

Body Language

Body posture and movements convey messages. Some body language can have a negative impact on the receiver. Examples include crossing the arms, shrugging the shoulders, tapping the fingers or feet, clenching the fists, and rolling the eyes. These communicate disagreement, lack of interest, disbelief, and impatience.

Positive body language conveys interest, caring, and the willingness to listen to the sender's message, even if there is disagreement. It encourages the sharing of information and promotes the exchange of honest messages. Positive body language includes the following:

- Looking at the other person
- Directing the body toward the other person
- Leaning slightly toward the person being addressed
- Holding the body in a relaxed position
- Nodding or verbalizing ("uh huh," "yes," "tell me more") occasionally to indicate acknowledgement
- Having open and warm facial expressions
- Approaching the patient, if standing at a distance
- Stopping the performance of tasks to give your full attention

Positive body posture communicates "I am focused on and paying attention to you and what you are saying." (See Figure 16–3.) Actions must match words. For example, if a patient wants to discuss a sensitive matter and the health care professional listens while facing toward the door, the message to the patient may be "I'm really in a hurry to leave." In another example, a health care professional wants to reassure a patient, but looks away nervously while speaking. The message will seem false and the patient will sense that important information, possibly negative, is being left unsaid. Establishing trust, an essential ingredient in

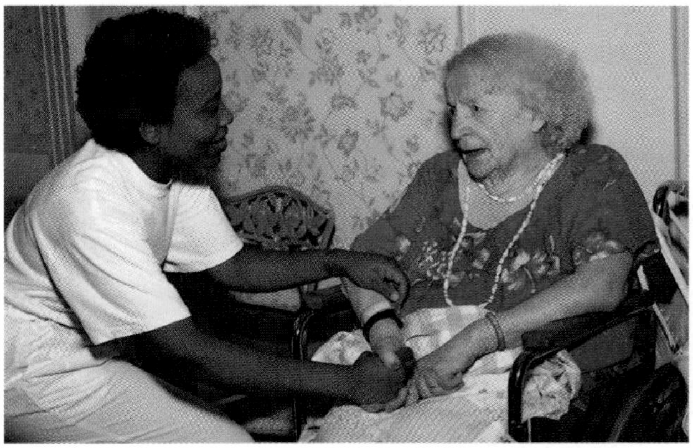

FIGURE 16–3 What positive body language is this health care professional demonstrating?

effective communication, requires that spoken and nonverbal communications match.

Facial Expressions

Facial expressions are an important form of nonverbal communication. The health care professional's expressions can be a source of reassurance or anxiety for patients, so it is important to learn to be aware of and control them. This can be difficult when dealing with situations that are challenging, unpleasant, or offensive. For example, you may feel very frustrated with the behavior of an angry patient. Efforts at calming the patient will be less effective if your face reflects signs of impatience and annoyance.

Patients look to the health professional for reassurance while receiving care, and facial expressions such as surprise or disgust can alarm them and undermine their faith in the services they are receiving. It is important not to react negatively to the sight of wounds or deformities and the smell of unpleasant odors. Patients are very sensitive to the reactions of health care professionals to these potentially worrisome and embarrassing conditions. The health care professional's face should reflect warmth, confidence, and interest in the welfare of the patient.

Gestures can help emphasize and enrich spoken messages. The use of **pantomime**, body movements that convey ideas or actions, can increase patient understanding. For example, acting out the movements a patient must make when performing an exercise can be used to demonstrate exactly what needs to be done. Pantomime is also an effective technique when patients cannot hear or understand the spoken word.

Gestures and facial expressions are helpful when patients cannot be attended to immediately. Acknowledging their presence conveys respect and creates good will. For example, if the medical receptionist is speaking on the telephone when a patient arrives for an appointment, the patient should be greeted with a smile, nod of the head, and quick hand gesture to indicate that he or she will be attended to shortly.

Use of Touch

The use of touch has become a difficult issue in health care today. Although a friendly pat or squeeze of the hand has been a traditional way of communicating care and interest, any touching that a patient considers to be inappropriate can lead to legal problems. It is essential that health care professionals always practice good judgment and use common sense. It is also important that they be aware that patients may have cultural preferences regarding touch, as discussed in Chapter 15. Many health care activities require entering personal space that is normally reserved for only the closest and most trusted people in the patient's life. It is important that patients be told what is to take place and why. Explain what they should expect to see, hear, and feel. For example, when administering an injection, the health care professional should inform the patient of its purpose, where it will be given, and what sensations might be experienced.

The health care professional should avoid touching areas that are considered sexual (buttocks, breasts, genital area) unless it is necessary when performing a procedure. Any unnecessary roughness, even done in a playful manner, can be interpreted as abusive and must be avoided.

Gestures and body movements that are either positive or neutral to one person may be unacceptable to others. As discussed in Chapter 15, health care professionals should be sensitive to the possibility of such differences, willing to learn about various cultural practices, and observant of patient reactions. If a patient seems uncomfortable with any contact that was intended to be a sign of caring or reassurance, seek clarification by stating your intention and asking if the gesture was unacceptable.

Physical Environment

The physical environment and how the health care professional is positioned in relation to the patient can affect the delivery of the message. Sitting behind a desk or standing over the other person projects a sign of authority or dominance. Other factors to consider include the following:

- Light sources: Can the patient see you clearly? Is there a glare on anything the patient is expected to see? Is light shining in the patient's eyes?
- Sounds: Can the patient hear you clearly? Are there unnecessary noises that are distracting? Should the television or radio be turned off?
- Privacy: Are there other people in the area who can hear the communication? If privacy is necessary, how can it be arranged? Are you speaking directly to the patient and only as loudly as necessary?
- Activity: Are you more focused on taking notes or entering data into a computer than on the patient?
- Comfort: Is the patient exposed or in an awkward position? Can communication wait?

Being aware of the effects of the environment and positioning on communication can help you deliver appropriate messages that achieve your intended communication goals.

Step Four: Listen to the Response

Listening is not passive, but an active process that requires the following:

- Concentration
- Attention
- Observation

Hearing and taking in words take place at a rate that is several times faster than the rate of speech. This is helpful when taking notes, but it also allows time for the mind to wander. Hearing too quickly can actually detract from engaging in **active listening**, which is characterized by focusing fully on what the speaker is saying. (Listening and trying to understand a message is also called "decoding.")

Effective listening can also be hindered by the receiver's reactions to what the sender is saying. For example, if the receiver strongly disagrees with the message, his or her mind may become occupied formulating mental arguments instead of listening carefully. Another common interference to listening is thinking about how one is going to respond when the speaker stops talking. The mind becomes engaged in self-talk and listening stops.

Good listening requires that receivers do not interrupt senders or complete messages for them. Allow enough time for senders to complete their messages. Encouraging remarks and gestures may be used as prompts: "I see," "Go on," or a nod of the head. Interrupting, however, can convey a lack of respect and impatience. It can also distort the sender's intended message, preventing important information from being conveyed. Effective listening skills can be developed. This is worth the effort because patients report that being listened to is a major determinant in their opinions of health care providers (Anderson, Barbara, & Feldman, 2007). Start by becoming aware of lapses in your attention. When a loss of focus is noted, bring your mind back to the speaker. With practice, internal interference and poor attention can be decreased. See Box 16–1 for a summary of good listening skills.

BOX 16–1

Summary of Good Listening Skills

Clear your mind of distractions

Face the sender

Focus your full attention on the sender

Maintain eye contact as appropriate for the culture

Turn off "self-talk"

Do not make value judgments about what you hear

Mentally note anything that needs clarification

Do not interrupt

Periods of silence can be a meaningful component of communication. The purpose of health care encounters is not to maintain a steady stream of conversation, but to help patients solve their health problems. Silence allows time for thought and reflection. It also provides a chance to observe the nonverbal communication that often takes place during silence. In addition, some cultures have a high respect for the value of silence. Allowing periods of silence may feel awkward at first, but they can be a valuable tool in promoting good communication.

Empathy

Good listening skills are necessary to achieve **empathy**, which means making an effort to understand another person's thoughts, feelings, and behavior. To experience empathy is to look at the world from the other person's viewpoint. The old expression "Walk a mile in my shoes" is a good description of the concept. Put another way, empathy states,

"I'm available to walk this road with you" (Tamparo & Lindh, 2008, p. 63). Empathy is a critical component of health care communication because it helps the health care professional understand and therefore more effectively address the needs of each patient. Practicing empathy allows each person to be considered as an individual.

Assumptions cannot be made about other people. This is especially true today when patients come from a variety of age groups and cultural backgrounds. Older adults, who make up a significant portion of today's patients, have a whole set of life experiences very different from those of their children and grandchildren. What seems common sense to one person may in fact make no sense to another. Health care professionals must understand the patient before they can help, and understanding only comes when they pay close attention to what patients say and do.

Empathy includes communicating that you are aware of the other person's feelings. Sharing in this way demonstrates care and respect. It can help relieve the loneliness and anxiety often experienced by patients and encourage them to feel safe about sharing feelings and discussing concerns. Empathy should not be confused with **sympathy**, which means feeling sorry for or taking pity on the other person.

Step Five: Offer Feedback and Seek Clarification

Feedback is a method by which the receiver can check his or her understanding of what the sender has said. Did the message come across as the sender intended? All of us have had the experience of believing we understood a message perfectly, only to discover later that we had misinterpreted it. Obtaining feedback helps avoid misunderstandings. Feedback also lets the speaker know that he or she has communicated effectively and therefore offers encouragement to continue.

Here are four ways to obtain feedback:

1. **Paraphrasing** The receiver rewords the sender's message in the receiver's own words and then asks the sender for confirmation.

   Example "I understood you to say that you have experienced these headaches every day for the past two weeks. Is that correct?"

2. **Reflecting** This is similar to paraphrasing, but prompts the receiver to either complete or add more detail to the original message.

   Example "You say that it's difficult for you to do the exercises the therapist has recommended because ___________." (Pause and allow time for response.)

3. **Asking questions** Request clarification and additional information. Many words, such as "difficult," "painful," and "a lot," have different meanings for people. In health care, the skillful use of questions can help patients describe their conditions more clearly. Accurate diagnoses and appropriate treatments depend, in part, on the clarity and completeness of information supplied by the patient.

   Example "What symptoms are you experiencing when you say you are feeling terrible?"

   Questions can be used to check the receiver's understanding of important information. Instead of asking if the receiver understands, ask a question whose answer will demonstrate understanding.

   Example "Can you list for me the three steps you'll take when giving your son his medication?"

   Open-ended questions, discussed earlier, can be used to encourage patients to talk about their values and beliefs. Although it is not the role of the health care professional to make value judgments about patients, what is learned can help you better understand the behavior and motivations of patients and find ways to meet their needs.

   Example "Why do you say that you deserved to have the accident?"

   This question may help in understanding why a patient is making no effort to perform the exercises that will assist in recovering from injuries.

4. **Requesting examples** Examples can help to more clearly explain and fill in meaning.

   Example "Tell me about the kind of situations in which you feel lightheaded."

   Establishing clear channels of communication by using feedback also helps maintain good relationships with coworkers and supervisors. Developing competence as a health care professional requires monitoring personal progress and learning from mistakes. Feedback can be an important tool for fostering professional growth. For example, Rosie's supervisor informs her that a report she has prepared is "unacceptable." Rosie can request more specific feedback by asking questions such as "What did I do or not do that made my performance on this task unacceptable?" and "Can you tell me exactly what it is that makes the report unacceptable?" These questions will encourage the supervisor to be specific and provide details from which Rosie can learn. If Rosie were to say "I don't know what you mean" or "I don't understand," the supervisor might not provide her with useful information. (See Figure 16–4.)

Step Six: Evaluate the Encounter

The purpose of evaluation is to determine whether the communication goals have been met. This can be demonstrated by either the response or behavior of the receiver. If the goal was not met, the following questions are examples of guidelines for identifying the difficulty:

- Did I clearly state my messages?
- Did I present them at a level appropriate for the receiver?
- Did I listen actively?
- Which part of the message was misunderstood?

The evaluation process actually continues throughout every communication encounter. A good communicator constantly checks for understanding by listening, observing, and asking for feedback as needed. Adjustments can then be made as needed.

Some communication goals are achieved over time, and the evaluation must be delayed. For example, if cardiac patient Heinrich Mueller is instructed about improving his eating habits, it may be weeks before the dietician finds out if he understood and was motivated to follow the low-fat eating plan. Another example of a long-term communication goal is making an effort over time to improve relationship with a coworker.

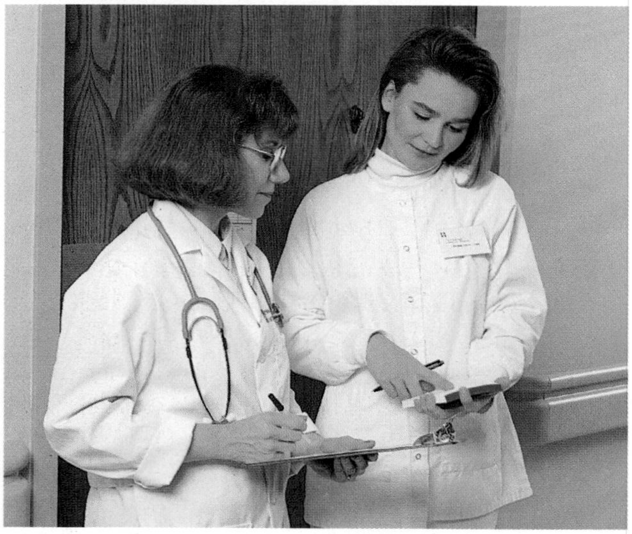

FIGURE 16–4 Good communication between members of the health care team is essential for providing good patient care.

Fascinating Facts

- Between 70% and 80% of our waking hours are spent in some form of communication: approximately 30% speaking and 45% listening.
- The average person speaks at 125 to 175 words per minute and can understand 400 words per minute.
- After listening to a 10-minute presentation, the average person retains 50% of what was said. After 48 hours, retention drops to 25%.

OVERCOMING COMMUNICATION BARRIERS

Obstacles known as **barriers** sometimes block communication. Barriers include the following:

- Language differences
- Cultural influences
- Defense mechanisms (see Chapter 15)
- Physical distractions
- Sensory impairments
- Medication effects
- Pain

Identifying and overcoming barriers require the use of empathy, observation, questions, and feedback. Specific techniques can be employed and extra time allowed in order to promote effective communication.

Patients Who Are Terminally Ill

Patients who are dying have reported that the loneliness they encounter is worse than the prospect of death itself (Purtilo & Haddad, 2007). As the dying

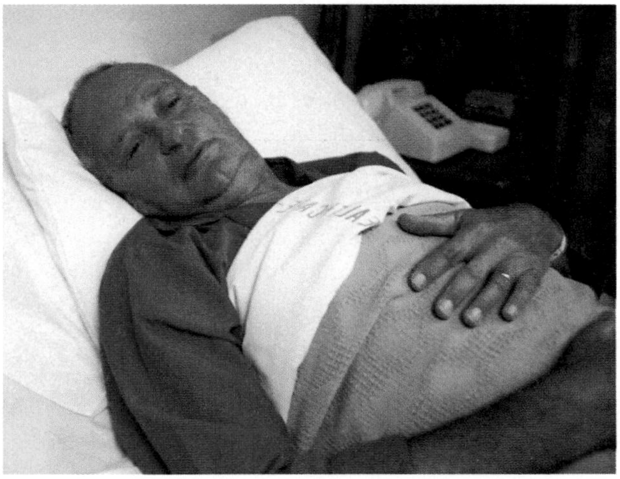

FIGURE 16–5 Dying patients often suffer from loneliness and feelings of isolation.

process advances, they may receive fewer visits and feel abandoned and cut off from the outside world. At the same time, many believe that they are given less attention than patients for whom "there is hope." (See Figure 16–5.) Some health care professionals view death as a failure of the system to help the patient. Others find it difficult to deal with because it brings up issues about their own mortality. It is important to come to terms with these difficult subjects in order to be truly effective and helpful when caring for terminally ill patients.

Terminally ill patients may have strong needs to share their fears and concerns, and health care professionals can serve as their major remaining links with life. Some patients want to talk about death and their desire to complete unfinished life tasks. The health care professional can improve the quality of this final phase by seeking, rather than avoiding, opportunities for communication. Be willing to listen and show that you care. Patients who cannot speak or respond may still be able to hear, so maintain oral communication. For example, greet the patient and explain what you are doing. Do not speak as if the patient is not in the room. (Home Care Institute, 2009). (See Chapter 8 for a discussion of death and dying.)

Thinking It Through

Craig Segal is a recently graduated licensed vocational nurse (LVN) who has been hired at an oncology clinic in his home town. Craig works with patients who are dealing with a potentially fatal disease. This is difficult because he has known many of them and their families for many years. He finds himself wondering how he can best communicate with patients and their families. Craig wants them to know that he cares and wants to be of assistance, but he is not sure how to approach what he believes to be emotional topics and finds himself keeping conversation to a minimum.

1. How can Craig use the steps of the communication process to help him feel more confident about communicating with patients?
2. Which techniques do you think he might find most effective?

Patients Who Are in Pain, Medicated, Confused, or Disoriented

Patients who are in pain, medicated, confused, or disoriented often have difficulty communicating. Health care professionals can assist them by taking extra time and following these guidelines:

- Identify yourself and say the patient's name.
- Maintain eye contact.
- Speak slowly and clearly in a moderate pitch of voice.
- Use simple language. Avoid slang and expressions that do not mean exactly what they say.
- Keep each message short and to the point. For example, do not give a series of instructions or ask more than one question at a time.
- Give the patient time to respond.
- Use touch if the patient is comfortable with it.
- Try to schedule interactions when patients are in the least amount of pain.
- Repeat the message as needed, without changing the content or words.
- Review the content with the patient to assess retention of the message.
- When appropriate, give the patient written information that can be referred to later.

(*Source:* Adapted from *Nursing Assistant: A Nursing Process Approach,* (9th ed.), by B. Hegner, E. Caldwell, & J. Needham, 2003, Clifton Park, NY: Delmar Cengage Learning.)

Patients with Alzheimer's Disease

In addition to causing memory loss, Alzheimer's disease decreases the ability to communicate, both in understanding others and expressing oneself orally. Patients may also exhibit difficult behavior, such as shouting, name-calling, hitting, and pushing. Health care professionals must be compassionate and patient, stay calm, and try not to take this behavior personally. The Alzheimer's Association (2015) offers the following suggestions for improving communication:

- Do not confront, argue, or try to reason with the patient.
- Give short, one-sentence explanations.
- Agree or distract with a different subject when what the patient says does not make sense or is repetitive.
- Respond to the patient's feelings rather than the words.
- Offer suggestions instead of corrections. For example, if a patient mistakes her brother for someone else, say, "I think this is your brother Gordon."

Patients Who Are Depressed

It is not uncommon for patients with serious conditions, such as cancer, to be depressed. This is usually a temporary condition, as opposed to **clinical depression**, but it can result in feelings of distress and can interfere with the patient's functioning and ability to communicate. Health care professionals should show compassion for all patients, but it is especially important to let depressed patients know: "I am here for you." "I'm glad to listen." At the same time, realize that these patients may respond negatively to everything you say. Specific suggestions for communication include the following:

- Invite, but do not force patients to talk about their fears, concerns, and how they are feeling.
- Listen carefully without judging.
- Offer hope, but do not advise them to "Cheer up" or "Be positive."
- Allow for silence.

(*Source: Adapted from American Cancer Society.* Caring for the patient with cancer at home. Depression. http://www.cancer.org/treatment/treatmentsandsideeffects/physicalsideeffects/dealingwithsymptomsathome/caring-for-the-patient-with-cancer-at-home-depression)

Patients Who Are Anxious

In addition to depression, anxiety is a common experience for many patients. Even a visit to the dentist can bring on anxiety for patients who fear needles, pain, or embarrassment about the condition of their teeth. Anxious patients may have difficulty focusing and responding, so exercise patience. Be empathetic and reassuring. At the same time, do not trivialize the patient's feelings by telling him or her, "It's silly to be anxious" or "There's nothing to be afraid of." Clearly, for the patient, the situation is fearful. Instead, try the following suggestions:

- Maintain a calm environment.
- Monitor the patient's anxiety level and respond accordingly.
- Keep messages simple.
- Stick to one topic to make it easier for the patient to follow.
- Use feedback to ensure the patient understood your message.

(*Source:* Home Care Institute, 2009.)

Patients Who Have Hearing Impairments

Hearing loss affects a significant number of Americans, as illustrated by the following statistics:

- Approximately 13% (30 million) Americans over age 12 have hearing loss in both ears.
- Who has disabling hearing loss?
  - 2% of adults 45 to 54 years old
  - 8% of adults 55 to 64 years old
  - 25% of adults 65 to 74 years old
  - 50% of adults age 75 or older
- About 2 to 3 out of every 1000 children in the United States are born deaf or hard of hearing.

(*Source:* National Institute on Deafness and Other Communication Disorders, http://www.nidcd.nih.gov/health/statistics/pages/quick.aspx)

When initiating conversation, especially with older adults, carefully observe the receiver and use appropriate feedback to check for understanding. It is important not to assume that people can hear just because they are not wearing a hearing aid or do not ask you to speak up. In fact, it is reported that only 30% of adults over age 70 who could benefit from using hearing aids actually wear them. Also, many people who experience hearing loss are unaware of

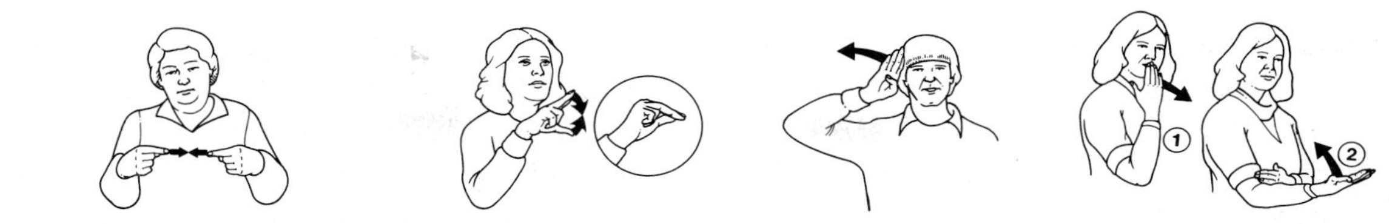

FIGURE 16–6 Sign language is a means of communication for many people who are hearing impaired.

it because it can happen gradually over the years or they are embarrassed to admit it. Following are signs that a person may have difficulty hearing:

- Leaning forward and turning the head
- Asking you to repeat information
- Failing to hear when not facing the speaker
- Not responding to you when you ask a question or finish speaking

American Sign Language (ASL) provides a means of communication for people with significant or complete hearing loss. It consists of hand movements and shapes, facial expressions, and corresponding body postures to convey meaning. (See Figure 16–6.) Partly due to the difficulty experienced in trying to communicate with people who have normal hearing, many hearing-impaired individuals consider themselves to be members of a unique cultural group they refer to as "deaf culture" (Gallaudet University, n.d.).

The following suggestions can improve communication with the hearing impaired:

- Position yourself close to the receiver and speak face to face.
- Remove or turn off sources of noise.
- Have the light source directed to your face.
- Make sure your mouth is visible to the listener.
- Keep your hands away from your face.
- Say the person's name before beginning the conversation.
- Determine if the person hears better in one ear than the other.
- Introduce the general topic of the conversation.
- Speak distinctly and do not mumble.
- Speak slowly, but naturally.
- Do not shout or exaggerate words. This can make it even more difficult for the person to understand.
- Maintain a low to moderate pitch of voice.
- Use short sentences.
- Watch for signs of comprehension.
- Do not change the subject without warning.

(*Source:* Alexander Graham Bell Association, 1996; University of California San Francisco Medical Center, n.d.)

When necessary, video services with ASL interpreters are available for communication with deaf patients.

Patients Who Have Visual Impairments

Patients who have visual limitations need special consideration, too. They do not have visual clues with which to orient themselves physically. With 70% of the meaning of communication being conveyed nonverbally, it is understandable that the visually impaired person experiences special communication challenges. Here are some ways to assist visually impaired patients:

- Start all communication by announcing your presence and identifying yourself.
- Before starting a procedure, describe any equipment to be used and its position in relation to the patient.
- As you proceed, explain what will be done and where you will be touching the patient.
- Explain what noises the patient will hear.
- Give clear and complete directions. For example, say, "Raise your left arm directly in front of you to a 45-degree angle," not "Raise your arm like this," or "Lift your arm."
- Let the patient know when you are leaving the area.
- If the patient is to leave, give specific instructions about doorways and other landmarks

and obstacles, such as uneven surfaces, that the patient will encounter.

- Give extra verbal information to describe anything that would usually be expressed through facial expressions, gestures, head nods, and other movements.

(*Source:* Adapted from *Nursing Assistant: A Nursing Process Approach*, (10th ed.), by B. Hegner, E. Caldwell, & J. Needham, 2003, Clifton Park, NY: Delmar Cengage Learning.)

Patients Who Have Speech Impairments

Patients may be unable to speak because of an injury or a stroke. The condition may be temporary, such as when on a ventilator or using an artificial airway. Patients who are unable to express themselves can become anxious, frustrated, and even panicked. Communication can be aided by the use of pantomime, pictures and drawings, writing, and specially designed communication boards that have the most common patient requests to which they can point.

Aphasia is a condition in which individuals have trouble saying (and/or writing) words correctly. Problems vary from having difficulty finding the correct word to saying whole sentences that do not make sense. The main cause of aphasia is stroke. It may also be the result of loss of brain function, as happens with Alzheimer's disease. Here are some ways to improve communication for people with aphasia:

- Remove noise and distractions.
- Use adult language. Do not treat patients as if they were children.
- Ask yes and no questions.
- Give clear choices for possible answers.
- Use visual cues. (See Figure 16–7.)
- Encourage the patient to communicate with you through gestures and drawings.
- Check for understanding.

Patients Who Are Angry

Anger is the emotional response of displeasure or extreme annoyance to a perceived wrong. The loss of personal control experienced due to illness or injury, worries about the expense of health care, and the inconvenience of having to wait for service can all result in patient anger. Anger can also be caused by problems unrelated to health care, such as family difficulties or the loss of a job.

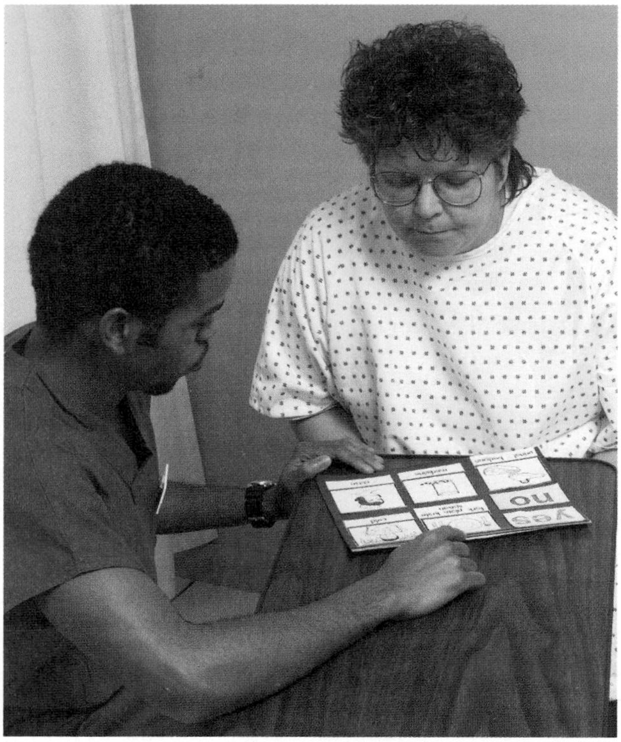

FIGURE 16–7 Picture cards help enable communication with patients who cannot speak or who do not speak English.

When dealing with an angry patient, try to determine the cause. In many cases, the anger is not the fault of the health care professional. Recall the defense mechanisms discussed in Chapter 15. Anger may be a form of displacement in which the patient is unable to direct anger at the real cause. If, however, you discover that you have done something to upset the patient, apologize sincerely and try to establish good communication aimed at meeting the patient's needs. The following guidelines are helpful when dealing with angry patients:

- Never respond in anger or argue with the patient.
- Remain calm and courteous.
- Listen attentively to the patient's concerns.
- Offer a sincere apology, if necessary.
- Do not raise your voice.
- Be aware of your body language. Look at the patient.

- Express concern and interest, not annoyance.
- Answer the patient's questions.
- If you cannot resolve the problem, discuss it with your supervisor or other appropriate person.
- If the patient is cursing or being verbally abusive, state politely that you are willing to listen but will not tolerate cursing or threatening language.
- Ask for help from a coworker or security, if necessary.

Patients Who Do Not Speak English

Imagine yourself as a tourist in a country whose language you do not speak and where the health care practices are different from those of the United States. You are involved in an accident and taken to a hospital where no one speaks English. You cannot explain your needs, the location of your pain, or ask questions about your condition. The treatments are different from anything you have ever experienced.

The fear and confusion experienced in this scenario are similar to those of some immigrants and non–English-speaking patients in the United States. Health care professionals can demonstrate compassion and care for these patients by learning at least a few common phrases of the major languages spoken in their community. In addition, the following ideas are helpful when working with non–English-speaking patients:

- A smile is a universal sign of good will.
- Determine if the patient speaks or understands any English at all.
- Find out if an English-speaking family member or friend is available to help. (Be sure that the patient agrees to have the other person involved so that confidentiality is not violated.)
- Speak slowly and clearly.
- Do not raise your voice. It will not help the other person understand.
- Use simple words and sentences.
- Do not use slang or expressions that may be misunderstood.
- Try repeating your message in different words.
- Use gestures and pantomime to demonstrate what you need the patient to do.
- Write the message.
- Use pictures, if available. (See Figure 16–7.)
- Request the services of an interpreter, if necessary. In addition to on-site, face-to-face interpreting, there are telephone and video services that enable health care providers to communicate with patients who speak other languages.

Hispanics, at 54 million, make up the largest population in the United States who may speak a language other than English. Of these, more than 38 million speak Spanish at home (U.S. Census Bureau, September 8, 2014). Although many Hispanics speak English as well as Spanish, a significant number do not. If a patient speaks a little English, take care not to assume that health care communication will be understood. Health care professionals who are likely to work with Spanish-speaking patients can better help patients by learning a few words and phrases. See Appendix 2 for a list of conversational and health-related phrases.

SPECIAL APPLICATIONS OF COMMUNICATION SKILLS

There are a variety of special applications of communication skills in health care work. Each application requires the use of specific techniques.

Telephone Communication

The telephone often provides the first means of contact between patients and health care facilities. The impression that patients, other professionals, and the general public receive at this time influences their perception of the facility and helps set the tone for all future communication. It is essential that caring, interest, and competence be projected to callers.

Employers report that the inability to properly handle telephone calls is a major weakness among new hires. The health care professional who develops excellent telephone skills is a valuable asset. It is a mistake to take these skills for granted or consider them to be unimportant.

The quality of the voice is an important factor in all types of oral communication, but it is especially significant when speaking on the telephone. The receiver has no visual clues and must depend on words and voice to understand the message.

The following guidelines can help create a telephone manner that is both welcoming and professional:

- Identify yourself.
- If necessary, ask permission to place the caller on hold.
- Speak clearly and pronounce words correctly and distinctly.
- Speak at a moderate rate of speed. When giving instructions or directions, speak more slowly.
- Strive for a pleasant tone, not too high-pitched.
- Project warmth, friendliness, and caring.
- Smile as you speak unless it is inappropriate in the situation, as in a call for emergency help.
- Put expression in your voice. Avoid speaking in a monotone.
- Allow appropriate periods of silence to give the other person an opportunity to speak.
- Never chew gum or eat when speaking on the telephone.

The Health Insurance Portability and Accountability Act (HIPAA) guidelines regarding patient confidentiality apply to telephone messages. Protected information, such as test results, cannot be given to anyone except the patient to whom the information applies. It is important, therefore, to determine the identity of the person with whom you are speaking. While it is acceptable to leave reminders of appointments or requests to call on answering machines, never leave messages that contain confidential information.

Patient Education

Many patients today are taking more responsibility for their own health. They want to know about preventive measures, such as diet and exercise, to avoid disease and injury. Patients have questions about the many television commercials they see promoting prescription drugs and other health aids. And many have searched the Internet for information about their symptoms and conditions, sometimes obtaining information from advertisers that may or may not coincide with their health care provider's professional opinion.

More hands-on care is being performed by patients themselves as a result of the decreasing length of hospital stays. The complex diagnostic and treatment procedures can be frightening for patients. For example, surgical technologists may be called upon to talk with patients who are anxious as they face surgery. Patient education by caring individuals has been shown to positively influence postoperative recovery (Frey & Ross, 2008). For these reasons, a significant portion of your time as a health care professional may be spent on patient education. See Table 16–2 for examples of categories of patient education topics.

Providing effective patient education can be one of the most satisfying responsibilities of health care work. Education requires the application of many general communication concepts. Its purpose is to provide knowledge and skills that lead to a change in patient behavior. The steps in the communication process described in this chapter can be adapted to provide a process for delivering patient education:

1. Set educational goals.

   Educators call these **learning objectives** and create them to describe what students will be able to do as a result of the instruction. Examples of goals for patients include the following:

   - Self-administer insulin injection following correct procedure
   - Follow a daily physical exercise program

Table 16–2 Examples of Patient Education Subject Categories

Category	Examples
Promote wellness	Hygiene Nutrition Exercise
Prevent illness	First aid Safety Immunizations Management of risk factors
Restore health	Orientation to treatment Introduction to staff Information about the illness Self-care practices
Improve coping skills	Stress management Grief counseling Community resources

Source: Adapted from Fundamentals of Nursing: The Art and Science of Nursing Care (6th ed.), by C. Taylor, C. Lillis, & P. LeMone, 2006, Philadelphia, PA: Lippincott-Raven Publishers.

- Identify medication side effects that require calling the physician

2. Create the instructional message.

   This means deciding how the instruction will be provided. As with any other communication, it is based on the patient's needs and current condition. When creating effective instruction, additional facts about the patient should be determined:

   - Level of knowledge: What does the patient already know about the topic? It is frustrating to be given information that either repeats what is already known or is too advanced for the patient to understand.
   - Preferred learning style: Ask patients whether they learn best by listening, seeing, or doing. (See Chapter 1 for more information about learning styles.)
   - Motivation: How important does the patient believe the information to be?
   - Ability to learn: Is the patient able to acquire and retain new information at this time?

     Use nontechnical language that patients are likely to understand. Break information into sections and relate it to something the patient already knows. Finally, try not to give too much information at one time to avoid overwhelming the patient.

3. Deliver the instruction.

   Instruction can be delivered in a variety of ways. In order to address the various learning styles of patients and to reinforce the material presented, use as many methods as possible:

   - Oral explanations, presented to either an individual or a group
   - Audiovisual materials such as videos, diagrams, and charts
   - Written materials such as instructional sheets, lists, informational reports, pamphlets, reprints of journal articles (See Chapter 17 for information about creating written documents.)
   - Discussion groups
   - Demonstrations of procedures, exercises, self-care techniques
   - Computerized instruction such as CDs, DVDs, interactive software programs, and information available on the Internet (See Chapter 18 about computer uses in education.)

4. Listen.

   Encourage patients to ask questions as material is presented and then listen carefully to find out what they do not understand and what they want to know.

5. Check for understanding (use feedback and seek clarification).

   Ask patients to summarize what they have learned or to explain how they will apply the new information. If appropriate, have patients demonstrate what they learned. They must be able to perform the task without prompting. Allow them to repeat the task as necessary to demonstrate mastery.

6. Evaluate.

   - Were the instructional goals met?
   - Does the patient appear to understand the instruction? Is the patient able to repeat information or satisfactorily demonstrate the skills?
   - Does the patient achieve the results intended by the instruction?

Presentations to Groups

You may not expect to give formal speeches as a health care professional, but there may be occasions when it is necessary to talk to a group. Examples include explaining home care procedures to a patient's family members, giving a report at a professional meeting, and demonstrating a new procedure to coworkers. Developing the ability to organize and present information orally can increase your effectiveness in helping others.

It is important to plan in advance what you are going to say, even when the audience is a small, informal group. Patient health may depend on the clarity of the presentation. The following strategies can help improve its effectiveness:

- Be clear about the purpose and most important points.
- Determine the needs and level of understanding of the audience.
- Organize material so it is easy for the audience to follow.

- Avoid jumping from topic to topic or adding unnecessary information that can be confusing.
- Speak at a moderate rate.
- Prepare notes or a checklist to prevent forgetting important points.
- Look at the audience while you are speaking.

Gossip and Patient Privacy

Gossip is unnecessary conversation, often negative, about people who are not present. It serves no constructive purpose and should always be avoided. Gossip about one's coworkers can disrupt the harmony of the health care team and compromise the quality of the patient care delivered. If it involves the inappropriate sharing of patient information, it can result in a lawsuit. (See information on patient confidentiality in Chapter 3.) Any type of gossip is a time-waster and cannot be justified in the busy schedules maintained by health care facilities. If a coworker tries to engage you in gossip, the following techniques may be helpful:

- Explain that you believe such conversation is unfair to the subject of the gossip. ("I don't think we know enough about the situation to discuss it," or "I don't think it's fair to talk about people behind their back.")
- State that you believe it is inappropriate for discussion. ("You know, I really don't feel comfortable talking about that.")
- Change the subject. ("What I really need to talk to you about is...")

Take care that private patient information is not included in social conversations with coworkers. Avoid making comments in public areas that might be overheard by the patient's friends or family members. Even sympathetic remarks such as, "I feel so bad. My favorite patient, Mr. Phillips, was just diagnosed with lung cancer," can be damaging if overheard. Patient names, along with personal information, should not be used during telephone conversations that can be heard by others. For example, when transferring a telephone call from the front desk, say "A patient is calling to follow up as you requested," *not* "Mr. Sanders is calling to get the results of his HIV test." If patient information is shared with another health professional in the patient's presence, it is best to include the patient in the conversation. Being "talked about," even by health care professionals discussing the patient's condition, can cause anxiety. Patients want to be acknowledged as individuals and not made to feel like "cases."

Thinking It Through

Robin Winters, the dental hygienist with Dr. Castro, wants to create a patient education program to teach effective dental home care and nutritional practices. Her patients range from toddlers to the elderly. They come from a variety of cultural backgrounds. Some speak English as a second language.

1. What should Robin take into consideration when planning a patient education program?
2. What types of methods would you suggest she use?
3. How can she check for patient understanding?
4. How can she evaluate the effectiveness of her program?

WEB ACTIVITIES

Go to your workbook and complete the exercises for this chapter.

SUGGESTED LEARNING ACTIVITIES

1. Make a poster that illustrates the six steps in the communication process.
2. Observe people as they communicate. What communication techniques are they using? Do they appear to be effective? Why or why not?
3. Apply what you have learned in this chapter to your everyday life. Use the listening techniques when communicating with your instructors, friends, and family members.
4. Practice asking different types of questions and using feedback in your everyday encounters.
5. Create a list or chart of various forms of nonverbal communication.
6. Look for examples of nonverbal communication in your daily life. List the instances when the

nonverbal message does not seem to match the verbal message.

7. Mentally monitor your telephone conversations over the next week. Note the conversations you find most pleasant and those that are most unpleasant. Explain why in each case.
8. Create a teaching situation with a friend or family member. Apply the education process presented in the chapter and describe the results.

WEB ACTIVITIES

The Focusing Institute
www.focusing.org

Point to the "Focusing and..." tab. On the drop-down menu, click on "Medicine." Scroll down the page and click on "Listening and Focusing: Holistic Health Care Tools for Nurses, Joan Klagsbrun, Ph.D." Read the article and then discuss how you can apply active listening and focusing to your future occupation.

Effective Communication

Using the term "effective communication techniques," conduct an Internet search. Review at least three articles and choose one you think contains helpful methods for the health care professional. Write a summary of one of the articles and try out at least two of the methods in your daily communications.

Aging Resources of Central Iowa
www.agingresources.com

Click on "Resources" at the top of the page. Scroll down to "PDF Documents" and open the document "Communicating with Older Adults." Read the online booklet to learn about the characteristics of aging and ways that health care professionals can work more effectively with older patients.

Health Literacy Consulting
www.healthliteracy.com

In the search box, enter "humor." You will see a list of health literacy articles. Click on "Adding a Dose of Humor to Your Patient Teaching." Do you agree that humor can be an effective communication tool when working with patients? Explain why or why not.

REVIEW QUESTIONS

1. Why is effective communication an important factor in health care delivery?
2. How does communication affect patient well-being?
3. What are the six steps of the communication process?
4. What are four types of questions? Give an example of each.
5. What is *nonverbal communication*? Give three examples.
6. What is the meaning of *active listening*?
7. What is the meaning of *empathy*? Why is it important in health care?
8. What is *feedback*? How can its use improve communication?
9. What are five common barriers that can interfere with communication?
10. Describe two specific considerations or techniques when communicating with patients who are:
    a. Terminally ill
    b. In pain or medicated
    c. Diagnosed with Alzheimer's disease
    d. Depressed
    e. Anxious
    f. Hearing impaired
    g. Visually impaired
    h. Speech impaired
    i. Angry
    j. Unable to understand English well
11. What are eight ways to project a professional impression when speaking on the telephone?
12. What are six steps for developing and delivering effective patient education?
13. What are five ways to improve presentations given to groups?
14. Explain how to handle situations at work that involve gossip.
15. Why is it unacceptable to discuss patients with anyone who is not involved in the patient's care?

APPLICATION EXERCISES

1. Refer to The Case of the Coder Who Lacked Confidence at the beginning of the chapter. What would you recommend that Jenny do in order to increase her communication skills?
2. Compare and contrast how you would initiate communication with each of the following patients. Include your communication goal, what information you would need to gather about the patient, and important factors to consider in preparing your message.
   a. You are a medical assistant. The patient has a severe hearing impairment. She is seeing the physician for a routine physical examination.
   b. You are a dental hygienist. The patient is 5 years old and terrified of the dentist's office.
   c. You are a physical therapist assistant. The patient is a well-to-do man in his 50s. He is furious about having had to wait for 20 minutes while you finished working with your previous patient.

PROBLEM-SOLVING PRACTICE

Josie has a new job at an imaging center conveniently located near her home. She loves working with the patients and applying what she learned in her radiology classes. But the manager of the center has poor supervisory skills and the staff constantly complains and gossips about the woman and sometimes about each other. Everyone seems to be taking sides. How can Josie use the five-step problem-solving process to help her improve her work situation?

SUGGESTED READINGS AND RESOURCES

Colbert, B. (2006). *Workplace readiness for health occupations* (2nd ed.). Clifton Park, NY: Delmar Cengage Learning.

Kelz, R. (1999). *Conversational Spanish for health professionals* (3rd ed.). Clifton Park, NY: Delmar Cengage Learning.

Milliken, M. E., & Honeycutt, A. (2012). *Understanding human behavior* (8th ed.). Clifton Park, NY: Delmar Cengage Learning.

Munoz, C., & Luckmann, J. (2005). *Transcultural communication in nursing* (2nd ed.). Clifton Park, NY: Delmar Cengage Learning.

National Federation of the Blind. www.nfb.org

National Institute on Deafness and Other Communication Disorders. www.nidcd.nih.gov

Practicing Spanish—Medical Spanish. www.practicing-spanish.com

Tamparo, C., & Lindh, W. (2008). *Therapeutic communications for health care* (3rd ed.). Clifton Park, NY: Delmar Cengage Learning.

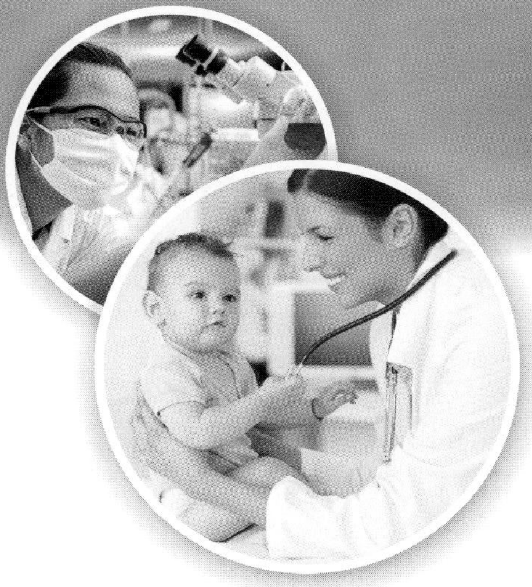

Chapter 17

Written Communication

OBJECTIVES

Studying and applying the material in this chapter will help you to:

- Explain why the ability to write clearly and correctly is an important skill for the health care professional.
- Describe effective techniques for planning and organizing written documents.
- Use correct spelling and grammar in all written communication.
- Explain how to write, format, and send effective business letters.
- List what should be included in meeting agendas and minutes.
- Describe techniques for creating effective written patient education materials.
- Discuss the proper handling of written documents to protect patient confidentiality.
- List ways to improve proofreading skills.

KEY TERMS

agenda
block letter
consonant
contraction
cross-training
etiquette
grammar
independent clause
justified
modified block letter
quotation
salutation
semi-block letter
suffix
syllable
vowel
word processing

The Case of the Surprised Therapist

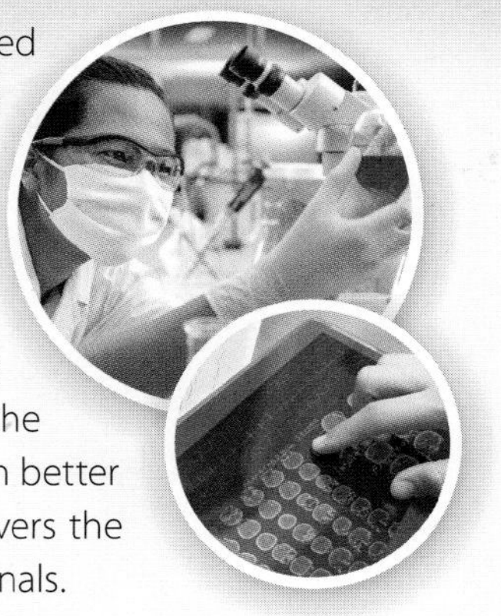

Al Trent was recently hired by Cathy Barnes, a physical therapist in private practice. When Al started work, he imagined that his tasks would consist mainly of working with patients. He was surprised when Cathy asked him to help her with several special projects that required good writing skills. She is active at both the local and state level of two professional organizations. Believing that professional organizations are important for the promotion of physical therapy, she has encouraged Al to become active and has requested his help in preparing agendas and reports for the meetings. Cathy has also asked him to prepare written instruction sheets for patients to use when doing exercises at home. Although there is an administrative assistant who does the billing, bookkeeping, and other clerical tasks, Cathy believes that Al's physical therapy education better qualifies him for writing materials that are directly related to physical therapy. This chapter covers the basics of effective written communication that may be required of today's health care professionals.

WRITTEN COMMUNICATION: A VITAL LINK IN HEALTH CARE

The quality of modern health care delivery depends heavily on the completeness and accuracy of written communications prepared by health care professionals. Many kinds of documents are created daily. They range from notes made in a patient's medical record to technical reports to formal business letters. The type of writing done by each health care professional depends on his or her specific occupation and employment circumstances. However, even workers who spend most of their time providing hands-on patient care may prepare written documentation and may be required to write an occasional letter or patient instruction sheet. Writing skills are used when preparing resumes, cover letters, and letters inquiring about employment opportunities. Health care professionals who decide to pursue additional education may find themselves assigned research papers and other writing assignments. The ability to write clearly and correctly is a mark of professionalism and increases the health care professional's value and promotional opportunities.

Written documents provide important links among the many professionals and facilities that make up the web of care for today's patients. However, while the growth in specialty services raises the level of care, it also increases the chances for miscommunication and lost information. Consider the communication trail created during the routine annual exam of Mrs. Kardinski, a 55-year-old patient of Dr. Landau:

1. Dr. Landau's administrative medical assistant, Denise Carter, sends Mrs. Kardinski a *reminder letter* to encourage her to make an appointment for her annual physical exam.
2. On the day of the appointment, Denise locates the patient's *file* for the clinical medical assistant, Lachelle Hayes.
3. Lachelle updates the *medical record* with Mrs. Kardinski's weight, blood pressure, and other vital signs.
4. Lachelle adds further notes to the *medical record* at the direction of Dr. Landau during the exam.
5. Dr. Landau signs *request forms* for routine tests to be performed at other facilities.
6. Mrs. Kardinski visits an off-site lab to have blood drawn for routine tests, and the lab sends the results in a *report* to Dr. Landau's office.
7. Mrs. Kardinski then visits an imaging center for a mammogram, and the center sends a *report* to Dr. Landau's office.
8. The cytology lab that examines the Pap specimen sends a *report* to Dr. Landau's office.
9. All reports are normal, so Denise sends a *letter* to Mrs. Kardinski, notifying her of the results.
10. Denise sends a *statement* to Mrs. Kardinski's insurance company.

Mrs. Kardinski's routine visit involves at least 10 written documents that contain essential information for ensuring that she receives consistent and appropriate care. (Even information that is sent electronically is entered in words and sentences that must be correct. This need for accuracy includes the spelling of medical terms which, if incorrect, can result in errors and misunderstandings.) Appropriate care depends on the smooth flow of clearly and accurately prepared written communications among health care providers and between them and their patients.

THE COMPONENTS OF GOOD WRITING

Good writing is characterized by logical organization and attention to detail, including spelling, grammar, and format. In addition to helping ensure good patient care, complete and accurate written documents are viewed by many as the sign of a competent professional. Writing that contains errors and is poorly presented reflects negatively on the quality of the individual as well as on the facility. Patients may question the competence of the facility to deliver quality health care if written documents are sloppily prepared, contain spelling errors, and are difficult to understand.

Organizing Content

All types of written communication, whether they consist of one paragraph or several pages, must be organized in a way that is easy for the reader to follow and understand. Unlike oral communication, in which the speaker can request feedback and make necessary adjustments, written communication must stand on its own. Writers cannot use nonverbal language to enhance and emphasize their messages.

The steps for organizing written content described in this section are designed as a guide for creating all types of written communication. The specific techniques used and the time spent on each are determined by the type of document being prepared. For example, a short memo might take 10 minutes to plan and write, whereas a research report could take more than a month and require attention to each step in the process. Whatever the length of a document, good writing requires that consideration be given to planning and organizing.

Preparing to Write

1. Determine the purpose for writing.
   - Inform
   - Persuade
   - Gather information
   - Encourage action

   It is possible to have more than one purpose. A patient information sheet about physical exercise, for example, may be designed to provide information about the health benefits of exercise *and* encourage patients to participate in regular physical activity.
2. Generate ideas for content based on the purpose of the document.
   - List as many ideas as come to mind. Write down everything you already know about the topic.
   - Gather facts. Sources include professional journals, books, publications from professional organizations, and credible websites. (See Chapter 18 for information on evaluating the quality of sites.)
   - Talk with others. Get content information from experts. Ask potential readers what they want to know.
3. Consider the reader's:
   - Knowledge of the subject matter
   - Reading level (age, native language, level of education)
   - Interest in the subject
   - Reason for needing the information

   It is appropriate to use medical terminology and abbreviations in writing that is directed to health care professionals because, as the "language of medicine," your message will be more clear and specific. This is why mastering medical terminology is important for health care professionals. At the same time, this language can confuse patients who do not have a background in health care. It is also important to know that

Thinking It Through

For each of the documents involved in Mrs. Kardinski's routine visit, discuss the possible consequences for the patient and health care providers if it were:

1. Written inaccurately
2. Sent to the wrong facility or person

some abbreviations are unacceptable because they can confuse even health care professionals. (See Chapter 4.)

The tone, which is the writer's attitude toward the topic, must be appropriate for the situation. Tone is expressed through the writer's choice of word. The following two sentences basically say the same thing, but notice the difference in tone:

- You must be here on time.
- We would appreciate it if you could be here on time.

The tone should be adapted to the circumstances. Take the example of collection letters for late payment. A long-time patient who always pays medical bills promptly but is currently experiencing financial difficulties might receive a different letter than the one directed to a patient with a history of late payments.

4. Organize the content.

The material should flow in a way that makes sense to the reader. The traditional structure of a written document includes three parts:

- Introduction—State the topic and purpose. Interesting facts and questions can be used to attract the reader's attention.
- Body—Fully develop the topic or message. Provide supporting facts and information. Ways to present information include:
    - Examples and illustrations
    - Description, using specific details
    - List of steps in a process
    - List of reasons
    - Grouping of items into categories
- Conclusion—Summarize the information contained in the body. Effective endings include restating the purpose or pointing out how the facts given support the purpose.

Starting to Write

The task of writing can be simplified by using one of the following organizing techniques. Even short documents can be improved by making a few notes before preparing the "real thing."

- Create a formal outline. Use letters and numbers to create a detailed outline, which is fleshed out when you begin to write. (See Figure 17–1 for an example.)
- Create an informal outline. Omit letters and numbers. Simply list major ideas and indent supporting ideas.
- Draw a diagram, also known as a mind map, using circles and lines to connect major and supporting ideas. This is especially helpful for visual learners, who may also want to use colors to clarify the relationships of ideas. Figure 17–2 shows how the information contained in the formal outline in Figure 17–1 looks in mind map form.

Many professional writers suggest writing the first draft as quickly as possible when starting to write a long document. Content, rather than grammar

Using an Outline to Organize Content
Subject: Hepatitis B

I. Introduction
  A. Threat to health
  B. Vaccine available
II. Symptoms
  A. Loss of appetite
  B. Fatigue
  C. Nausea
  D. Headache
  E. Fever
  F. Jaundice
III. Transmission
  A. Contact with virus
    1. Sexual contact
    2. Blood
    3. Body fluids
      a. Vaginal secretions
      b. Semen
      c. Fluids from body cavities
      d. Sputum
IV. Treatment
  A. Dietary measures
    1. Decrease dietary fat
    2. Low protein
    3. Small, frequent high-calorie meals (if nausea present)
    4. Decrease fluids (if retaining)
  B. Bed rest
V. Prevention
  A. Hepatitis B vaccine for employees at risk for exposure
  B. Standard precautions
    1. Handwashing
    2. Gloves
    3. Personal protective equipment
    4. Proper handling of needles
    5. Proper disposal of hazardous waste

FIGURE 17–1 Sample of formal outline to organize content for writing.

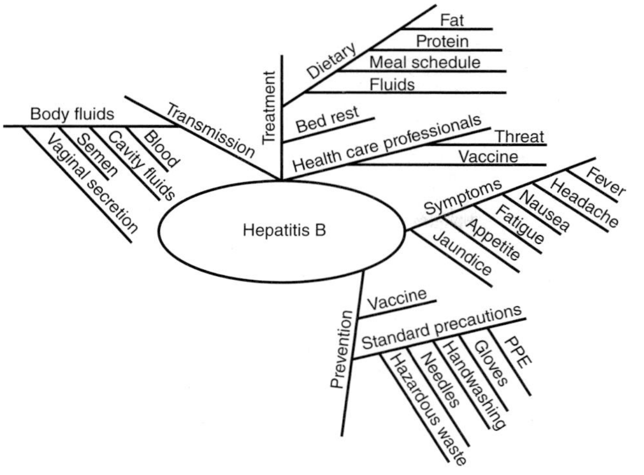

FIGURE 17–2 Some visual learners find mind maps to be a helpful way to organize content.

and spelling, should be emphasized at this time. Creativity can be lost when the focus is on detail. Trying for perfection on the first draft can be so intimidating that the writer becomes overwhelmed. The final draft, however, should have perfect spelling and grammar.

Spell Your Way to Success

Spelling errors in medical documents can have serious consequences. Apart from giving the impression of carelessness, misspelled words can cause confusion that negatively affects patient care. As discussed in Chapter 4, many medical terms can present difficulties because they were borrowed from Latin and Greek, are long, have silent letters, or have spelling that is similar to other words with different meanings. A medical dictionary, either printed or computerized, is a good tool for the medical professional. Online medical spell checkers are also available and can be located by entering the search term "online medical spell checker" into a search engine, such as Google or Bing. There are also a number of online medical dictionaries, including one at medlineplus.gov, a service of the National Library of Medicine.

If you are ever in doubt about the spelling of any word, take the time to check it. Not doing so is negligent. There are many tools available to assist with proper spelling:

- General English dictionary. If English is your second language, you may also need a bilingual dictionary.
- Medical dictionaries, available in print, online, and as an app
- Word books for health care specialties
- Online dictionaries
- Spell-checkers on **word processing** software (programs for creating written documents on a computer). These are available for general English and medical vocabulary. Do not depend on spell-checkers to catch all errors, because the computer cannot identify words that are spelled correctly but used incorrectly. For example, "to" is spelled correctly, but is incorrect if you meant to write "too" or "toe."
- Pharmaceutical reference guides, such as the *Physicians' Desk Reference* (PDR), available online at www.pdr.net

Spelling Tips

Everyday English, as well as medical spelling, can be challenging, but it is well worth the time and effort necessary to achieve mastery. Here are a few suggestions for improving spelling:

1. Learn the major spelling rules listed in Table 17–1. Each rule governs the spelling of many words and prevents having to learn to spell each word individually.
2. Memorize words that are look-alikes, exceptions to the rules, or ones you usually misspell. Try a method that complements your learning style. (See Chapter 1.)
   - Write each word several times.
   - Spell each word out loud several times.
   - Make flashcards for practice and self-quizzes.
   - List words on a wall chart and place it where you will see it often.
   - Create rhymes or associations. For example, the sentence "He was vain about owning a big van" might help distinguish between "vain" and "vein."
   - Create a personal dictionary of words with which you have trouble. This can be handwritten or stored electronically. Review the list regularly.
3. Review troublesome words regularly for mastery. See Table 17–2 for a list of frequently misspelled words that are commonly used in health care.

Table 17–1 Major Spelling Rules

Rule	Examples
Place *i* before *e* except after *c* or in words in which the *ei* sounds like ay. *Exceptions:* seize either weird height foreign leisure	relieve receive weight
Drop the final silent *e* before adding a **suffix** (word ending) that begins with a **vowel** (the letters *a, e, i, o, u*). Keep the *e* if the suffix begins with a **consonant** (all letters except *a, e, i, o, u*).	care → caring care → careful achieve → achievable achieve → achievement
Change the final *y* to *ie* when adding *s* or *d* when the *y* is preceded by a consonant.	laboratory → laboratories dry → dried
Double the final consonant when adding a suffix if all the following conditions are met: 1. The final consonant is preceded by a vowel. 2. The suffix begins with a vowel. 3. The word is only one **syllable** (part of a word that has a single spoken sound) or the final syllable is stressed.	sit → sitting commit → committed
Add *k* to words ending in *c* before adding suffixes that begin with *e, i*.	panic → panicking, panicked
Add *s* to make most words plural.	patient → patients X-ray → X-rays
Add *es* to make the plural form of words that end in *s, sh, ch, x*.	abscess → abscesses dish → dishes crutch → crutches suffix → suffixes
Add *s* to make the plural form of words that end in *o* if it is preceded by a vowel. Add *es* if *o* is preceded by a consonant.	ratio → ratios tomato → tomatoes
Some words that were borrowed from other languages, mainly Latin and Greek, keep their original plural forms, which do not use the letter *s*.	diverticulum (singular) → diverticula (plural) (pouch in mucous membrane lining) curriculum (singular) → curricula (plural)

Table 17–2 Commonly Misspelled Words

abscess	eligible	maneuver	rhythm
absence	eliminate	miscellaneous	schedule
accidentally	embarrass	necessary	scissors
accommodate	emphasize	negligence	secretary
accumulate	encourage	negligible	seize
address	enthusiastic	neighbor	seizure
aggravate	environment	noticeable	separate
analyze	equipped	occasionally	severely
appropriate	equivalent	occur	significance
assistant	especially	occurrence	similar
association	exaggerate	often	strategy
behavior	exercise	pamphlet	strictly
belief	exhausted	parallel	substantial
beneficial	experience	particular	succeed
business	extremely	patience	success
cafeteria	fatigue	persistent	surprise
caffeine	February	physically	sympathy
calendar	fluctuation	physician	technique
cancel, canceled	foreign	pneumonia	temperature
column	forty	possession	thorough
commitment	fourth	practical	though
communicate	fragile	precede	tongue
comparative	friend	prejudice	transferred
cooperate	government	privilege	typical
correspond	harass, harassment	proceed	urgent
criticism	height	prominent	vacuum
criticize	intelligence	psychiatry	vague
decision	judgment	psychology	vegetable
deficiency	knowledge	qualified	Wednesday
definitely	knowledgeable	quantity	weight
describe	label	questionnaire	writing
disease	laboratory	recommend	
efficiency	license	reference	
eighth	maintenance	resuscitate	

Source: Adapted from Delmar's Comprehensive Medical Assisting: Administrative and Clinical Competencies, *by W. Lindh, M. Pooler, C. Tamparo, & J. Cerrato, 1998, Clifton Park, NY: Delmar Cengage Learning.*

4. Set weekly goals. Challenge yourself to learn a certain number of new words. Create self-quizzes and give yourself small rewards for perfect scores.

Grammar at a Glance

Every language has a set of rules that determines proper word order, sentence construction, punctuation, and capitalization. Collectively these are referred to as **grammar**. The use of correct grammar is a sign of a good education, competence, and professionalism. As representatives of the facilities in which they work, health care professionals need to achieve a level of grammar that gives a favorable impression of both them and their employers.

The following sections are designed to provide a quick review of English grammar. If you are unsure about your knowledge of grammar, plan to take an English class, purchase educational software, or locate a workbook with review exercises. Time spent now can make a significant difference in your professional life. A good grammar reference book will be useful now and on the job. Most word processing software programs have grammar-checkers. It is the authors' experience, however, that more than half the suggestions made by the grammar-checker in one popular word processing program are incorrect.

Capitalization Rules

Capitalizing correctly is an important mark of good written English. The following conditions require capitalization:

- First word in a sentence
- Proper names of people, countries, organizations, companies, products, holidays, and so on
- Names of months and days of the week
- Medical acronyms: AIDS, ECG
- Titles used with a person's name: Dr. Castanedo, Mrs. Cranston
- First word of a **quotation** (words written exactly as spoken): The patient asked, "Why do I need this surgery?"

Punctuation Rules

Punctuation marks help the reader understand written messages. Incorrect or missing punctuation can lead to confusion and distorted meanings. Here are guidelines for the most common uses of punctuation marks:

1. The *period* is used at the end of a sentence and after some abbreviations.

   Examples Respiratory therapists must have good technical skills.

   Dr. Hansen is a noted thoracic surgeon.

2. The *comma* is used:

   a. To join two **independent clauses** (parts of a sentence that can stand on their own as complete sentences) joined by *and, but, or, nor, for, so, yet*

   Example Brushing the teeth after each meal is important, but flossing is also necessary.

   b. To separate three or more words or phrases that appear in a series

   Example The three energy nutrients are carbohydrates, fats, and proteins.

   c. At the end of an introductory group of words

   Examples When the patient arrived at the office, he was having trouble breathing.

   Efficient and well organized, Dr. Bancini's office staff rarely got behind schedule.

   Buried under piles of papers, Mrs. North's medical chart was nowhere to be seen.

   d. Around inessential phrases that describe or add information

   Examples The patient, who lives in my neighborhood, came to the clinic on Monday. (*Phrase adds interesting but unnecessary information.*)

   The physician who specializes in pulmonary disorders agreed to see the patient this afternoon. (Phrase adds important information about the physician.)

   e. To set off transitional expressions: *however, therefore, for example, in other words, as a matter of fact*

   Examples Practicing sterile technique, for example, is an important skill for surgical technologists.

   Giving medical advice, however, can be done only by the physician.

   f. With dates and addresses

   Examples The clinic first opened on June 2, 1985, in Omaha, Nebraska.

   The nearest hospital is located at 417 Santa Clara Road, San Diego, California.

3. The *semicolon* is used:
   a. Between independent clauses that are *not* joined with connecting words such as *and, but, or, nor, for, so, yet*

   Example The physician referred Mr. Denton to a physical therapist; his leg requires special exercises to regain strength and range of motion.

   b. Between independent clauses joined by transitional expressions such as *also, besides, finally, furthermore, for example, in conclusion, on the contrary*

   Example Good health is influenced by proper nutrition; also, exercise plays an important role.

4. The *colon* is used:
   a. At the end of an independent clause that introduces a list or a quotation

   Example The major functions of the integumentary system include the following: provide protection from the external environment, control body temperature, and maintain homeostasis.

   b. Between independent clauses when the second clause explains, illustrates, or expands on the first

   Example The clinic director called a staff meeting: he wanted to discuss the new guidelines for reporting accidents in the lab.

   c. After the **salutation** (greeting) in a business letter

   Example Dear Dr. Phillips:

5. The *apostrophe* is used:
   a. To create the possessive form of a noun

   Example The nurse's stethoscope lay on the counter.

   b. To indicate the **contraction** (combining) of two words

   Example It's a busy day at the clinic. (It's = It is)

6. Quotation marks are used:
   a. To enclose direct quotes (exact words of a speaker)

   Example "I need you to help me turn Mrs. Sands," said Nurse Ames to the CNA.

   b. Around titles of magazine and newspaper articles, chapters in books, stories, songs, and poems. (Note: titles of books, plays, movies, and names of magazines and newspapers are put in italics—*like this*—or underlined.)

Using More than One Punctuation Mark

- Always place periods and commas inside quotation marks.

  Example This month's journal had an interesting article titled "Postoperative Pain in Knee-Replacement Patients."

- Place exclamation and question marks inside quotation marks unless they apply to the entire sentence.

  Examples When Dr. Pedersen told Mr. Watson that his cholesterol was lower as a result of the new medication, the patient exclaimed, "That's great news!"

  Have you read Chapter 10, "Infection Control"?

> **Fascinating Facts**
>
> Computer grammar-checkers are helpful for catching common grammatical errors, but they do not replace proofreading by the writer. According to a study by Diana Hacker, author of *A Writer's Reference*, grammar-checkers flagged only 20% to 50% of the run-on sentences in a sample. (A run-on sentence consists of two independent clauses that are not joined with a connecting word, a construction that is incorrect in English. Example: I saw Dr. Anderson, he was in a hurry and couldn't answer my question.)

Writing Numbers Correctly

The general rule when using numbers in sentences is to write them out as words when:

- They consist of only one or two words (Note: Hyphenate compound numbers from twenty-one to ninety-nine.)
- They are the first word in a sentence

Otherwise, they are written as figures. See the following examples:

- There were five patients waiting to see the doctor.
- There were 25,000 cases reported last year in the United States.
- Twenty-five thousand new cases were reported last year in the United States.

In technical writing, such as that used in health care, using figures rather than writing out words for numbers is sometimes preferred. Check the preferences for your specific profession and facility. The American Psychological Association (APA) and the American Medical Assocation (AMA), for example, publish style manuals. They have their own rules for writing numbers as figures or words. Figures are also used in the following situations:

- When expressing time with a.m. or p.m. (am and pm are also correct)

  Example Your next appointment is scheduled for 3:15 p.m. on Monday, January 12, 2015.

  Otherwise, write the numbers out in words.

  Example Mr. Hashimoto's surgery is scheduled to begin at eight o'clock in the morning.

- Percentages

  Example The range of normal hematocrit (volume percentage of red blood cells in whole blood) values for newborns is 45% to 60%. (The word *percent* may also be spelled out.)

- Temperature

  Example His temperature was below normal at 97.6 degrees.

- Fractions and decimals

  Examples A quart is equal to ¼ gallon.

  The specific gravity (weight compared to equal volume of water) of normal urine ranges from 1.003 to 1.035.

Writing Titles Correctly

Use standard abbreviations if the title appears immediately before or after names (never in both places).

Dr. Joanna Carter	*or*	Joanna Carter, MD (Doctor of Medicine)
Dr. Esteban Alvarez	*or*	Esteban Alvarez, Ph.D. (Doctor of Philosophy)
Dr. Mary O'Leary	*or*	Mary O'Leary, D.D.S. (Doctor of Dental Surgery)

Periods have traditionally followed abbreviations for titles. However, usage varies and periods are often omitted, except for the abbreviation Dr. Use the form preferred by your employer or professional organization.

BUSINESS LETTERS

A trend in health care employment today is **cross-training** employees. This means that they learn to perform tasks in addition to those traditionally performed by individuals with their job titles. For example, more administrative tasks are being required of health care professionals who provide direct patient care. The ability to write business letters correctly is a necessary skill for an increasing number of occupations.

Business letters create an important link between health care providers and their patients and colleagues. The following types of letters are commonly used in health care:

- Appointment: Reminds a patient of the date and time of the next appointment
- Recall: Requests a patient to call and make an appointment
- Collection: Requests a patient to pay a bill
- Follow-up: Summarizes reports regarding test results, outlines further treatment needs
- Consultation: Requests another professional to examine a patient

Thinking It Through

Karin McFarland is the office manager for Drs. Kern, Wilkes, and Ruiz. She recently hired a new medical receptionist, Wanda Belini, whom patients like for her warm, friendly personality. Wanda has excellent telephone skills and good judgment about handling calls appropriately. Karin is concerned, however, about Wanda's writing skills. The short documents such as memos and meeting announcements that she has prepared have contained spelling and punctuation errors. Karin believes that Wanda is a valuable asset to the office and wants to help her improve.

1. Why is it important for memos and meeting announcements to be written properly if they are only seen by people who work in the office?
2. What might Wanda do to improve her writing skills?
3. What impact might Wanda's poor writing skills have on her future career if she does not improve them?

- Explanation: Provides an excuse from work or school, explains special needs for patient accommodation
- Inquiry: Requests information about products or processes
- Special occasion: Accepts an invitation or sends regrets, offers congratulations
- Announcement: States new office hours or other policies, announces new associate or retirement of staff member

Using Form Letters

Many letters are sent out repeatedly with the same information. Creating form letters can save time. With today's word processing software, it is possible to personalize form letters and print them without the telltale signs of repeated passes through the copy machine. The patient's name and address can be entered, and personal notes included within the text. Form letters should be personally signed whenever possible.

Writing Effective Letters

Effective business letters are courteous, clear, and direct. Getting to the point, without being abrupt, is a sign of respect for the reader's time. Although they should be businesslike, letters to patients should never be so formal as to seem uncaring. The message of a letter is organized in the same way as for other types of writing:

1. State the purpose in the introduction.
2. Develop ideas in the body. Provide necessary information and explanations. Use an appropriate tone. For example, a collection letter might be written using a firm tone.
3. Summarize, and state what you want the reader to do.

Carefully proofread all letters for content, grammar, and spelling. A letter that contains even a single error is not considered mailable.

Business Letter Formats

Certain traditions govern the appearance of business letters. Like dressing appropriately for a business occasion, the correct use of a prescribed letter format is a sign of proper business **etiquette** (manners). Remember that the quality and appearance of correspondence represent the level of professionalism of the sender.

The three most commonly used letter formats are block, modified block, and semi-block. The main difference between the formats is how the lines of text are **justified** (lined up with the margins).

- **Block letter**: All lines are flush (lined up evenly) with the left margin. This is the most efficient format to use because it eliminates the need for extra keystrokes to indent the lines. (See Figure 17–3.)
- **Modified block letter**: All lines are flush with the left margin except the date, closing, and signature. These begin just to the right of the center of the page. (See Figure 17–4.)
- **Semi-block letter**: The same as block, except that the first line of each paragraph is indented five spaces and the subject line begins just to the right of the center of the page. This format is considered the least formal of the three. (See Figure 17–5.)

Preparing Letters for Mailing

When a letter requires more than one sheet, use a piece of plain matching paper (without the information about the sender and receiver) for the second page. The correct way to fold a completed letter depends on the size and type of envelope used. (See Figure 17–6.) Proper delivery is ensured if the envelope is addressed according to the following guidelines:

- Write the address in all uppercase (capital) letters.
- Do not use punctuation in the address.
- Use the zip code. Add the additional zip + 4 code when possible.
- Do not write in the lower-right corner.
- Include a complete return address in the upper-left corner.

See Figure 17–7 for an example of a correctly addressed envelope.

MEMOS

Memos are written to share information within an organization. Examples of typical memo topics include policy changes, staff schedules, explanations

WINSTON LEWIS, MD
2501 CENTER STREET
NORTHBOROUGH, OH 12345

NORTHBOROUGH
FAMILY MEDICAL GROUP

Date Line	January 12, 20___ (approximately 15th line)
Inside Address	Jeremy Brown, MD (approximately 20th line) 111 S Main Blossom, UT 10283-1120 (double-space)
Salutation	Dear Dr. Brown: (double-space)
Subject Line	Blossom Medical Society Meeting (double-space)
	Thank you for inviting me to speak at the Blossom Medical Society Meeting on June 15, 20___. As requested, my topic will describe using MRI scans to make more accurate diagnoses without resorting to invasive procedures. I will send you the exact title of my speech by next Friday. (double-space)
	Please have your office manager send me information about the number of participants expected, the time of the meeting, location, and any other details that will assist me in preparing my speech.
	I will write or call if I have any additional questions. (double-space)
Complimentary Closing	Yours truly,
	Winston Lewis, MD (4-5 line spaces)
Keyed Signature	Winston Lewis, MD (double-space)
Reference Initials	WL:jg (double-space)
Enclosure Notation	Enclosure: Handout on MRI

FIGURE 17–3 Block style letter format. The contents of a standard business letter are labeled.

L

WINSTON LEWIS, MD
2501 CENTER STREET
NORTHBOROUGH, OH 12345

NORTHBOROUGH
FAMILY MEDICAL GROUP

January 12, 20___ (approximately 15th line)

Jeremy Brown, MD (approximately 20th line)
111 S Main
Blossom, UT 10283-1120

Dear Dr. Brown:

Blossom Medical Society Meeting

Thank you for inviting me to speak at the Blossom Medical Society Meeting on June 15, 20___. As requested, my topic will describe using MRI scans to make more accurate diagnoses without resorting to invasive procedures. I will send you the exact title of my speech will by next Friday.

Please have your office manager send me information regarding the number of participants expected, the time of the meeting, location, and any other details that will assist me in preparing my speech.

I will write or call if I have any additional questions.

Yours truly,

Winston Lewis, MD

Winston Lewis, MD

WL:jg

Enclosure: Handout on MRI

FIGURE 17–4 Modified block style business letter format.

WINSTON LEWIS, MD
2501 CENTER STREET
NORTHBOROUGH, OH 12345

NORTHBOROUGH
FAMILY MEDICAL GROUP

January 12, 20___ (approximately 15th line)

Jeremy Brown, MD (approximately 20th line)
111 S Main
Blossom, UT 10283-1120

Dear Dr. Brown:

Blossom Medical Society Meeting

Thank you for inviting me to speak at the Blossom Medical Society Meeting on June 15, 20___. As requested, my topic will describe using MRI scans to make more accurate diagnoses without resorting to invasive procedures. I will send you the exact title of my speech will by next Friday.

Please have your office manager send me information regarding the number of participants expected, the time of the meeting, location, and any other details that will assist me in preparing my speech.

I will write or call if I have any additional questions.

Yours truly,

Winston Lewis, MD

Winston Lewis, MD

WL:jg

Enclosure: Handout on MRI

FIGURE 17–5 Semi-block style business letter format.

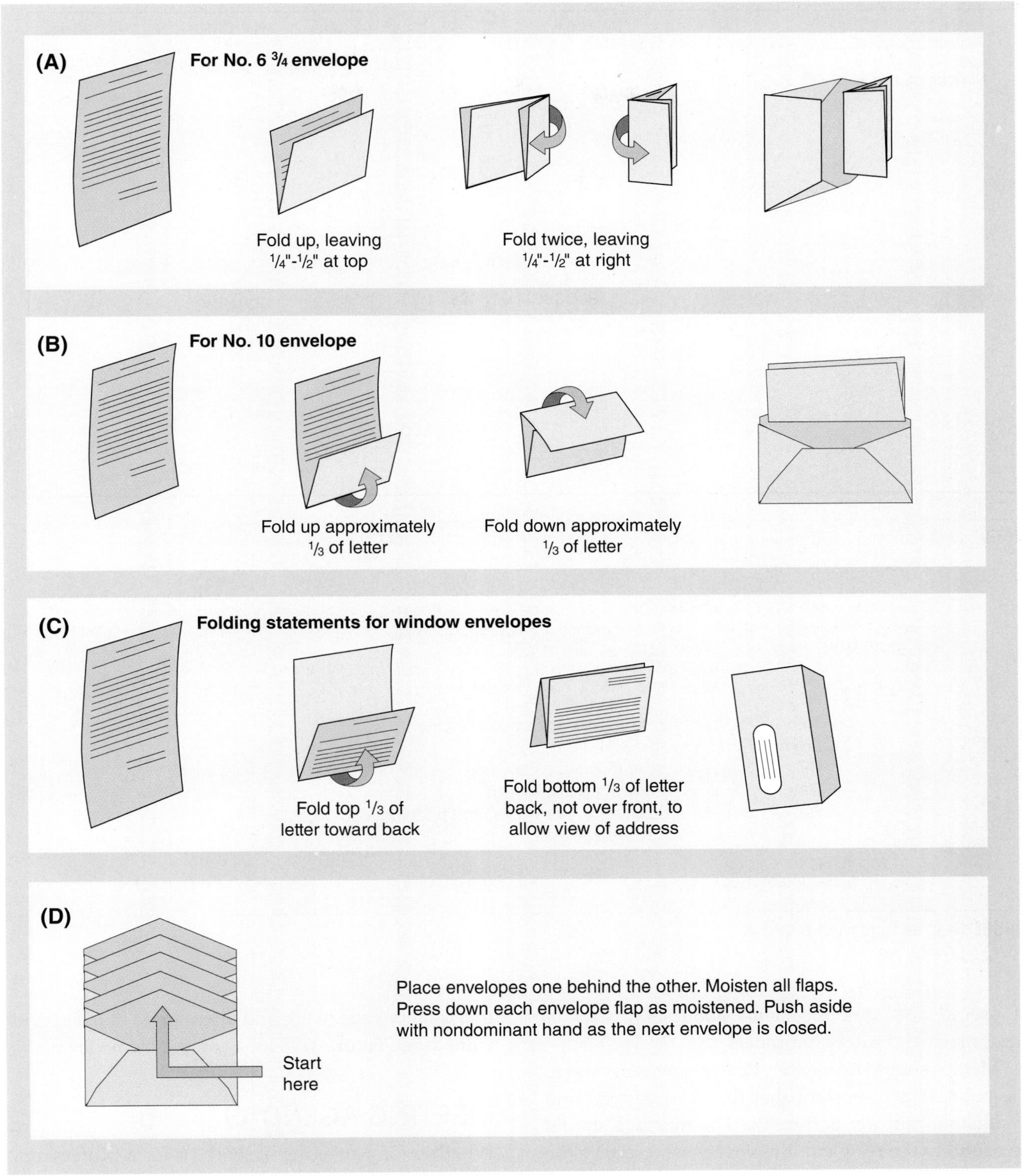

FIGURE 17–6 Proper methods for folding business letters for mailing.

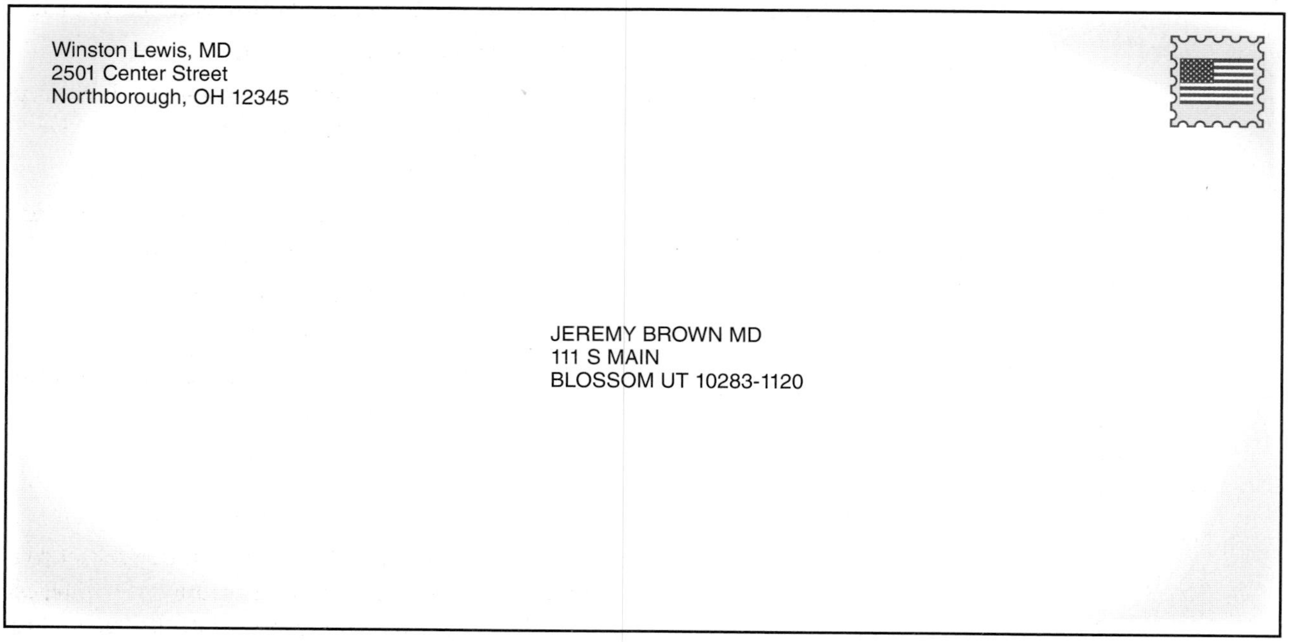

FIGURE 17–7 Correctly addressed envelope.

Wilsonville Orthopedic Clinic

MEMO

To: Person(s) to whom the memo is being sent
From: Person sending the memo
CC: Names of other individuals to whom a copy of the memo is being sent
Date: Date memo is written and/or sent
Re: Subject of the memo. Helps recipient prioritize and organize memos if they are saved

Body of message here

FIGURE 17–8 Sample memo format.

of procedures, announcements about new staff or equipment, and safety reminders.

Memos should be written clearly, concisely, and to the point. It is important that they can be read and understood quickly and easily. The message should be useful to the recipient. Employees who receive too many memos begin to ignore them. All suggestions regarding memos pertain to both paper and electronically sent memos (emails).

Prepare memos with the same care given to outgoing letters. The quality of memos can set the tone for work standards at a facility. Poorly prepared memos and other internal documents can send the message that quality paperwork and attention to detail are not valued. See Figure 17–8 for a sample memo format.

MEETING AGENDAS

Whether for a meeting at work or for a professional organization, the health care professional may be called upon to prepare a meeting agenda. An **agenda** lists what is to take place at a meeting. Agendas promote efficiency by helping attendees prepare in advance and by keeping meetings focused on what needs to be discussed and accomplished. A good agenda should include the following:

Thinking It Through

Kendra Washington is the administrative assistant for Dr. Benson, the director of an inner-city community clinic. The clinic depends on charitable contributions for a significant portion of its operating funds. Dr. Benson has asked Kendra to draft a letter to past and potential contributors in anticipation of the clinic's annual fund-draising drive. The purpose of the letter is to explain the progress of the clinic over the last year and how it contributes to the community. The most important part is to ask the recipient to make a donation. Kendra knows that the organization and wording of the letter are important in order for it to be effective.

1. What must Kendra consider when deciding how to write this letter?
2. What steps should she take to plan its content?
3. What tone do you think would be most appropriate? Explain.
4. If she decides to use a form letter, how could it be personalized for the recipients?

1. Date of the meeting
2. Start and end times
3. Exact location
4. Topics to be discussed
5. What attendees should bring, if applicable
6. Guest speaker(s), if applicable

MINUTES OF MEETINGS

Minutes provide written documentation of what happens at meetings. They serve several purposes:

- Inform those who did not attend about important decisions and announcements that took place.
- Create a record of facility business. Document, for regulatory and accrediting purposes, that specific items were discussed.
- Serve as a guide for the next meeting's agenda.
- Provide a resource for future reference and a reminder of decisions made.
- The following items are commonly included in minutes:

1. Date and time the meeting is called to order
2. Members present and absent
3. Acceptance of previous minutes, including any corrections or additions
4. Announcements
5. Short write-up of discussions, decisions made, and conclusions agreed on
6. Date and time of next meeting
7. Time of adjournment
8. Signature of the person preparing the minutes and of the chairperson

PATIENT EDUCATION MATERIALS

High-quality written materials are an important part of effective patient education, introduced in Chapter 16. Written materials are appropriate for providing information on many topics:

- Diets
- Exercises
- Medications
- Postoperative instructions
- Preparing for a diagnostic test
- Self-exams
- Tips for quitting smoking
- Wound care

Whether the content is original information or material borrowed from other sources, it should be verified for accuracy. Organize the material in an easy-to-follow format. Bulleted or numbered lists may be easier for patients to follow than solid text. Create a logical order. For example, when listing possible postoperative complications, start with the most serious. Clearly indicate which ones require notifying the physician. When explaining the steps of a procedure, list them in the order in which they are performed.

Write at a reading level that is appropriate for patients. Avoid technical language that may be confusing or misunderstood. Use diagrams to illustrate important points or procedures. Use a larger-than-standard font size for patients with poor eyesight. Keep clear master copies so that repeated copying does not result in poor-quality print. An even more effective way is to maintain computerized patient information and education files. Doing so makes it easier to keep materials up to date with medical advances and facility policies. The materials can even be edited to meet the individual needs of patients. Good sources for patient education information include the National Library of Medicine (Medline Plus) at http://medlineplus.gov and the Mayo Clinic at www.mayoclinic.com.

CONFIDENTIALITY OF WRITTEN MATERIALS

All written materials containing patient information must be secure from the sight or possession of any unauthorized person. As discussed in Chapter 3, patient confidentiality must be respected at all times. Seemingly innocent documents, such as appointment reminder letters, are considered confidential if patients' names are visible. These, along with similar written materials, should never be left out where they can be seen by other patients, vendors, or other office visitors.

PROOFREADING WRITTEN WORK

All written work should be proofread for content, grammar, punctuation, spelling, and appearance. It is easy to overlook errors, because most people read more than one word at a time. The brain, reading for content, fills in missing letters and even whole words. Here are some tips for proofreading effectively:

- Reread the document to verify content. Check all facts for accuracy.
- Check the organization of the material. Does it make sense? Does it flow well?
- Read aloud. Listen for odd-sounding phrases and words.
- Check spelling by reading backward, word by word. This way, you concentrate on the appearance and spelling of words rather than on the meaning.
- Use the spell-checker feature on the computer. (However, as cautioned previously, do not depend on the spell-checker to catch all errors.)
- Print out documents created on the computer if you find it easier to read material on paper than on the screen. It is worth using extra paper and printer ink to ensure that documents are well written and accurate.
- If you are unsure about any aspect of a document, ask a qualified person for help.
- Have your written work checked as required by your facility.

See Box 17–1 for a list of items to check when reviewing written work.

BOX 17–1

Written Communication Checklist

____ Appearance: margins, formatting, print quality

____ Completeness: all information filled in

____ Accuracy: numbers, dates, facts verified

____ Grammar

____ Punctuation

____ Capitalization

____ Corrections done properly

____ Confidentiality protected

Fascinating Facts

The following examples show why it is sometimes difficult to catch spelling errors. Our brains, as Live Science explains, are "code-cracking machines."

For emaxlpe, it deson't mttaer in waht oredr the ltteers in a wrod aepapr, the olny iprmoatnt tihng is taht the frist and lsat ltteer are in the rghit pcale. The rset can be a toatl mses and you can sitll raed it wouthit pobelrm.

S1M1L4RLY, YOUR M1ND 15 R34D1NG 7H15 4U70M471C4LLY W17H0U7 3V3N 7H1NK1NG 4B0U7 17.

(Source: Breaking the Code: Why Yuor Barin Can Raed Tihs, by N. Wolchover, 2012, Live Science, http://www.livescience.com/18392-reading-jumbled-words.html.)

WORKBOOK PRACTICE

Go to your workbook and complete the exercises for this chapter.

SUGGESTED LEARNING ACTIVITIES

1. Quiz yourself on the spelling of the words in the list of frequently misspelled words.
2. Start your own personal dictionary for words you misspell. Dedicate time each week to studying and mastering these words.
3. Collect samples from health care facilities of nonconfidential written documents, such as instruction sheets, form letters, and office policies. Compare their quality and look for examples that illustrate good written communication.
4. Pay attention to writing styles as you read your textbooks, magazine and newspaper articles, and novels. Identify characteristics you believe make writing effective. Start a scrapbook of good examples.

WEB ACTIVITIES

Purdue University's Online Writing Lab

http://owl.english.purdue.edu

Click on the "Purdue Online Writing Lab"; then "General Writing" at the top of the subjects listed on the left side of the screen. Choose one or more of the following sections: Mechanics, Grammar, and/or Punctuation. Review at least five topics and complete and check the accompanying exercises.

Study Guides and Strategies

www.studygs.net

Scroll down the page to "Guides: Writing and Vocabulary." Explore the topics to find 10 ideas you think might help you improve your writing.

Capital Community College

http://grammar.ccc.commnet.edu/grammar/

Explore the many topics available and report on what you learn.

REVIEW QUESTIONS

1. What are three reasons why every health care professional should develop good writing skills?
2. What are the four steps to take when planning a written document?
3. Why is it important that the health care professional use correct spelling and grammar?
4. Compare and contrast the three major business letter formats.
5. How should the content of an effective business letter be organized?
6. What should be done to ensure that business letters are delivered properly to the addressee?
7. What items should be included when preparing meeting agendas?
8. What items should be included when writing the minutes of a meeting?
9. What are five strategies for preparing effective written materials for patient education?
10. How can patient confidentiality be protected when handling written documents?
11. What are five good proofreading techniques?

APPLICATION EXERCISES

1. Refer to The Case of the Surprised Therapist at the beginning of the chapter. Explain what Al can do to ensure that the agendas, reports, and instruction sheets are written effectively and correctly.
2. Dental assistant Tanya Lucas is the chair of the program planning committee for her local professional organization. She has written the letter in Figure 17–9 to Dr. Samantha Speares, a local dentist, inviting her to speak to the group.
   a. Should Tanya send her letter as written to Dr. Speares?
   b. If not, explain what she should do to make it "mailable." Apply what you learned in this chapter about spelling, capitalization, punctuation, and letter formats.

Tanya Lucas, RDA
943 Castro Lane
Oakland, CA 94662

January 11, 2016

Dr. Samantha Speares, D.D. S.
Speares Pediatric Dentistry
7920 Glenwood Circle
Oakland, Ca 94662

Dear Dr. Speares,
On behalf of the Oakland Dental Assistants Society, I would like to invite you to speak to our group about pediatric dentistry. Many of our members are interested in working with children, they are thinking about working in pediatric dentistry and would like to know more about it. It would definately be a priviledge to have you as our speaker.

The meeting will be held on Febuary 18, 2016, at seven o'clock P.M. at the Town and Country hotel located at 2275 Scenic Road Oakland. I sincerely hope you can attend. Please call me or our secretary, Diana LaMer at (510) 123-4567.

Sincerely,

Tanya Lucas
Program Committee Chair

FIGURE 17–9 Letter Tanya has written to Dr. Speares.

PROBLEM-SOLVING PRACTICE

Teresa is in an associate's degree program studying to be a respiratory therapist. She is having difficulty with her English composition class. Teresa spends a lot of time writing her papers, but is disappointed when the instructor returns them marked up with many grammar and spelling errors. How can Teresa use the five-step problem-solving process to improve her writing skills?

SUGGESTED READINGS AND RESOURCES

Capital Community College Guide to Grammar and Writing. http://grammar.ccc.commnet.edu/grammar/

Hacker, D. (2010). *A writer's reference* (7th ed.). Boston, MA: Bedford/St. Martin's.

National Library of Medicine: Medline Plus Medical Dictionary. http://medlineplus.gov/

Purdue University's Online Writing Lab. http://owl.english.purdue.edu

Study Guides and Strategies. www.studygs.net

Terryberry, K. (2005). *Writing for the health professions*. Clifton Park, NY: Delmar Cengage Learning.

Villemaire, D., & Villemaire, L. (2006). *Grammar and writing skills for the health care professional* (2nd ed.). Clifton Park, NY: Delmar Cengage Learning.

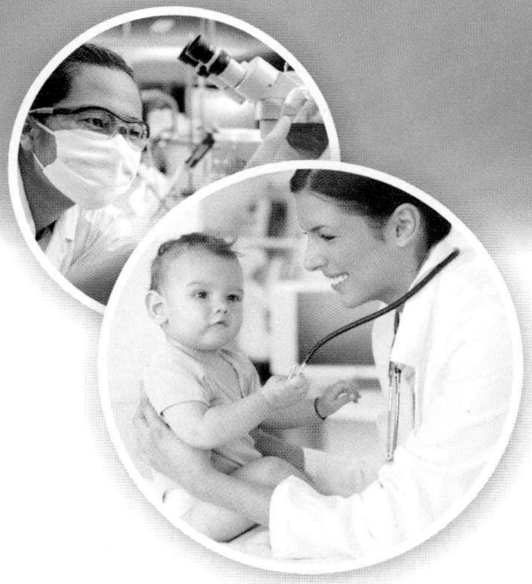

Chapter 18

Computers and Technology in Health Care

OBJECTIVES

Studying and applying the material in this chapter will help you to:

- Explain why it is important for today's health care professional to be computer literate.
- Describe how computers and technology are applied in the following areas of health care:
- Information management
- Electronic health records
- Creation of documents
- Numerical calculations
- Diagnostics
- Treatment
- Patient monitoring
- Research
- Education
- Communication
- Explain the difference between computer hardware and software.
- Describe how to properly handle and maintain hardware components.
- Identify and describe the two major types of data storage.
- List six important guidelines for using computers effectively.
- Explain precautions that the health care professional can take to ensure computer security.
- List ways that the health care professional can acquire computer skills.

KEY TERMS

application program
artificial intelligence
bioinformatics
CD-ROM
central processing unit (CPU)
cloud storage
computer literate
computer virus
database
downloaded
electronic mail
electronic spreadsheet
expert systems
fiber optics
fields
file
gateways
hard drive
hardware
Internet
key words
lasers
networks

(continues)

KEY TERMS (continued)

peripheral
plagiarism
point-of-care charting
RAM
record
search engine
site license
software
style manual (writing)
telemedicine
virtual communities
Web directories

The Case of the Therapist Who Wants to Add to Her Computer System

Carol Lindstrom has maintained a physical therapy practice in a small community for more than 30 years. Her interpersonal communication skills are excellent, and she is known for her ability to motivate her patients to reach their highest physical potential following accidents and surgeries. Carol recognizes the worth of computers to her practice and has a system capable of word processing, bookkeeping, and accessing the Internet. Her assistant, Graciela, uses the computer mainly for correspondence and billing. Carol is aware that she and Graciela could be using computer technology in additional ways both to make the practice more efficient and to better help patients. Carol discusses this with Graciela and assigns her the task of investigating additional computer applications. This chapter includes a discussion of the many ways that computers are being used to provide enhanced services to patients.

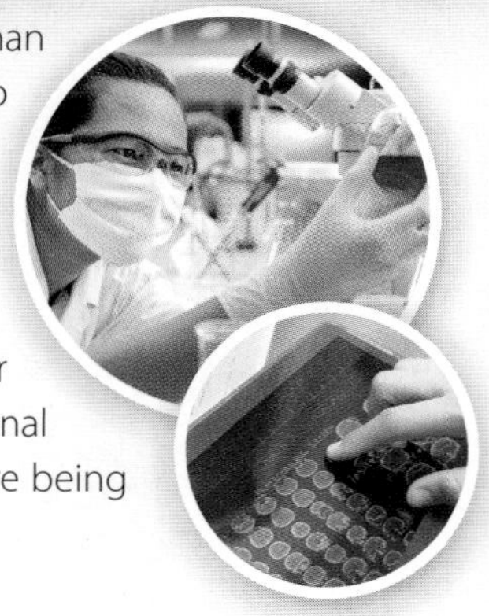

COMPUTERS IN HEALTH CARE

Computers and their applications have influenced every aspect of modern health care. From patient check-in procedures to diagnostics and research, technology is changing the way that health care is delivered. All health care professionals now function as information managers, and the ability to use computers has become an essential part of health care competency.

Computers perform three major types of operations:

1. Store huge amounts of data
2. Calculate, manipulate, organize, and retrieve data quickly and accurately
3. Enable high-speed communication

Harnessing the capabilities of the modern computer relieves workers from having to perform repetitious tasks. Mathematical calculations and organizational tasks involving enormous amounts of data can be completed quickly and accurately. Additions, revisions, and corrections to, as well as deletions from, documents can be made quickly and easily. Changes and updates are immediately available to those who need them. Information can be accessed simultaneously by many people.

We can see more clearly the impact of computers on health care by following one patient, Mr. Johnson. Mr. Johnson was mowing his lawn on a Saturday afternoon when he experienced chest pains and nausea. His wife took him to the emergency department at nearby Ames General Hospital. The following list includes some of the many ways that computer technology was used during his stay at Ames:

1. Mr. Johnson was seen by a physician immediately, because of the possibility that he was suffering a myocardial infarction (heart attack). Mrs. Johnson gave information about Mr. Johnson and their health insurance coverage to the admitting clerk, who entered it on the hospital's *computerized patient record system*.
2. An electrocardiogram (ECG, a diagnostic method used to measure the heart's electrical activity) was performed on Mr. Johnson. The results were interpreted by a *computer* and produced on a paper printout for qualified personnel to read and review.

3. Dr. Sanchez, the cardiologist on duty, examined Mr. Johnson and decided to admit him to the hospital for observation. He dictated his observations, which were then *word processed* by a hospital transcriptionist for entry into the medical record.
4. A room was scheduled for Mr. Johnson using the hospital's *computerized scheduling program*.
5. Orders for medications prescribed by Dr. Sanchez were sent via a *computer network* to the hospital pharmacy.
6. A hospital pharmacy technician used a *pharmaceutical software program* to compare the new medications with those that Mr. Johnson was already taking to check for possible drug interactions.
7. All supplies used for Mr. Johnson's hospitalization were tracked on a *computerized inventory system*. This information was used for reordering supplies and preparing billing statements.
8. Mr. Johnson's blood pressure and pulse were intermittently monitored at preset intervals by *computerized equipment* at his bedside.
9. Mr. Johnson is diabetic and the nursing assistant took his blood sugar level before meals and at bedtime. She used a handheld piece of equipment called a glucometer that has *computer components* for testing blood and storing the readings.
10. Mr. Johnson's blood and urine samples were sent to the laboratory for processing. As soon as the tests were completed, the results were entered and available on *computer* for the staff to review.
11. Mr. Johnson's charge nurse entered nursing notes about his care and condition directly into the *computerized medical record system* to enable ready access for his health care team.
12. When Mr. Johnson was discharged, he was given instructions about diet and exercise that had originally been created with *word processing software*.

The health care professionals who provided direct care for Mr. Johnson or provided support services needed to be **computer literate**. This means having the knowledge and skills to efficiently perform the computer tasks required of them, as well as a basic understanding of how computers work and what types of health care applications are currently available. The type and number of computer-related tasks performed by health care professionals depend on their specific occupations and factors such as the size of the facility in which they work. Duties range from simple data entry to interpreting diagnostic test results. Employees in small facilities sometimes need to have a wider variety of computer skills than those in larger facilities, which have computer specialists on staff. For example, a dental receptionist in a single-dentist office may be asked to research and purchase a computer system to upgrade the administrative functions of the office. Large facilities, such as hospitals and groups of associated clinics, have information technology departments with specialized staff who purchase and maintain the computer systems. They may also design and program customized software. Figure 18–1 illustrates the flow of information in a medical practice management system. As you look at the flow chart, consider how computerizing data increases the accuracy and efficiency for health care providers.

Information Management

Keeping track of huge amounts of data is a challenge in the health care world. Having quick access to information is necessary for tasks such as selecting appropriate courses of treatment, preparing reports for regulatory agencies, and justifying insurance bills. A major role of the computer is storing and making this information easily accessible in useful formats.

A **database** is a collection of information organized in a structured way. Databases can be set up by the user with application software that can be purchased at a relatively low cost. For example, a small medical office might use a software program to develop a database of all active patients served by a specific insurance company. Many vendors today sell medical record and practice management software designed for small offices. Some have been created for particular specialties, such as pediatrics. Complex databases for large facilities may be created by computer programmers to meet the specific needs of the facility. See Box 18–1 for other examples of health care databases.

The basic structure of a database is the key to its usefulness. Each collection of related data is called a **record**. For example, the data about each individual

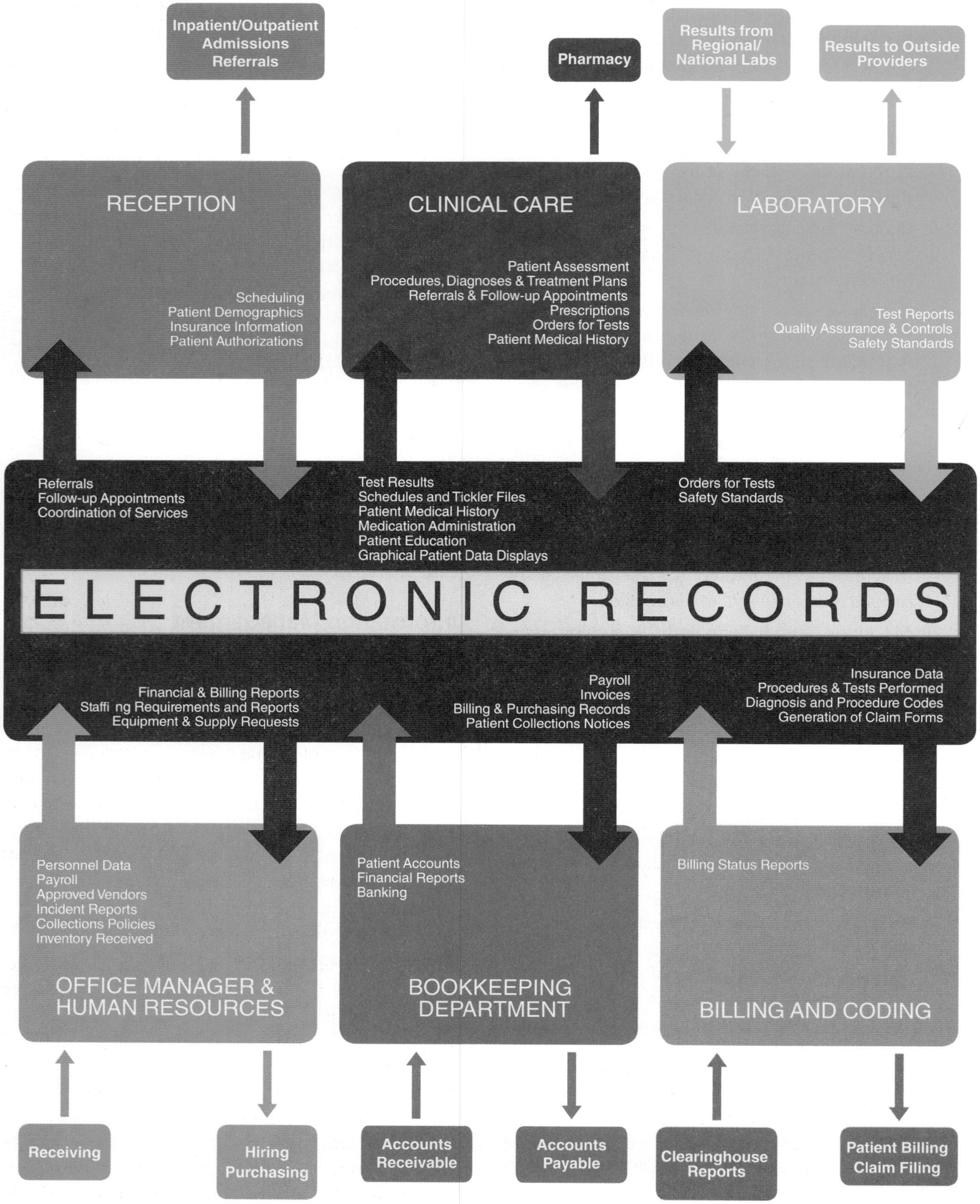

FIGURE 18–1 Information flow in an integrated computerized management system for an ambulatory care setting.

BOX 18–1

Examples of Health Care Databases

Disease profiles

Insurance company records

Inventory management

Mailing lists

Patient records

Personnel records

Pharmaceutical records

Production reports

Research projects and results

are grouped together in a separate record. These data are entered into **fields**. Suppose that a computerized patient record contains 15 pieces of demographic information, such as name, address, telephone number, occupation, and insurance company name. Each record is called a **file**.

Computerized databases have many advantages over paper filing systems. The following features make them especially useful in health care information management:

- Records can be retrieved quickly and easily.
- Records can be sorted, accessed, and reported in many ways. For example, patient records can be organized alphabetically by last name, grouped by zip code, grouped by insurance company, or listed chronologically by date of last visit.
- Information can be accessed by more than one person at the same time.
- Additions and changes can be entered easily.
- Reports can be generated as needed.
- Quality improvement studies can be conducted. (See Chapter 23.)

Many health care professionals are responsible for entering data on forms that are displayed on the monitor. Some forms use abbreviations or numerical codes to identify the various fields. The data are converted into a readable form, such as the computerized medical history and physical examination in Figure 18–2.

Accuracy is critical when entering data. Patient diagnoses, treatment plans, and billing are negatively affected by incorrect data. Carefully review and verify all input. If an error is made when inputting data, be sure that only the intended sections are erased. Reconstructing records can be difficult and time-consuming and can be the cause of inconsistent patient care and legal problems. (See Figure 18–3.)

Health care professionals who function as information managers may be required to design and create databases. In these cases, it is important to carefully study the information needs of the facility. A computerized database is valuable only if it serves the needs of the users.

Thinking It Through

Tyler is an occupational therapy assistant who works for Kelly Graziano, an occupational therapist with a private practice that specializes in hand therapy. In addition to assisting patients with their therapy and making splints, Tyler is helping Kelly computerize the administrative activities of the office. He wants to create a system to track the vendors used by the practice to supply equipment and materials. Use the following questions to help him design a useful database:

1. How can the database be organized?
2. What data would be useful in each record?
3. How will the database make it easier to order supplies?
4. What reports might be useful for the practice? How often should they be generated?
5. How would such a system help Kelly with the financial management of her practice?

Electronic Health Records

Electronic health records (EHRs), also called electronic medical records (EMRs), described in Chapter 19, are based on database technology. Once kept on paper and maintained in file folders, they filled rows of shelves and many file cabinets in health care facilities. In the last several years, the U.S. government has promoted the use of computerized records as a way to make health care safer, more efficient, and more cost effective. To encourage computerization, the Centers for Medicare and Medicaid Services (CMS) periodically offered financial incentive programs for professionals and facilities to use electronic records

Patient: Leo McKay
Date of Birth: 01/22/44
Visit Date: 04/01/__

Chief Complaint: Abdominal pain
History: Has been ill over the last 2 weeks with progressively worsening abdominal pain.
Review of Symptoms: Patient denies the following:

- Chest pain, Chest pressure, Chest heaviness, Circulation problems, Palpitations, Rapid heartbeat Irregular heartbeat, Ankle swelling
- Cough, Phlegm, Coughing up blood, Shortness of breath, Wheeze, Change in exercise tolerance
- Burning or pain on urination, Difficulty starting or stopping urination, Dribbling after urination Incontinence of urine, Blood in urine, Cloudiness of urine
- Change in appetite, Unexpected weight loss, Nausea, Vomiting, Difficulty Swallowing, Belly pains, Gas pains, Change in bowel habit: change in frequency, shape, color, consistency, size of stool; Blood Mucus, or Slime, Rectal pain or discomfort, Hemorrhoids
- Skin rash, New or changing moles, Excess bruising or bleeding
- Mouth sores, Denture problems, Sinus drainage or stuffiness, Facial pain
- Panic attacks, Anxiety, Depression, Sadness, Seizures, Problems with concentration or memory, Disturbance of sleep, Insomnia, Early wakefulness
- Dizziness, Fainting, Lightheadedness on standing, Headaches, Vision problems, Hearing problems, Numbness or tingling in arms or legs, Weakness in arms or legs

Medications:

Drug	Dose	Freq.	Started
none			

Medical Problem List:

Problem	When Dxd	Active?
Peptic Ulcer	1985	no

List of Surgeries:

Surgical Procedure	When
none	

Family History: Parents deceased, father died of heart attack, mother of breast cancer.
Social History: Divorced, no children
Habits: Smokes 2 ppd, Several beers daily
Allergies: Penicillin

Physical Examination

GENERAL: Well developed and well nourished gentleman in no distress. No jaundice, cyanosis, clubbing, or edema.
VITALS: Weight = 192, Temp = 97.6, Pulse = 78, BP = 152/88
HEENT: Normocephalic and without evidence of trauma, tympanic membranes and external auditory canals are normal. Pharynx and mouth are normal.
NECK: Supple, no masses or thyromegaly.
NODES: No cervical nodes palpable. No axillary or inguinal adenopathy.
CARDIOVASCULAR SYSTEM: Heart sounds: no murmurs, rubs or gallops, carotids with good upstrokes, no bruits heard. Peripheral pulses including radials, brachials, and femorals intact. Posterior tibial, and dorsalis pedis pulses intact.
RESPIRATORY SYSTEM: Resps 16/min, trachea central, expansion, fremitus, resonance, and breath sounds normal.
ABDOMEN: Soft, no masses, organomegaly, or tenderness. No loin or costo-vertebral angle tenderness. Inguinal canals are intact without herniae. Bowel sounds active.
GENITOURINARY: Penis without lesions or discharge, scrotum, testicles, epididymis and cords all normal
RECTAL: no masses, tenderness, or hemorrhoids. Soft brown stool in vault. Prostate normal in size, and shape without nodules or tenderness.
MUSCULOSKELETAL SYSTEM: Joints with full ROM, no joint tenderness or swelling. Muscle bulk symmetric and normal.
SKIN: Without masses, skin tags, rash, blisters or ulcerations. Nails are normal without splinter hemorrhages.
NEUROLOGICAL SYSTEM: Alert and oriented to place, person, and time. Communicates with good word recognition and appropriate word usage. Cranial nerves and spinal nerves grossly intact.

Assessment and Plan

Problem	Plan/Status
Abdominal pain	Reports about two weeks of epigastric and retrosternal chest pain radiating up and to the left. Episodes of pain occur usually during the day and last for 3-4 hours. No associated dyspnea, palpitations, sweats, dizziness. No nausea, vomiting or diarrhea. No blood in the stool. To get barium swallow, CBC, Chem 7 and UA.

follow-up appointment: 3 days
Mark Woo MD

FIGURE 18–2 Sample computer-generated medical history and physical examination.

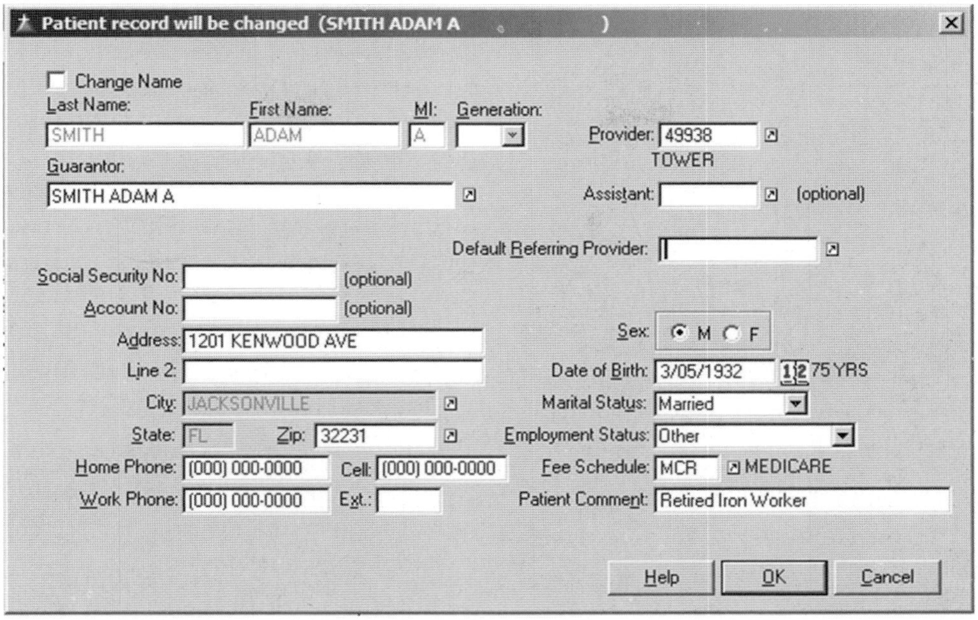

FIGURE 18–3 Example of a computerized patient registration record.

(CMS, 2015). Recently the use of EHRs by both physicians and hospitals has increased significantly as seen in the following statistics. As of 2013:

- 78% of office-based physicians had adopted some form of EHR system
- 59% of hospitals had adopted an EHR system with advanced functionalities
- 39% of physicians shared information electronically with other providers (U.S. Department of Health & Human Services [DHHS], 2014)

At the same time, work is still needed to create a health system that enables nationwide information exchange. This will enable increased care coordination for patients, as well as improving clinical quality and ensuring patient-record privacy and security (DHHS, 2014).

A major consideration in a national effort to create EHRs is to coordinate the variety of companies creating the software. To be truly effective, hospitals, clinics, physicians, and other providers must be able to share information. For example, the emergency department that treats an individual who becomes ill on vacation out of her home state should be able to access her medical records. However, systems from different manufacturers are often unable to "talk" to each other. As an example, the clinic in one Western city has a system that cannot communicate with the records system used by the hospital across the street in which many clinic physicians have hospital privileges.

Some health care providers, including physicians, have resisted adopting EHR technology. Reasons cited include the following barriers:

- Time needed to select and learn to use a new product
- Cost of implementing the system
- Lack of computer and keyboarding skills
- Concern about the security and privacy of patient records
- Worry about interrupting the physician–patient relationship by entering data into a computer instead of fully focusing attention on the patient (Ajami & Bagheri-Tadi, 2013).

In spite of these barriers, it is generally agreed that EHRs have the potential to improve health care efficiency, reduce errors, and help lower health care costs. Health care professionals should expect to see the introduction of EHR systems in the workplace if they are not already there. They should be prepared to learn to adapt to new methods, learn to use new software, and participate in the ongoing overhaul of how health care is organized and documented.

Creation of Documents

The importance of accurate and professional-looking documents was discussed in Chapter 17. Computers are excellent tools to help create high-quality written material. Word processing software converts the computer into a "super typewriter" that gives the user the capability to create customized documents that are error-free. Written materials of all types—letters, reports, forms, and newsletters—can be produced with word processing software. See Box 18–2 for examples of word processed documents found in health care. Software programs are available that enable the user to perform the following functions:

- Design the appearance of text and documents
- Edit, correct errors, and check spelling and grammar
- Store documents for later use
- Print and send documents by email, fax, or direct connection to other computers

Desktop publishing software is related to word processing software. It enables the user to easily combine text and graphics to create attractive newsletters, brochures, calendars, announcements, and so on. Presentation software carries documents a step further. Users can create slides to project from a computer, usually a laptop, onto a screen. Digital slides are commonly used for making professional presentations and for teaching.

Voice dictation software, a form of voice recognition software, converts spoken words to text. Increasing numbers of health care providers are using this technology for patient charting, reports, and standardized forms. Information that is dictated appears on a screen and the speaker can edit it as needed. Another type of software allows the speaker to complete the dictation and then sends the text to a professional medical transcriptionist for final editing. Voice dictation software has improved in accuracy over the past several years and has several advantages over traditional transcription services, which rely on handwritten documents from health care providers:

- It eliminates the problem of illegible or difficult-to-read handwriting.
- Reports tend to be more complete, as individuals can speak faster than they can write.
- The turn-around time for a complete, printed report is much faster.
- It is nearly as accurate, with one study showing it to be within 1.2 percentage points.
- The cost is considerably less.

BOX 18–2

Using Word Processing in Health Care

Announcements
Business letters
Home care instructions
Information sheets for patient education
Medical reports
Memos
Newsletters
Payment collection notices
Research reports

Spreadsheets

Electronic spreadsheet software permits the user to apply the computer's ability to perform high-speed calculations of numerical data. Spreadsheet software provides a worksheet that consists of intersecting rows and columns that form squares called cells. Numbers and formulas (instructions for performing calculations) are entered into the cells. To create a simple budget using spreadsheet software, the user enters the amounts of income and expenses and the formulas for the desired calculations. A formula may have several steps. The budgeting example would allow the user to calculate monthly income by adding all income and subtracting all expenses.

Accounting and financial management were two of the first computer applications in both business and health care. Electronic spreadsheets provide the basis for billing and accounting programs. In addition to speed and accuracy, these programs allow changes to be reflected throughout the spreadsheet. For example, if the cost of a clinic's rent increases, the effect on income can easily be calculated. All numbers affected by the change in rent will automatically be adjusted. Changes or corrections that might take a person hours to recalculate can be accomplished in seconds.

Computers have significantly changed patient billing methods. Amounts to be billed are not only calculated electronically, but they are also sent electronically to payers instead of being mailed. Starting in the year 2000, all Medicare and Medicaid claims had to be submitted electronically. Standardized codes have been developed that correspond to various diagnoses and treatment procedures. (See Chapter 22 for more information about medical codes.) The computer matches the codes for various procedures to a fee schedule and prepares bills. Computerized billing is easier and more accurate than bills prepared manually. Additional numerical codes that identify specific insurance companies can be entered so that bills are automatically prepared in the proper format.

The high speed of computer calculations also enables the user to employ "if…then" scenarios to explore a variety of options. Questions such as the following can be posed:

- "If the number of patients visiting the clinic continues to grow at the current rate, how many full-time medical assistants will be needed next December?"
- "If we finance the purchase of new medical equipment at 6.5% interest, how much will the total cost be if the repayment period is three years? Five years?"

This type of information assists in delivering high-quality patient care and making sound business decisions. Electronic spreadsheet programs are also able to create graphs and charts that illustrate numerical concepts and statistics. (See Figure 18–4.)

Thinking It Through

Ellie Myers has been entering patient billing data into the computer as part of her work as the administrative assistant and bookkeeper at Chandler Sports Medicine Clinic. The last week has been difficult for Ellie, because she has out-of-town relatives staying at her house and she is dealing with a variety of family problems. She is usually able to concentrate on her work but has been so tired the last few days that it has been difficult for her to fully focus on the details of data entry.

1. What might be the consequences if Ellie makes the following types of errors?
   a. Enters the wrong medical procedure codes on a bill to an insurance company
   b. Sends an appointment letter to the wrong patient
   c. Directs laboratory test requests to the wrong lab
   d. Enters the wrong numbers for expenses in the computerized accounting program
2. What would you recommend that Ellie do to protect against making mistakes of this kind?

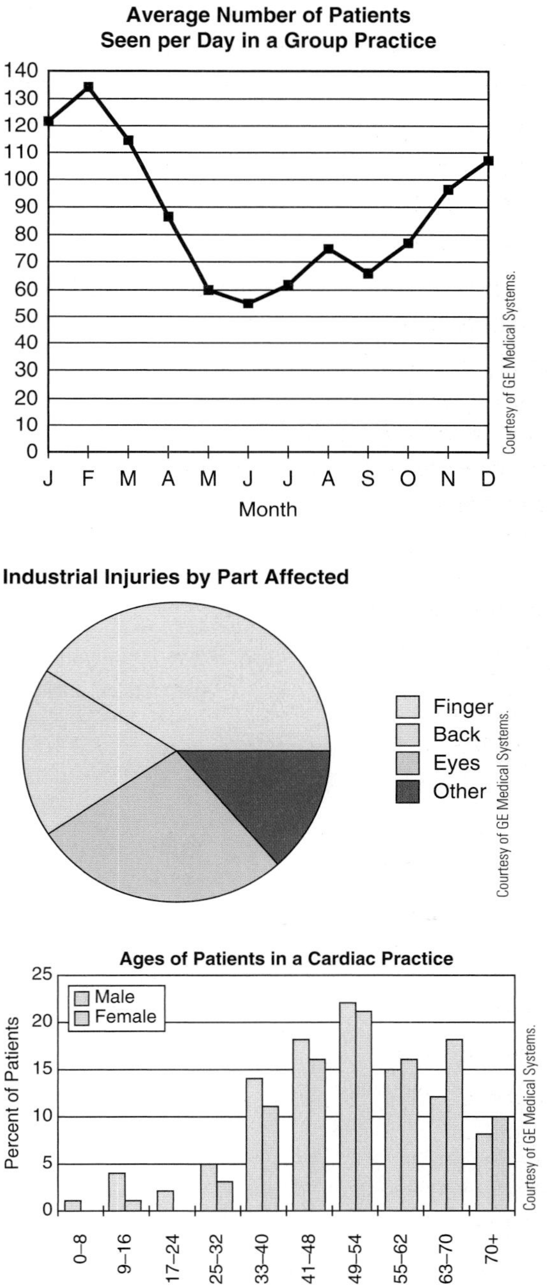

FIGURE 18–4 Graphs and charts can be easily created using computer software.

As with databases, it is critical that data entered into the spreadsheet be accurate. One incorrect entry can affect hundreds of numbers. Carefully check all electronic spreadsheet entries.

Diagnostics

Many types of diagnostic tools are available as a result of the computer's capacity to manipulate data and perform high-speed calculations. For example, blood and other body fluids can be tested and analysed quickly and accurately. Diagnostics is an area in which technology has advanced rapidly.

Diagnostic Imaging

The computer's ability to mathematically convert thousands of measurements into images has encouraged the growth of technology that permits the viewing of soft tissues not possible with traditional X-rays. Safer and more efficient ways of seeing the inner workings of the body continue to be developed and implemented in modern medical facilities. (See Table 18–1 and Figures 18–5, 18–6, and 18–7.)

The practice of dentistry has been improved by the introduction of safer methods of X-ray. Digital X-rays can now be taken, in which a small electronic chip is placed in the patient's mouth and an image sent to a computer. Viewed on the monitor, it can be enlarged, studied, and then stored in the patient's electronic record. The patient is exposed to a smaller amount of radiation than with traditional X-rays.

Table 18–1 Diagnostic Imaging Techniques

Procedure	How it Works	Examples of Use
Computed tomography (CT)	X-rays are taken from many angles. Measurements of the density of tissues are converted to cross-sectional views.	Evaluate soft tissues for presence of disease and conditions, such as blood clots, fractures, and tumors
Magnetic resonance imaging (MRI)	Patient is placed in a magnetic field. The activity of hydrogen atoms in tissues is measured and converted into cross-sectional images.	View tumors clearly View brain structure and abnormalities See movement in the body, such as blood flow
Positron emission tomography (PET)	A radioactive substance is injected into the patient and detected by a scanner, resulting in three-dimensional images.	Determine how brain is functioning; used with Parkinson's and Alzheimer's disease, epilepsy, cancer Can study effects of drugs on the brain and on some forms of mental illness
Ultrasonography	High-frequency sound waves hit tissues and organs and bounce back as echoes. The signals obtained are used to create images.	View movement Used when X-rays might cause harm, as with a fetus Examine organs Detect tumors, aneurysms, and blood vessel abnormalities
Electrical impedance tomography (EIT). Still considered experimental, but being used by research groups in hospitals	Conducting electrodes are attached to the skin. Electrical currents are measured to detect differences in tissue.	Proposed for: Monitoring lung function Detecting skin and breast cancer Producing images of the brain to locate hemorrhages, areas with inadequate blood supply, and sources of epileptic seizures

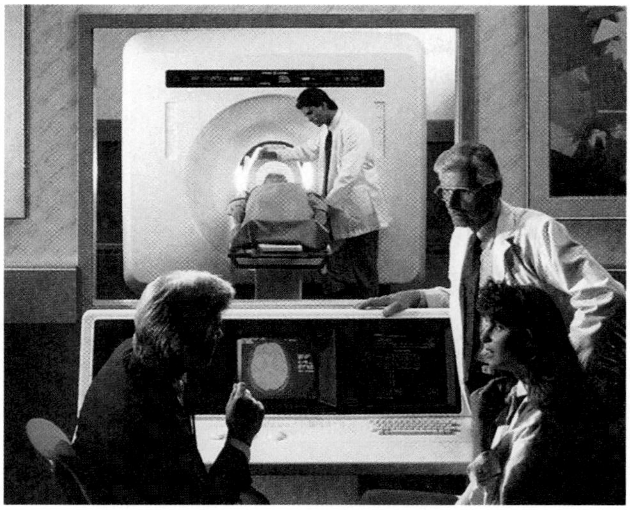

FIGURE 18–5 For magnetic resonance imaging (MRI), the patient is placed in the center of a large magnet.

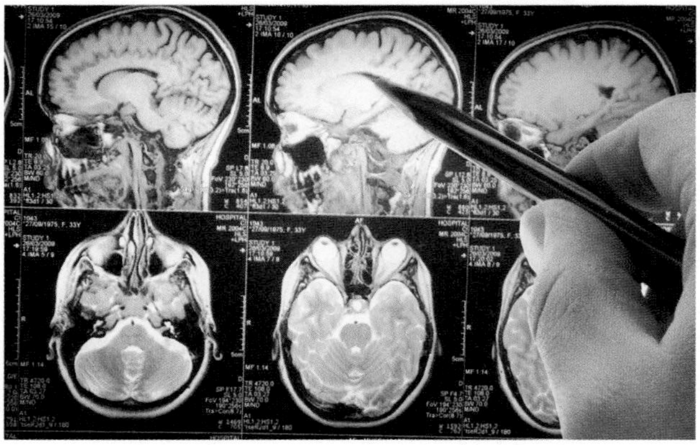

FIGURE 18–6 MRI images of the brain.

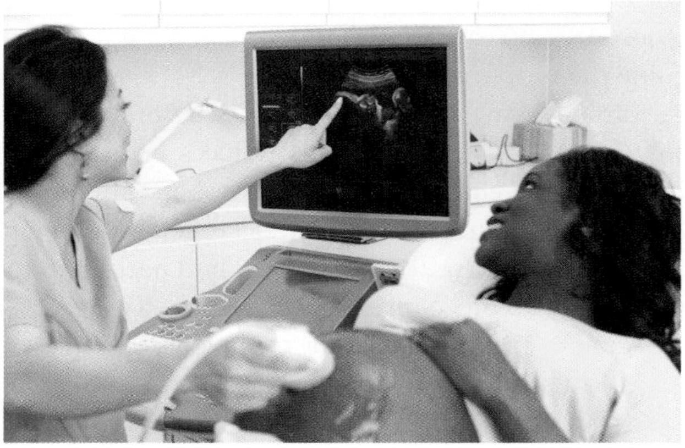

FIGURE 18–7 Ultrasonography is a safe procedure to use during pregnancy to determine the size, position, sex, and possible abnormalities of the fetus.

Fiber Optics

Fiber optics is a technology that involves the use of hair-thin cables to transmit data. This technology has applications in diagnostics, treatment, and the high-speed transfer of medical data. In dentistry, tiny fiber-optic cameras moved within the mouth create images that are projected onto a screen. Both the dentist and patient can see areas that are otherwise very difficult to access. Patient understanding of necessary dental procedures is greatly enhanced.

The use of fiber optics for both viewing and working inside the body has increased the safety of surgery. A tiny camera, inserted through a narrow tube, projects images along the cable onto a screen, allowing the physician to see the inside of the body without having to make a large incision. If surgery is required, tiny instruments are introduced through other tubes and the procedure is guided by images on the screen.

Remote Diagnostics

Technology enables information to be transmitted to nearly every corner of the earth. This ability is being applied to diagnose patients in remote locations who cannot be examined by a health professional face to face. Web-connected devices capture and communicate information to health care providers who can assess the data, give treatment advice, and subsequently follow up on the patient's condition. In addition to medical data, such as vital signs, voice and video can be transmitted. Common users of remote diagnostics include the military, airlines, and shipping companies. In addition to remote locations, clinics and hospitals are using remote connections to diagnose and monitor patients in their homes.

New uses of this technology are continually being created. Examples of what is currently available include the following:

- Web-connected stethoscope that transmits heart and lung sounds
- Device that transmits data while a patient is sleeping at home to diagnose sleep apnea (disorder in which breathing stops and starts)
- Blood pressure cuffs that transmit information to a health care provider so medication can be adjusted if needed

Fascinating Facts

PiiX is a wireless, water-resistant sensor developed by Corventis that sticks to a patient's chest, monitoring heart rate, respiratory rate, bodily fluids, and overall activity. It transmits these data to a central server for analysis and review by both physician and patient. The designers are working to generate algorithms that can analyze the data and predict when a patient is on the verge of heart failure by comparing trends in his or her vital signs against other cases.

(Source: PSFK Presents Future of Health: Remote Diagnostics. http://www.psfk.com/2010/08/future-of-health-remote-diagnostics.html.)

Expert Systems

Expert systems are a form of **artificial intelligence**, a very sophisticated technology that makes decisions based on real-life situations. Health care providers use these systems to help them diagnose and treat specific conditions. One of the first successful systems, MYCIN, was developed at Stanford University in the early 1970s. Its purpose was to help identify bacterial infections of the blood and cerebrospinal fluid and recommend appropriate antibiotics. The system operated by asking a series of questions. The answers narrowed down the choices by matching symptoms with information that was stored in the database. Although the system outperformed the diagnostic skills of the medical school faculty, it never had widespread use. This was because computer technology had not advanced sufficiently to support efficient use of MYCIN. It had to be used as a stand-alone system and could not be connected to any other system. In fact, physicians at that time did not have personal computers and a MYCIN session could take 30 minutes to complete. Other concerns at the time involved ethics and legalities: If the system made an error, who would be responsible? The example of MYCIN demonstrates how good ideas must sometimes wait until other technology catches up.

Today, there are many clinical decision-support systems (CDSS) that use artificial intelligence to assist with diagnoses and treatments:

- ATHENA Hypertension Decision Support System: Up-to-date information and medical guidelines for managing hypertension (high blood pressure)
- CEMS (Clinical Evaluation and Monitoring System) Mental Health Decision Support System: Assistance in diagnosing and treating psychiatric and mental conditions
- GIDEON (Global Infectious Diseases and Epidemiology Network): Support for diagnosis and treatment of infectious diseases
- HepatoConsult: Assistance in diagnosing liver and biliary tract disease
- TherapyEdge–HIV: Decision support system for treating human immunodeficiency virus (HIV)

Artificial intelligence, although intended to make computers behave like humans, is intended to *assist* health care professionals, *not* take the place of trained individuals. The reliability of expert systems varies, and they are never to be substituted for human input and decision making.

Treatment

Many new methods of treatment are based on computer technology. Patients have benefited from new applications that range from robotics to the computer's ability to quickly sort and match data.

Robotic surgery is an advanced method of surgery that benefits patients by increasing accuracy and using minimally invasive procedures. As with expert systems, robots are not intended to replace humans. In fact, surgeons must receive special training and guide every movement made by the robot. The success of this type of surgery depends on the expertise of the "human partner."

Sophisticated cameras provide surgeons with high-resolution, three-dimensional images. Sophisticated robots can be matched to the surgeon's voice and follow oral commands. This enables surgeons to perform procedures at a distance as they watch a monitor and guide the movements of the robot. Robotic surgery is performed using micro-tools and therefore requires only very small incisions. This reduces healing time as well as the chance of infection. Robotic surgery is currently used in many types of surgery, including cardiac, gynecological cancers, head and neck cancers, and urological procedures. (See Figure 18–8.)

Another treatment technology involves the use of **lasers**, focused light rays that can cut and remove tissue. Lasers are guided by computerized measurements to make precise incisions. A common use is for corrective eye surgery. Laser procedures are also used to remove diseased tissue and to treat bleeding blood vessels.

Image-guided surgery is based on a nearly three-dimensional mapping system that combines

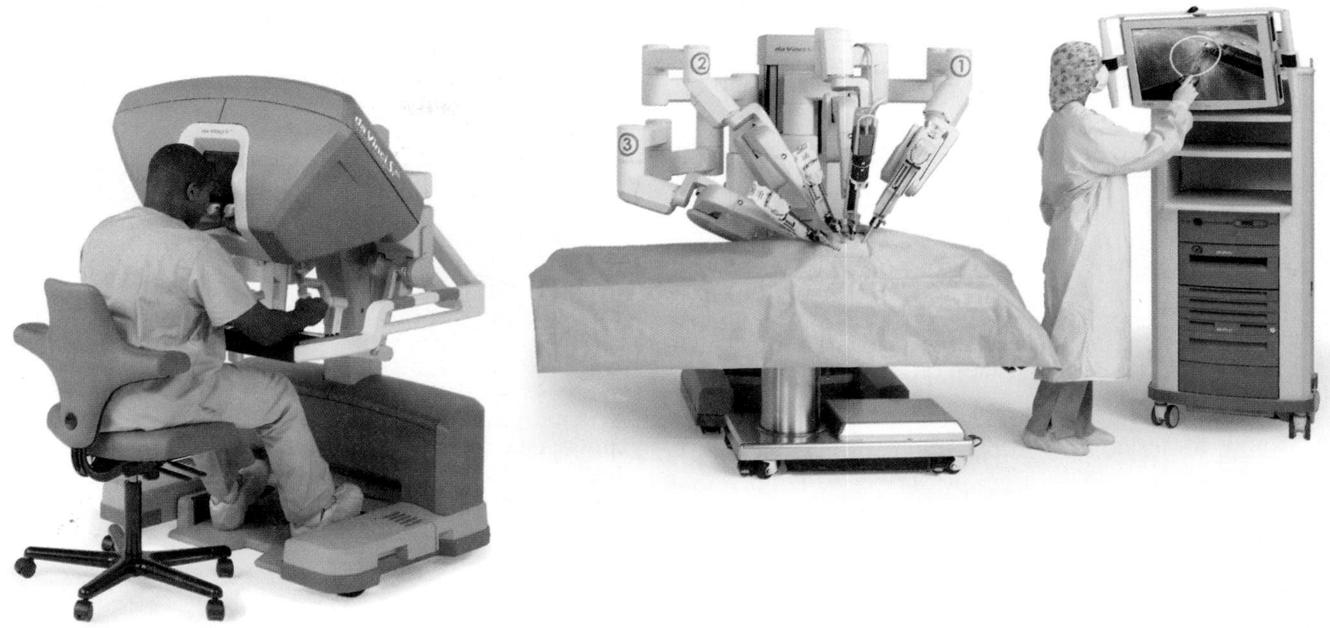

FIGURE 18–8 Surgeons are now able to work with robotic equipment to perform procedures that are less invasive and safer for patients than traditional surgery.

computed tomography (CT) with real-time information about the exact position of surgical instruments using infrared signals. This makes surgery more accurate and is especially useful when previous surgeries have changed the usual formation of a patient's body part, such as can happen with nasal surgery. As with robotic surgery, image-guided surgery tends to be less invasive and more accurate.

Computer-modeling capabilities assist plastic surgeons in reconstructive and cosmetic surgery. Many dentists employ computerized images to make perfectly fitting crowns.

Rehabilitation

Computer technology has helped people with disabilities live more independently. Commands that can be activated with the touch of a button or pad, the voice, or simply by eye contact with the monitor allow the control of household functions. These include turning lights and appliances on and off, answering the telephone, and controlling room temperature.

Computer-aided design has contributed to improvements in prosthetic devices. For example, artificial legs can be designed that more exactly fit the physical characteristics of the individual. Tiny microprocessors can be inserted in prosthetics to improve their movement and to allow them to be better controlled by the user. In another application, computer technology enables the electrical stimulation of muscles that no longer receive stimulation from the brain through the nervous system. Scientists are even developing ways to enable brain function to operate prosthetic devices, enable paralyzed individuals to move by using their thoughts.

Fascinating Facts

Stephen Hawking, one of the world's most brilliant thinkers of the last several decades, is significantly paralyzed and has lost his ability to speak due to a motor neuron disease. He continues to communicate with the world, including giving lectures, by means of computer technology that "reads" his facial movements and creates both text and speech through a synthesizer. Currently, SwiftKey, a London-based company, is developing the means to *predict* what Hawking *plans* to say, based on his history of writing and speaking. This technology has nearly doubled the rate at which Hawking can communicate.

(Source: How Stephen Hawking Is Using SwiftKey to Communicate Twice as Fast, by P. Sawyers, 2014, VB News. http://venturebeat.com/2014/12/02/how-stephen-hawking-is-using-swiftkey-to-communicate-twice-as-fast/)

Pharmaceuticals

Computers have improved many aspects of the dispensing of pharmaceutical products. Drugs, including anesthetics, are accurately measured and dispensed through computer-controlled devices. The chance for error is decreased, as well as the potential for abuse by health care professionals.

MEDI-SPAN, for example, sells commercial database products that assist in the prescribing of safe, effective medications. It contains information about drug–drug and drug–food interactions. It also has updates on the latest drug releases and those that are pending approval and information to help patients understand their drug therapy. The U.S. Food and Drug Administration publishes postmarket drug safety information for both patients and health care providers. This information is available at www.fda.gov/Drugs/DrugSafety.ClinicalTrials.com is a registry of federally and privately supported clinical drug trials being conducted in the United States and around the world.

Adverse drug incidents, estimated at one million annually, harm or cause the death of thousands of patients each year. These incidences include dosage errors, patient allergies, and dangerous drug interactions. One technology that shows promise to prevent these errors is the computerized physician order entry (CPOE) system. In this system, the prescribing provider enters medication orders into a computer that contains patient information, standard dosages, drug interactions, and so on. The system uses these data to check the appropriateness of an order before sending it to the pharmacy. Although research suggests that CPOE systems could reduce errors by 85%, not all hospitals have adopted them; and even some that have implemented CPOE do not keep the systems up to date, thus making them partially ineffective.

The FDA Adverse Event Reporting System (FAERS) is a database that contains information on adverse event and medication error reports submitted to the Food and Drug Administration. A system for tracking such errors has been developed and is involved in pilot testing in several states. It is hoped that the system, called MEADERS (Medication Errors and Adverse Drug Event Reporting System), will help prevent these occurrences, thus representing a significant positive contribution to patient care.

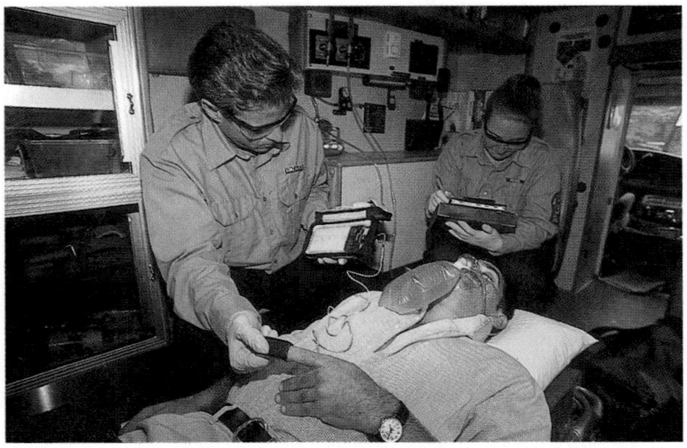

FIGURE 18–9 Pulse oximeters use computer technology to monitor a patient's pulse and determine the oxygen level in the blood.

Patient Monitoring

Physiological monitoring systems employ computer technology to oversee critical body functions, such as heart and respiratory rates. Alarm systems may be connected to various types of monitoring systems to advise health care personnel when patients need intervention. (See Figure 18–9.) Obstetrical monitoring of the fetus during a woman's labor has become a standard procedure.

In addition to performing actual physical measurements, computer systems enable health care professionals to enter and track data for charting and recordkeeping. For example, bedside terminals and mobile computers, such as laptops, allow keyboard entry of information, such as vital signs, dispensing of medications, fluid intake and output, and other information about care. Many systems, known as **point-of-care charting**, allow information to be entered from the patient's home or hospital bedside.

A growing number of health care facilities, including dental offices and medical clinics, now use small computer units (laptops) for charting and all types of recordkeeping. In many hospitals, for example, laptops on carts are rolled into patients' rooms. Nurses and other personnel enter all patient data, including vital signs, test appointments and results, and medications into a hospital-wide system. Laptops, tablets, and smart phones are increasingly being used for patient monitoring, in addition to communication and on-the-spot research. Some facilities have internal websites that can be accessed from any location. Physicians who cannot get to the hospital can review patient data, look at X-rays and test results, and recommend treatments from anywhere in the world.

Computerized devices are also used by home health professionals, such as nurses and physical therapists, to record patient notes and progress. This information is then transmitted electronically into the patient's health record. Making sure that data are entered accurately when working in the field is extremely important.

Many specialized devices have been developed to assist health care professionals in tracking patient recovery. For example, a camera connected to a computer allows hand therapists to store and compare photographs of the patient's hand taken over time. This aids in evaluating the effectiveness of the treatment plan.

Research

Learning and keeping up to date with medical advances has been made easier by computerized resources. The National Library of Medicine, through MEDLINE/PubMed, contains over 24 million citations to journals and books (National Center for Biotechnology Information).

Literature databases are like giant indexes, containing references to specific journal articles, books, and research reports. Each entry is accessible in various ways, such as the following:

- Preassigned key words that describe the content
- Words in the title
- Name of author(s)
- Name of journal
- Publication date

Other specialized databases are available in addition to MEDLINE. One of potential interest to health care learners is the Cumulative Index to Nursing and Allied Health Literature (CINAHL). It contains more than 3.2 million records from over 3000 journals. Two other large, specialized indexes of interest to health care professionals are the Educational Resources Information Center (ERIC) and PsychINFO.

In addition to providing published information, databases can serve medical researchers by their capacity to sort and match data. The term **bioinformatics** refers to the organization of biological data into databases applying information technology and computer science. Such databases make information easily available to scientists all over the world. Sharing information in this way contributes significantly to scientific progress.

Fascinating Facts

In March 2015, ClinicalTrials.gov listed 186,339 studies taking place in 50 states and 188 countries.

The Human Genome Project is an example of bioinformatics. Begun in the late 1980s and completed in 2003, it was an international effort to collect the results of investigations relating to human genes (one of the biological units of heredity). The goal of the project was to identify all the approximately 20,000 to 25,000 genes in human DNA and store this information in an organized manner. Gene therapy is an exciting area of medical research that uses the results of the project. In this therapy, a "normal" gene is inserted into a cell to replace an "abnormal," disease-causing gene.

Pharmaceutical research has benefited from the computer's ability to sort and match the results of thousands of tests carried out to explore the effectiveness and safety of new drugs. Results can be obtained more rapidly and sent to the Food and Drug Administration for review. This is decreasing the time needed to obtain approvals for new products.

Education

Computers offer new ways to learn for learners, health care professionals, and patients. Distance education is becoming more widely available. This is a method of accessing courses over the Internet that enables learners to take a wide variety of courses in their own homes at times convenient for them. As discussed in Chapter 14, this is a way for health care professionals to earn continuing education units, as well as to keep up on the latest developments in their career fields.

Sound, voice, and interactive components make computer learning an effective way for learners to proceed at their own pace. The Internet, CD-ROMs, and DVDs allow storage of vast amounts of reference information. Entire sets of encyclopedias are now available online or on a single disk. Medical reference books, including specialized dictionaries, have also been placed on disks and online. It is now possible to have access to an extensive reference library even if space is limited. Wireless reading devices, such as Amazon's Kindle and Apple's iPad, can hold thousands of pages, offering a convenient, mobile method for downloading and reading books in electronic form.

A.D.A.M. is an example of how the power of the computer can be harnessed to help students learn. Designed to teach anatomy, it is an interactive resource that contains a multimedia encyclopedia, more than 3000 illustrations, and three-dimensional images that can be rotated (A.D.A.M. Education, 2014).

Computerized simulations provide scenarios that allow learners to interact. A realistic situation is presented, followed by questions and opportunities for learners to suggest appropriate action. The computer responds to the student's input, either indicating its correctness or requesting more information. Virtual reality technology, in which reality is simulated as closely as possible, enables individuals to practice procedures before working on patients. These include inserting needles and performing surgical tasks. Virtual reality provides opportunities for surgeons to practice entire operations before working on actual patients. This opportunity is especially helpful with very complex and delicate procedures.

Many professional licensing exams are now administered by computer. In the past, many exams were offered only once or twice a year and graduates had to wait until they were scheduled. Some testing programs now individualize the exams by selecting each question based on the response given for the previous question. Test-takers who answer all questions correctly may pass the exam with fewer total questions. An example of this type of test is the National Council Licensure Exam (NCLEX), which is administered to registered nurse candidates.

Patients, too, can learn about their health conditions, self-care, and prevention techniques using the Internet. Credible, user-friendly websites, such as Medline Plus, offer dozens of articles, slide shows, and illustrations to inform health care consumers. Some hospitals make it possible for patients to obtain computerized health information.

Communication

Computer technology has greatly expanded the ways in which people can communicate. **Networks** consist of computers that are linked together so they can share information or output devices, such as printers. Networks enable communication among the staff of one clinic or among a group of thousands of individuals world over. An example of a simple networked system is five linked computers in a small medical office. Patient records are shared, and all staff members use the same printer. A large facility may have hundreds of computers linked together that carry out many of the functions described in this chapter. The Internet is the ultimate networked system, consisting of billions of computers located all over the world.

The Internet

The **Internet** began as a method for government authorities to communicate in case of nuclear attack. It has rapidly grown to become a principal means of communicating, conducting business, shopping, learning, securing needed information, and socializing.

Using the Internet for Research

Health care professionals can benefit from the Internet in many ways. Consider the case of Mark, a recently graduated nurse, who is hired by an orthopedic surgeon who specializes in joint replacements. Mark wants to learn more about these procedures and decides to see what he can find on the Internet. In one afternoon, he locates the following resources:

- Articles in medical journals
- Information produced by and about companies that manufacture artificial joints
- A newsgroup in which patients who have had joint replacement surgery share their experiences
- Articles in popular magazines, such as *Newsweek*
- A list of medical facilities and surgeons in the United States who specialize in joint replacement
- Government reports about the effectiveness of artificial joints
- Email addresses of university researchers who are experimenting with new types of artificial joints
- A medical bookstore that takes orders over the Internet

Mark was successful in finding information because he knows a number of ways to look for what he wants:

1. **Web directories** organized into broad topics. There are directories for health topics, such as Highlight Health Web Directory (www.highlighthealth.info).
2. **Gateways** are similar to Web directories in that they contain links to other websites that contain

specific kinds of information. For example, Medline Plus (http://medlineplus.gov), a service of the U.S. National Library of Medicine and the National Institutes of Health, has organized links under major headings that include "Health Topics," "Drugs and Supplements," and "Dictionary." The Riley Guide (www.rileyguide.com) is a gateway to hundreds of websites containing information about resumes, interviewing, and other job-search topics.

3. **Search engines** are programs that look through millions of documents, organized as databases, to locate **key words** the user provides. Mark entered the key words "artificial joint" to begin his search. A number of search engines are available, such as the following:
   - Google: www.google.com
   - Windows Live Search: www.bing.com
   - Yahoo: www.search.yahoo.com

The major search engines allow you to be more specific by specifying phrases that must appear exactly as you enter them. In Mark's case, if he enters the words *artificial joint*, a search engine will find documents that contain both these words—but not necessarily together. (Search engines are becoming better at recognizing these types of common phrases.) Using the advanced search function, or by enclosing the phrase in quotation marks, Mark increased his chances of finding useful websites.

It is important for learners to remember that they must cite (give the source of) information taken from a website and used in a report or paper just as they would for material taken from a book or journal article. Copying information word for word from a Web source or using materials such as images without permission is **plagiarism**. There are several ways to correctly cite and list Web sources, just as there are different ways to organize a bibliography or reference list. Check with the appropriate **style manual** or your instructor to learn the preferred form.

Evaluating Internet Sources

At this time, material placed on the Internet is not regulated. Anyone can say anything and make any claims. Not all information is reliable. Much of it consists of personal opinions or is motivated by the desire to sell products. Health care professionals must take care to determine the reliability of any information taken from the Web. There are thousands of health-related websites, and many of them were created by reliable organizations. The following guidelines are designed to help evaluate sites:

- Identify the source: Universities and government agencies tend to be reliable sources of information. Research and professional organizations, if not organized for the purpose of selling specific products, may also be reliable—for example, the American Heart Association and the American Association of Medical Assistants. The ending of a website address gives information about the sponsor. (See Table 18–2.) It should be noted here that commercial websites can be good sources of information. Many large corporations provide nonbiased information.
- Determine the author: Is the person an expert in the field? Does he or she have appropriate education and credentials? Is the purpose of the material to share information or report research findings? Or to persuade readers and sell ideas or products?
- Check for accuracy: Is a reference given for the information? Is the reference from a reliable source?
- Verify important data: Cross-check statistics and other numerical data.

Table 18–2 Identifying Website Sponsors

Type of Sponsor	Website Address Extension	Example
Educational institution	.edu	University of Michigan, www.umich.edu
Government office or agency	.gov	National Institutes of Health, www.nih.gov
Professional organizations	.org	American Cancer Society, www.cancer.org
Businesses, corporations, and other commercial organizations	.com	Merck & Co., Inc. (pharmaceuticals) www.merck.com

- Look for signs of quality: Are the ideas well supported? Is the spelling accurate and vocabulary used correctly?
- Check for currency: Is the information recent and up to date?

Electronic Mail

Electronic mail, also known as email, is a means of creating and sending messages from one computer to another, using the Internet system of networks. Email has become a standard professional communication tool. It provides a way to quickly send documents, such as memos, announcements, and reports to one or more persons. Some physicians and other health care providers are using email as an efficient means of communicating with patients.

It is important that email messages be clear and accurate, just as with any written material. The growing popularity of email means that some people receive dozens of transmissions daily. Keeping messages brief and to the point is considered a professional courtesy. Proper email communication is known as "netiquette."

> **Fascinating Facts**
>
> Mount Sinai Hospital in Toronto has taken advantage of iPhone® technology to develop an app called VitalHub that pulls together data from the hospital's 66 different applications. The new system includes patient records, test results, vital statistics, and medical research literature. Physicians use the system to quickly view all the information they need to make fast, accurate decisions about patient care. Using the iPhone®, everything can be accessed remotely, as well as on-site. For example, before arriving at the hospital a physician can review a patient's chart, see what drugs he is on, identify another drug that might benefit the patient, and then quickly check for possible drug interactions.
>
> *(Source: iPhone in Business: Mt. Sinai Hospital, www.apple.com/iphone/business/profiles/mt-sinai/.)*

Files created in other programs can be sent with an email message. For example, a report created in MS Word can be sent as an "attachment" to an email message without rekeying the document. This provides a convenient and economical way to send, review, revise, and return documents and share useful information. Suppose that two respiratory therapists in different states are working together to write a journal article. Using email attachments, they can send updated drafts of their work to each other for review. Sharing research findings is another example of collaboration made easier through the ability to exchange documents electronically.

It is important for health care professionals to understand that it is not appropriate to conduct personal email correspondence or explorations on the Internet at work. Be aware that email messages may be stored in the form of backup files that belong to the employer. Employers have the right to read and monitor any messages sent through their computers by any employee. Many organizations have increased their monitoring of employee activity on the Internet. Using work hours to write unflattering messages about the boss and to order personal care products are invitations for trouble on the job. They may be cause for disciplinary action and can even lead to dismissal.

Social and Professionals Networking Sites

Social networking websites, such as Facebook, have become popular "meeting places" for individuals to connect with friends and share personal news. These sites can provide the means to stay in touch with family, friends, and in the case of learners, with former classmates. In this way, they can help you network when it comes to the job search or when looking to change jobs throughout your career. A word of caution: Posting unflattering images of yourself, intended to be funny or entertaining, may be a harmful career move. This is because employers are increasingly checking social networking sites when considering applicants for employment. Showing yourself in a situation that demonstrates poor judgment, lack of respect for others, or other unfavorable characteristics could prevent you from being hired. In extreme circumstances, it can be cause for dismissal from a job.

In addition to Facebook, there are dozens of networking sites, many serving to link people around the world who share common interests, such as music and travel. One large specialty website is LinkedIn, which promotes professional networking. Its profile page emphasizes a member's employment history and education rather than personal information.

The company reports that many of its members are employment recruiters.

Telemedicine

The American Telemedicine Association defines **telemedicine** as "the use of medical information exchanged from one site to another via electronic communications to improve a patient's clinical health status" (American Telemedicine Association, 2015). Transmission devices may include two-way video, smart phone, email, and various wireless tools. The medicine practiced by telemedicine is the same as that practiced in face-to-face consultations. Its major advantage is that it provides expert medical help to patients in remote areas, such as farms far from towns, war zones, and wilderness areas. It is also increasingly used where convenience, rather than distance, is the issue. As discussed previously, patients can be monitored while remaining in their homes. A physician can send patient information to a colleague halfway around the world to obtain an opinion about a rare condition. Because images can be transmitted electronically, X-rays and other images can be sent for analysis. One hospital emergency department in Oregon sends CT scans of patients admitted during the night to Australia to be interpreted if there are no radiologists on duty at the hospital.

Telemedicine is especially helpful for the following functions:

- Allowing patient access to specialists who are located at a distance
- Communicating vital signs from home to allow monitoring at a health care facility
- Checking pacemaker function and performing ECGs over telephone lines
- Performing physical exams from a distance
- Providing more comprehensive emergency care by linking emergency medical professionals in the field and during patient transport with physicians

Although telemedicine has become an important part of health care delivery, there are three major obstacles to its expanded use:

1. Not all facilities, especially those in remote areas, have adequate infrastructure to support the necessary high-speed wireless technology.
2. State licensing laws sometimes prohibit the exchange of medical practice across state lines, even when done electronically.
3. Not all health care professionals are comfortable with the technology (American Telemedicine Association, 2015).

In spite of these obstacles, telemedicine offers exciting possibilities for patients everywhere. For example, the California company InTouch has developed a robot to which a variety of medical devices can be connected. The information obtained can be transmitted to far-away locations. The "head" of the robot is a screen that enables all participants to see one another and communicate directly (InTouch Health, 2015). Other patients who may benefit from telemedicine in the near future are those in developing countries that lack sophisticated imaging equipment. Bioengineers have developed a way to separate the imaging machines that gather data from the more expensive components that process that data and create the images. In this way, health care providers can use the less expensive image-gathering equipment and send the data, via cell-phone technology, to the much more expensive computer located in an industrialized country.

Telepharmacies

Telepharmacies allow the dispensing of drugs at sites other than pharmacies. Instructions for prescriptions are sent to a computerized dispensing unit. The unit prepares and releases the exact dosage. Safety features are built into the system to prevent incorrect types and amounts of drugs from being dispensed. This technology is especially useful in medical facilities that are located far from commercial pharmacies.

In North Dakota, telepharmacy technology provides services to thousands of rural customers from a pharmacist physically located at a central pharmacy site. Using video conferencing technology, the pharmacist communicates with the customer and a registered pharmacy technician who prepares the drug for dispensing. The pharmacist performs a drug utilization review, prescription verification, and patient counseling just as he or she would do if present in person. North Dakota was the first state to pass rules that allow retail pharmacies in remote locations to operate without a pharmacist on location (North Dakota State University, 2010). Since 2001, when South

Thinking It Through

Robin Winter, a dental hygienist, is working on creating a patient education program to teach effective dental home care and nutritional practices. Her patients range from toddlers to the elderly.

1. Describe how Robin can use computers and a variety of applications in her patient education program.
2. How can she apply the principles of patient education described in Chapter 17?

Dakota implemented telepharmacies, several states have passed legislation that enable telepharmacies to serve outlying populations.

Virtual Communities

Virtual communities consist of individuals who use the Internet to communicate and share information. Both health care professionals and patients can share information and experiences about specific health conditions. Chronically ill, bedridden, and disabled patients use the communication capabilities of the computer to break from the isolation that often results from these conditions. (See Figure 18–10.) There are at least four ways that this can be accomplished:

Fascinating Facts

As of March, 2015, there are more than 100,000 newsgroups in operation with more being added every day.

1. Chat rooms allow participants to correspond in real time, using typed messages. Many groups are organized to create communities of individuals who share similar interests, including chat rooms dedicated to health issues.
2. Mailing lists, also known as email discussion groups, are automated systems that distribute email on specific topics. Subscribers can respond to the emails they receive. Their responses are sent to all other subscribers. There are mailing lists for thousands of topics. LISTSERV®, a mailing list server, has almost 60,000 mailing lists in its catalog at www.lsoft.com/catalist.html.

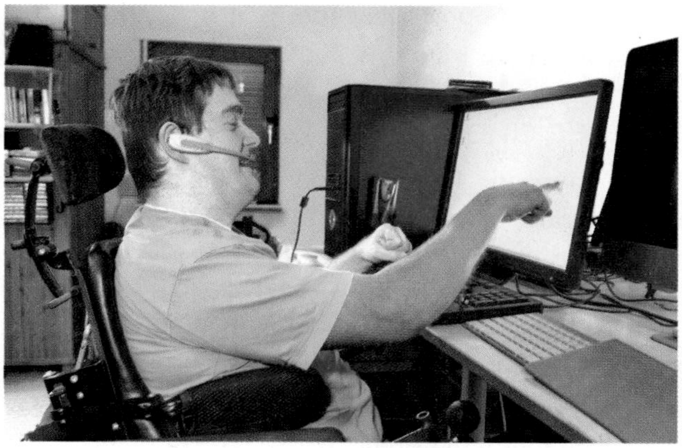

© Belushi/Shutterstock.com.

FIGURE 18–10 Computers allow disabled people to more easily connect with the outside world and communicate with others.

3. Newsgroups provide opportunities for participants to contribute information and comment on items submitted by others. They are organized by subject and range from general topics to specific local issues. Newsgroups can be accessed using the "newsreader" available on most Web browsers. A directories of newsgroups is available at http://groups.google.com/groups/dir.
4. Web forums are online discussion groups. Thousands of groups are available. Google maintains a list of groups at http://groups.google.com.

COMPUTER BASICS

Although it is not within the scope of this text to teach computer operations, certain fundamental concepts are introduced to guide learners who are not familiar with the basic terms and components of computer systems.

Computer Hardware

All computers, whether small laptops that fit into a briefcase or large mainframes that run the operations of a hospital, have physical components in common. These are known as **hardware** and consist of the following:

- **Central processing unit (CPU)** Located inside the computer, the CPU has three major functions:
  1. Manages all operations
  2. Performs calculations and manipulate data (facts)
  3. Stores program instructions and data

- **Peripherals** Equipment that allows the user to interact with the CPU. Common devices that allow the input of data include the following:
  1. Keyboard
  2. Mouse, trackball (built into keyboard), track pad, and trackpoint (small eraser-like protrusion on keyboard)
  3. Scanner
  4. Microphone

Following are the three most common output devices:

1. Monitor
2. Printer
3. Speakers

Laptop computers, used in many health care settings, combine the CPU and peripherals (except the printer) into one compact unit. Wireless technology, widely used today, enables computers to communicate with their peripherals and with other computers without the use of physical wiring.

Caring for Hardware

The physical components of a computer system require regular care. Health care professionals should exercise the same care for them as for other medical equipment used on the job. All components of the system contain delicate parts and must be handled gently. A mouse, for example, should never be brought down sharply onto a hard surface. Wires and cables should not be jerked or pulled. Spilled liquids can permanently damage the inner workings of electronic equipment. Dust and food crumbs can also cause problems. For example, salt crystals attract moisture, so salty snacks should not be eaten over the keyboard.

Regular maintenance will help ensure the continued operation of computer equipment:

- Clean monitor screen with an antistatic cloth. Do not use a commercial glass cleaner.
- Vacuum keyboards periodically with a handheld vacuum cleaner or attachment.
- Wipe plastic and metal cases with a soft, damp (not wet!) cloth.
- Clean printers according to manufacturer's instructions. Dust that collects on the moving parts can cause smears and fuzzy print.
- Use dust covers when equipment is not in use.
- Read all directions carefully when using and caring for computer components. Follow the manufacturer's recommendations.

Storing Information

The **hard drive** is a storage device located inside the computer, out of the user's view. All types of work can be saved on the hard drive: letters to patients, medical records, accounting reports, and research articles. Today's computers can store huge amounts of data.

Occasionally hard drives cease functioning properly and become inaccessible to the user. This is known as a "crash" and can be caused by a number of factors, including problems with electrical power supplies. To protect against the loss of important data, all work should be saved in at least one other place. This is called "backing up files" and is an essential habit to develop. There are several ways to back up files, such as using a different section of your hard drive, a Zip drive, an external hard drive, or a flash drive. Increasingly popular is **cloud storage** in which data is backed up by a service that may span several servers and locations. Determining what will work best with your computer and learning to save your data will pay off if your data are ever destroyed.

Computer Software

Software programs contain instructions that enable computers to function. Hardware components cannot perform a single operation without the direction of software. An **application program** is a type of software that performs a specialized task, such as patient billing, performing diagnostics, or word processing. Some software provides information, such as entire medical dictionaries that can be loaded onto the computer. Many software programs are available off the shelf, such as the following:

- Norton Internet Security: Antivirus and antimalware program
- Microsoft Word: Word processing program
- Excel: Spreadsheet program
- Medi-Soft and Medical Manager: Integrated medical office management programs
- Taber's Cyclopedic Medical Dictionary: Comprehensive medical dictionary available on the Web and for mobile devices

CD-ROM discs contain the setup files for application programs. They can store many times more data than the diskettes that were used in the past. Entire medical dictionaries and encyclopedias are available on a single CD. Newer computers allow their users to copy data onto a CD, commonly called "burning a CD." Today, many applications can be downloaded from the Internet and CDs are gradually being phased out as storage devices.

In addition to off-the-shelf application programs, software engineers custom design systems to meet the specific needs of their clients.

Apps

Apps, which stands for applications, are small computer programs usually designed to be used on mobile devices, such as smart phones and tablets. There are currently more than 500,000 apps available for the iPhone alone. They are able to perform almost any task and include many apps that are specific to health care such as the following:

- Micromedex: Contains drug reference information
- New England Journal of Medicine: Includes articles, images, and videos
- Critical Link: An emergency medical information resource for use in areas that lack emergency medical services
- UpToDate: An evidence-based clinical decision support resource

USING COMPUTERS EFFECTIVELY

You can increase the effectiveness of computers as work tools by using good work habits such as the following:

- Verify the accuracy of all data entered: When working on a large system, incorrect entries can negatively affect the work of others as well as the welfare of patients. Many medication errors in hospitals are the result of incorrect data entry. Health care work demands accuracy to ensure high-quality patient care, as well as compliance with regulatory agencies.
- Always back up work: Save work to the hard drive periodically. The computer workspace, called **RAM**, stores data only while the computer is on. If power is interrupted, any work not saved will be lost. Many software programs allow you to save work automatically at regular intervals. When a task or work session is completed, back up all files as discussed earlier. Computers can break down, and emergencies can occur.
- Stay legal: It is against copyright law to install software that has been installed on another computer unless it is specifically allowed and stated by the manufacturer. Purchase and register needed programs. **Site licenses** that give permission to install software on more than one computer can be purchased for programs that will be loaded on more than one computer at a facility. Never bring personal software to load onto the workplace computer.
- Keep up with advancements: Software is continually updated with new versions that offer additional features. Many updates are available at reduced prices for owners of previous editions. New websites, offering an increasing number of products and services, appear daily.
- Do not panic: Computers are still a relatively new technology, and the complexity of today's systems results in occasional glitches. It is almost impossible to damage computer hardware through normal use. If the computer does not understand a command, an error message will appear on the screen. These error messages can sound rather serious, but the worst thing that can usually happen is that work performed since it was last saved—either by the user or automatically by the program—is lost and must be redone. As discussed earlier, this can be avoided by regularly saving work. This said, entire system crashes do occur and thus there is a need to back up your files.
- Be flexible: When large facilities update or change their computer system, the transition can be stressful. During the first few days after "going live," it can seem as if the new system adds more work instead of more efficiency. It can take staff members time to learn and adapt to the changes. Fortunately, software analysis, design, and support are continually improving and making information technology easier for everyone to learn and use.
- Avoid injury: Prolonged use and improper positioning can result in physical injuries. See Chapter 9 for information about reducing the risk of workplace injuries, such as carpal tunnel syndrome, related to computer use.

COMPUTER SECURITY

The very characteristics that make computers useful in health care can also be a cause for concern. For example, the increased accessibility to patient records also increases the risk of breaching patient confidentiality. The need to protect privacy has been addressed by the federal government. Several major laws, such as the Electronic Communication Privacy Act of 1986, provide protection against unauthorized access or interception of data communications. The privacy of medical records is specifically addressed in the Health Insurance Portability and Accountability Act (HIPAA) implemented in 2003. (HIPAA is discussed in Chapter 19.)

There are simple precautions the health care professional can take to help ensure computer security. If assigned a password to gain access to a computer system, never give it to anyone else, even a coworker. Unauthorized users can destroy or falsify data, add hours to their payroll records, or illegally transfer funds. Entries can often be tracked to the password used. The following simple practices will increase computer security:

- If passwords are chosen rather than assigned, do not use something obvious, such as a nickname.
- Close files containing private information before leaving the work area.
- Do not allow patients or other unauthorized persons to wander into the area where data entry is taking place.
- Shred discarded printouts before throwing them in the trash.

Computer viruses are a threat to computers. Viruses are programs that contain instructions to perform destructive operations, such as scrambling and erasing files and preventing the computer from operating normally. Viruses can get into the hard drive from "infected" CD-ROMs and files that are **downloaded** (transferred onto the computer) from the Internet. A common means of transmitting harmful programs is by clicking on links contained in emails from unknown sources.

It is not always obvious that a virus is present because the instructions may have been programmed to activate at a future date. All computers are susceptible to viruses. Entire organizations have been shut down by viruses downloaded from the Internet when employees opened email messages.

The following practices will help prevent viruses from infecting workplace computers:

- Do not open email messages or download files from unknown parties.
- Do not use your work email address for personal correspondence.
- Use purchased software to load application programs, not copies secured from friends or other outside sources.
- Use antivirus software and keep it updated to protect against new viruses that are continually being created.

Wireless technology has its own security threats. When using public Internet access ("hot spots"), do not enter private passwords to websites or personal data, such as credit card numbers. Office as well as home computers that use wireless technology should be secured so that strangers cannot piggyback (use your wireless service for free) or, under certain conditions, monitor your computer activity or access your directories and files.

MAINTAINING THE HUMAN TOUCH

Although computers have become part of everyday life, there are still people who are not familiar or completely comfortable with this new technology. They complain that they feel like a number in a vast system over which they have little control. This perception may result in feelings of intimidation and annoyance. In fact, some physicians have resisted the implementation of EHRs because they have difficulty focusing on a patient, maintaining eye contact, and observing the patient's body language, while simultaneously entering data into a computer.

The health care professional should strive to provide a personal interface between patients and machines. Do not let the computer become a barrier. Those responsible for inputting patient data should extend a friendly greeting before beginning the data entry process. Look up and make eye contact periodically. If it is not obvious to the patient, explain what information you are entering and why. Make appropriate comments to convey a sense of caring to the patient. Communicate verbally and nonverbally that the patient is more important than the machine.

Health care professionals should also be prepared to respond to patients' concerns about the privacy of

Thinking It Through

Stacey Petersen is the admitting clerk at a large urban hospital. The patients served come from a wide variety of cultural and economic backgrounds. Much of Stacey's work involves collecting and entering patient data into the hospital's computer system. Although most patients are comfortable with this procedure, some find it intimidating or are uneasy about "just what is being put into the computer." Of particular concern to Stacey are elderly patients from cultures in which health care is very personalized and where practitioners are well known to the patient.

1. What can Stacey do to help these patients feel more at ease?
2. How can a lack of understanding on the part of patients about the health care system affect the way they deal with health problems?

their medical records, identity theft, and the possibility of errors being entered on computers.

LEARNING MORE ABOUT COMPUTERS

Learning more about the capabilities and operation of computers can increase the efficiency and job satisfaction of the health care professional. Opportunities for promotion may be increased. The many ways to increase computer knowledge and skills include the following:

- Take classes
- Read the manuals that come with hardware and software
- Work through tutorials and help menus included with software programs
- Take tutorials available on the Internet
- Explore the various functions of software programs
- Read some of the many books that are available for all levels of users
- Research topics on the Web

Finding effective ways to learn about computers will help you keep up with a rapidly advancing technology that will continue to change the nature of health care.

WORKBOOK PRACTICE

Go to your workbook and complete the exercises for this chapter.

SUGGESTED LEARNING ACTIVITIES

1. Find out what types of computer classes are available at your school and in the community that are appropriate for your needs.
2. Explore health-related websites such as Medline Plus, Web MD, and the Mayo Clinic. List the address and give a brief description of each. (Add these to the webliography started for Suggested Learning Activity 4 in Chapter 14.)
3. Look for health-related mailing lists and groups on the Internet.
4. Visit a health care facility to learn about how computers are used for diagnosis, treatment, and administration.
5. Interview someone who is working in a health care field of interest to you. How are computers used in this field? How much work does this person perform using computers or computerized technology? What computer skills are considered essential to be successful in this occupation? Which skills will increase promotional opportunities? Write up a short report of your findings.

WEB ACTIVITIES

American Telemedicine Association
www.americantelemed.org

Choose three case studies to read. Write a "news report" about the benefits of telemedicine using examples from the case studies.

Medical Library Association
www.mlanet.org

Click on "For Health Consumers"; then on "Find and Evaluate Health Information." Write a brochure or fact sheet explaining how to evaluate websites. Then explore at least three of the "Top Health Websites" and write a brief description of each: the kind of information available on the site, ease of use, and one fact or idea that you learned while reviewing the site.

Healthcare Cost and Utilization Project
www.hcup-us.ahrq.gov/overview.jsp

Explore the use of databases to gather and organize data about hospital admissions and stays to enable research on health policy issues.

Technology in Health Care

Do a Web search using the phrases "technology in healthcare" and "using computers in healthcare," then choose at least four websites to explore and report on.

Study Guides and Strategies
www.studygs.net

Under the headings "Guides: Internet" and "Online communicating" click on "Netiquette." Using what you learn, create a poster or brochure outlining the principles of good electronic communication.

REVIEW QUESTIONS

1. Why is it essential for today's health care professional to be computer literate?
2. List at least two computer applications for health care in each of the following areas:
   a. Information management
   b. Creation of documents
   c. Numerical calculations
   d. Diagnostics
   e. Treatment
   f. Patient monitoring
   g. Research
   h. Education
   i. Communication
3. What is the difference between computer hardware and software?
4. What are five ways to properly handle and care for computer hardware?
5. What are six guidelines for using computers effectively?
6. How can the health care professional help ensure the security of computerized records?
7. What are three ways the health care professional can learn more about using computers?

APPLICATION EXERCISES

1. Refer to The Case of the Therapist Who Wants to Add to Her Computer System at the beginning of the chapter. Based on what you learned in the chapter, list new ways that Carol can use computer technology in her practice.
2. The students in an Introduction to Health Care class have just completed their study of the application of computers in health care. The course was an overview, and the students have been thinking about how they will use computer technology in their work. For each of the following students, suggest potential applications and the skills they should acquire for on-the-job success.
   a. Craig Kingman, paramedic
   b. Otis Brownwell, radiologic technician
   c. Christine Abbott, surgical technologist
   d. Marta Singh, registered nurse
   e. Jaime Bustamante, medical assistant

PROBLEM-SOLVING PRACTICE

Grace has been the medical assistant in a small clinic for many years. She performs both clinical and administrative duties. The two physicians in the clinic want to explore using telemedicine and other new technologies, as well as updating the office computer system. They have asked for Grace to be involved. She feels she has enough to do with the medical assisting duties and does not have time to help, nor is she really interested in having to learn a lot of new things. How can Grace use the five-step problem-solving process in this situation?

SUGGESTED READINGS AND RESOURCES

American Telemedicine Association. www.american-telemed.org

Human Genome Project. http://web.ornl.gov/sci/techresources/Human_Genome/publicat/primer2001/primer11.pdf

National Library of Medicine's Visible Human Project. www.nlm.nih.gov/research/visible/visible_human.html

PubMed. www.ncbi.nlm.nih.gov/pubmed

Robotic Surgery. www.nlm.nih.gov/medlineplus/ency/article/007339.htm

Study Guides and Strategies—Online Learning/Communicating. www.studygs.net

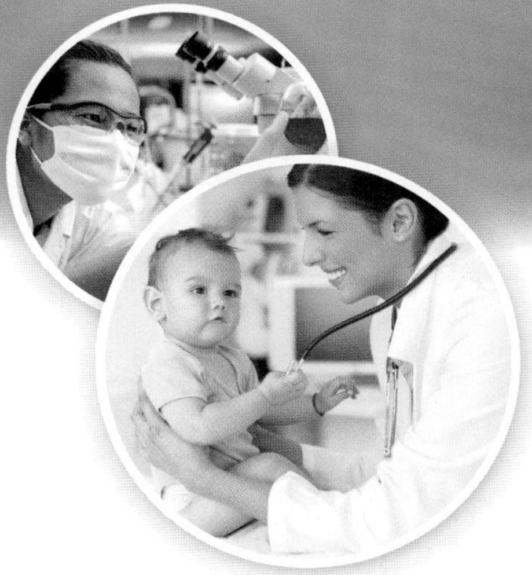

Chapter 19

Documentation and Medical Records

OBJECTIVES

Studying and applying the material in this chapter will help you to:

- State the primary responsibility of the health care professional regarding HIPAA regulations.
- List and explain the purposes of medical documentation.
- List the characteristics of good medical documentation.
- Explain the proper method for correcting errors on medical records.
- List the various sources of information that may be found in a medical record.
- Describe three different formats used for progress notes.
- Discuss the advantages and disadvantages of each progress note format.
- Discuss the advantages of an electronic health record (EHR) coordinated system.
- Describe what information would be included in a personal health record (PHR)

KEY TERMS

charting
chief complaint
electronic health record (EHR)
HIPAA (Health Insurance Portability and Accountability Act of 1996)
medical documentation
medical history
medical record
personal health record (PHR)
plan
progress notes
SOAP

The Case of the Therapist Who Hates to Write

Joseph Lane, a respiratory therapist, enjoys working with patients and the technical aspects of his profession. But he has never enjoyed paperwork and dislikes writing documentation following the treatment he administers. His notes are hurriedly scribbled, and other health care professionals find them difficult, if not impossible, to read. In this chapter the importance of accurate, complete, and legible documentation will be stressed. Inaccurate, incomplete, and illegible charting has consequences for patient care, jeopardizes regulatory compliance, and presents legal risks.

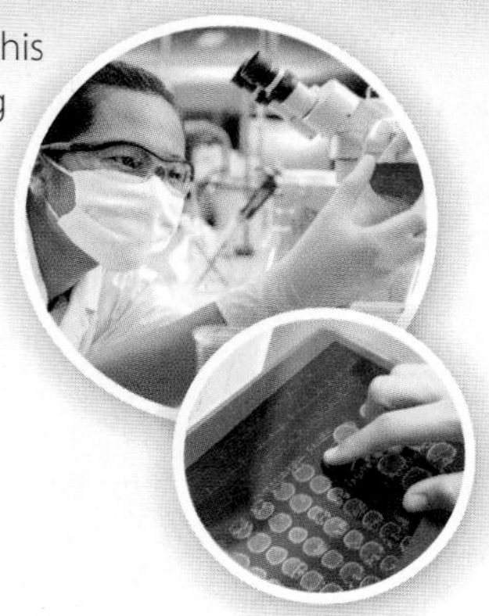

HIPAA

HIPAA—the **Health Insurance Portability and Accountability Act of 1996**—has been mentioned in previous chapters of this book. But due to its importance, it is worth expanding on the provisions of this act that relate to medical records and documentation. HIPAA mandated significant changes in the legal and regulatory environment governing the provision of health benefits, the delivery of and payment of health care services, and the privacy and security of individually identifiable, protected health information (PHI) in written, electronic, and oral formats. It is the Privacy and Security Rules that are of greatest significance within the framework of this discussion. The Privacy Rule gives the patient specific rights related to his or her medical record, such as the right to request:

- Access to and copies of the medical record
- An amendment to the medical record
- An accounting of disclosures of PHI
- A limit on information about himself or herself that is provided in a hospital directory

The Security Rule has administrative, physical, and technical safeguards. The following examples pertain to electronic PHI:

- Administrative safeguards: Developing security policies and procedures regarding use of electronic health records (EHRs); training the entire workforce on implementation of these policies and procedures
- Physical safeguards: Preventing unauthorized viewing of computer terminals by positioning them in appropriate locations, and not propping open doors that may allow unauthorized access to private work areas
- Technical safeguards: Following good password policies, and logging off the computer when stepping away

A health care professional must at all times be aware of and protect the privacy of the patient's record. If you are working with paper charts, it is important not to leave them lying around where others can view them. If you are working with computerized records, your computer must be locked before leaving the station to prevent others from casually viewing the record. Many computers are located in traffic areas and a privacy screen placed over the monitor prevents others from reading the material unless they are directly in front of the monitor. Remember that patients' medical information belongs to them and them alone. No one else has a right to that information, regardless of the relationship, without the consent of the patient. If a patient is unable to handle his or her own health care decisions, then a power of attorney should be on record specifying who has the authority to receive information and make the decisions. This limitation of access also applies to health care professionals. If you are not actively involved in a patient's care, you do not have a right to access that patient's chart. You also do not have a right to access a coworker's chart or a family member's or friend's chart. Breaking any of the HIPAA regulations could

Thinking It Through

Ms. Shing Chun works in a clinic. The provider asks her to call Mrs. Yang and tell her the labs were normal and that a new medication has been sent to the pharmacy for her. When Ms. Chun calls, Mr. Yang answers and says his wife is not home, but he can take a message. Ms. Chun tells him to tell her the labs were normal and a new medication was sent to the pharmacy. Mr. Yang asks what tests were run and what medication was ordered. Ms. Chun declines to answer the questions by explaining that it is confidential information.

1. Did Ms. Chun break any HIPAA regulations?
2. If the labs had been abnormal, should she have handled it differently?

result in a corrective action that could include the following:

- Notification of the federal government if there is an incident involving a Medicare patient
- Notification of the individual patient whose PHI was illegally accessed, used, or disclosed
- Corrective action, up to and including termination, for the individual health care professional responsible for the incident

MEDICAL DOCUMENTATION

Medical documentation refers to notes and documents that health care professionals add to the medical record. For example, patient statistics and information about care, results of tests performed, the patient's diagnosis written by a physician, treatments received, and medications given are the types of information that are commonly included in medical documentation.

A **medical record** refers to the collection of all documents that are filed together and form a complete chronological health history of a particular patient. A medical record is also commonly referred to as a medical chart, patient chart, or patient record. Recording observations and information about patients is known as **charting**.

Many health care professionals are responsible for some aspect of charting. Tasks may include the following:

- Recording demographic information about new patients
- Interviewing patients and filling in the medical history form
- Recording vital signs (e.g., temperature, blood pressure)
- Noting comments made by the patient
- Making notes on the patient's record as dictated by the physician, dentist, or other professional
- Recording any procedures performed
- Transcribing notes or dictation from other professionals into the medical records

Purposes of Medical Documentation

Complete and accurate medical documentation is critical in providing consistent patient care. It is the lifeline of communication that supports the coordination of care. Information included in the medical record is a significant source of data on which other health care professionals can base their approach to the patient.

In addition to ensuring good patient care, medical documentation serves other important purposes:

- Provides legal protection: Medical records are legal documents that are admissible as evidence in court. In the case of a malpractice lawsuit, for example, documentation provides proof of what has taken place with the patient. Only through written documentation can tests, procedures, and treatment be proven to have occurred. In the world of health care, "If it isn't documented, it isn't done."
- Helps ensure compliance with regulatory agencies: These include governmental bodies and accreditation organizations such as the Joint Commission on Accreditation of Healthcare Organizations (JCAHO). Participation in certain programs, such as Medicare, requires that specific documentation guidelines be strictly followed.
- Improves cost control: Proper documentation prevents repetition and the performance of unnecessary procedures. It also helps ensure that appropriate preventive measures, early intervention, and correct procedures are performed.

- Decreases denials from insurance companies: The need for care and proof that it is provided by appropriate personnel are supported by documentation.

Fascinating Facts

Subpoenas, in malpractice lawsuits, frequently arrive a year or more after the care was given and documented. When called to testify, most health care professionals do not even recall the patient or the care given and must rely entirely on their own documentation.

Characteristics of Good Medical Documentation

- Complete: All requested information must be included. Each entry must include the date and signature of the appropriate health care personnel. Charting should be completed as soon as possible to prevent the omission of important information.
- Concise and factual: A lot of words are not better than a clear concise statement. Never use the chart to record guesses or opinions. State only what has been observed, done, or heard. If you are quoting a patient's statements, use quotation marks. For example, "I feel a sharp pain in my left leg every time I try to walk."
- Properly identified: The patient's name and identifying numbers should be visible on every page. It is critical that the record match the patient so that correct entries are made.
- Legible: Notes that cannot be read are useless. They do not serve their purpose of providing continuity of care. Furthermore, they present a liability and cause for negative legal and regulatory outcomes.
- Uses correct spelling, terminology, punctuation, and grammar: Poorly written documentation can be easily misinterpreted and gives the appearance of carelessness when the record is reviewed by others.
- Clearly and objectively expressed: Important details are correctly noted: temperature, size, amounts (fluids, drainage, medication, etc.). The words used are not subject to misinterpretation, such as "small," "a lot," and so on. Notes should be limited to what is observed. For example, write "ate 25% of the meal" rather than "ate poorly."
- Does not duplicate findings: Some facilities use graphic sheets on which the blood pressure, temperature, pulse, and respiratory rate are recorded. If so, it is not necessary to repeat this information in the written record. When a finding is abnormal, it may be repeated in the written record along with the associated action taken or treatment given to correct the problem. The record would then also include a follow-up assessment of how the patient responded to the action or treatment.
- Uses abbreviations only if approved and listed in the facility's policy manual: This reduces the possibility of misunderstandings if the abbreviation used has several different meanings. For example, does "pt" stand for patient, prothrombin time, physical therapy, or part-time?
- Shows time and date of all entries: Accurate and chronological charting presents a picture of how

Thinking It Through

Juanita is a registered nurse (RN) who works for a home health agency. She enjoys the work, because she really cares about each of her patients and likes getting to know them as individuals. She tries to spend a little extra time on each home visit, chatting with them about their families, interests, pets, and so on. With more patients being released to their homes rather than to rehabilitation or other settings, her case load has increased. Juanita finds that sometimes she does not have time to complete all her charting until late in the evening. Sometimes she is not able to get to it until the following morning. She tries to complete it while eating breakfast before leaving for another day of rounds.

1. Discuss the possible consequences of Juanita's current work habits in terms of legal compliance and reimbursement.
2. Discuss any changes you would recommend.

the patient appears over time. If charting is not done in a timely manner, another health care professional may record an event with a time that occurred after the action that you intended to chart. The only option then is to write "late entry" and then chart, but this out-of-sequence information can still create confusion for others. (See Figure 19–1.)

- Signed by the proper person: Never sign for someone else or have anyone sign the charting you have done. Recording false information is a serious offense and should not be done under any circumstances.
- Completed without leaving empty lines: All charting that begins after the previous signature and runs to the next signature belongs to the latter entry. If an empty space or line is left above the entry and signature of the health care professional, it is possible for someone else to chart information that now becomes part of the other health care professional's entry. (See Figure 19–2.)
- Never entered in advance of the medication or procedure: Chart only after the event has occurred, never before, in anticipation of doing it. For example, if a nurse charts that medications were given and then is suddenly called away, the other health care professionals will assume that the medications were given, and the patient will not receive the proper medications he or she needs for treatment.
- Written with black or blue ink (or as specified by the facility): Pencil is *never* acceptable.

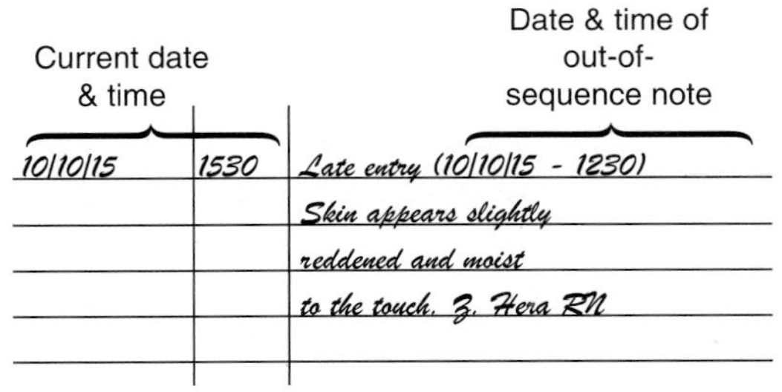

FIGURE 19–1 Sample of a late entry in charting.

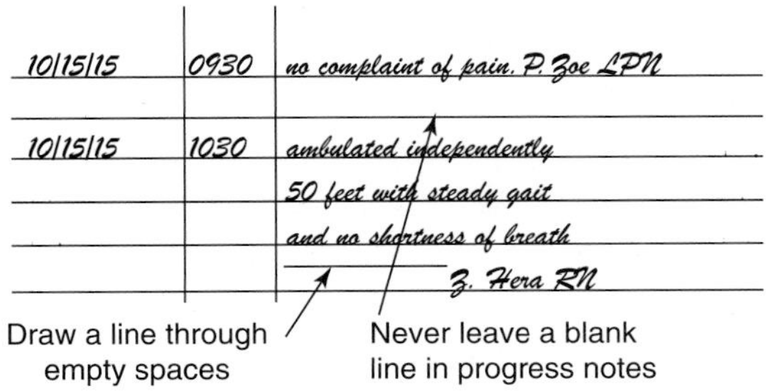

FIGURE 19–2 Never leave empty lines in charting.

Making Corrections on Medical Documentation

Medical records cannot be corrected in a way that covers up what was originally written. To do so can give the appearance that the records have been illegally altered and negates their value as legal records. Never use correction fluid (such as White-Out), erase, or use correction tape over errors. Observe the following practices:

1. Draw a single line through the error. The original entry must still be legible.
2. Write in the correct information where there is the most space: above, below, or following the original entry.
3. Note the error as required by your facility. For example, "M.E." may be used for "mistaken entry"; "correction" or "corr" may be acceptable. Be sure to learn the specific requirements for notations, and never create your own or assume that the facility will use the ones presented in textbooks. Regulatory agencies differ in the terms accepted, and it is important to carefully follow their guidelines.
4. Date and initial the correction.
5. If an error is made while typing or word processing a document, you may correct it as you work. If it is discovered later, correct it by hand, following steps 1 to 4 as described here. (See Figure 19–3.)

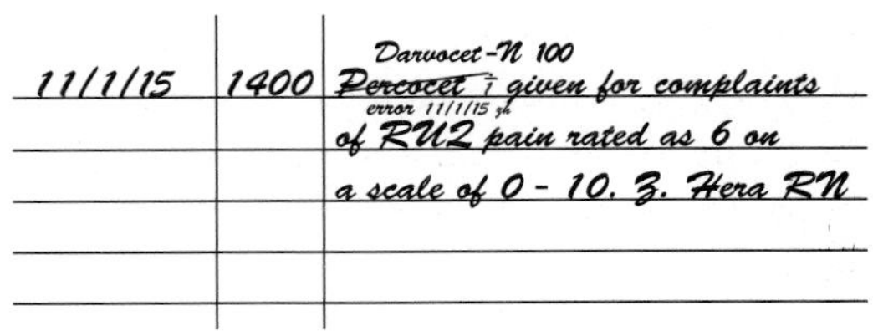

FIGURE 19–3 Sample of how to make a correction in charting.

CONTENTS OF THE MEDICAL RECORD

The medical record will be organized according to facility policy, and the health care professional is expected to maintain the integrity of the record by following all policies and procedures. Many physician offices will have a continuous chronological record format, but in large health care facilities there may be a *source-oriented* approach. This approach divides the record into different sections separated by tabs for each health care specialty. This has the advantage of making it easy to find specific information related to a specialty, but has the disadvantage of increasing the difficulty of seeing the overall view of the patient because many sections need to be referred to for the complete picture. In a source-oriented charting format, the chart may be separated into the following sections:

- History and physicals (H&P) and consultations: Typed or handwritten reports on the initial findings of all physicians seeing the patient. The primary physician will do a complete **medical history**, which includes a personal, familial, and social history. The personal history includes the patient's past medical problems and surgeries, allergies, current problems, assessment of each body system (see Chapter 20), and medications. The familial history lists medical problems of relatives that may indicate a tendency for the patient to develop these problems. The social history includes use of tobacco, alcohol, and illegal drugs. The suspected diagnosis and plan for further assessment and treatments are also included in the medical history. Consultations occur when the primary physician asks another physician to see the patient for further evaluation of a specific problem. Some facilities have transcription services in which the physician dictates the detailed findings and then the transcriptionist types from the taped message. This is then placed in the chart for the physician to review and sign.
- Physician's orders: Written record of all orders for medications and treatments prescribed for the patient
- Diagnostic tests: Any report that includes findings obtained in an attempt to diagnose or monitor the progress of patients, such as the results of laboratory tests, X-rays, and electrocardiograms (ECGs)
- Admissions: Completed forms and consents that deal with the admission process
- Surgical procedures: Consents for and reports related to any surgical procedures performed
- Graphics: A graphed format for blood pressure, temperature, pulse, and respiratory rate; may also have spaces for height and weight
- Flow sheets: Forms for specialty needs, such as monitoring blood sugar levels or measurements of a wound as it heals. Many specialty fields create forms specific to their needs (Figure 19–4)
- Medication record: Includes all medications administered by health care professionals at the facility
- **Progress notes**: Written chronological statements about a patient's care. For example, each time a physician sees a patient he or she will make an additional note to update findings and plan for the care of the patient. Therapists (e.g., physical, occupational, and speech therapists) and other services (e.g., social workers, chaplain services) will note what was done and their assessment of results. Nurses will record what treatments they perform, the patient's response, and any abnormal assessments, and plans for intervention. In large facilities, the physician, therapists, and nurses may have different sections of the chart in which to record their documentation.

When filing forms, reviewing charts, or charting, always verify that the correct form is in the chart by checking that the patient's name is on each document.

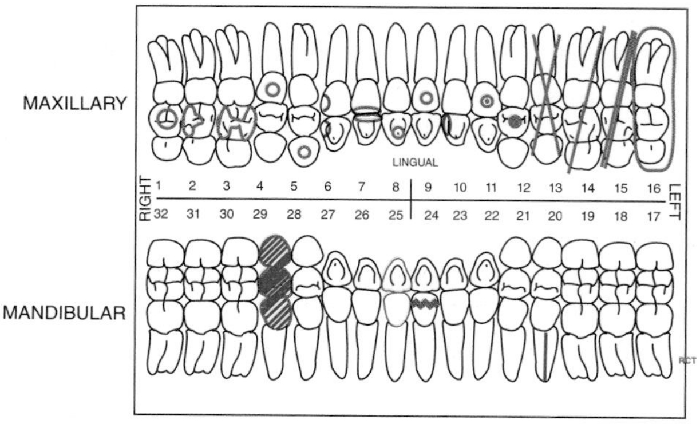

FIGURE 19–4 Sample dental form that uses symbols to record conditions as they occur over time with an individual patient.

Thinking It Through

Sally Jones is an administrative medical assistant for Dr. Yin, an orthopedist in a single-physician office. Sally takes great pride in the appearance of all her work, particularly patient records. She neatly corrects any mistakes made with white correction fluid and is pleased at how tidy the files are. Sally is shocked when Dr. Yin is sued by a patient and loses the case. Dr. Yin's attorney reports that the patient's medical records were largely at fault for the loss of the case.

1. What do you think happened?
2. How might Sally's handling of patient records have contributed to the loss?
3. What recommendations would you make to avoid this type of problem in the future?

An incorrectly filed form can lead to misunderstandings and errors. When filing or adding additional blank forms to the chart, always place them in the correct section in chronological order. The forms within each section will be chronological. The most current is usually on top, depending on facility policy.

Sometimes a patient's chart becomes too thick, and another file on the patient is started. This is referred to as "thinning a chart." A note is then made in the new chart that an older file exists for this patient. When requesting charts, always make sure that you have all the charts on the patient for review.

The security of records is the responsibility of each health care professional. Never leave charts or the content of charts lying around for unauthorized individuals to see. Specific rules and regulations dictate who can be given copies of the chart and what procedure must be followed to request copies. Ask your supervisor for these guidelines and follow them without exception.

Progress Notes

The progress notes make up the written record of every aspect of a patient's relationship with the health care providers. They are the primary tool used to record, communicate, and coordinate the care given to the patient. Careful documentation is a critical skill for the health care professional. Before charting, it is important for the health care professional to take a moment to organize his or her thoughts. For example, health care professionals can ask themselves what they observed while working with a patient, what has been done for the patient, and what the patient's response was to any interventions. It is important to always address the primary problem that required the assistance of health care services.

There are several ways to organize progress notes. It is the responsibility of health care professionals to learn the formats used at the facilities in which they work. Examples of common approaches are presented next.

Problem-Oriented Charting

Problem-oriented medical records are organized around the patient's health problems. After the initial assessment is completed, a list of problems and related plan of care are identified, and then all subsequent charting refers back to this problem list. If new problems develop, they are added to the list and dated. If a problem is treated and no longer exists, it is marked as resolved and dated. The advantage of this approach is that all health care professionals focus their charting on the same problems. The disadvantages of this approach are difficulties in keeping the problem list up to date and the possibility that patients may be seen more as problems to be resolved than as individual human beings.

The format for charting of each problem is known as **SOAP**. These letters stand for the following components of the documentation:

S—Subjective: This is information that is sensed and reported by the patient. Known collectively as symptoms, they describe how the patient feels as a result of a disease or injury. It is best to record the patient's own words as closely as possible. Use quotation marks when noting exact words. The **chief complaint** is the reason the patient is seeking medical care and is included in the subjective section of the record. Significant patient behavior, such as missed appointments, failure to follow directions, and statements about discontent with treatments, should also be included in this section.

O—Objective: This information includes the observations of health care personnel. Included are measurements, such as temperature and blood pressure; lab test results; description of a wound; color, temperature, and moisture of skin; and how a patient walks (gait). These observations are known as signs.

A—Assessment: The assessment is the health care professional's impression of what is wrong with the patient, based on the signs and symptoms.

P—Plan: The **plan** documents the procedures, treatments, and patient instructions that make up the patient care. (See Figure 19–5.)

A variation of the SOAP charting is SOAPIE. The S, O, and A have the same meanings as just described. The P and the additional letters stand for the following:

P—Plan: What is planned for tests and treatment?

I—Interventions: What interventions are actually carried out?

E—Evaluation: Evaluation of the interventions. What were the results? Was the treatment effective?

Narrative Charting

Narrative charting includes detailed written notes on all aspects of care. It includes routine care, normal and abnormal findings, and any other information related to the patient's plan of care. The advantage to this approach is that the health care professional can use his or her own approach to describe the patient and the care given. The disadvantage is that it is often time-consuming and results in an extensive written record that is difficult to read through to find specific information. (See Figure 19–6.)

Problem List

Date Opened	No. Problem	Identified By	Date Resolved
1/15/15	#1 Angina related to coronary artery disease	B. Meed M.D.	
1/17/15	#2 Impaired mobility due to weakness of right lower extremity secondary to old stroke (1998)	Z. Hera RN	

Plan of Care

Date	Problem
1/15/15	#1 Angina related to coronary artery disease GOAL: Prior to discharge patient will be able to ambulate 300 feet with no angina PLAN: Gradually increase walking distance & pace after starting on new medication regimen

Progress Note

2/5/15	1700	Problem #1
		S: states "I had no pain in my chest when I walked twice around the floor."
		O: skin cool & dry. B/P 120/76 p. 84
		A: increasing walking distance with no angina
		P: continue to increase walking distance as long as stays angina free.
		Z. Hera RN

FIGURE 19–5 Sample of a problem-oriented progress note.

11/15/15	1800	Alert and oriented x3. No complaints of pain. Vital signs normal. Ate 100% of dinner. —— Z. Hera RN

FIGURE 19–6 Sample of a narrative progress note.

Charting by Exception (CBE)

Charting by exception is an abbreviated format. Only abnormal findings are noted. This requires a well-defined understanding of the normal findings that are used for a comparison. If no abnormal findings are found, then no written notes are required. The advantage in this approach is that it saves time and that the problems are easily identified by reviewing the notes. The disadvantage is that it is problem oriented, so the preventative or wellness aspects of care are not included. (See Figure 19–7.)

Computerized Charting

In Chapter 18, the multiple uses of computers in health care were introduced. The impact of computers on the health care professional includes the trend toward computerization of charting. This trend accounts for the most significant changes in patient care documentation. Facilities that do not currently

Clear lung sounds are normal and would not be charted. Rales are the exception to the normal.

12/5/15	2200	Rales noted in both lung bases. Will call Dr. Johnson to notify of change in condition —— Z. Hera RN

FIGURE 19–7 Sample of a charting by exception progress note.

have computerized systems will likely have them in the future as the hardware and software become more affordable. When the decision to computerize charting is made, facilities have three options:

1. Purchase a computerized program package and use without modification
2. Purchase a computerized program package and pay for modifications to the system to meet the facility's specific needs
3. Develop a computerized program package for their own individual needs

The choice of options is greatly influenced by identifying the needs of the facility versus the cost involved in the purchase and implementation of the program. These options are listed from least to most expensive. The most common decision by a facility is to choose option number 2. Most computerized programs are not specific enough for the individual needs of the facility, but trying to design a customized version is both very costly and time-consuming. In addition, most facilities do not have the in-house expertise to design such a sophisticated program. The vendor and facility enter into a contract that details the cost of any modifications.

The decision to change to computerized charting has far-reaching effects. One of the main challenges is the training of personnel on the new system. Change creates increased stress in an already stressful environment. Time, training, support, and patience will be required by all involved in the transition. Some of the advantages and disadvantages of a computerized system are listed here.

Advantages:

- Improved legibility of charting
- Anticipated decreased recording time and costs and fewer errors
- Improved communication among health care team members
- Greater access to medical data for patient care, education, research, and quality improvement
- Records easily transmitted to different sites for various health care professionals to have access to information

Disadvantages:

- Possible system breakdown
- Cost of converting to a computerized system
- Potential problems with patient confidentiality—anyone with the correct code can access files

Previously in this chapter, the proper way to correct errors in handwritten documentation was discussed. Errors can also occur in computerized charting. As long as the chart is open, changes can be made. But once the chart is closed it cannot be reopened and corrections made in the prior note. The proper way to correct an error is to reopen the chart and note that a correction is being made to a prior charting entry and include the correction. The date and time stamp is automatically included by the computer system.

Other helpful features a computerized system may have are "copy and paste" and "smart phrase" functions. These features have the ability, with only a few key strokes, to add extensive text to your document. Both features can save a great deal of time when charting commonly performed actions as much of the information does not have to be retyped. It also leads to problems if not used with caution. Information that is copied and pasted from a previous entry should be modified to demonstrate updated content with relevance for that date. Although inserting a smart phrase that details the entire procedure you may be preparing to perform can be very advantageous, blanks frequently need to be filled and findings relevant to the process added to personalize the entry. Leaving the information unaltered, without modification, can misrepresent the patient's condition or the care provided during the encounter.

ELECTRONIC HEALTH RECORDS

Electronic health record (EHR) systems, also called electronic medical records (EMRs), are computerized information and coordination systems used by health care systems. As discussed in Chapter 18, these systems can go far beyond the core charting to include systems that coordinate with laboratory, radiology, pharmacy, admission-discharge-transfer functions, and tools to allow data exchange with aggregate reporting systems. For example, when a patient registers at the front desk, the computer shows the arrival time. This notifies the back office personnel to bring the patient back to the exam room and take the patient's vital signs. The provider can review the patient's past history, current medications, and recent labs. During the visit the provider can record his or her findings; order any new medications, labs, or other tests; and place referrals. After the visit the patient can go to the lab, pharmacy, radiology, or other area as the orders are already in the computer.

The computerized systems can also include many informational and safety tools. Such tools have many uses: Medications ordered can be compared to any previous orders to assess for compatibility problems; extensive libraries of information can be accessed for provider research and clarification of recommended treatment protocols; and documents that detail what has been ordered, future appointments, and any screening tests that are due, can be printed out for patients to take home. If the system is tied to a patient education databank, educational materials can be printed out for patients to refer to later. This helps reinforce information that may have been missed or forgotten when explained verbally at the visit.

An additional feature of many systems is the ability to scan documents to be included on the computer. This allows for other forms of written material presented by the patient or a family member to be included in the computerized system if deemed helpful.

As long as the patient stays within the same health care system where all departments can access the same computer system, this information would be available to the various departments via computer. But if the patient transfers to another health care network, a written request would be required to send a hard copy of the documents to the new facility. This can prove frustrating for the patient and time-consuming for the health care professionals as each new provider needs to enter all the data into his or her own system. For example, individual medical offices usually have a system designed for their own use, only. Thus, it is possible that a patient may have an internist, a cardiologist, an ophthalmologist, and one or more other specialists involved in his or her care, and each will use a different software system. In the case of multiple separate providers with different computer systems, this would require each patient to set up a personal ID and password for each different computer system so they can access their health data or email their provider. However, the provider cannot access another provider's system, which can result in a breakdown in communication between providers.

PERSONAL HEALTH RECORD

Personal health records (PHRs) are documents created and maintained by individual patients to help them communicate with various health care providers. Due to the mobility of individuals and the frequent changes in health care providers and insurance groups, it is recommended that each individual keep a PHR to ensure greater continuity of care. When patients bring their own PHR with them it benefits both the provider and the patient. It helps prevent the patient from forgetting information and also minimizes long delays on the provider's end in requesting the information from a prior source.

The type of information frequently provided in a PHR includes the following:

- Demographics, such as name, address, and contact information
- Emergency contacts
- Name, specialty, and contact information of previous health care providers
- Insurance provider(s)
- Medical directives, living will, organ donation, and so on
- General medical information: height, weight, blood type, vital signs, and so forth
- Allergies and drug sensitivities
- Current conditions and date of diagnosis
- Previous surgeries, including date and results
- Medications (prescription and nonprescription)
- Immunizations and when last received
- Any relevant health care visits, such as hospitalizations, other specialists or therapists
- Pregnancies
- Medical devices
- Foreign travel
- Family history information

WORKBOOK PRACTICE

Go to your workbook and complete the exercises for this chapter.

SUGGESTED LEARNING ACTIVITIES

1. If you are currently working in a health care facility, review the written or computerized documents and evaluate the documentation. Why are the examples good or poor? Can you get a real picture of that patient by reading the chart? Remember to follow HIPAA guidelines and access only those records that you are working with as part of your designated work assignment.
2. Write samples using the three formats of progress notes presented and then check them against the characteristics of good documentation. If you make an error, remember to make the corrections according to accepted guidelines.
3. Work with another student to identify a specific situation that may occur in your health care specialty area. Then both write a documentation and compare the results.
4. Prepare a personal health record (PHR) with your health information following the guidelines presented in the text regarding the type of content to be included.

WEB ACTIVITIES

Seer Training Modules
www.training.seer.cancer.gov

Search for "Medical Record" and click on "Composition of a Medical Record." Review the material and take the quiz to check your comprehension.

Capterra
www.capterra.com

This site contains some of the top electronic medical records software. Click on "browse software," then click on "electronic medical records." Choose two to three programs and view their profiles. Compare the features listed for each program and determine which one you feel would be the most helpful in the field you are interested in pursuing.

All Nurses
www.allnurses.com

Search for "Nurses Notes: Guidelines on what not to chart" then click on the link to that source. Identify three that you previously did not know.

REVIEW QUESTIONS

1. What are the main features of the Health Insurance Portability and Accountability Act of 1996 (HIPAA)?
2. What are five major purposes of medical documentation?
3. What are five characteristics of good medical documentation?
4. How should errors be corrected on medical records?
5. What information is typically found in a medical record?
6. What are three different formats used for progress notes?
7. What are the advantages and disadvantages of each progress note format?
8. What are two advantages and two disadvantages of an electronic health record (EHR)?
9. What is a personal health record (PHR) and why is it important for an individual to have one?

APPLICATION EXERCISES

1. Refer back to The Case of the Therapist Who Hates to Write.
    a. What are the possible consequences of the therapist's approach to charting?
    b. What characteristics of good charting is he not following?
2. Ms. Henrietta Jenkins, a nursing assistant at an ambulatory clinic, is helping Mr. Wilkins off of the examining table. Mr. Wilkins suddenly feels faint,

his legs give out from under him, and he falls to the floor. Ms. Jenkins notes that Mr. Wilkins never lost consciousness, but he is confused and asks where he is. She notes a 2- by 3-centimeter red mark on his forehead. His vital signs are B/P 100/60, T 98.6, P 92, R 20 (B/P, blood pressure; T, temperature; P, pulse; R, respirations). The physician examines Mr. Wilkins, finds no other injuries, and notes that he is no longer confused. Another set of vital signs are taken: B/P 124/80, P 78, R 18. Mr. Wilkins states he is feeling fine and leaves without further incident.

a. What would be documented using problem-oriented charting?
b. What would be documented using narrative charting?
c. What would be documented using charting by exception?
d. What additional information, if any, would be needed to complete the progress notes using each of the three charting formats?

PROBLEM-SOLVING PRACTICE

Katrina Cabrillo has always hated the idea of computers. She realizes that the Internet and email are useful for other people, but thinks they are not necessary for her job. Recently she learned that her facility will be computerizing its charting, and she is horrified. She is so anxious that she has difficulty sleeping at night. Using the five-step problem-solving process, determine what Katrina can do about the fact that her facility will have computerized charting within the next year.

SUGGESTED READINGS AND RESOURCES

Krager, D., & Krager, C. H. (2008). *HIPAA for health care professionals*. Clifton Park, NY: Delmar Cengage Learning.

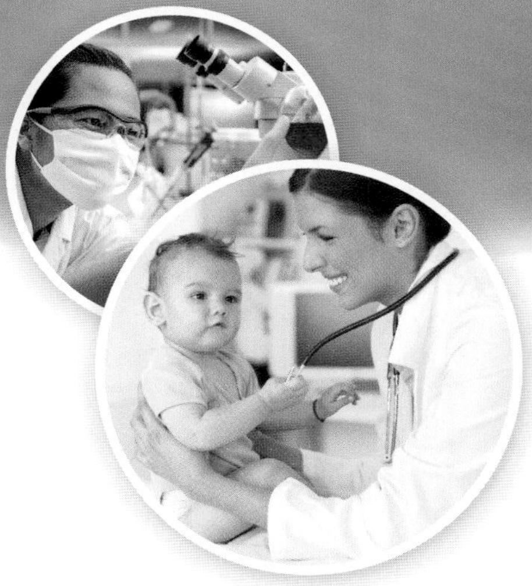

Unit 7

Health Care Skills

This page intentionally left blank

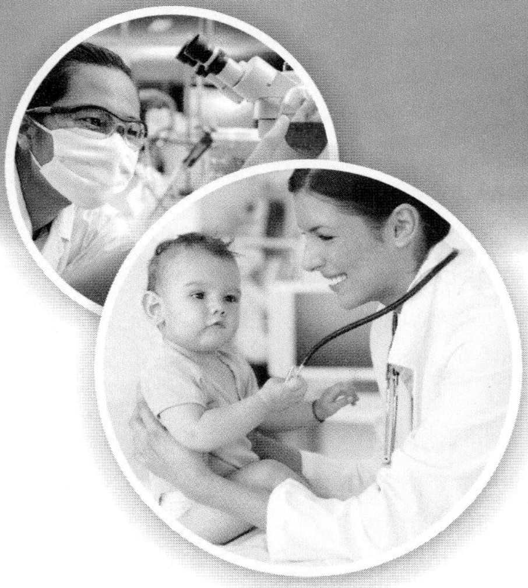

Chapter 20

Physical Assessment

OBJECTIVES

Studying and applying the material in this chapter will help you to:

- State the purpose of a history and physical (H&P) and indicate what data the provider will obtain.
- Discuss variances from normal for each of the body systems.
- Discuss the value of using a pain scale.
- Define what actions are included in the activities of daily living (ADLs).
- Correctly take the vital signs (temperature, pulse, respirations, and blood pressure).
- Describe how the presence of an apical-radial deficit is determined and what it means.
- Measure the height and weight of a patient.

KEY TERMS

afebrile
apnea
bradycardia
bradypnea
Cheyne-Stokes
dyspnea
eupnea
exhalation
febrile
hypertension
hypotension
inhalation
orthopnea
orthostatic (postural) hypotension
pulse deficit
pulse points
respiration
sphygmomanometer
stethoscope
tachycardia
tachypnea
vital signs

The Case of the Unreported Observations

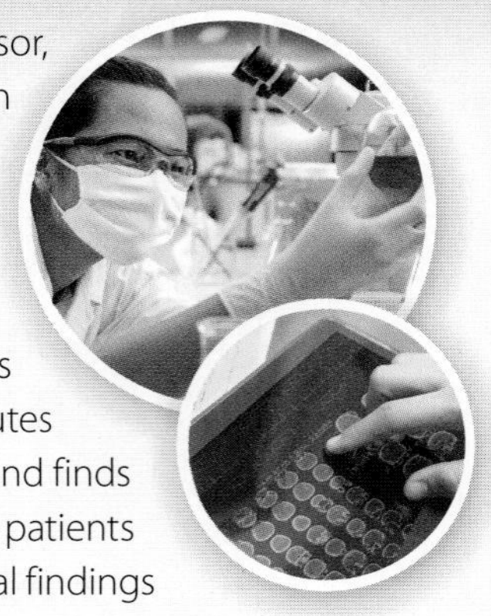

Mrs. Becker, age 83, arrives on time as usual for her appointment with Dr. Myers. Carrie Winsor, medical assistant, notes that Mrs. Becker seems unsteady as she walks across the room. When asked if she is all right, Mrs. Becker's answer is slightly garbled, but she states, "I must just be getting old." When Mrs. Becker speaks, Carrie notes a sweet, fruity smell that she thinks must be mouthwash. Carrie thinks Mrs. Becker seems depressed, but then thinks that she would be too if she had all the physical problems the patient has had with her diabetes, especially now that she has recently been diagnosed with renal failure and has started on dialysis. Dr. Myers is running behind with his appointments, and Carrie knows that it will be at least another 30 minutes and informs Mrs. Becker. Carrie continues with her other tasks, until she hears a sudden sound and finds Mrs. Becker on the floor and unconscious. This chapter will discuss how to objectively observe patients and how important it is for the health care professional to observe and promptly report abnormal findings to his or her supervisor so that early detection and treatment can be initiated.

GENERAL ASSESSMENT

The physician (or other primary care provider) takes a history and performs a physical exam on patients when they are seen for the first time or when they are admitted to the hospital. This is called the history and physical, commonly referred to as the H&P. As discussed in the previous chapter, the physician then either writes the findings in the patient's chart or enters them into the computer. If the facility is not computerized, the provider may have the option of dictating the notes for someone else to type up and place in the chart. When the typed information is placed in the chart, the physician must review it for accuracy and then sign the document.

An accurate and thorough H&P is very important, because it provides the data on which the physician bases the initial diagnosis and treatment. The H&P consists of the following information:

- Date: The day on which the H&P is actually done.
- Demographic data: Include age, sex, race, place of birth, marital status, occupation, and religion.
- Source of referral: Often one physician refers a patient to another because of that individual's expertise in a specific area; if so, it will be stated as such.
- Chief complaint(s): The primary problem from the patient's view—why the patient is seeking medical care.
- History of present illness: Includes when the problem first started; how frequently it occurs; how long it lasts; description, location, and severity of symptoms; if they are aggravated by any specific activities; if anything relieves the problem; if any treatments have been tried; and their effect on the symptoms.
- History: Includes the general state of the patient's health and any previous physical or psychological illnesses, accidents, injuries, surgeries, and hospitalizations.
- Current health status: Includes a list of allergies and immunizations; normal activity level and diet; current medications (prescription and over the counter); if tobacco, alcohol, or illegal drugs are used; if any environmental or safety hazards are present; and if there are any sleep pattern disturbances.
- Family history of illness: Includes the age and health or cause of death of parents, siblings, spouse, and children. The physician will also ask if any family members have or are experiencing similar symptoms. The family history of specific diseases or conditions is also included (e.g., diabetes, heart disease, high blood pressure, cancer).
- Psychosocial history: Includes the home situation and support structure (family and friends) and any significant information that may affect the care of the patient.
- Review of all systems: Includes height, weight, vital signs, and a review of each body system. When a complete physical assessment is done,

it is commonly referred to as a head-to-toe assessment, which indicates that all systems are being evaluated. It can also indicate a method that some health care professionals use to organize their assessment. The following survey is based on assessment of an adult patient. When working with children (pediatrics), the approach will vary depending on the child's age and condition (e.g., when assessing young children, it may be more appropriate to start with the feet instead of the head; also normal findings will vary based on the age of the child). After assessing orientation, the process would include an examination in the following order:

1. Head
2. Neck
3. Upper extremities
4. Chest (respiratory and cardiac systems)
5. Abdomen (digestive, urinary, and reproductive systems)
6. Lower extremities

The musculoskeletal, integumentary, nervous, endocrine, vascular, and lymphatic systems are relevant to the entire body and are assessed as one moves along the body.

The information obtained during the H&P is considered the *baseline*. The baseline information is important to determine how the patient is progressing in relationship to how he or she was at a particular point in time. It is important for the health care professional to review the H&P because this information will increase the understanding of the patient's condition.

Noting Variances from Normal

A critical function of the health care professional is to be able to discriminate between normal and abnormal conditions and situations. Learning to observe patients, their symptoms, and their actions and asking appropriate questions provide vital information that can be used by other health care professionals and the physician in the care of the patient.

The observational skills needed are based on a thorough understanding of normal anatomy and physiology. Once the meaning of normal is understood, it is an easy step to identify abnormal situations. A health care professional who observes an abnormal condition should immediately report the finding to his or her supervisor. Remember, though, that some patients begin with problems noted in the H&P. In this case, it is more valuable to compare a change in condition to this baseline.

Any change in a patient's condition may indicate a worsening of the condition, an improvement, a new problem developing, or a need for a change in treatment. The health care professionals who interact with and observe a patient over time may provide valuable information that the physician may not detect during relatively brief visits with the patient. It is for this reason that strong assessment skills are needed by all health care professionals whose responsibilities include interaction with patients.

Before continuing with the material presented in this chapter, it is important to note the distinction that is made when using the term *assessment* versus *observation* and *data collection. In the health care workplace, the term* assessment *is restricted to activities performed by licensed health care professionals. When unlicensed health care professionals ask questions and make observations, it is called* data collection. This distinction in no way negates the value of data collection. It is often the data collected by the unlicensed health care professional that guides licensed personnel to do further assessments.

General Survey

A problem with dividing the body into systems for the purpose of study is that health care professionals sometimes forget to look at the patient as a whole. To prevent this from happening, the health care professional should develop the habit of first performing a general survey of the patient. This means looking at and listening to the patient to secure an overall impression of presentation. It is important to note the normal findings in addition to the abnormal. How does the patient appear? What is the general impression you get from the patient? Another advantage of this approach is that it provides information about which area to focus on if time is limited. When doing a general survey, the health care professional should look for answers to the following questions:

- What is the overall impression of the patient? Does he or she appear strong and healthy looking or weak and ill?
- What is the posture? Is the patient walking normally with a straight and erect posture or is he or she stooped or limping? Is there paralysis present?

- Are there any signs of distress? Is the patient moving and communicating freely or is there difficulty breathing, face wincing in pain, sweating or trembling, or holding part of the body (hand over area or rubbing area on body may indicate pain)?
- What is the body proportion and size? Is the body proportionate and normal in size or is there a noted disproportion, such as very thin or obese, tall or short?
- What is the color of the skin? Is the skin normal in tone or pale, flushed (reddish), jaundiced (yellow), or cyanotic (gray, dusty, or blue)? In non-Caucasian patients, the nail beds, whites of the eyes, and mucous membranes should be examined for color changes.
- Are any odors noted from body or breath? For example, is there a sweet or fruity smell to the breath (may be untreated diabetic or severe restriction of food intake)? Alcohol breath?
- What is the character of speech? Does the patient speak clearly and normally or is speech hesitant, slurred, fast, or slow?
- What are the vital signs (temperature, pulse, respirations, and blood pressure)? During these procedures, which are discussed later in the chapter, you will be touching the patient's skin. This provides the opportunity to note the skin for temperature changes and moisture (warm, cold, dry, moist); shaking the patient's hand upon greeting also provides an opportunity to note the skin temperature and moisture.
- What is the height and weight? Has there been a recent gain or loss?
- What is the level of consciousness? When patients have a diminished level of consciousness, it is necessary to note the extent of the problem, so comparisons can be made that indicate whether the patient is getting better or worse. Areas to note are:
    - Orientation: What is their best verbal response? Are they oriented to time (can tell you what day it is and what time), place (can tell you where they are), and person (can state their name)? Are they confused, inappropriate, or incomprehensible, or is there no response?
    - If there is no verbal response, note whether the eyes open spontaneously, or perhaps only to speech or to pain, or there is no response.
    - What is their best motor response—do they obey commands, move only in response to pain, or is there no response?

Using appropriate communication skills is necessary when working with patients. How we communicate verbally and nonverbally often determines the quality of the response we get when interviewing patients. Refer back to Chapter 16 to review special communication skills.

Psychosocial Observations

When performing a general survey, both the physical and psychological aspects of the patient need to be considered. When incorporating a psychosocial status of patients, along with a general survey, the following questions can guide the health care professional:

- Emotional status: What are the emotional responses? For example, is the patient anxious, angry, depressed, indifferent? Are the facial expressions appropriate to what is being discussed?
- Mental status: Is the patient's behavior appropriate for his or her age? What is the attention span? Does the patient ask appropriate questions? Can the patient recall information and incorporate new information?
- Appearance: Is the patient dressed appropriately for the weather? Well groomed? Does the patient have good personal hygiene? (This may give clues on emotional status or ability to care for self.)

Physical Observations

Skills frequently used during physical assessment are inspection, palpation, percussion, and auscultation.

- Inspection: Using the senses of vision, hearing, and smell for observation of patient condition
- Auscultation: Listening to sounds inside the body with the aid of a stethoscope (e.g., lungs, heart, and bowel sounds)
- Palpation: Using the hands and fingers on the exterior of the body to detect evidence of abnormalities in the various internal body organs
- Percussion: Using the fingertips to lightly tap on the exterior of the body to determine position, size, and consistency of underlying structures

The preceding skills will be briefly introduced in the following sections as they relate to each of the systems presented earlier in Chapter 7. The health care professional should chart the normal and the abnormal findings, so a complete picture of the patient can be documented. Palpation and percussion of the body will not be covered, as these are more advanced skills. As health care students progress through their educational programs, additional and more advanced skills will be introduced that are specific to their specialties. Examples of advanced skills that may be performed by licensed health care professionals will be listed, but not expanded on, because they are beyond the scope of this text.

Musculoskeletal

- Is there any discomfort with movement (pain, muscle spasms, stiffness)?
- Is the gait (manner of walking) normal or altered? Observe the posture.
- Observe muscle strength: Can the patient turn in bed without assistance; does the patient complain of weakness; is walking done with or without assistance?

Examples of advanced skills are inspection of joints for any swelling or deformity, assessment of the range of motion (ROM) of joints in which discomfort is experienced, and assessment of the amount of counter-resistance (pulling against an examiner's pull) to a force that a patient can maintain.

Integumentary

- Status of skin: What is the color and temperature (warm or cold), hair distribution? Note whether dry or moist.
- Are there any cuts, scrapes, swelling, rashes, incisions, or bruises on the skin?

Circulatory

- What are the vital signs?
- What is the weight? Has there been a recent unexplained gain or loss of weight?
- Is there any pain in the extremities? Where does pain occur; how is pain relieved (resting, elevation, or placing extremity in dependent position); does it occur at night; how far can the patient walk before leg pain occurs (claudication distance)?
- Palpate peripheral pulses for quality and strength. (Pulse points are presented later in this chapter.)
- Inspect extremities for swelling.
- Observe capillary refill: Pinch the patient's fingertip and let go, then watch how long it takes for the nail bed to become pink again. The nail beds of patients with poor circulation to the extremities will take longer to return to a pink color. Use fingers/toes if nail beds are discolored or too thick to detect color changes.
- Inspect for neck vein distension: With the patient in erect or sitting position, inspect the neck for distension of the jugular veins; normally there is no distension of neck veins when in an erect position.
- Observe for activity intolerance: Does the patient report fatigue, palpitations (pounding felt in heart), or syncope (fainting) when engaging in any activities of daily living?

Examples of advanced skills include palpating the calf area for tenderness; using dorsiflexion (movement of the foot backward at the ankle) to check for pain in the calf, an indication of possible clots in the leg; auscultating breath and heart sounds, and using a Doppler probe if pulses are nonpalpable.

Respiratory

- What are the respiratory rate and rhythm?
- What colors are the skin and mucous membranes?
- Is there obvious difficulty with breathing? Is there any chest pain when breathing?
- Is there a cough? Productive (coughing up mucus) or nonproductive? If productive, what is the color (clear, white, yellow, green, red) and consistency (thin, thick, frothy) of the mucus?
- If the patient is experiencing difficulty breathing, when does this occur? Is there **dyspnea** (difficulty breathing) on exertion? Does the patient use accessory muscles to assist breathing (lifting shoulders on inspiration, retraction of abdominal muscles with respiration, flaring of nostrils)? Is the chest unusually large and rounded in shape? (This is called a barrel chest and may indicate an underlying chronic respiratory condition.)
- Check for cyanosis: Do the skin or nail beds appear cyanotic? The skin of a Caucasian patient who is receiving adequate oxygen is pink; in dark-skinned patients, a problem with

oxygenation is noted by looking at the nail beds, lips, and mucous membranes of the mouth.

- Does the patient have **orthopnea** (i.e., does the patient breathe easier in a sitting versus a standing position)?

Examples of advanced skills are auscultation and percussion of the lungs, determining if the chest expansion is symmetrical or asymmetrical, and determining which accessory muscles are used for breathing.

Digestive

- What is the size and contour of the abdomen? Is the abdomen round, flat, or distended? Soft or hard?
- Has there been a change in bowel pattern or color or consistency of stools?
- When was the last bowel movement?
- Is there any abdominal discomfort? How is it relieved? What aggravates it?
- Have there been any sudden changes in weight and appetite?

Examples of advanced skills are auscultation of bowel sounds in all four quadrants and palpating for tenderness and masses.

Urinary

- What is the appearance of the urine (clear or cloudy, yellow or some other color)?
- Is there any burning when the patient urinates? Any urgency (sudden, strong desire to urinate), hesitancy (having the urge to urinate but difficulty getting started), or frequency (urinating more often than normal)?
- Does the patient have nocturia (the need to get up during the night to urinate)? If so, how often?
- Is the patient ever incontinent (unable to retain urine)? If so, does it occur all the time or only when coughing, laughing, or sneezing?

Examples of advanced skills are palpation and percussion of the bladder.

Eyes and Ears

Eye

- Are there any complaints of discomfort in the eye (pain, foreign body sensation, itching or irritation, fatigue)?
- Are there any complaints of visual disturbances—floaters or spots, loss of vision, tunnel vision (loss of peripheral vision), flashes of light, halos around lights, blurred vision, diplopia (double vision), curtain or veil over visual field, difficulty with color discrimination, photophobia (hypersensitivity to light)?
- Is there redness, swelling, drainage, tearing, or squinting when attempting to read printed material, or crusting of eyelashes?

Examples of advanced skills include using an ophthalmoscope to examine the internal structures of the eye, examining the movement of eyeballs and eyelids, and assessing the reaction of pupils to light (see later section).

Ear

- Is there any drainage from the ear?
- What is the patient experiencing (e.g., feeling of fullness; unusual sounds, such as popping or cracking when yawning or swallowing; heart beating in ear; tinnitus [ringing in the ears])? If a child is having discomfort in the ear, he or she is most likely to demonstrate it by rubbing the ear and crying.
- Does the patient use a hearing aid? Does the patient have a cochlear implant? The cochlear implant is an electronic device that can help provide a sense of sound to a person who is profoundly deaf or severely hard of hearing. The implant consists of an external portion that sits behind the ear and a second portion that is surgically placed under the skin.
- Hearing acuity: Is there difficulty hearing in one ear or both? Does the patient show behaviors consistent with diminished hearing, such as turning the head and leaning closer when spoken to or frequently asking for statements to be repeated? Many patients compensate for a hearing loss by reading the lips of the speaker. To prevent this from disguising hearing loss, the health care professional can speak while standing behind the patient or when the patient's back is turned.

Examples of advanced skills include using an otoscope to look inside the ear canal to examine the internal structures and conducting various hearing tests.

Nervous

- Is there any numbness or tingling?
- Many types of abnormal data already discussed may indicate a neurological problem, such as changes in skin temperature or color, impairment of mobility, and problems with emotional or mental status.

Examples of advanced skills are testing the reflexes, conducting a neurological exam to determine the strength and movement of extremities, and cranial nerve testing. Another commonly used assessment technique is to test the response of the pupil to light. Normally, the pupils are equal in size and shape and constrict symmetrically when exposed to a light source. Variances from this normal response may indicate neurological damage.

Endocrine

The endocrine system has such wide-ranging effects on the body that no additional questions are listed here. The most common problems with the endocrine system (i.e., diabetes and thyroid disorders) are usually identified in the evaluation of the other systems.

Female Reproductive

- Does patient menstruate? If so, how often, how long, and are there any problems related to this? When did menses (menarche) begin?
- Is there any pain, discharge, itching, or discomfort with the vagina or genitalia? Any lumps in the breasts or discharge from the nipples?
- Has the patient undergone any surgeries, such as hysterectomy (removal of uterus), oophorectomy (removal of ovary), mastectomy (removal of breast), or cesarean section (surgical delivery of the baby through an abdominal incision)?

Male Reproductive

- Is there any discharge from or are sores noted on the penis?

Pain Evaluation

Pain is subjective, and there is no test to confirm it in an objective manner. The best approach is to use a pain rating scale. Most facilities use this approach, and it helps to make the patient's level of pain easier to compare. The patient is asked to rate his or her pain on a scale of 0 to 10. Zero is no pain, and 10 is the worst

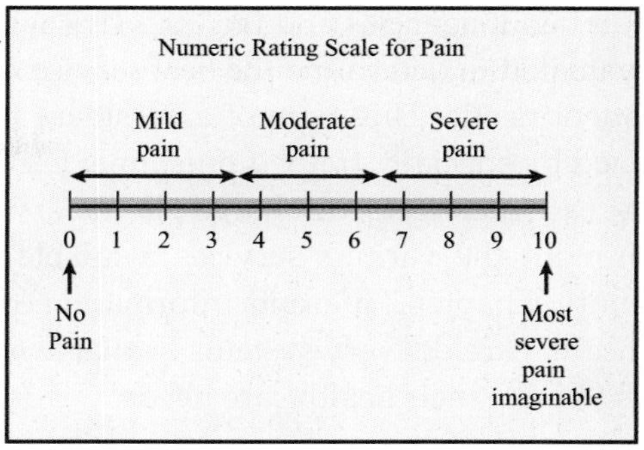

FIGURE 20–1 Visual analog scale for rating pain.

pain the patient can imagine. (See Figure 20–1.) Each time a pain rating is done, the same scale is used. For example, if a patient reports pain to be 7 and then, after pain medication, reports it has dropped to 2, this is a good indication of the effectiveness of the medication. But if it has only dropped to a 5 or 6, this would indicate that the pain medication regimen needs to be reevaluated. It is also important to note any nonverbal cues that may indicate pain, such as limping, favoring an area, moaning, restlessness, and wincing.

If the patient is cognitively unable to rate his or her pain using a numeric scale, there are several visual representations that can be used. Refer to www.oucher.org and http://wongbakerfaces.org to view two such options. This is especially helpful for young patients (3 years or older) to communicate how much pain they are having as they can point to the face that best describes how they are feeling.

ADL Evaluation

Activities of daily living (ADLs) are the actions done on a regular basis to meet physical needs. These include bathing, eating, toileting, shopping, doing laundry, cleaning the house, paying bills, dressing, turning in bed, getting out of bed, and ambulating (walking). Conditions that affect the ability to perform ADLs may be temporary or permanent. For example, patients recovering from a recent surgery may temporarily not be strong enough to care for themselves, but a patient with a major and permanent spinal cord injury will never regain full function.

There are many diseases and conditions that diminish the patient's ability to perform these activities. When a patient is unable to perform his or her basic ADLs, help must be arranged. Family and friends are often able to assist, but if this is not possible, there are a number of agencies and facilities that will need to be evaluated to determine the best service for specific patient needs. This type of assessment is often performed by specially trained personnel (e.g., social workers, case managers, discharge planners) who are familiar with the various services available in the community. Chapter 2 presents information on some of the health care delivery systems available to assist patients to meet their health care needs.

VITAL SIGNS

The term **vital signs** refers to taking a patient's temperature, pulse, respiratory rate, and blood pressure. (See Table 20–1.) Taking the vital signs provides important information on the status of the patient. When referring to the temperature, pulse, and respiratory rate of a patient, it is common to use the abbreviation TPR. The abbreviation for blood pressure is B/P.

Vital signs have normal ranges. Readings that fall below or above normal may indicate a problem that needs further assessment. Comparing new readings with previous readings can provide information about whether the patient is improving or not. It is necessary to follow specific procedures to obtain accurate results; however, be aware that the procedures as outlined in this chapter may vary somewhat in different clinical settings. Never estimate or assume that the readings are the same as before, because inaccurate results can cause the wrong health care decisions to be made, which can jeopardize the patient's health.

Temperature

The body functions to maintain its temperature within a range that is best for maintaining homeostasis. If the body gets too warm, it will feel hot, begin to sweat, and cause a sense of thirst to be experienced. Sweating is a normal cooling system of the body. The intake of fluids assists in the sweating process, as well as in the replacement of lost fluids. If the body gets too cool, the skin will feel cool, and shivering will start as a way to increase metabolism through muscular activity. The normal average temperature varies with the route used to obtain the temperature. Readings obtained from the oral (mouth) and aural (ear) routes have the same range, but those from the rectal and temporal artery routes normally run a degree higher, and the axillary (under the arm) runs a degree lower. (See Procedure 20–1.) Other factors that affect the temperature are age of the patient (temperature control in younger patients is less stable and normal readings run higher than in adulthood), time of day (early morning readings are typically the lowest), and pregnancy (readings are higher). The temperature also varies depending on the temperature of the room, amount of clothes being worn, and number of blankets used while in bed. There are also normal variations among patients. Always refer to the patient's chart to review prior readings for comparison.

Electronic, tympanic (aural), chemical-dot, and temporal artery (infrared technology) are different types of thermometers available today. (See Figures 20–2a–d.) An *electronic thermometer* and *tympanic thermometer* will have a disposable plastic probe that is placed on the thermometer prior to use and discarded after each use. The temporal artery thermometer is rolled across the forehead and can be cleaned with alcohol between uses. There is also an infrared thermometer that does not require contact with the skin. It is swiped across the forehead and the reading appears within a second. Follow the manufacturer's instructions for the proper use, care, and

Table 20–1 Vital Signs

Procedure	Purpose	Page
Temperature	Measures how much heat is in the body. An elevation may indicate that an infection or other disease process is present	420
Radial Pulse	Measures how fast the heart is beating when felt at the wrist	426–427
Apical Pulse	Measures how fast the heart is beating by listening over the heart with a stethoscope	428
Respirations	Measures how fast the patient is breathing	430
Blood Pressure	Indicates how hard the heart is working to distribute blood to all parts of the body	433–434

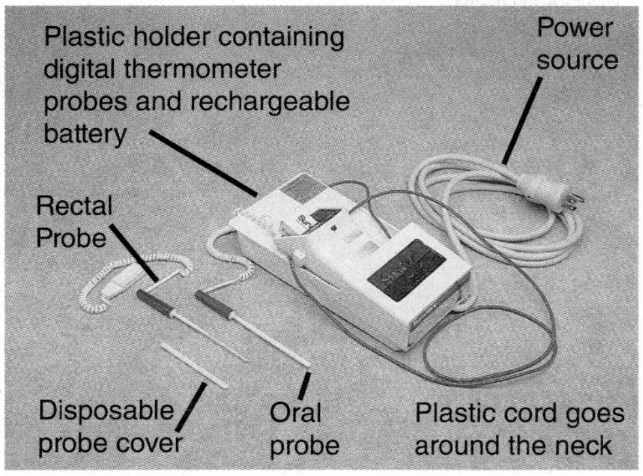

FIGURE 20–2a Electronic thermometers have a plastic probe that is placed on the thermometer and discarded after use. The temperature is read on a digital display.

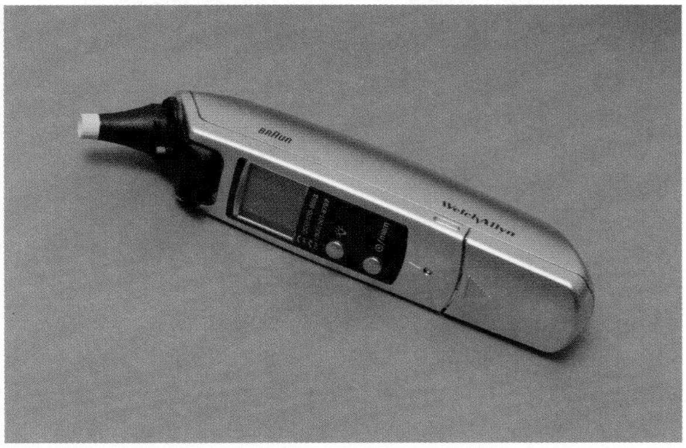

FIGURE 20–2b Thermo-scan tympanic thermometer.

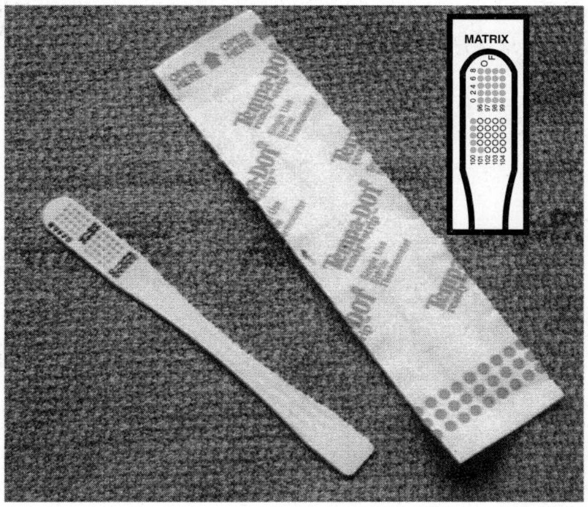

FIGURE 20–2c Chemical-dot thermometers change color in response to the temperature of the body.

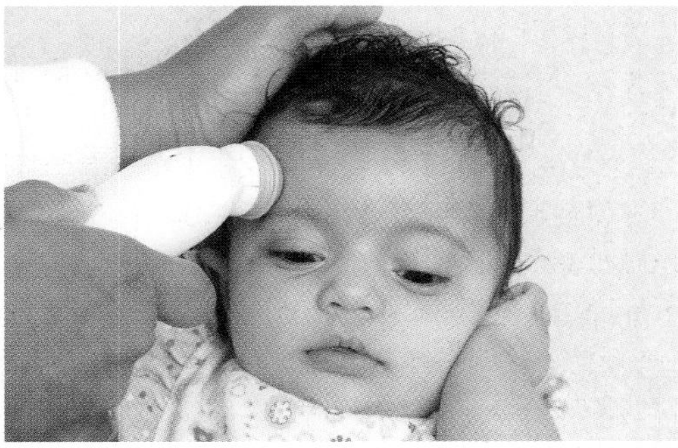

FIGURE 20–2d Temporal artery thermometer is used by sliding it across the forehead. The temperature is read on a digital display.

PROCEDURE 20–1

How to Take a Temperature

Always Observe Standard Precautions

ROUTE

Oral

Normal Range (Adult)

97.6°F–99.6°F (36.5°C–37.5°C)

Procedure

1. You will need a clean electronic thermometer with oral probe and something to record the results on.

   Precautions: Do not use this route if the patient is a mouth breather; is unable to keep mouth closed around the thermometer; has had surgery or an injury to nose or mouth; is confused, unconscious, prone to seizures, has oxygen or a nasogastric tube; is too young; or is for any other reason unable or unwilling to follow directions.

2. Verify that the patient has not taken any food or fluid by mouth, smoked, or chewed gum in the last 30 minutes.

   Precautions: This will result in an inaccurate reading.

3. Clean with alcohol and when dry, apply temperature probe sheath.

4. Ask the patient to open mouth.

(continues)

PROCEDURE 20–1

How to Take a Temperature

(continued)

5. Place thermometer under the tongue on either side, as close to the midline as possible.

   Precautions: The thermometer must be placed close to the fleshy area where the tongue attaches in order to get an accurate reading. If it is placed too far to either side, it may result in an inaccurate reading (low).
6. Instruct patient to close lips around thermometer but not to bite down on it.
7. Leave it in place until unit signals a final reading (see manufacturer's instructions).
8. Remove thermometer and read digital display.
9. Immediately record your findings.
10. Remove temperature probe sheath and dispose of properly. Clean thermometer with alcohol.

ROUTE

Axillary

Normal Range (Adult)

96.6°F–98.6°F (36°C–37°C)

Procedure

1. You will need a clean electronic thermometer, with oral probe and something to record the results on.

   Precautions: This is the least accurate method, but is often used when the oral route is not appropriate and an aural thermometer is not available.
2. Clean with alcohol and when dry, apply temperature probe sheaf.
3. Remove clothing from patient's shoulder and arm.
4. Ensure that axillary area is dry, wiping with dry towel if necessary.

   Precautions: Moisture can cause an inaccurate reading.
5. Place thermometer in the center of the armpit and place arm across the abdomen and close to side of body.

   (See Figure 20–3.)

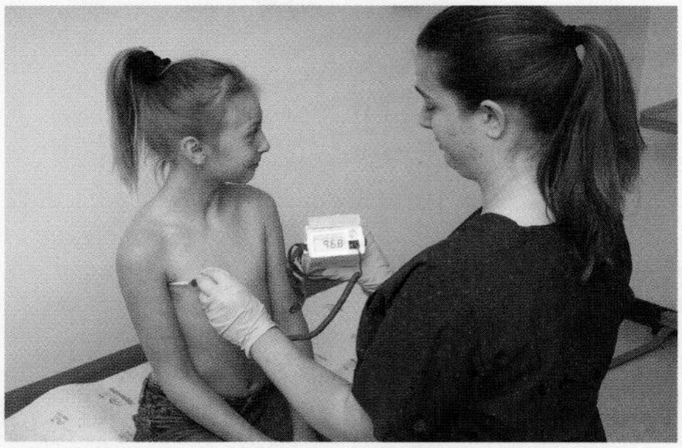

FIGURE 20–3 To take an axillary temperature, place the bulb of the thermometer into the center of the armpit and hold arm close to body.

6. Leave it in place until unit signals a final reading (see manufacturer's instructions).
7. Remove thermometer, read the digital display.
8. Immediately record your findings.
9. Remove temperature probe sheath and dispose of properly. Clean thermometer with alcohol.

ROUTE

Rectal

Normal Range (Adult)

98.6°F–100.6°F 37°C–38°C

Procedure

1. You will need an electronic thermometer with rectal probe (used only for rectal temperatures) and something to record the results on.

   Precautions: The rectal route is often inappropriate for infants and young children. Policies regarding its use vary among facilities.
2. Clean with alcohol and when dry, apply temperature probe sheaf.

   Precautions: Do not use this method if patient has diarrhea, has had recent surgery or injury to the rectum or prostate, or has had a recent myocardial infarct (heart attack).

(continues)

PROCEDURE 20–1

How to Take a Temperature

(continued)

3. Ensure that adults are in a side-lying position with top leg flexed forward.
4. Lubricate thermometer.
5. Insert thermometer into the rectum (1 inch for children, and 1½ inches for adults).

   Precautions: Never force the thermometer into the colon.
6. Leave it in place until unit signals a final reading (see manufacturer's instructions).
7. Hold tip of thermometer while in place.

   Precautions: The thermometer must be held in place to prevent damage to rectal tissue or loss of thermometer into rectum.
8. Remove thermometer and read digital display.
9. Immediately record your findings.
10. Remove temperature probe sheath and dispose of properly. Clean thermometer with alcohol.

ROUTE

Aural (Tympanic)

Normal Range (Adult)

97.6°F–99.6°F 36.5°C–37.5°C

Procedure

1. You will need an aural thermometer and something to record the results on.
2. Place disposable probe on the thermometer.

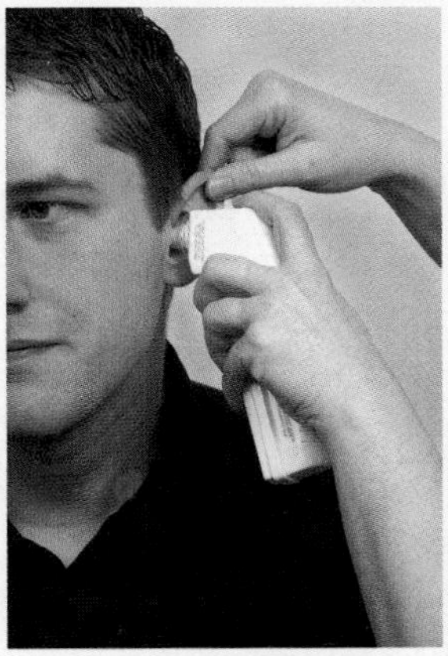

FIGURE 20–4 Taking a patient's temperature with a tympanic (aural) thermometer.

   Precautions: Follow manufacturer's instructions.
3. Stabilize the patient's head.
4. In children younger than 1 year, gently pull the ear straight back; in children older than 1 year and adults, pull the ear back and up.
5. Insert probe into ear canal until you obtain seal. (See Figure 20–4.)
6. Press scan button. (Results are obtained within seconds.)
7. Immediately record results.
8. Properly dispose of probe.

ROUTE

Temporal Artery (Infrared)

Normal Range (Adult)

98.6°F–100.6°F 37°C–38°C

Procedure

1. You will need a temporal artery thermometer, alcohol wipes, and something to record the results on. Clean thermometer with alcohol and let dry before using.

   Precautions: Considered very accurate. Other sites that can be used are the femoral, axillary, and behind the ear; check manufacturer's directions regarding any restrictions.
2. Remove perspiration from forehead, remove hat, push back hair from forehead.

   Precautions: Moisture (perspiration) on the forehead causes cooling, which results in inaccurate results. Hair or hat on the forehead can raise the temperature and cause inaccurate results.
3. Center probe on the forehead (midline), press scan button and slowly move it across forehead to the temple area hair line.

   Precautions: Moving it too quickly can result in inaccurate results.
4. Immediately record results.
5. Clean probe with alcohol wipe, let dry, and return to holder.

   Precautions: Must be dry to work effectively.

cleaning of this equipment. When using *chemical-dot thermometers,* do not remove them from their protective covers in advance because they will begin to react to the room temperature. Be sure to follow directions supplied by the manufacturer. Always remember to follow standard precautions and facility policies regarding cleaning of equipment when working with patients.

Note: Glass mercury thermometers are not used in health care settings. They have been phased out due to concerns about mercury toxicity. Encourage your patients to switch to electronic thermometers for home use as there are a number of reliable, inexpensive brands on the market. Inform the patient that disposal of their mercury thermometers requires special handling and they should contact a hazardous waste collection facility for instructions. If they improperly dispose of products containing mercury, they may break and release mercury vapors. These vapors are harmful to their health and the environment.

When temperature is within the normal range, patients are said to be **afebrile**. When it is elevated above the normal range, they are **febrile**. An *intermittent fever* means that the temperature rises and falls. It can become elevated and then return to normal or even below normal. A *continuous fever* stays elevated over a prolonged period.

Media Link

Learn more about how to take a temperature using chemical-dot, digital, and tympanic thermometers by viewing the Thermometers, Digital/ Electronic Thermometers, and Tympanic Thermometers videos on the Online Resources. The videos show a medical assistant (MA) in an office setting demonstrating the proper technique.

A fever is a defense mechanism against microorganisms. In an effort to kill the invading microorganisms, the body triggers the muscles to shiver, which increases metabolic activity and further increases the temperature. When the febrile episode subsides, it is accompanied by profuse sweating that acts as a cooling mechanism. When the sweating episodes occur at night, they are called night sweats. It is common for intermittent fevers to occur at night.

Thinking It Through

Mr. Hulchanski calls the physician's office and speaks with Becky Smith, the medical assistant. Mr. Hulchanski has had recent surgery and was instructed to call the office in one week to report how he is doing. Mr. Hulchanski reports that he is feeling fine and that the surgical incision looks like it is healing well. He says the only thing that he has noticed is that when he awakens in the morning, his pajamas and linens are soaked. Becky asks if he has been running a fever, and he states that he has routinely taken his temperature several times during the day and it has been normal. In fact, he states that he is sure he is not having a fever because he actually feels chilled at times. Becky states that she is glad to hear that he is doing so well and to call back if any problems develop.

1. Becky documents "patient reports he is doing well and will call back if any problems develop." Is this the correct note to make in the chart? Why or why not?
2. Did Mr. Hulchanski report any variances from the norm?
3. What could possibly be happening to Mr. Hulchanski?

If the health care professional notes signs that may indicate that the temperature is rising, such as that the body feels warmer than normal to the touch or the patient is shivering, he or she should take the patient's temperature at this time. If the patient is sweating profusely, it means that the fever has broken and is coming back down to a lower temperature.

Pulse

When the heart contracts and forces blood out of the heart and into the arteries, it creates a pulsing sensation that can be felt by the health care professional at certain points in the body. There are a number of locations where an artery comes close enough to the surface of the skin and where it passes over a firm surface (e.g., bone) that it can be felt. (See Figure 20–5.) These major **pulse points** are as follows:

- Temporal: Located on either side of the forehead.
- Carotid: Located on the front side of the neck on either side of the trachea (never massage this

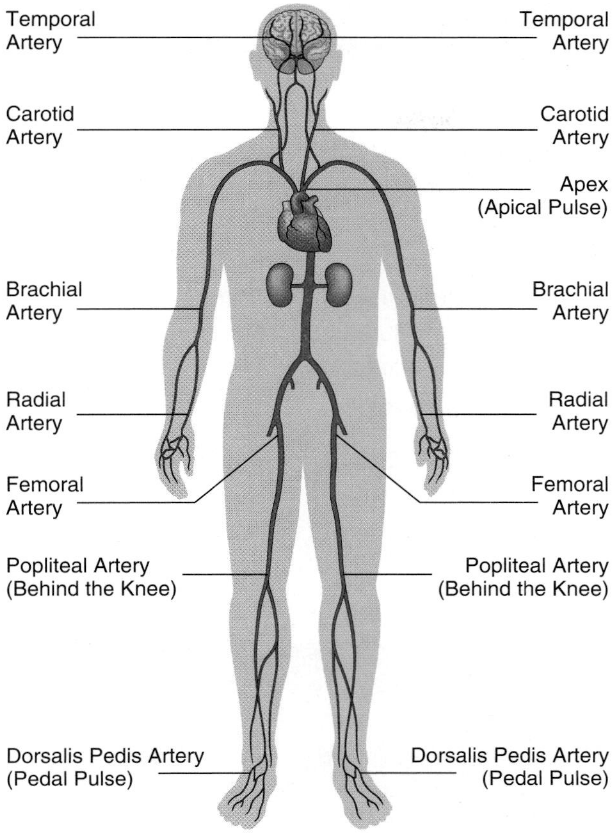

FIGURE 20–5 Location of pulse points that can be felt on the body.

area or compress both carotids at the same time when taking a pulse; massages can trigger a sudden slowing of the heart rate, and compressing both carotids can decrease the blood flow to the brain).

- Brachial: Located in the inner side of the antecubital space (crease created when elbow is bent)
- Radial: Located in the wrist (thumb side); most commonly used site
- Femoral: Located in the inner aspect of the crease where the upper thigh joins the trunk of the body
- Popliteal: Located behind the knee
- Dorsalis pedis: Located on top of the foot arch

When taking a pulse (Procedure 20–2), three observations are made:

1. Rate: The rate is the number of beats that occurs in 1 minute.
2. Rhythm: When the beats occur at even intervals, it is called a *regular rhythm*. If they do not occur at regular intervals, it is called an *irregular rhythm*. It is also possible to have a recurring pattern with an irregular rhythm. For example, there may be a beat missed every two beats, and this happens consistently. This pattern is called

PROCEDURE 20–2

How to Take a Radial Pulse

Always Observe Standard Precautions

STEPS	RATIONALE
1. You will need a watch with a second hand and something to record the results on.	As a health care professional, you should at all times have a watch with a second hand, a pen, and notepaper with you. A water-resistant watch with a large face for ease in reading is recommended.
2. Locate the radial pulse by gently but firmly pressing on the thumb side of the wrist until an indented area is felt. This is where the pulse is located. Use two or three fingers to feel the pulse. (See Figure 20–6.)	The health care professional always uses the fingers and never the thumb in taking a patient's pulse. The thumb has a pulse of its own, and if the thumb is used, the worker's own pulse may be mistaken for the patient's.
3. Place the patient's hand on his or her chest. (See Figure 20–7.)	This makes it easier to count the respirations after the pulse is taken because the health care professional can feel the rise and fall of the chest.

(continues)

PROCEDURE 20–2

How to Take a Radial Pulse

(continued)

STEPS	RATIONALE
4. Count the pulsations you feel in a 60-second period.	Counting the heart rate for a full minute increases the accuracy of the result. If the pulse is strong, regular, and within the normal range, you can count the pulsations for 30 seconds and multiply times two for the 1-minute reading.
5. When you complete the procedure, leave your fingers on the pulse, and count the respirations.	See Procedure 20–4.
6. Immediately record your findings.	Getting in the habit of writing down the actual numbers, instead of relying on your memory, will prevent errors.

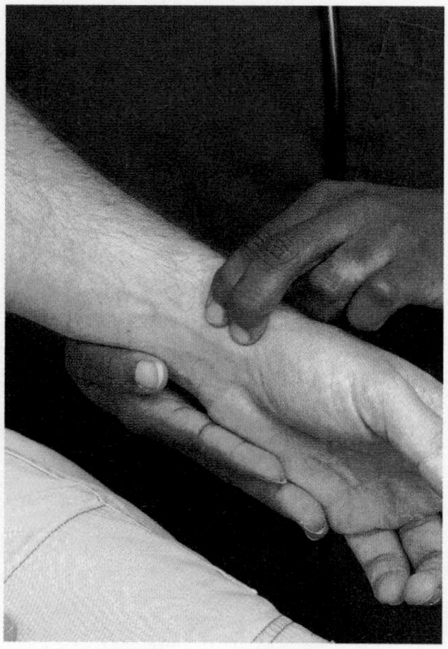

FIGURE 20–6 To take a radial pulse, place two or three fingers in an indented area on the thumb side of the wrist.

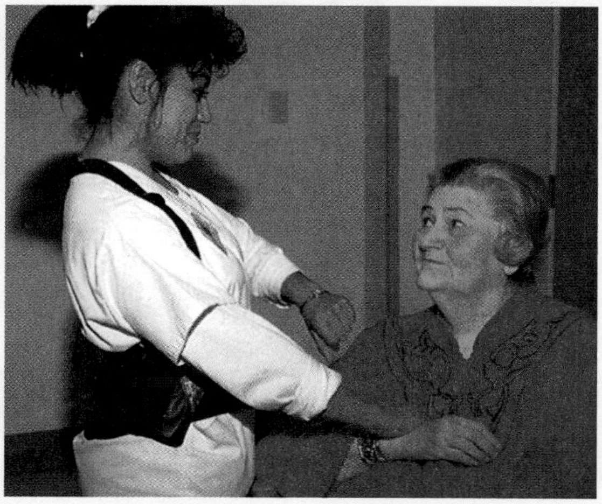

FIGURE 20–7 Positioning the patient's hand over the chest makes it easier to count the respirations without the patient's awareness.

a *regular irregular rhythm*. If there is no pattern to the irregular rhythm, then it is called an *irregular irregular rhythm*.

3. Pulse volume (strength of the beat): This describes the character of the beat. It may be described as weak, strong, thready (very fine and scarcely perceptible), or bounding (higher intensity than normal, then disappears quickly).

Another method for taking the pulse is to take an *apical pulse*. This method requires the use of a stethoscope. (See Figure 20–8.) A **stethoscope** is an instrument that amplifies sound and allows a health care professional to hear sounds from within the body. The stethoscope is placed over the apex of the heart, and the beats are counted as they are heard. The sound heard through the stethoscope as "lub-dub"

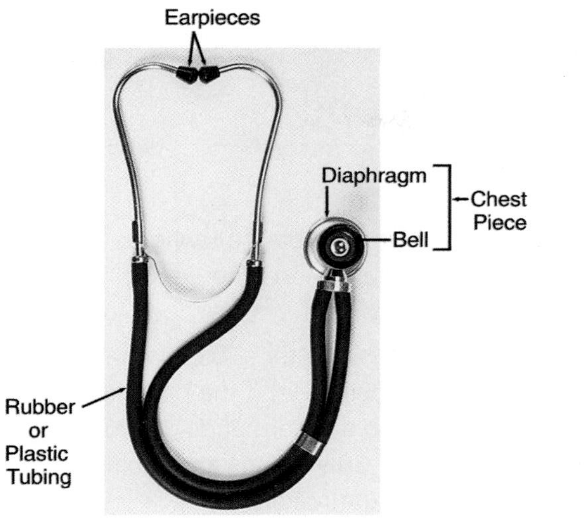

FIGURE 20–8 The parts of a stethoscope.

represents one beat. (See Procedure 20–3.) The "lub-dub" actually includes the sounds of the various valves opening and closing as the blood flows through the heart's chambers. Sometimes the physician will order an apical pulse, but often this is not specified and the choice of pulse point is left up to the judgment of the health care professional. An apical pulse should be obtained when there is an irregular rate, on cardiac patients, when the radial pulse is difficult to palpate, and with infants and young children.

When the pulse rate is abnormally low, it is called **bradycardia**. For example, in an adult patient, a rate of less than 60 beats per minute would be called bradycardia. When the pulse rate is abnormally high, it is called **tachycardia**. For example, in an adult patient, a rate of more than 100 beats per minute would be

PROCEDURE 20–3

How to Take an Apical Pulse Using a Stethoscope

Always Observe Standard Precautions

STEPS	RATIONALE
1. You will need a stethoscope, a watch with a second hand, and something to record the results on.	As a health care professional, you should at all times have a watch with a second hand, a pen, and notepaper with you. A water-resistant watch with a large face for ease in reading is recommended.
2. Wipe the earpieces and diaphragm of stethoscope with alcohol wipes, and inspect the stethoscope prior to use.	If the earpieces have wax in them, remove wax prior to use, so the sound will not be diminished; do not use a stethoscope that has cracks or tears in the tubing because it may lead to inaccurate results.
3. Verify that the diaphragm side is where the sound will be heard.	The end of the stethoscope can be turned to switch between the diaphragm (high pitch) and the bell (low pitch) side (refer back to Figure 20–7); some stethoscopes have only a diaphragm, then no adjustment is needed.
4. If the diaphragm is cold to the touch, rub it against your clothing or hand until it is warm.	A cold instrument placed on the skin creates a very uncomfortable sensation for the patient.
5. Place earpieces into your ears, with the earpieces pointing forward.	This directs the sound into the ear canal at the correct angle.
6. Place the diaphragm of the stethoscope directly on the skin, over the apex of the heart, and hold it with gentle but firm pressure.	If placed over clothing, sounds caused by the stethoscope rubbing on the clothing may be misinterpreted as beats.

(continues)

PROCEDURE 20–3

How to Take an Apical Pulse Using a Stethoscope

(continued)

STEPS	RATIONALE
7. Instruct the patient to breathe normally.	The patient may think you are trying to listen to their lungs and start to breathe deeply, which can alter the heart rate.
8. Count the beats you hear in a 60-second period.	Counting the heart rate for a full minute increases the accuracy of the result. If the pulse is strong, regular, and within the normal range, you can count the pulsations for 30 seconds and multiply times two for the 1-minute reading.
9. When you are done, leave the stethoscope in place and count the respirations.	See Procedure 20–4.
10. Immediately record your findings.	Getting in the habit of writing down the actual numbers, instead of relying on your memory, will prevent errors.

called tachycardia. The pulse rate is affected by many factors, including the age of the patient (Table 20–2), certain medications and disease conditions, physical activity, fever, and pregnancy.

Another procedure that the health care professional may be asked to assist with is a pulse deficit assessment check. This requires two health care professionals. One will take the pulse at one of the pulse points (usually radial), and the other will simultaneously take the apical pulse. (See Figure 20–9.) This is always taken for a full minute and must be coordinated to start and stop at the same time. If there is a difference between the two readings, it is called the **pulse deficit**. For example, if the apical rate is 100 and the radial is 80, the apical–radial pulse deficit is

Table 20–2 Pulse Rates at Various Ages

Age	Average Pulse	Normal Range
Newborn	140	120–160
Infant	110	80–140
Toddler	105	80–130
Preschool Child	100	74–120
School-Age Child	95	70–110
Adolescent–Adult	80	60–90

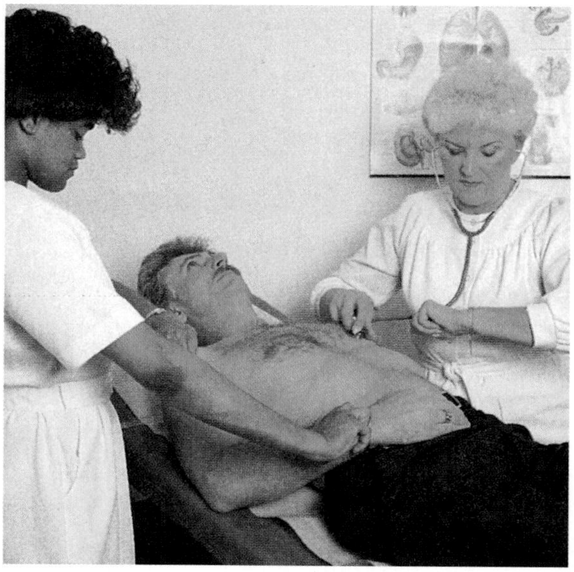

FIGURE 20–9 To determine a pulse deficit, one person counts the apical pulse while a second person counts the radial pulse.

20 beats. The deficit represents the number of cardiac beats that do not reach the radial artery. Normally, there should be no pulse deficit.

An apical–radial deficit can be present in a number of cardiac conditions. For example, the heart may not contract with enough force for a pulse to reach the extremity, or the heart may be beating so rapidly that not enough blood can enter the heart on each beat. When doing an apical–radial pulse reading, the reading will be the same or the apical will be higher. It is not possible to get a radial pulse reading that is higher than the apical reading.

Media Link

Learn more about how to take apical, radial, and apical–radial pulses by viewing the TPR and BP, Radial Pulse, and Apical Pulse videos on the Online Resources. The videos show a medical assistant (MA) in an office setting demonstrating the proper technique.

Respirations

Respiration refers to the process of moving air into and out of the lungs. When air is taken into the lungs it is called **inhalation** (inspiration), and there is a corresponding expansion of the chest as the lungs fill. When the air is expelled back out of the lungs, it is called **exhalation** (expiration), and there is a corresponding deflation of the chest cavity as the lungs empty. One full cycle (inhalation and exhalation) is called one respiration. Normal breathing is called **eupnea** and should be within the normal range, unlabored, and have an even rhythm. If the respiratory rate is above the normal range, it is called **tachypnea**, and if below normal it is **bradypnea**.

Three observations are made when taking the respiratory rate (Procedure 20–4):

1. Rate: This is the number of respiratory cycles that occur in 1 minute.
2. Rhythm: Both the respirations and the intervals between them should be evenly spaced; when there is a temporary absence of respirations, it

PROCEDURE 20–4

How to Count Respirations

Always Observe Standard Precautions

STEPS	RATIONALE
1. You will need a watch with a second hand and something to record the results on.	As a health care professional, you should at all times have a watch with a second hand, a pen, and notepaper with you. A water-resistant watch with a large face for ease in reading is recommended.
2. After you finish counting the pulse, leave your fingers in position (if taking the radial pulse) or keep the stethoscope on the chest (if taking the apical pulse), and count the respirations.	Because the respiratory rate can be consciously altered, it is important that the patient not know when you are counting the respirations. Do not tell the patient that you are now counting the respirations, or the rate may not be accurate. The health care professional can also feel the chest rise and fall by leaving the arm on the chest or the stethoscope in place.
3. Count the number of respirations taken in 1 full minute.	One respiration is a complete cycle that includes inhalation and exhalation.
4. Immediately record your findings.	Getting in the habit of writing down the actual numbers, instead of relying on your memory, will prevent errors.

Table 20–3 Respiratory Rates at Various Ages

Age	Normal Range
Infant	30–60
Toddler	20–40
Preschool Child	22–34
School-Age Child	18–24
Adolescent–Adult	16–20

is called **apnea**, and the length of the interval should be timed. Report any periods of apnea to your supervisor. **Cheyne-Stokes** is a particular breathing pattern with a period of apnea that can last for 10 to 60 seconds, which is then followed by a gradually increasing depth and frequency of respirations.

3. Respiratory effort: Breathing should occur through the nose, be unlabored, and be without sound; report to your supervisor if you note that the patient shows extra effort during breathing or if any sounds are heard (e.g., wheezing, gurgling, or other sounds). Also note the depth of the breathing, such as shallow, normal, or deep.

Many factors can affect the respiratory rate, but if the rate is outside the normal range, has an irregular rhythm, or is labored, report it to your supervisor. Factors that can affect the rate are age (Table 20–3), illness, drugs, exercise, and emotions. Because the respiratory rate can be consciously altered, it is important that the patient not know when you are counting the respirations. The best approach is to place the patient's arm across his or her chest to take the pulse and then, when completed, leave your fingers on the radial pulse while counting the respirations. This is also an appropriate time to note the color of the nail beds. They should be pink; if they are cyanotic, report this to the supervisor immediately.

Media Link

Learn more about how to take a respiratory rate by viewing the Respiration video on the Online Resources. The videos show a medical assistant (MA) in an office setting demonstrating the proper technique.

Blood Pressure

Blood pressure (B/P) is written as two numbers separated by a slash—for example, 120/80 or 140/90. The first number is referred to as the *systolic pressure* and is the highest pressure in the cardiovascular system. The second number is the *diastolic pressure* and is the lowest pressure in the cardiovascular system. (See Table 20–4 for a definition of adult blood pressure categories.) If the patient's reading falls below normal, it is called **hypotension**. If the reading is above normal, it is called **hypertension**.

Another way of correlating the reading of the B/P is to think of a normal cardiac cycle. As previously described, when listening to the heartbeat, the examiner hears a "lub-dub" sound. The "lub" sound occurs as the heart chambers are contracting at their maximum force to push the blood out of the heart and into the arteries. This is the systolic phase of the heart. The "dub" sound is when the heart relaxes and is refilling with blood. This is the diastolic phase of the heart.

Two pieces of equipment are needed to take a manual blood pressure: a stethoscope and a sphygmomanometer. A **sphygmomanometer** is an instrument that records the blood pressure in millimeters (mm) of mercury (Hg). The health care professional may encounter different types of recording devices.

Table 20–4 Blood Pressure Categories for Adults (18 Years of Age or Older)

Category	Systolic (Top Number)	Diastolic (Bottom Number)
Normal	Less than 120	Less than 80
Pre-hypertension	120–139	80–89
Hypertension (High Blood Pressure)		
Stage 1	140–159	90–99
Stage 2	160 or higher	100 or higher
Hypertensive Crisis	Higher than 180	Higher than 110

Source: www.heart.org.

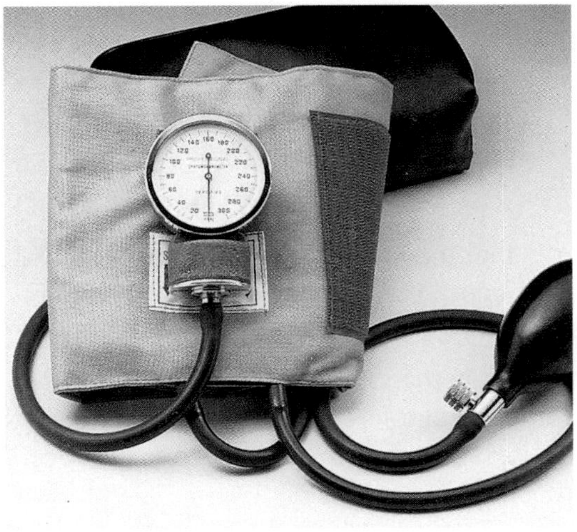

FIGURE 20–10a Dial (aneroid) sphygmomanometer.

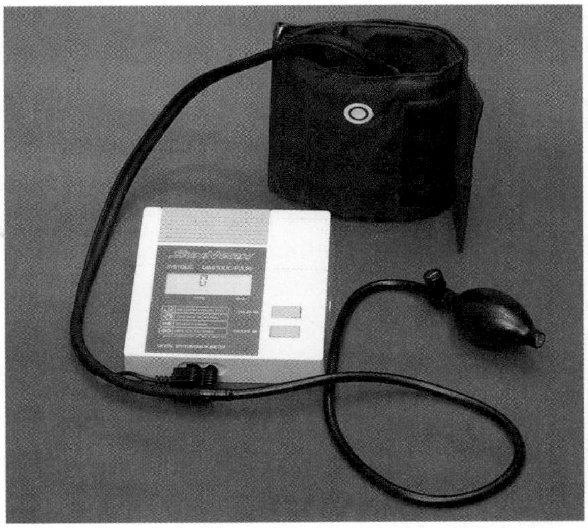

FIGURE 20–10b Digital sphygmomanometer.

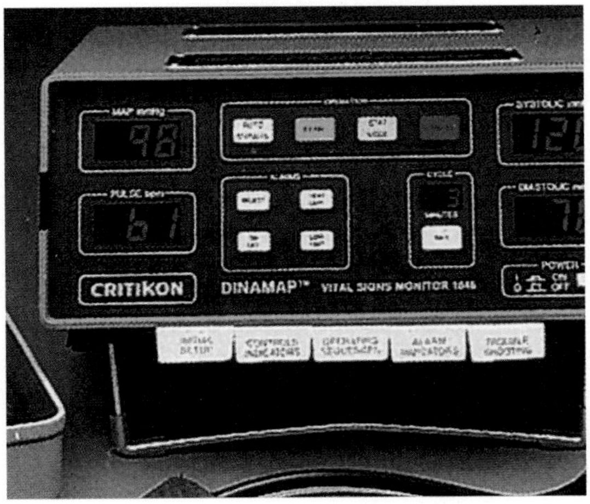

FIGURE 20–10c Electronic sphygmomanometer.

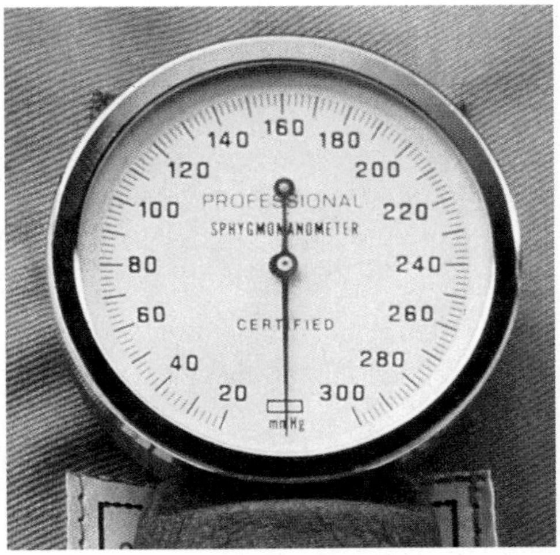

FIGURE 20–11 The gauge of a dial (aneroid) sphygmomanometer. Systolic and diastolic readings are recorded as even numbers.

(See Figures 20–10a–c.) Some units show pressure on a circular dial and others as digital numbers. The circular dials are calibrated so that each mark represents 2 mm Hg. (See Figure 20–11.) Electronic sphygmomanometers (see Figure 20–10c) take the blood pressure and pulse automatically and display the readings on a digital screen. (Once the cuff is placed on the arm, the machine can be programmed to automatically take readings at specific intervals.)

It takes repeated practice to master the skills for accurate manual blood pressure measurement. See Procedure 20–5 for the steps in taking a blood pressure reading.

When working with a manual sphygmomanometer, it is necessary to close the screw to inflate the cuff and to loosen the screw to release the air. Some health care professionals have difficulty remembering if turning the screw to the left or right will close or open the valve. It may be helpful to remember the saying "righty tighty, lefty loosey." This means that if you turn the screw to the *right* (as you look straight down at it) the valve will *tighten* and the cuff can be inflated. Turning the screw to the *left loosens* the screw, and air escapes.

The blood pressure cuff must fit correctly to get accurate results. Patients with very large or small

PROCEDURE 20–5

How to Take a Manual Blood Pressure

STEP	RATIONALE
1. You will need a stethoscope, a sphygmomanometer, and something to record the results on.	To verify that the sphygmomanometer is calibrated correctly, check that the dial is resting at zero prior to use.
2. Verify that the cuff is the correct size for the patient and that the valve is closed to allow for inflation of bladder.	The bladder in the cuff needs to cover at least 80% of the circumference of the arm and clear the antecubital space by 1 to 1½ inches to give accurate results.
3. Place the patient in a relaxed lying or sitting position, remove the clothing from the arm, and position the arm at heart level. Instruct the patient not to talk during the procedure.	Rolled-up sleeves can constrict the arm and alter the results; talking can interfere with hearing the readings correctly (it may also be necessary to turn off the television or radio).
4. Locate the pulse of the brachial artery in the inner aspect of the antecubital space, and place the arrows on cuff over this area.	Placing the stethoscope directly over the brachial artery will give the strongest sound.
5. Place your fingers on the radial artery and inflate the cuff until you can no longer feel the pulse. Note the reading and add 30 to it. For example, if the dial reads 120 when the radial pulsation ceases, add 30 to equal 150.	To get an accurate reading, it is necessary to pump the cuff to 30 mm Hg higher than the anticipated systolic pressure. This is the amount of inflation you will use when the blood pressure is taken.
6. Deflate the cuff by opening the screw. Wait at least 30 seconds.	Repeated inflation on the same arm in rapid succession will give inaccurate results.
7. Place the stethoscope in your ears and place the diaphragm over the brachial artery. Press gently.	The stethoscope diaphragm should be in full contact with the skin surface but not be pressed too hard.
8. Close the screw and inflate the cuff to the predetermined amount (from the example given earlier, this would be 150 mm Hg).	Never guess how high to inflate the cuff based on previous readings; check each time.
9. Slowly release the screw so the cuff deflates evenly (about 2 mm Hg at a time), and listen for the first sound of the pulse returning to the brachial artery. Make a mental note of the reading.	If the cuff is deflated too rapidly, the health care professional may not hear the first beat until a lower number is reached; the first sound heard from the brachial artery is the systolic pressure.
10. Continue allowing the cuff to deflate until you no longer hear any sounds from the brachial artery.	The health care professional will continue to hear a pulsing sound until it ceases, which is the reading for the diastolic pressure.

(continues)

PROCEDURE 20–5

How to Take a Manual Blood Pressure

(continued)

STEPS	RATIONALE
11. Continue to listen for any return of sounds from the brachial artery for an additional 20 to 30 mm Hg.	Some patients have what is called an auscultatory gap, where the beat of the brachial artery will again be heard. Note the new beginning and ending beats and chart the findings. For example, if you first heard beats at 170, the beats ceased at 120, then resumed at 100, then ceased again at 60, you would chart B/P 170/60 with auscultatory gap between 120 and 100.
12. Open the screw completely and let the cuff deflate rapidly.	The procedure is completed, and many patients do not like the tightness created by the cuff being inflated.
13. Remove the stethoscope from your ears and the cuff from the patient's arm and immediately record your results in even numbers only (manual B/P) along with which arm was used.	Getting in the habit of writing down the actual numbers, instead of relying on your memory, will prevent errors.
14. If you are unsure of the blood pressure reading and want to recheck it, use the other arm or wait several minutes before using the same arm.	Repeated blood pressure attempts can cause inaccurate results.

upper arms may need a larger cuff or a pediatric cuff. An inflatable bladder is located within the outer covering of a cuff and should be long enough to cover 80% of the circumference of the arm. (See Figure 20–12.) The width of the cuff should fit comfortably below the armpit and extend no farther than 1 to 1½ inches above the antecubital space.

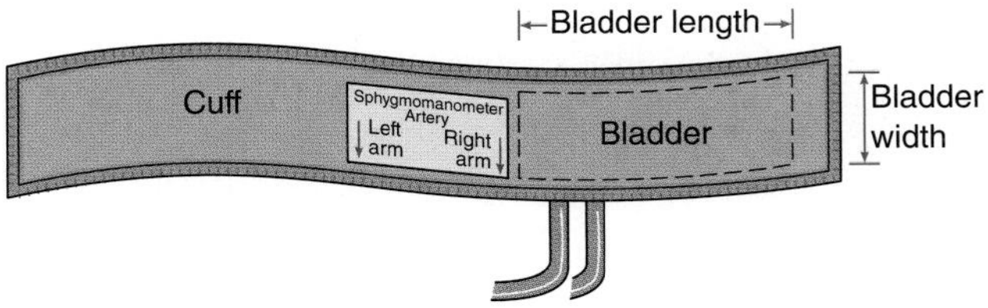

FIGURE 20–12 The blood pressure cuff must fit correctly to get accurate results. The bladder should cover 80% of the circumference of the patient's arm. Position arrows on the cuff over the brachial artery.

Blood pressure is affected by many factors, including the age of the patient (Table 20–5), certain medications and disease conditions, physical activity, the position of patient, and emotions. In fact, blood pressure is so variable in response to different factors that a diagnosis of hypertension is never made on just one reading. When patients visit the physician's office, they may feel anxious, and this causes the

Table 20–5 Blood Pressure at Various Ages

Age	Average B/P	Normal Range
Infant	70/42	60/20–94/56
Toddler	90/60	80/50–100/70
Preschool Child	100/54	84/50–110/60
School-Age Child	110/72	90/56–120/80
Adolescent–Adult	120/80	90/60–140/90

blood pressure reading to be higher than normal. Most physicians will want to see several high readings over time, when the patient is lying down in a resting position, before they conclude that the patient has high blood pressure.

White coat syndrome is a term that was coined to describe a situation in which patients' blood pressure readings are high in the provider's office but otherwise in the normal range. Even patients with diagnosed high blood pressure may have higher readings in the provider's office. The correlation is seldom this clear cut, however, the anxious emotions felt in the provider's office can also apply to other situations. If blood pressure is only occasionally high, it is not as dangerous as when it remains elevated most of the time. The patient may or may not actually feel anxious at the time (this mechanism appears to occur at a subconscious level). There are two concerns when considering white coat syndrome:

1. Patients may put themselves in this category and dismiss the need for treatment, as they feel it only occurs in that particular situation.
2. The high reading in the provider's office is assumed to be the patient's usual pressure and the patient is overtreated.

The best solution to this problem is for the patient to purchase his or her own blood pressure machine, take the blood pressure at home, and keep a record of all recordings. Taking this record to the next office visit will assist the health care provider in determining the best course of action.

When a patient's cardiovascular system is unable to make rapid changes to accommodate changes in position, he or she will experience a condition call **orthostatic (postural) hypotension**. Normally, when a person rises to a standing position, the blood vessels in the lower extremities constrict and the blood pressure increases to maintain adequate flow of blood to the brain. When that does not occur, the blood pools in the lower extremities and the blood pressure drops quickly, which results in a lack of oxygen to the brain. The patient experiences lightheadedness and may even pass out. This can also occur when a person has been on bed rest and is getting up for the first time, has recently had surgery, or is on certain medications. Patients with low blood pressure or low pulse rates are also prone to this problem.

When working with patients, always be on the alert and implement measures to ensure their safety. Have the patient get up slowly to allow more time for the cardiovascular system to adjust to the change in position. To assist the physician in diagnosing this problem, the health care professional may be asked to obtain a lying, sitting, and standing B/P. To do this, the health care professional takes a blood pressure reading with the patient lying down, then leaves the blood pressure cuff in place, instructs the patient to sit up, and rechecks the blood pressure. The same routine is repeated for the standing position. Check your facilities' policies because some specify the exact time interval required between the subsequent blood pressure measurements when performing this procedure. Also remember to ensure the patient's safety at the time of the test by monitoring during changes of position to prevent injury if he or she gets dizzy or passes out.

Media Link

Learn more about how to take a blood pressure by viewing the Blood Pressure and Taking a Patient's Blood Pressure videos on the Online Resources. The videos show a medical assistant (MA) in an office setting demonstrating the proper technique.

Thinking It Through

Ms. Sanchez is a nursing assistant at an acute care hospital in her hometown. Her supervisor has requested that she take Mr. Jordan's vital signs. When she enters the room, she introduces herself to Mr. Jordan and informs him that she will be taking his vital signs. He asks what she means by vital signs. He also tells her that he was hospitalized after having a myocardial infarction two days ago. She notes that he is receiving oxygen and has an IV line in his left arm.

1. What are vital signs?
2. Which arm should be used to take the blood pressure? Why?
3. What route should be used to take the temperature? Why?
4. Should the pulse be taken radially or apically? Why?
5. What three observations should be made when taking the pulse?
6. What three observations should be made when taking the respiratory rate?

At certain times the arm cannot be used for blood pressure readings. Do not use the arm if surgery was performed on it, the patient has had a mastectomy on that side, a hemodialysis shunt (surgically created vascular access) is present in the arm, or if there is an intravenous (IV) infusion running into the arm (fluids running through a tube into a cannula placed in a vein). Patients who have a shunt for the purpose of dialysis can never have blood pressures taken on that arm. If neither arm is available for taking a blood pressure (e.g., burns to both arms), the popliteal artery can be used. A large blood pressure cuff will be required that fits around the thigh. Follow the same blood pressure procedure as with the brachial artery, but place the stethoscope behind the knee to use the popliteal artery.

HEIGHT AND WEIGHT

Height and weight measurements are routinely taken as part of the patient's chart when he or she visits the physician's office or is admitted to a health care facility. The height measurement for an adult does not need to be repeated once it is recorded in the patient's chart, because it will not vary. An exception to this may be elderly patients with severe osteoporosis. When this condition is present, the height will actually decrease as they age. For younger patients, it is important to take both the height and weight. Growth charts used to record the measurements show the normal ranges for various ages. When the readings fall outside the normal ranges, it will alert the physician to potential problems requiring further evaluation. Refer back to the Suggested Learning Activities in Chapter 8 for the website that contains growth charts.

The weight will vary with a change in the patient's condition and with certain medications (e.g., diuretics). How frequently the patient is to be weighed is ordered by the physician or may be determined by your supervisor. Weight loss or gain may indicate a loss or gain of fat, muscle, or fluid. Patients with kidney or cardiac conditions often have problems with fluid balance and are weighed to determine the effectiveness of their medical regimen. When a patient starts to retain fluid, it will be seen on the scale long before it is visible on the body in the form of edema (swelling caused by excess fluid in the tissues of the body).

When a patient has edema or ascites (fluid accumulation in the peritoneal cavity), additional measurements may be indicated. Measuring the ankles or abdominal girth (around the abdomen) gives objective data on the patient's condition when results are compared to previous readings.

Various scales are available for measuring weight. Following are some of the most common:

- Standing balance scale: The scale must be balanced prior to use, and the patient must be able to stand upright in a steady position without holding on to anything or anyone. The weights on the bars are then moved until the bar balances at the center point. The height can be obtained at the same time by extending the height bar. (See Figures 20–13a–c.)
- Chair and wheelchair scales: Some chairs come equipped with a scale so the patient can sit while the weight is being taken. Another method is to place the patient in a wheelchair and then push it onto a scale, but in this case the wheelchair needs to be weighed while it is empty and its weight subtracted from the total weight of the patient in the chair to get the actual weight of the patient. (See Figure 20–14.)

Fascinating Facts

- The Centers for Disease Control and Prevention's National Center for Health Statistics reports that as many as 50 million Americans have hypertension. The prevalence of hypertension is 17% among white women, 26% among white men, 37% among black women, and 44% among black men 35 to 45 years old. In persons older than age 65, the incidence of high blood pressure is almost the same among men and women. In this age group, about 63% of whites and 76% of blacks will develop hypertension.
- Hypertension is called the silent killer because there are few if any symptoms, but if left untreated, it can lead to a heart attack, stroke, embolism, and kidney failure.
- In 90% to 95% of the cases, hypertension has no known cause. This type of high blood pressure is known as essential hypertension. In rarer cases, high blood pressure can result from other illnesses, such as kidney or adrenal gland problems. That type of high blood pressure is called secondary hypertension.

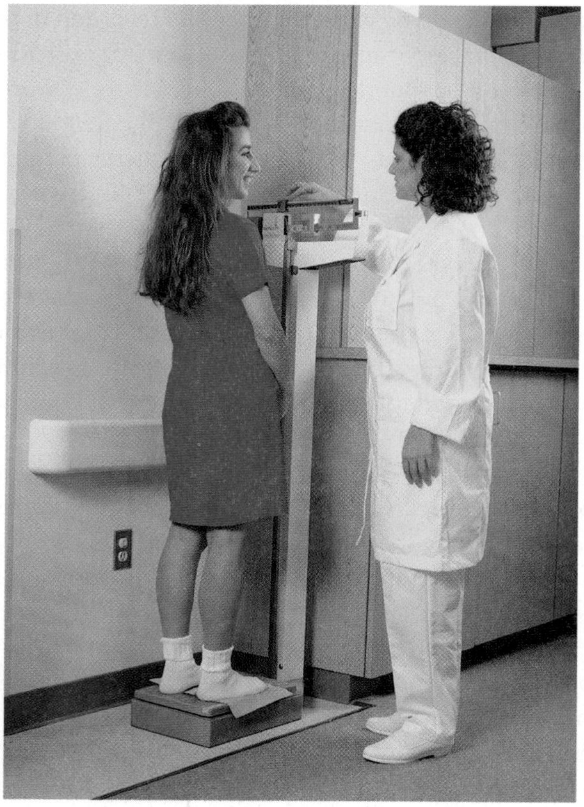

FIGURE 20–13a The patient should stand unassisted on the scale, with the feet centered on the platform and slightly apart.

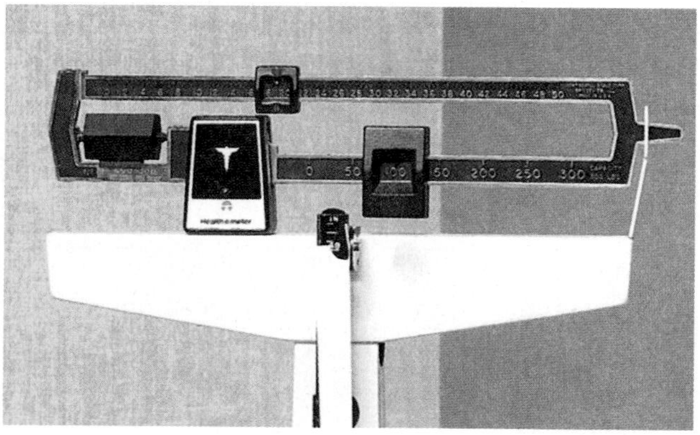

FIGURE 20–13c Adjust the weights on the balance bar until the bar balances at the center point. The combined total of the top and bottom bars is the weight of the patient.

- Mechanical lift scales (Figures 20–15a–b): Patients unable to move on their own can have a sling positioned under them and then be lifted off the bed to obtain their weight.
- Bed scales: Some hospital beds now come equipped with a scale. The advantage is that

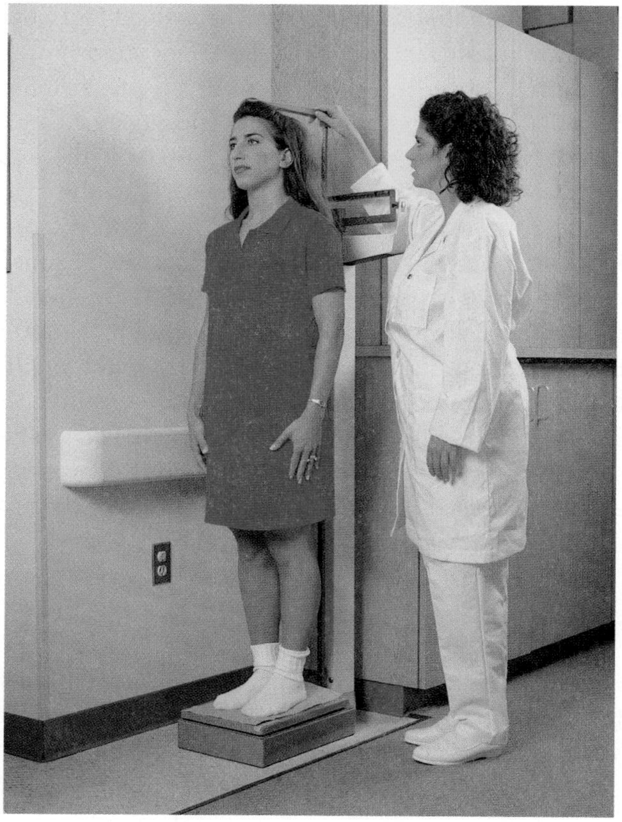

FIGURE 20–13b The patient should stand as erect as possible while height is being measured.

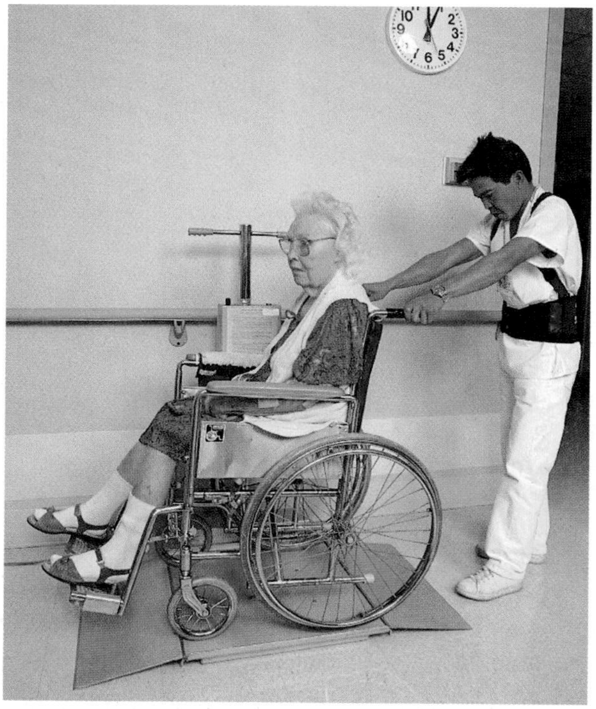

FIGURE 20–14 Subtract the weight of the wheelchair from the total weight of the patient sitting in the wheelchair.

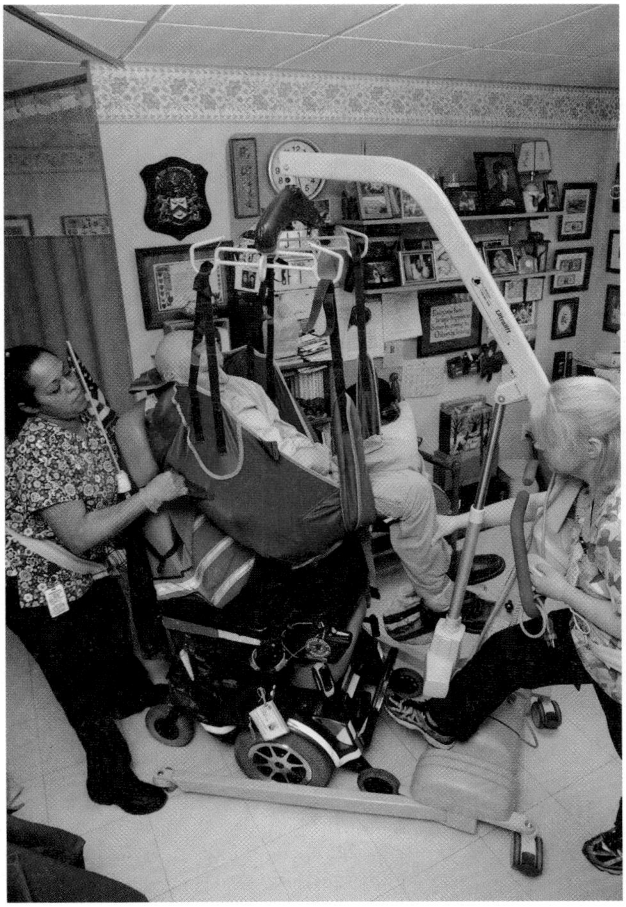

FIGURE 20–15a Chair-style mechanical lift with scale.

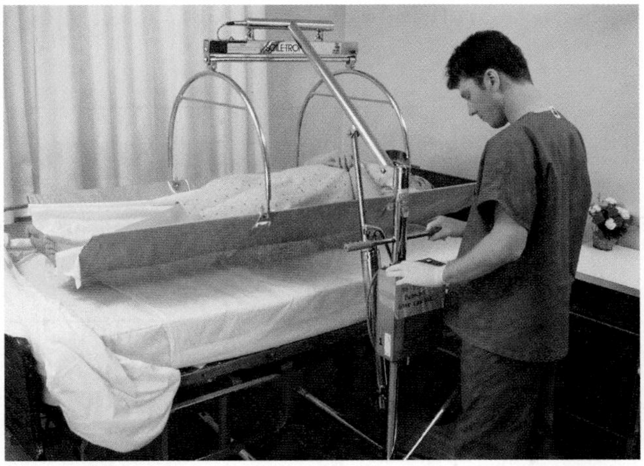

FIGURE 20–15b Bed-style mechanical lift with scale.

the patient does not have to be moved to take a weight. The patient lies in bed, and the scale is activated while a digital display shows the weight. Remove any excess items from the bed before weighing the patient.

Following certain guidelines when weighing patients will ensure more accurate results. These guidelines are listed in Box 20–1.

If a patient is unable to stand for a height measurement, the measurement will need to be taken when the patient is lying down. Place the patient flat on the bed or examining table in a straight aligned position. Then place a mark at the top of the head and one at the bottom of the heels. Measure the distance between the marks and record it as the height. This method is also used with infants and children who are unable to stand.

Many facilities are now using a body mass index (BMI) to determine if the patient is at a healthy weight. The BMI measures the relationship between weight and height. BMI ranges are not absolute indicators but can serve as a guide to patients to demonstrate if they are at a health risk due to their weight. An inaccuracy occurs when the individual is very muscular or has lost a lot of muscle mass. See Figure 20–16 for BMI ranges for adults.

BOX 20–1

Guidelines for Weighing Patients

- Weigh patients at the same time every day; the recommendation is to weigh patients first thing in the morning, after they empty their bladder and before they eat or drink.
- Use the same scale each time.
- Balance the scale before use, if indicated.
- Have the same amount of clothes on the patient each time and remove the shoes.
- Maintain the safety of the patient at all times by monitoring for signs of unsteadiness that could result in a fall.

WORKBOOK PRACTICE

Go to your workbook and complete the exercises for this chapter.

ARE YOU AT A HEALTHY WEIGHT?

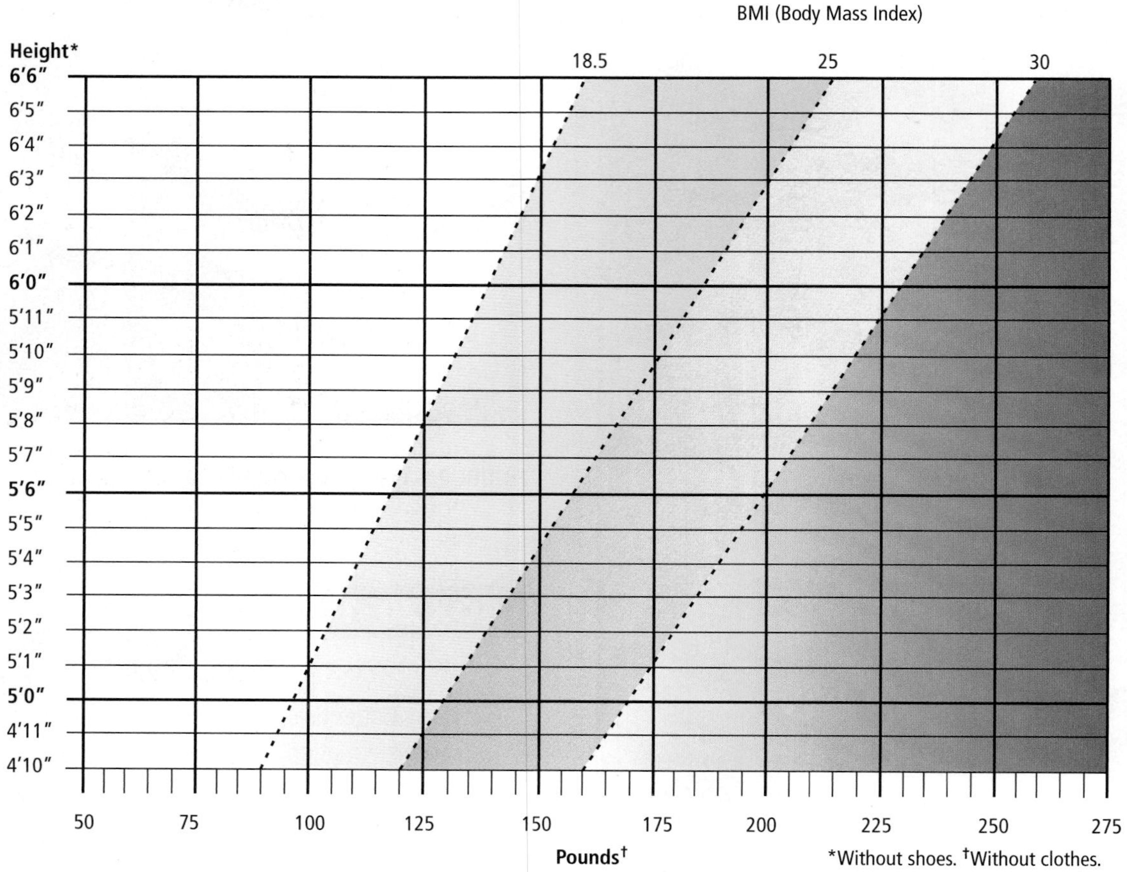

BMI measures weight in relation to height. The BMI ranges shown above are for adults. They are not exact ranges of healthy and unhealthy weights. However, they show that health risk increases at higher levels of overweight and obesity. Even within the healthy BMI range, weight gains can carry health risks for adults.

Directions: Find your weight on the bottom of the graph. Go straight up from that point until you come to the line that matches your height. Then find your weight group.

Under weight: below 18.5

Healthy Weight: BMI from 18.5 up to 25 refers to healthy weight.

Overweight: BMI from 25 up to 30 refers to overweight.

Obese: BMI 30 or higher refers to obesity. Obese persons are also overweight.

Source: *Report of the Dietary Guidelines Advisory Committee on the Dietary Guidelines for Americans*, 2000.

FIGURE 20–16 Body mass index (BMI) chart.

SUGGESTED LEARNING ACTIVITIES

1. Identify the information included in a history and physical for yourself, a family member, or a friend, and write the information down in a chronological and organized manner.
2. Perform a head-to-toe evaluation on yourself and write the results in a narrative documentation format (refer back to Chapter 19).
3. Next time you experience pain (e.g., headache, stub your toe), assess your level of pain on a scale of 1 to 10. Then note how this level changes over time, until it is completely gone (level 0).

4. It will take time to develop the ability to feel a pulse, to hear the apical heartbeat, and to hear the blood pressure. Practice on yourself and your family to assist you in developing the needed sensitivity in your fingertips to feel these variations and in your ears to hear the sounds with a stethoscope. Closing your eyes to help focus all of your attention on your fingertips or ears may be a helpful technique to use when practicing.
5. Find all the pulse points on your body.
6. Find your BMI. (See Figure 20–16.) Based on this information, use the five-step problem-solving process to develop a plan for improvement. Then, even if you are in the normal weight range, evaluate whether you are at a peak aerobic level or your flexibility and strength could be improved.

WEB ACTIVITIES

Wikipedia
http://en.wikipedia.org/

Search for "Activities of Daily Living" and click "GO." How does this site define ADLs? Scroll down to see how the difference between Basic and Instrumental ADLs is defined. Summarize your findings and thoughts on these definitions.

National Heart Lung and Blood Institute
www.nhlbi.nih.gov

Search for "Blood Pressure." Identify five healthy habits to prevent or control high blood pressure. How many adult Americans have high blood pressure? Report on three of the nine types of medications used to treat high blood pressure and how they work to lower blood pressure.

Everyday Health
www.everydayhealth.com

Click on "Hypertension" under Health A-Z in the menu bar. Read an article of interest and write a one-page report.

American Heart Association
www.heart.org

Search for "low blood pressure." How is it defined? What would indicate a need for concern?

REVIEW QUESTIONS

1. State the components that comprise a history and physical.
2. What does the phrase "noting variances from the normal" mean?
3. Why is it a critical function for the health care professional to be able to discriminate between normal and abnormal conditions and situations?
4. What are sample questions to be asked to evaluate each of the body's systems?
5. What does it mean to use a pain ratings scale?
6. What are activities of daily living (ADLs)?
7. What are the different types of equipment for taking a temperature?
8. What is an apical–radial deficit?
9. How do the vital signs vary over the life span?
10. What are the steps in taking an accurate TPR and B/P?
11. What problems may be indicated by a rapid weight gain in a patient?

APPLICATION EXERCISES

1. Refer back to The Case of the Unreported Observations and answer these questions.
   a. What variances from the normal was Mrs. Becker displaying?
   b. What are the possible outcomes of the patient losing consciousness and falling?
   c. How could Carrie have handled the situation differently?
2. Mr. Hussar, a 76-year-old patient, walks into the physician's office for his regular checkup. Mr. Hussar seems to be limping slightly as he approaches the desk to sign in for his appointment. Mrs. Jacobs, the receptionist, inquires how he is doing, to which he replies, "Fine." Mrs. Jacobs always looks forward to seeing Mr. Hussar because he is usually so cheerful and talkative, but she is disappointed when he just takes a chair in the waiting room to wait for the doctor. She notes

that Mr. Hussar is not as neatly dressed as usual, nor as well groomed.

a. Is there an alteration in the patient's gait?
b. What value will being able to "note variances from the normal" provide? What knowledge is needed to be able to determine a variance from the normal?
c. Are there any physical variances? If so, what are they?
d. Are there any psychosocial variances? If so, what are they?

PROBLEM-SOLVING PRACTICE

Allen Burns gets a reading of 94/60 when taking a patient's blood pressure. Using the five-step problem-solving process, determine what Allen should do with this finding.

SUGGESTED READINGS AND RESOURCES

Bickley, L. S., & Hoekelman, R. A. (2012). *Bates' pocket guide to physical examination and history taking* (7th ed.). Philadelphia, PA: Lippincott Williams & Wilkins.

Estes, M. E. Z. (2011). *Health assessment & physical examination* (5th ed.). Clifton Park, NY: Delmar Cengage Learning.

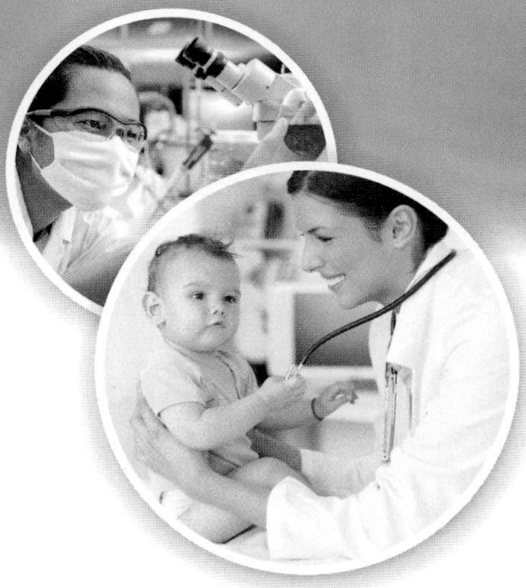

Chapter 21

Emergency Procedures

OBJECTIVES

Studying and applying the material in this chapter will help you to:

- Explain when first aid should be administered.
- Discuss how the Good Samaritan Act protects the rescuer.
- State the golden rule of first aid.
- Understand the seven steps to follow that will protect both the victim and the rescuer when an emergency occurs.
- Identify when CPR should be performed.
- Identify illnesses and injuries that may require first aid, including their signs and symptoms and treatment.
- Demonstrate the proper application of slings and spiral, figure-eight, and finger wraps.

KEY TERMS

anaphylactic shock
cardiopulmonary resuscitation (CPR)
closed fracture
external bleeding
first aid
frostbite
golden rule
Good Samaritan Act
hemorrhage
hyperthermia
hypothermia
internal bleeding
joint dislocation
Medic Alert
open fracture
rescue breathing
rescuer
sprains
strains (muscle)
sucking wound
victim
wound

The Case of the Out-of-Control Party

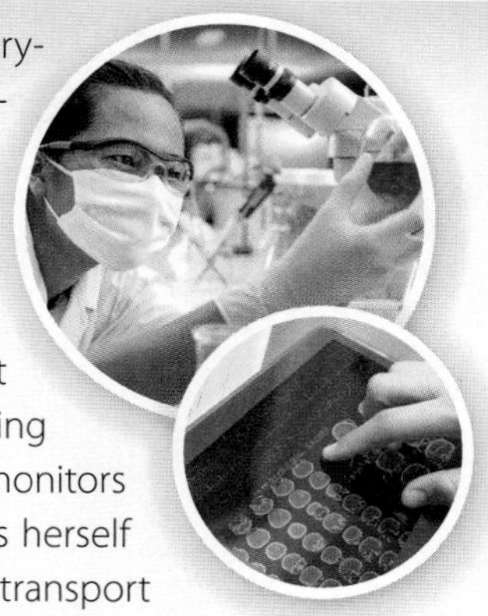

Josephine Robbins is a nurse at a local hospital. She lives in a nearby apartment complex and is trying to tune out loud noises coming from a party in the next complex. The noise seems to escalate, then she hears someone shout, "Oh my God, he stabbed him," and then there is silence. She calls 9-1-1, gets dressed, and goes to see if it is safe to offer assistance. After deeming it safe, she enters and sees the victim lying on the couch, unconscious. His respirations are shallow and rapid; his skin is pale and cold to the touch; and his lips, earlobes, and fingertips have a bluish tinge. The victim has a 2-inch cut on the left side of his chest where a knife is still inserted, but it is currently not bleeding. There is, however, a great deal of blood in the kitchen area, on the living room carpet, and on the victim's clothing. Josephine does her assessment, gives first aid, and monitors the victim's condition until the paramedics arrive. When the paramedics arrive, she introduces herself and gives them a report of observations and care given. The paramedics continue the care and transport the victim to the hospital. In this chapter, you will learn how to approach emergency situations and how to give appropriate first aid measures to assist victims.

EMERGENCY SITUATIONS

First aid refers to providing emergency care to an accident victim or to someone who has suddenly become ill. The goal of first aid is to provide care to minimize the effects of the injury or illness until the victim can be treated by a physician.

The American Red Cross recommends that all persons take a first aid and safety course. The course covers what to do in an emergency, how to give first aid, and how to prevent accidents and injuries. The American Red Cross and the American Heart Association (AHA) recommend that everyone be trained in giving **cardiopulmonary resuscitation (CPR)**. CPR is administered when someone is not breathing and does not have a pulse. The ARC and AHA believe that many lives would be saved if more people were trained to give emergency care. More people trained in emergency care increases the chance that an injured person can start to receive care immediately rather than it being delayed until medical help arrives.

To encourage individuals to get involved in helping victims during an emergency, a law has been passed by most states called the **Good Samaritan Act**. This protects individuals from liability when they stop to assist someone who has been hurt or is ill. This protection covers acts that are within the ability of the person to provide as long as there is no gross negligence or willful intent to harm the victim. The Good Samaritan laws vary between states. Specific information should be requested from the local police department, the library, or an attorney. (See Box 21–1.)

BOX 21–1

Example of Good Samaritan Law as Written for the State of Arizona

Health care providers and other persons administering emergency aid are not liable. Any health care provider licensed or certified to practice as such in this state or elsewhere, or a licensed ambulance attendant, driver or pilot as defined in 41-1831, or any other person who renders emergency care at a public gathering or at a scene of an emergency occurrence gratuitously and in good faith, shall not be liable for any civil or other damages as the result of any act or omission by such person rendering the emergency care, or as the result of any act or failure to act to provide or arrange for further medical treatment or care for the injured persons, unless such person, while rendering such emergency care, is guilty of gross negligence.

Source: Arizona Good Samaritan Law, Article 4, Emergency Aid.

The **golden rule** in providing first aid is to "do no further harm." When a person goes into health care as a career, it is because of a desire to help others. When an emergency situation arises, it is natural to want to do anything and everything possible to assist the victim. The best way to be ready for this situation is to learn as much as possible about first aid and CPR. But it is also just as critical not to attempt anything you do not have the skills to perform. If the procedure needed is beyond your skill level, then immediately seek help. Getting the appropriate help for the victim can save a life.

Many people fantasize about having the ability to assist someone in an emergency. The thoughts are that the intervention performed saved a life, the rescuer is declared a hero or heroine, and the victim recovers and is very grateful. This indeed may be the situation, but another reality can also occur. Perhaps there is little that can be done to help, the victim is uncooperative, or all attempts at first aid fail, and the victim dies. Some accident sites can be extremely upsetting, and the images and sounds can continue to emotionally upset the Good Samaritan for some time after the event. If the outcome of assisting someone is less than ideal, then take satisfaction in knowing that you did the best you could to assist in a very difficult situation.

When an Emergency Occurs

When approaching an injured or ill person, there are certain steps to follow. These steps include actions that will protect the **rescuer** (person giving care), as well as the **victim** (person requiring care).

Assess the Environment

Before approaching the victim, assess the situation to determine if it is safe to approach. If there are loose electrical wires, the potential for a sudden fire or explosion, the smell of gas, or any other hazards that would put the Good Samaritan at risk, the appropriate course of action is to not approach, but to call for help immediately. If the victim is conscious, inform him or her that you will call for assistance and stay with them until help arrives. Most states have emergency medical services (EMS) that are reached by dialing 9-1-1 on a telephone. The person answering has been specially trained and will ask questions that should be answered as accurately as possible. EMS will want to know the name and location of the victim, what the nature of the emergency is, and what, if any, treatment has been given. The EMS personnel will send services as deemed appropriate, such as an ambulance, a fire engine, and the police. They may also be able to advise you on what to do to further assist the victim. Remember that your first priority is to keep yourself safe. If you take a risk and become a victim, too, then there is no one to call EMS. Assessing a situation is not done only once; the situation must be repeatedly monitored. For example, if there is smoke in the immediate area, is the amount increasing?

Obtain Consent to Treat

When approaching a stranger, identify yourself and your intent to give assistance. If the victim is conscious, permission must be obtained prior to administering care. If the victim is a child, determine if a parent or guardian is present, to obtain consent for care. If the victim is unconscious, consent is implied and first aid can be administered. Remember that victims have the right to refuse care, and this request must be respected. If consent for care is not given and it is obvious that care is required, immediately call EMS.

Try to Determine What Happened

Do not assume what might have occurred. If the victim is conscious, ask for information. Look around the environment for any clues that would assist in determining what care is needed. For example, if there is an empty bottle of pills or chemicals that may have been ingested, note what they are and inform EMS, because they may be able to give you directions on how to treat the victim immediately. Many people with specific medical conditions wear necklaces or bracelets or carry cards with them that contain important information that can assist you in determining what care to consider and also in informing the EMS about what type of help to send. This form of identification is called **Medic Alert**, and it may specify if the victim is diabetic, epileptic, or has specific heart problems. There may also be information about specific allergies that will be helpful for the personnel from EMS to know before administering medications. Another thing to determine is if there are other victims. Perhaps someone was thrown from the car or is in a different area than where you are located.

Follow Standard Precautions

Following standard precautions is essential in all situations that may result in the rescuer coming into contact with body fluids. Carry disposable gloves that can be put on prior to contact. Another valuable item to carry at all times is a barrier device for giving mouth-to-mouth resuscitation. These resuscitation devices have a mouthpiece with a one-way valve attached to a plastic shield that prevents the rescuer from getting saliva, blood, or vomit in his or her mouth. (See Figure 21–1.) Some of these devices are small enough to fold into a small pouch that is attached to a key chain. Information about the contents of a first aid kit can be obtained from the American Red Cross. A first

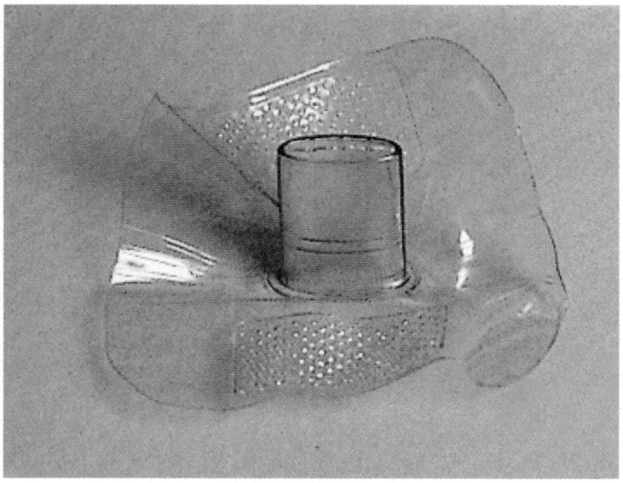

FIGURE 21–1 Portable barrier device to protect rescuer during resuscitation.

aid kit can be kept in the home, car, or office for ready access when needed.

Enlist the Help of Bystanders

Determine if there are others in the area who can assist in the care of the victim. If you are the most experienced person, then stay with the victim and instruct someone else to call EMS. Instruct those willing to help to do other tasks, such as rerouting traffic, keeping onlookers away from the scene, looking for clues as to what happened, or tending to other victims.

Never Move a Victim

A neck or back injury can be made worse or result in permanent paralysis if the victim is moved. The only exception to this rule is if the victim's life is in immediate danger if he or she is not moved. When it is absolutely necessary to move the victim, make every attempt to keep the spine in straight alignment. When turning a victim with a neck or back injury, turn the body as a unit to prevent spinal cord injury. If you move an injured extremity, support it during the move to prevent further vessel or nerve damage.

Stay Calm

A calm, reassuring manner in treating a victim will decrease the stress of the situation for the victim, others in the area, and you. Many people who feel they cannot handle certain situations are quite surprised to discover how effectively they can think and act in an emergency situation. If the scene is more than the rescuer can handle, the best thing to do is to call EMS immediately.

CARDIOPULMONARY RESUSCITATION (CPR)

An expectation of most health care employers is that all health care professionals will attend classes to maintain a current certification for performing CPR. These classes provide theory and hands-on practice on how to assist a victim in the following situations:

- Obstructed airway: Perform the Heimlich maneuver, a method that uses pressure to expel material that is stuck in the throat, preventing the victim from being able to inhale air.
- Not breathing: Perform **rescue breathing**, which is a technique in which the rescuer breathes for the victim.
- Not breathing and has no pulse: Perform CPR, which includes rescue breathing and doing compressions to the chest to stimulate cardiac blood flow for the victim.

Because the specific guidelines for CPR may be revised annually and the best approach to learning this material is to receive training from a CPR-certified instructor, the specific procedures are not presented in this text. It is highly recommended that every person be certified in CPR. It is of particular importance that all health care professionals and students obtain and maintain CPR certification.

Advanced certificates are also available. Advanced cardiac life support (ACLS) is available for health care professionals who take care of adults, and pediatric advanced life support (PALS) is offered for those working with children. Employers may require these classes as a condition of employment for physicians, specialty nurses, respiratory therapists, emergency technicians, and paramedics but they can also be taken by others. ACLS and PALS usually include a review of CPR, but their primary focus is advanced life support measures, such as interpretation of cardiac rhythms and the determination of the medications to administer for treatment in cardiac emergencies.

FIRST AID PROCEDURES

When approaching any victim to administer first aid, the first step is always to determine whether the victim is breathing and has a pulse. If not, CPR should be started.

CPR is always the first priority in an emergency. If the victim does not require CPR, then the next step is to assess the victim for any other problems that may need attention. Implementing proper first aid procedures can prevent further injury and assist in the recovery of the injured person. Discussed in the following sections are a variety of first aid procedures that are commonly used in medical emergencies.

Allergic Reactions

Allergic reactions can range from mild to life threatening. The reaction is the result of the body's defense mechanism being triggered by a normally harmless substance. An allergic reaction can be triggered by skin contact (e.g., lotions, poison ivy); ingestion (e.g., certain foods and drugs); inhalation (e.g., sprays and pollen); or injection (e.g., venom from insect and snakebites). Once an allergy has developed, it will often become more severe with each re-exposure. In the most extreme case, a condition called anaphylaxis occurs, in which the respiratory system swells to such an extent that air is prevented from entering the lungs. This is called **anaphylactic shock**, and if it occurs, death will follow if it is not treated immediately.

See Procedure 21–1 for first aid related to allergic reactions.

PROCEDURE 21–1

First Aid for Allergic Reactions

Always Observe Standard Precautions

CONDITION AND SIGNS AND SYMPTOMS	PROCEDURE	RATIONALE
Mild to Moderate Reaction *S/S*: Itching, hives, and flushed face. Swelling may involve the eyes, face, or tongue. The victim may be weak and dizzy and have nausea and vomiting.	• Be calm and reassuring in approach to victim.	• Anxiety increases the allergic reaction.
	• If there is an itchy rash, apply anti-itch lotion (e.g., calamine lotion) and cool compresses.	• Soothing the itch makes it less likely that the victim will scratch the area, which not only increases the intensity of the rash but may also cause an infection.
	• Try to determine the source of the allergic reaction.	• The victim can avoid it in the future.
	• A physician may recommend an over-the-counter medication (e.g., Benadryl).	• Taking an antihistamine can decrease the effect of an allergic reaction.
	• Call EMS if the condition worsens.	• It may advance to a severe reaction.
Severe Reaction *S/S*: ThThe mild to moderate reactions may be present, but they can quickly become more severe. In the worst cases that lead to anaphylaxis, there is	• Call EMS.	• Severe reactions can lead to anaphylactic shock.
	• If the victim has emergency allergy medication, help him or her administer it.	• Victims with known severe allergies may carry a kit for administering an injection to stop a reaction.

(continues)

PROCEDURE 21–1

First Aid for Allergic Reactions

(continued)

CONDITION AND SIGNS AND SYMPTOMS	PROCEDURE	RATIONALE
Severe Reaction (continued) difficulty breathing, wheezing, and tightness of the chest. The victim may have difficulty swallowing and become unconscious. Untreated anaphylaxis can lead to death.	• Do not give the victim anything by mouth if he or she is having difficulty breathing. • Do not place a pillow under the victim's head.	• It may enter the lungs and cause further breathing difficulties. • Elevating the head may close off the airway.
Bites and Stings (e.g., insects, spiders, scorpions, and snakes) *S/S*: Localized reaction to bite or sting may be seen, such as redness, pain, and swelling. There may be an obvious bite mark. An allergic reaction may occur as noted in the section on allergic reactions.	• Try to identify what bit or stung the victim.	• This will assist EMS personnel to treat victim.
	• Kill it if there is no risk to the rescuer, and keep it for identification.	• The rescuer's safety comes first, or there will be two victims and no one to call EMS.
	• If there is a stinger (e.g., from a honeybee), remove it by scraping it with your fingernail or a credit card.	• Do not use tweezers because it may force more venom into victim.
	• Do not forcibly remove a tick; instead suffocate it by covering it with a heavy oil (e.g., Vaseline, mineral oil), wait 30 minutes, then carefully remove it with tweezers, placing them as close to the mouth parts as possible (if all parts are not removed, seek medical attention).	• This decreases the chance of mouth parts remaining in the victim.
	• Call EMS immediately if a poisonous spider, scorpion, or snake has bitten the victim.	• The victim must receive the appropriate injection of antivenom without delay.
	• If an allergic reaction occurs, treat it as noted for allergic reactions.	• Same as for allergic reactions.
	• Stay with the victim for at least an hour.	• Sometimes reactions are delayed.
	• Clean the area with soap and water and apply antiseptic ointment.	• Cleaning helps to prevent infection.
	• Remove any confining clothing or jewelry.	• Clothing and jewelry act as a constricting band if swelling occurs.

(continues)

PROCEDURE 21–1

First Aid for Allergic Reactions

(continued)

CONDITION AND SIGNS AND SYMPTOMS	PROCEDURE	RATIONALE
Bites and Stings (continued)	• Apply a cold compress.	• This can decrease pain, swelling, and the spread of venom.
	• Have the victim lie still and keep the bite area below heart level.	• Lying still slows the rate at which the venom spreads.
	• Do not apply a tourniquet.	• A tourniquet cuts off blood to the extremity, may result in damage to tissues, and could result in the need for an amputation.
	• Consult with a physician to determine if any additional preventive measures should be taken.	• The victim may need additional treatment to prevent disease that may have been contracted through the bite or sting (e.g., tetanus, Lyme disease).
	• Instruct the victim to observe for infection (e.g., increased pain, redness, or swelling; discharge from the site, swollen glands, fever, flu-like symptoms, or red streaks coming from the site) and get medical help immediately if symptoms occur.	• Infections require follow-up care and treatment by a physician.

Bleeding and Wounds

Bleeding occurs when a blood vessel is damaged. Heavy bleeding is called a **hemorrhage**. Damage to the soft tissue of the body from violence or trauma is called a **wound**. **External bleeding** occurs when blood drains to the outside of the body through a break in the skin. If there is bleeding that occurs inside the body, it is called **internal bleeding** and is more difficult to detect. Suspect internal bleeding if the victim has a broken bone or has been hit forcibly (e.g., a car accident in which the victim hits the dashboard or steering wheel, is struck by an object, or receives other types of trauma to the head or body). If internal bleeding is suspected, the victim must have a medical evaluation.

When giving first aid to a victim who has a wound, the rescuer must clean the wound and protect it from further damage. If there is external bleeding that does not stop spontaneously, first aid will be required to stop the bleeding before the victim loses too much blood.

Bleeding can occur from a vein or an artery. *Arterial bleeding* is a brighter red and comes out in spurts with each heartbeat. This is a life-threatening situation and must be stopped as soon as possible. *Venous bleeding* flows evenly and can also result in a great deal of blood loss. Remember to follow standard precautions when caring for victims with wounds and bleeding.

A tourniquet (tight band placed around an arm or leg to stop bleeding) is rarely used in emergency care because it too often does more harm than good. It is used only as a last resort to save a life and may result in the loss of the limb below the injury. See Procedure 21–2 for first aid related to bleeding and wounds.

Bone, Joint, and Muscle Injuries

When a bone is broken, it is called a fracture. An **open fracture** is when the broken bone protrudes through the skin. A **closed fracture** is a broken bone that does not break the skin. When a joint becomes disconnected from its socket, it is called a **joint dislocation**.

Strains result from the sudden tearing of muscle fibers during exertion and are often referred to as pulled muscles. **Sprains** are torn ligament fibers that result in a loosening of the joint.

See Procedure 21–3 for first aid related to bone, joint, and muscle injuries.

PROCEDURE 21–2

First Aid for Bleeding and Wounds

Always Observe Standard Precautions

CONDITION AND SIGNS AND SYMPTOMS	PROCEDURE	RATIONALE
External Bleeding *S/S*: Blood coming from a wound. Weakness, confusion, or a decreasing level of consciousness may indicate excessive blood loss. Loss of function distal to the wound indicates damage to tendons or muscles. Loss of sensation distal to the wound indicates damage to the nerves.	• Call EMS if you suspect internal bleeding or if there is heavy external bleeding or other serious injuries.	• The victim will require medical evaluation and intervention.
	• Apply cold compresses to bruised areas.	• Bruising can be decreased as the cold constricts the blood vessels.
	• If there is bleeding from the leg or arm, elevate it above heart level (unless contraindicated by neck or back injury, or discomfort).	• Elevation of the extremity will decrease the pressure in the vascular system of the arm or leg and thus decrease bleeding.
	• Do not use a tourniquet.	• Cuts off blood to the extremity, resulting in damage to tissues and the possible need for an amputation.
	• To stop bleeding, apply direct pressure with a clean cloth or sterile dressing over the area. (See Figure 21–2.) If the rescuer needs his or her hands free to do additional first aid, a pressure dressing can be applied to decrease the bleeding. (See Figures 21–3a–e).	• Pressure slows the blood flow so body can use its natural clotting mechanism.
	• When the dressing becomes soaked with blood, do not remove it; instead place the new dressing on top.	• Removing the dressing may reinitiate or increase bleeding.

(continues)

PROCEDURE 21–2

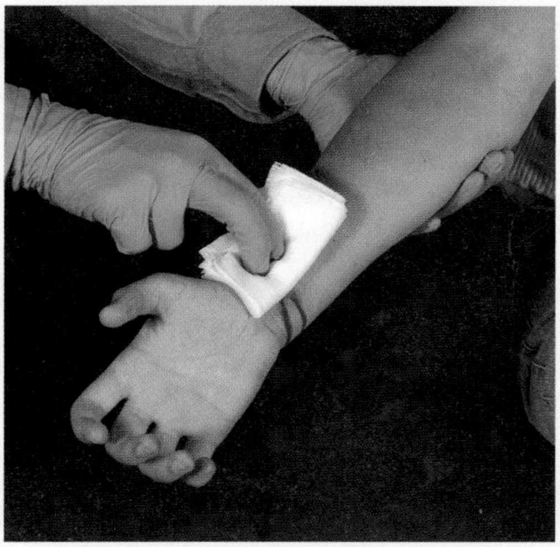

FIGURE 21–2 By using direct pressure and elevation, most severe bleeding can be controlled.

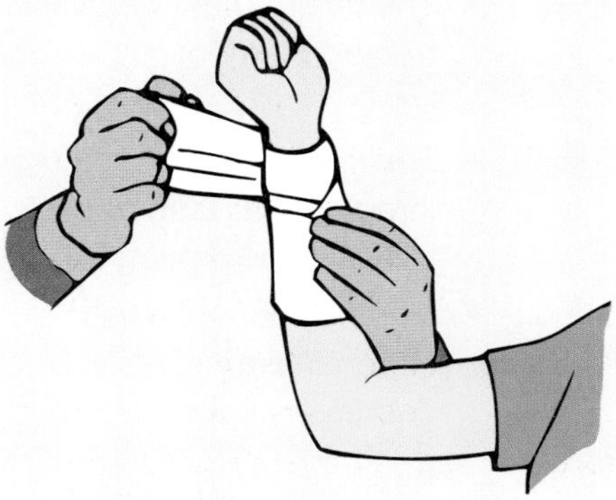

FIGURE 21–3a Maintain direct pressure and elevation when applying a pressure dressing. Do not remove previous dressing, but apply the pressure dressing over the previous dressing.

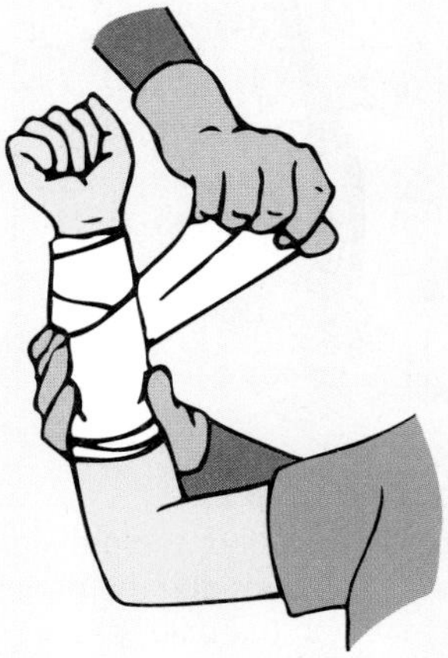

FIGURE 21–3b Wrap the roller bandage or long strip of cloth firmly around the wound. Overlap each rotation partially over the previous one to hold it securely in place.

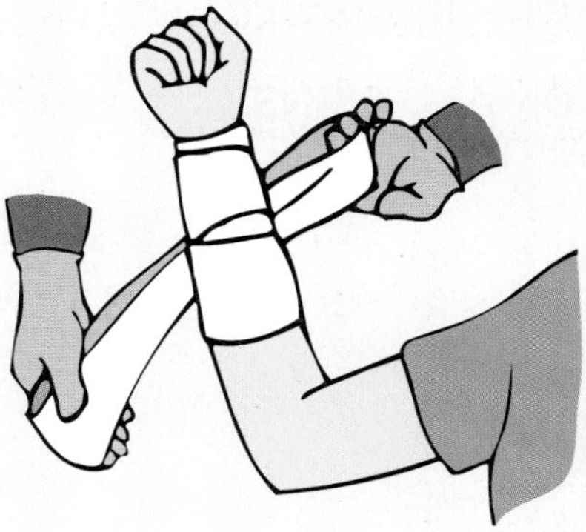

FIGURE 21–3c Split the end of the bandage into two strips.

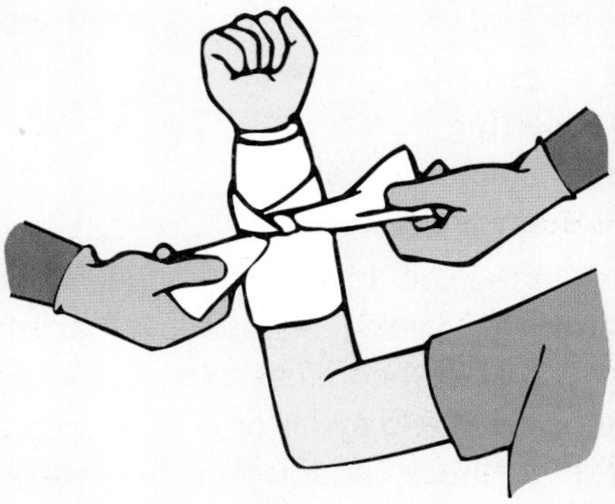

FIGURE 21–3d Tie the ends tightly into a knot right over the wound.

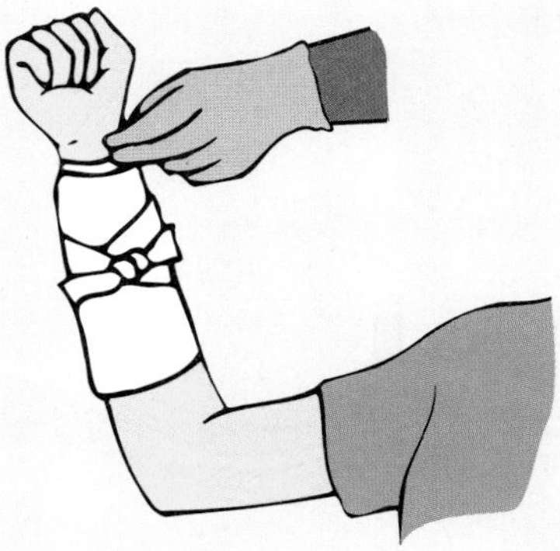

FIGURE 21–3e Check for circulation to verify that the dressing is not too tight. If there is no pulse or the fingers are turning bluish, loosen the dressing and rewrap it.

(continues)

PROCEDURE 21–2

First Aid for Bleeding and Wounds

(continued)

CONDITION AND SIGNS AND SYMPTOMS	PROCEDURE	RATIONALE
External Bleeding (continued)	• Do not look under the dressing to see if the bleeding has stopped.	• Lifting the dressing may reinitiate bleeding.
	• Do not apply pressure over an embedded object, the eye, or on a head injury if a skull fracture is suspected.	• This may cause further damage.
	• If bleeding from an arm or leg does not stop after 15 minutes of direct pressure, then use pressure-point bleeding control. (See Figures 21–4a–b.)	• This technique will decrease the flow of blood to the affected area.
Internal Bleeding Abdominal injuries can cause internal bleeding.	• Call EMS	• The victim must be evaluated and treated by medical personnel.
S/S: Blood in the vomit, urine, or stool, or from the vagina; distended abdomen; nausea; abdominal tenderness; signs and symptoms of shock. (See shock under Other Conditions.) Weakness, confusion, or a decreasing level of consciousness may indicate bleeding inside the skull that is causing pressure on the brain.	• Do not give the victim anything to eat or drink.	• The victim may need surgical intervention; food or drink may cause vomiting.
	• Place the victim on his or her back and elevate the knees with a pillow or blanket if there is abdominal discomfort.	• This position relaxes the abdominal muscles and decreases pain.
	• Keep the victim still and treat him or her for shock as needed.	• This is to prevent further injury.

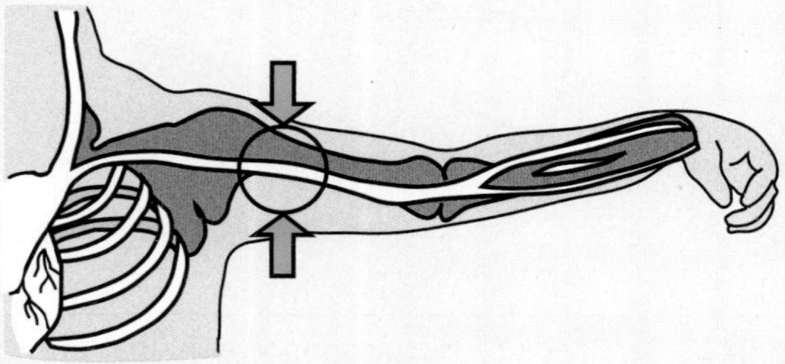

FIGURE 21–4a For an arm wound, the pressure point is on the brachial artery. It is located between the large muscles (biceps and triceps) on the inside of the arm. Press firmly with your fingers, until you no longer feel a pulse.

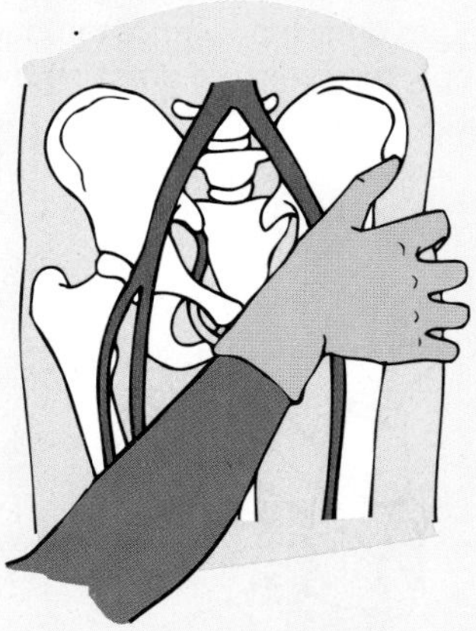

FIGURE 21–4b For a leg wound, the pressure point is on the femoral artery. It is located in the groin at the bend of the leg. Press firmly with the palm of your hand (or use both hands for more pressure) against the pelvic bone, until you no longer feel a pulse.

(continues)

PROCEDURE 21–2

First Aid for Bleeding and Wounds

(continued)

CONDITION AND SIGNS AND SYMPTOMS	PROCEDURE	RATIONALE
Internal Bleeding (continued)	• Stay with victim until medical assistance arrives.	• Give rescue breathing or CPR as needed.
Wounds *S/S*: Tear or open area anywhere on the body.	• Do not try to clean a large wound or remove any embedded objects.	• Cleaning can increase the bleeding and cause additional damage.
	• Remove any obvious loose debris from the wound.	• This decreases contamination of wound.
	• If an object is protruding from the body, do not remove it. (See Figure 21–5.)	• Removing the object may cause further damage or initiate bleeding.
Sucking Wounds *S/S*: Bubbling from any wound of the neck or chest; difficulty breathing.	• If the chest or neck has been punctured or if there is an object protruding from the chest or neck, note if there is any bubbling from the wound. If so, this is called a **sucking wound**, and it needs to be sealed as soon as possible.	• Bubbling is caused by air passing through a wound that has penetrated the respiratory system. The victim will be experiencing difficulty with breathing because air is escaping as he or she breathes.

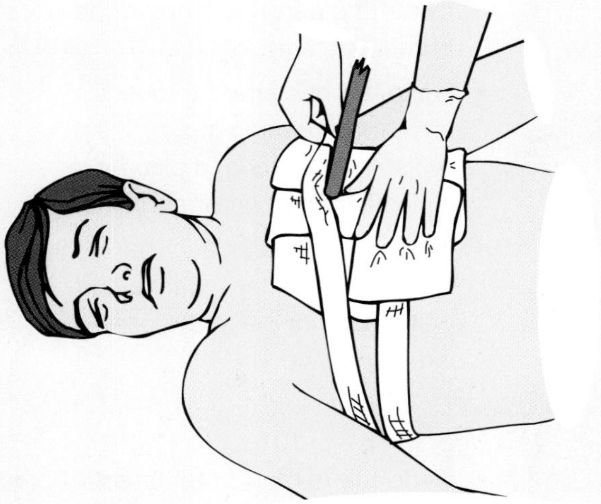

FIGURE 21–5 Never remove an object protruding from the body. Immobilize the object by placing dressings around the object and taping the dressing in place.

(continues)

PROCEDURE 21–2

First Aid for Bleeding and Wounds

(continued)

CONDITION AND SIGNS AND SYMPTOMS	PROCEDURE	RATIONALE
Sucking Wounds (continued)	• With a sucking wound, apply an airtight dressing (e.g., plastic wrap, tin foil, plastic bag, or other nonporous material) over the site. If you do not have nonporous material, you can use a regular gauze pad or clean cloth coated with petroleum jelly (i.e., Vaseline).	• An airtight dressing prevents the escape of air from the respiratory system.
	• When applying an airtight dressing, leave one edge untaped or unsealed.	• This allows trapped air to escape.
	• Do not move the patient unless absolutely necessary.	• Movement may cause further injury.
	• Do not give the patient anything by mouth.	• Surgery may be required.
Amputations *S/S*: Part of the body severed from its attachment (e.g., all or part of a finger, toe, arm, leg, nose, or ear).	• If an amputation of a body part occurs, save the severed part.	• It may be possible to reattach the amputated part after reaching the hospital.
	• After giving the appropriate first aid to the victim, try to locate the part if it is not in the immediate area.	• First aid for the victim is the first priority.
	• Once the body part is found, rinse it off, wrap it in a moistened cloth, and place it in a plastic bag or other container.	• A clean, moist body part is more apt to be successfully reattached.
	• If ice is available, place the bag in a container with ice and water. Do not place the part directly on ice.	• Lowering the temperature of the body part will extend the amount of time for successful reattachment. Direct contact with the ice will cause freezing and damage the tissue.
	• Write the name of the patient and the time of the accident on the container with the body part.	• This assists medical personnel at the hospital who will decide if reattachment is possible.
	• Make sure the amputated body part remains with the victim when he or she is transported to the hospital.	• This prevents unnecessary delays in locating the part.

Fascinating Facts

The National Center for Environmental Health (NCEH; www.cdc.gov/nceh/), which is part of the Centers for Disease Control and Prevention (CDC), reports the following statistics:

- Unintentional injuries were the fifth leading cause of death for all ages.
- Poisonings were responsible for 25% of the injury deaths, followed by motor vehicle traffic accidents at 17.5%, and firearms 17.4%.
- There were 34.4 million medically attended injury and poisoning episodes in the noninstitutionalized population.
- Home was the leading place of injury occurrence, accounting for 42% (24% in the home and 18% outside the home) of the respondent-reported nonfatal, medically attended injury episodes.

Thinking It Through

Marlow Barrons is a nurse on vacation in Alaska. After fishing all day, she and her friends are unloading their boat when an emergency call comes to the Coast Guard. She overhears them discussing that a professional fisherman has amputated his arm in the gears of his boat. She tells them she is a nurse and offers assistance. Her offer is accepted, she boards the Coast Guard boat, and they speed off to the site of the accident.

1. What signs and symptoms can Marlow anticipate seeing based on the report of the accident?
2. What type of first aid should she anticipate the victim will need?
3. Are there special considerations regarding the amputated arm?

PROCEDURE 21–3

First Aid for Bone, Joint, and Muscle Injuries

Always Observe Standard Precautions

CONDITION AND SIGNS AND SYMPTOMS	PROCEDURE	RATIONALE
Fractures and Joint Dislocations *S/S*: Pain, swelling, and loss of function. In an open fracture, a bone protrudes through the skin, creating a wound. If the joint is dislocated, the joint will appear deformed. Deformity may also occur with fractures.	• Immobilize the broken bone or dislocated joint using a splint or sling. (See Figures 21–6a–c). Do not move the victim until the affected limb is immobilized, unless there is no other option. If no medical supplies are available, look around for items that will work as an alternate splint (e.g., a thick twig or board could be used on each side of a leg or arm and attached with strips of cloth; a sweater could be used to make a sling for the arm).	• This prevents further injury.

(continues)

PROCEDURE 21–3

First Aid for Bone, Joint, and Muscle Injuries

(continued)

CONDITION AND SIGNS AND SYMPTOMS	PROCEDURE	RATIONALE
Fractures and Joint Dislocations (continued)	• Do not attempt to realign a misshapen bone or joint. Do not test for function.	• This may cause further injury to the tissues. For example, it could cause hemorrhage, nerve damage, or an embolus (a mass that travels through the body and can cause damage elsewhere by obstructing blood flow).
	• Do not give anything by mouth.	• The victim may require surgical repair of the bone.

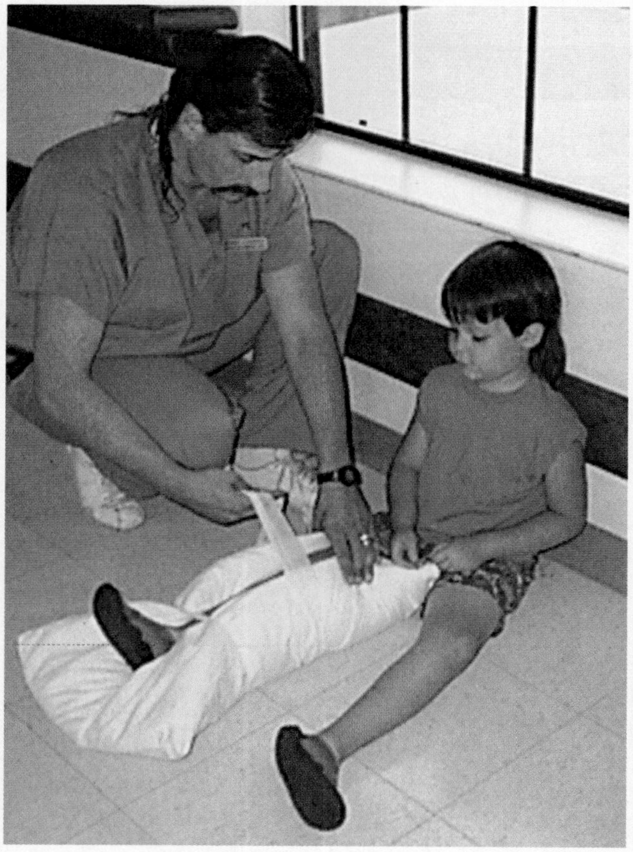

FIGURE 21–6a Splints should be long enough to immobilize the joint above and below the injured area.

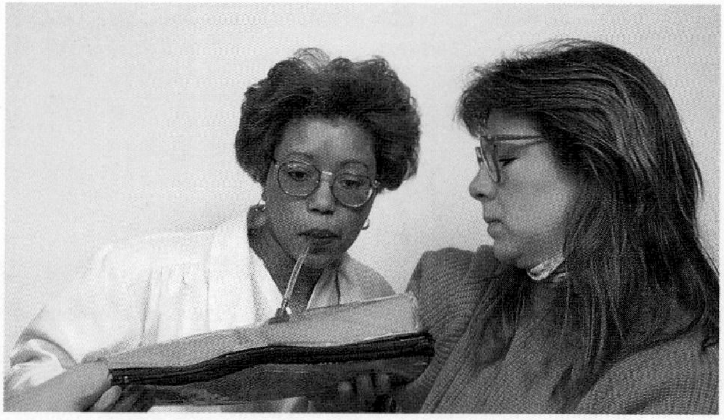

FIGURE 21–6b Some air splints are inflated by blowing into a nozzle. Care must be taken to avoid overinflating any splint. Always check for a pulse distal to the splint.

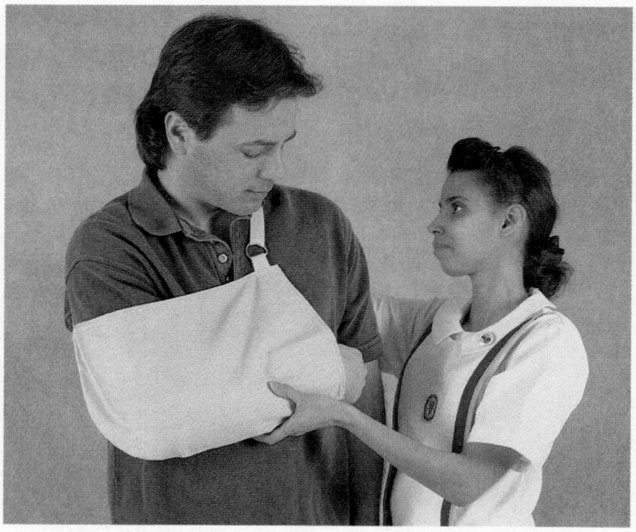

FIGURE 21–6c Commercial slings usually have a series of straps that extend around the neck and the trunk of the body.

(continues)

PROCEDURE 21–3

First Aid for Bone, Joint, and Muscle Injuries

(continued)

CONDITION AND SIGNS AND SYMPTOMS	PROCEDURE	RATIONALE
Fractures and Joint Dislocations (continued)	• If there is an open fracture, cover it with a dressing prior to immobilizing the area. Do not wash or attempt to remove anything from the area.	• The dressing prevents further contamination of the wound. Washing or removing anything from the area can result in further damage.
	• When immobilizing an area, leave it in the position in which you found it and make sure that the area above and below has extra support, so the injured area is immobilized.	• This prevents further injury.
	• Check for circulation below the injury to ensure that the splint is not too tight.	• Lack of circulation can result in damage to and death of the tissues.
Muscle Strain (Pulled Muscle) *S/S*: Sudden tearing sensation felt during exertion, followed by pain and swelling.	• Remove any constricting clothing or jewelry.	• Clothing and jewelry act as a constricting band if swelling occurs.
	• Apply cold compresses as soon as possible and repeat every 3–4 hours for 15–20 minutes.	• This decreases swelling.
	• Do not place ice directly on the skin.	• Freezing the skin causes tissue damage.
	• Elevate the limb.	• This decreases swelling.
	• Contact a physician if the pain is severe, if there is loss of function or impairment of circulation below the injury, or if the area is misshapen.	• The injury will need medical evaluation and treatment.
	• A physician may also recommend an over-the-counter anti-inflammatory medication.	• This decreases inflammation and swelling.
	• Rest the injured area for at least 24 hours. Do not use the injured area if pain occurs with movement.	• Rest allows the injury to heal and prevents further injury.
	• If there is no improvement, seek medical assistance.	• The injured area needs further evaluation.
Sprain *S/S*: Pain and swelling; loosening of the joint. Unless there is a complete tear, the joint will still function.	• Same as for muscle strain.	• Same as for muscle strain.

Injuries to Facial Structures

Injuries to the eyes, ears, and nose are common. Any eye injury should always be taken very seriously because it can involve the loss of vision. A blow to the ear can cause loss of hearing.

See Procedure 21–4 for first aid related to injuries of the facial structures.

Burns

Burns can occur from heat, radiation, chemicals, or electrical current. The severity of the burn is determined by the size, depth, and location of the burn. Minor burns are referred to as *superficial* or *first-degree burns* because only the top layer of the skin (epidermis) is involved. If the burn continues and extends beyond the superficial layer to the dermis, it is a *partial-thickness* or *second-degree burn*. (See Figure 21–7.) If the burn continues even deeper, it is a *full-thickness* or *third-degree burn*. (See Figure 21–8.) The amount of pain the victim reports does not necessarily reflect the severity of the burn because deeper burns can destroy nerve endings and be painless. (See Figure 21–9.)

When caring for burns, remember the following three steps:

1. Stop the burning.
2. Cool the burned area.
3. Cover the burned area with clean, dry dressings (apply loosely).

See Procedure 21–5 for first aid related to the various sources of burns.

When treating burn victims, always assess them for the possibility of damage to the respiratory system through inhalation of smoke or fumes from chemicals. The damage to the respiratory system can cause swelling that will prevent the victim from breathing properly. Look for discoloration around the nostrils or mouth as a possible indication. If it is likely that the victim has inhaled smoke or fumes (was in a smoky room, exposed to chemical fumes, or has discolored nostrils) but is not experiencing difficulty

PROCEDURE 21–4

First Aid for Facial Injuries

Always Observe Standard Precautions

CONDITION AND SIGNS AND SYMPTOMS	PROCEDURE	RATIONALE
Eye Injuries *S/S*: Tearing, redness, stinging, burning, or pain in or around the eye; sensitivity to light; and rapid blinking. Blows to the eye can cause internal bleeding and damage to the tissues.	• Do not press on the eye or allow the victim to rub the eyes.	• This prevents further injury.
	• If a foreign object is irritating the eye, flush the eye with a large amount of water.	• Loose particles will wash away in the water.
	• Do not use cotton swabs (e.g., Q-tips) or any instruments (e.g., tweezers) to try to remove objects from eye.	• Cotton sheds fibers that will get in the eye. Sharp instruments can cause further damage.
	• If the object is not flushed out and is embedded, do not attempt to remove it; instead cover both eyes with a dressing and await medical assistance.	• Trying to remove the object can create more damage. Covering both eyes decreases movement of the injured eye.

(continues)

PROCEDURE 21–4

First Aid for Facial Injuries

(continued)

CONDITION AND SIGNS AND SYMPTOMS	PROCEDURE	RATIONALE
Eye Injuries (continued)	• If there has been a blow to the eye, lay the victim flat, cover both eyes, and call for medical assistance.	• Laying the victim flat decreases loss of fluid from the eye. Covering both eyes decreases movement of the eyes.
	• If a "black eye" is forming, apply a cold compress to the area.	• A cold compress decreases bleeding by causing vasoconstriction (constriction of blood vessels).
Ear Injuries *S/S*: Bleeding or drainage from the ear, loss of hearing, earache, redness, bruising, or swelling around the ear. Ruptured eardrum causes severe pain.	• Do not block bleeding or drainage from the ear. If possible, lay the victim on his or her side with the injured ear down.	• Promoting drainage will prevent buildup of pressure in the ear that can cause more damage.
	• Do not attempt to clean inside the ear.	• This prevents further injury and contamination.
	• If an object is in the ear and clearly visible, place the victim's injured ear downward and gently wiggle the object with tweezers.	• This may dislodge the object, and it will fall out as a result of gravity.
	• Do not attempt to remove an object that is not visible. Seek medical assistance.	• This may push the object farther into the ear canal.
	• If ruptured eardrum is suspected, place a dressing over the ear. Seek medical assistance.	• This prevents contamination of the ear.
	• If an insect is in the ear, do not allow the victim to poke a finger into the ear. Have the victim hold his or her head with the ear pointing up. If medical assistance is not immediately available, the victim is very uncomfortable, and you are sure it is only an insect, place several drops of room-temperature oil into the ear (e.g., cooking oil, baby oil, mineral oil). Seek medical assistance.	• Putting an object in the ear may cause an insect to bite or sting. The insect may climb out on its own if given an opportunity. Oil will drown the insect, but can dangerously expand other objects that may be in the ear.

(continues)

PROCEDURE 21–4

First Aid for Facial Injuries

(continued)

CONDITION AND SIGNS AND SYMPTOMS	PROCEDURE	RATIONALE
Nose Injuries Most nosebleeds (epistaxis) stop on their own, but if not, first aid may be needed. *S/S*: Blood coming from the nostrils or running down the back of the throat. If the bleeding is from the back of the nose, there may be a feeling of fullness in the ears, coughing up blood, gagging, or choking due to blood in the back of the throat. A broken nose may look crooked.	• If there is an object lodged in the nostril, attempt to remove it by having the victim hold the other nostril and blow out the nostril with the object, or have the victim sniff some pepper to induce a sneeze. If this does not work, get medical help.	• This increases pressure behind the object to propel it out.
	• Do not put anything into the nostril to try to grab hold of the object.	• This may push the object in farther.
	• Instruct the victim to breathe through the mouth and not inhale through the nostril.	• This decreases the risk of blood entering into lungs.
	• If the nose may be broken, have the victim sit down, lean forward, and apply a cold compress.	• Leaning forward helps prevent blood from running down the back of the throat. A cold compress decreases bleeding by constricting blood vessels.
	• Do not attempt to straighten a broken nose, but seek medical assistance.	• This may cause further damage.
	• If the nose is not broken, attempt to stop the bleeding by instructing the victim to sit down and lean forward while applying pressure on the soft part of the nose. Maintain the pressure for at least 15 minutes, then release. If there is still bleeding, repeat the procedure for 15 more minutes. Then, if it has not stopped, seek medical assistance.	• Leaning forward helps prevent blood from running down the back of throat. Applying pressure decreases the blood flow and encourages clotting. If you cannot stop the bleeding, medical evaluation and treatment are needed.

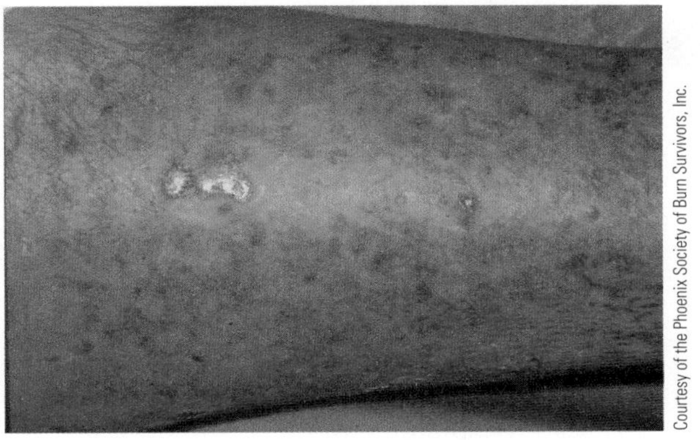

FIGURE 21–7 Second-degree or partial-thickness burn: The skin is wet, red, swollen, painful, and blistered.

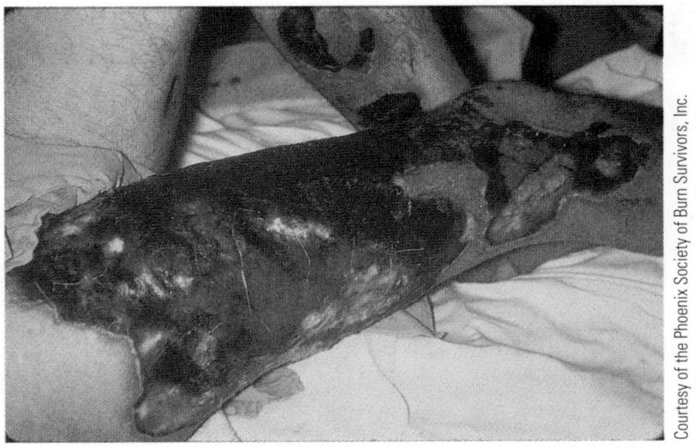

FIGURE 21–8 Third-degree or full-thickness burn: All layers of the skin, plus the fat, muscles, bone, and nerve tissues, are destroyed.

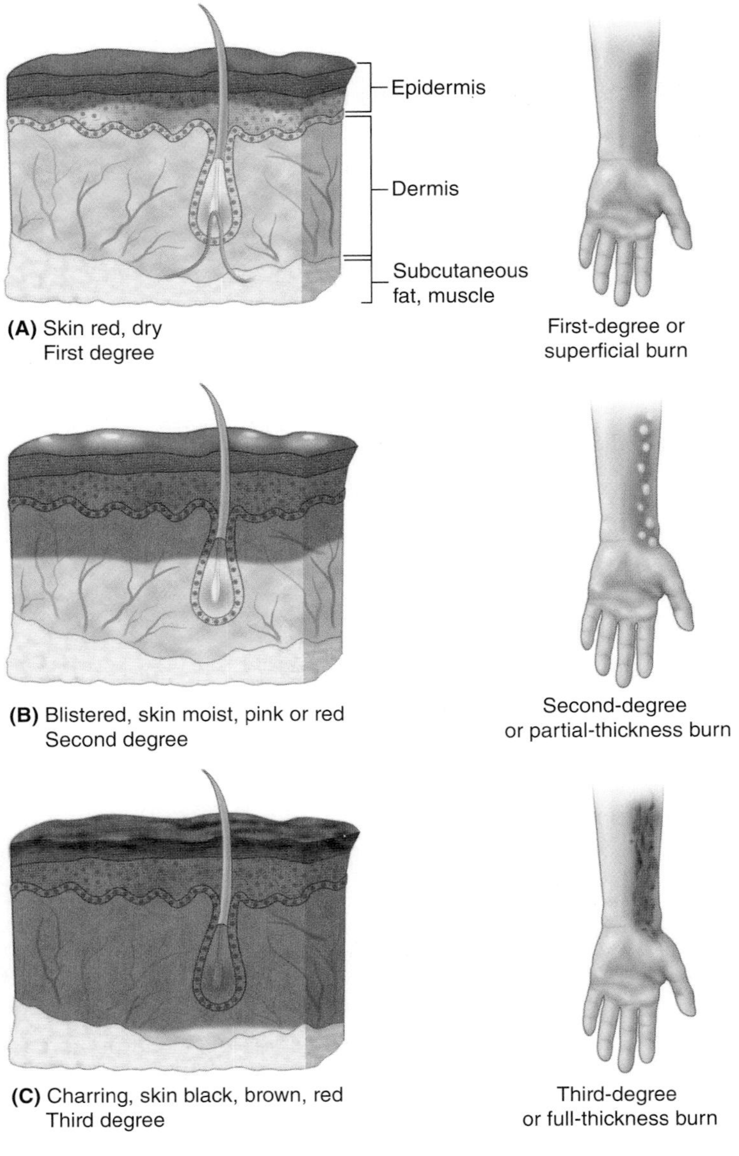

FIGURE 21–9 Types of burns.

PROCEDURE 21–5

First Aid for Burns

Always Observe Standard Precautions

CONDITION	PROCEDURE	RATIONALE
Heat (e.g., flames, hot liquids, or grease)	• Extinguish the fire (e.g., if the victim's clothing is on fire).	• This stops the burning.
	• Move the victim to a well-ventilated area if smoke is present. Move accident victims only when it is necessary to protect them.	• This protects the victim from damage to respiratory tract due to smoke inhalation.
	• When moving victims, maintain their body alignment.	• This prevents further damage in the event they may have a neck or back injury.
	• Run cool water over the burned area for several minutes or immerse the area in cool water (use a cool, wet cloth on areas that cannot be immersed and rewet as necessary by pouring additional cool water onto the cloth).	• This cools the burned area. Cooling should not be done if a burn is major or covers an extensive area, because it can dangerously lower the body temperature.
	• Do not apply ice except on a minor burn, such as a finger burned on the stove.	• This can freeze tissue and cause further damage.
	• Remove clothing from the burn area if possible, but if it is stuck to the burn, do not use force.	• Forcibly removing clothing will increase damage to tissues.
	• Do not break blisters.	• Blisters form a natural sterile protection to the area.
	• Cover the burn with a clean, dry cloth (use sterile, nonadhesive dressings if available).	• This covers the burned area to prevent contamination.
	• Do not apply any ointments to a severe burn.	• Ointments can hold the heat in, increasing the severity of the burn.
	• Apply a bandage loosely.	• This prevents pressure on the burn.
	• Do not use cotton as a dressing.	• Cotton adheres and leaves small fibers embedded in the wound.
	• Prevent chilling.	• Chilling is common with burns.
Radiation (e.g., sunburn)	• Move the victim so he or she is no longer exposed to the sun.	• This stops the burning.
	• Cool the burn as discussed earlier.	• Same as for heat burns.
	• Apply a dressing as discussed for heat burns.	• Same as for heat burns.
	• Prevent chilling.	• Same as for heat burns.

(continues)

PROCEDURE 21–5

First Aid for Burns

(continued)

CONDITION	PROCEDURE	RATIONALE
Chemicals Numerous household and environmental products cause burns when in contact with skin.	• Prevent any further contact of the victim with the chemical.	• If any chemical remains on the victim's clothing, it will continue to burn the victim; if possible, remove any clothing and jewelry exposed to the chemical.
	• Move the victim to a well-ventilated area if fumes are present. Move accident victims only when it is necessary to protect them.	• This protects victim from damage to the respiratory tract due to inhalation of fumes.
	• When moving victims, maintain their body alignment.	• This prevents further damage if the victim has a back or neck injury.
	• Flush the burn with large amounts of cool water and continue to do so until EMS arrive.	• This cools the burn.
	• Always flush away from the body.	• This prevents the chemical-laden water from touching unexposed areas of the skin.
	• If there is any chemical in the eyes, flush them continuously with cool water.	• Eyes are very sensitive to chemical burns, and vision may be lost if chemicals are not completely removed.
	• If only one eye is affected, flush from the inner aspect of the eye to the outer. (See Figure 21–10.)	• This prevents the chemical from getting into the other eye.
Electrical Current (electrical cords or lines and lightning)	• Do not touch the victim if he or she is still in contact with a live electrical wire (have the power turned off first).	• As the rescuer, you must protect yourself first. If you are unable to touch the victim, call EMS.
	• Do not cool the burn.	• Burns are not on the surface.
	• Apply a clean, dry dressing.	• This prevents contamination.
	• Prevent chilling and do not move the victim if possible, because other injuries may be present.	• There will usually be only a small burn area noted on the surface, but extensive internal damage can be present, caused by the current as it traveled through the body (look for an exit burn also).

(continues)

PROCEDURE 21–5

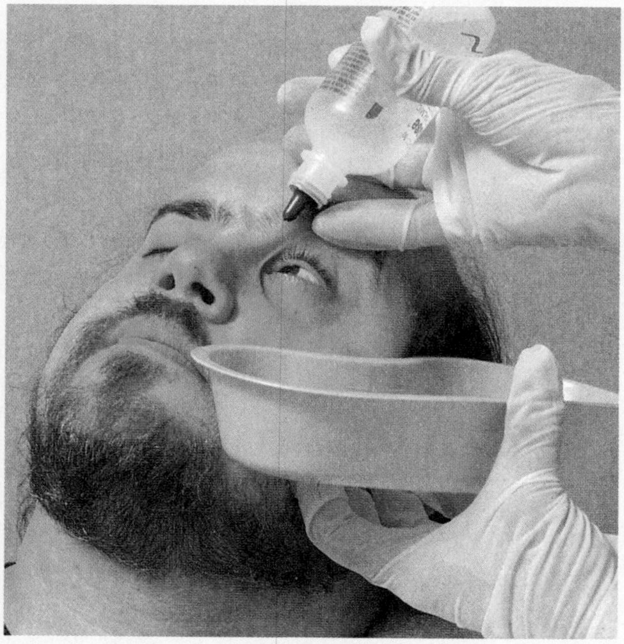

FIGURE 21–10 To flush an eye, hold the eyelid open and run the water from the inner part of the eye toward the outer part.

in breathing, do not dismiss the problem because the effects can be delayed for up to 24 hours.

Drug Abuse

"Drug abuse" refers to the misuse or overuse of any drug. These drugs may be legal or illegal, prescription or over the counter, and include any substance that alters how the body functions. For example, prescription and over-the-counter medications, caffeine, alcohol, nicotine, or any illegal drug preparation can cause life-threatening situations.

Another condition that can cause the need for medical intervention is when an addictive drug is taken and the body develops a craving for more of the drug. If the drug is not continued, the body will go through a process of withdrawal that can also create life-threatening situations.

See Procedure 21–6 for first aid related to drug overdose and withdrawal.

Poisoning

Poisoning most commonly occurs through ingestion and inhalation. Poisons that come in contact with the skin are treated similarly to burns that occur when caustic (destructive to living tissue) chemicals come into contact with skin. The procedure is to perform lots of flushing to remove the poison, while taking care not to get it on the victim's uncontaminated areas or on the rescuer's skin.

If you suspect poisoning, do not wait for signs and symptoms to develop; instead seek medical assistance immediately. Do not rely on the label's directions, because they may be incorrect. Instead call the poison control center or EMS because they can supply you with the information needed to immediately and most effectively treat the poison victim.

Identifying the source of the poison is important in determining the proper treatment for the victim. If the victim is unable to give any information (is a child, unconscious, or confused), look around for any clues as to the source of the poison (e.g., empty bottle or other container, source of fumes, traces of powders or liquids in the area, poisonous plants, and bystander information).

The most critical component of poisoning first aid is prevention. Because young children are the

PROCEDURE 21–6

First Aid for Drug-Related Problems

Always Observe Standard Precautions

CONDITION AND SIGNS AND SYMPTOMS	PROCEDURE	RATIONALE
Drug Overdose *S/S*: Behavioral changes, such as overexcitation, hallucinations, and agitation. There may be difficulty breathing, drowsiness, tremors, and excessive sweating. The size of the pupil is often smaller or larger than normal. Nausea and vomiting may occur. Seizures and unconsciousness may develop.	• Call EMS.	• The victim needs medical evaluation and intervention.
	• Try to determine what was taken, when, how much, and which route (e.g., oral, inhalation, injection). Be aware that it may have been more than one type or also combined with alcohol or other substances.	• This information will assist in determination of treatment.
	• If possible, collect samples of the drug and of any vomit for analysis.	• These samples can be analyzed to assist in determination of treatment.
Withdrawal from Addictive Drug *S/S*: Behavioral changes, such as extreme restlessness, hallucinations, depression, anxiety, and agitation. Tremors and cold sweats may occur. Nausea and vomiting may occur. Seizures may develop. The main focus of the victim may be to find some of the drug he or she is withdrawing from in order to alleviate the discomfort.	• Call EMS.	• Same as for drug overdose.
	• Try to determine what drug the victim has been taking.	• Same as for drug overdose.
	• Keep the victim safe and comfortable until medical assistance arrives.	• The victim may harm himself or herself when experiencing severe behavioral changes or if seizures occur.

frequent victims of accidental poisoning, it is essential to keep all harmful substances locked in cabinets or out of the reach of children. Remember that children can be quite inventive in using furniture to climb up to reach desired objects, so using a locked cabinet is the preferred approach.

Poisoning by ingestion can be caused by many common products found around the home, such as cleaning agents, yard care products, cosmetics, medications, paints, plants, car fluids, personal care items, and spoiled food or contaminated water. Inhalation dangers include sources of poisonous fumes, such as gas leaks, automobile exhaust, and chemical fumes.

See Procedure 21–7 for first aid related to poisoning.

Temperature-Related Illness

Exposure to excessive cold can cause cold-related injuries. If the skin begins to freeze, it is called frostbite.

PROCEDURE 21–7

First Aid for Poisonings

Always Observe Standard Precautions

CONDITION AND SIGNS AND SYMPTOMS	PROCEDURE	RATIONALE
Ingestion (swallowing) *S/S*: Vary widely depending on the substance ingested and how it affects the various systems. For example, gastrointestinal (GI) symptoms may include nausea, vomiting, diarrhea, abdominal pain, or loss of appetite. The skin may be pale, and the victim may feel dizzy, weak, irritable, or drowsy. There may be pain while swallowing or burns or residue around the mouth. There may be seizures or complete loss of consciousness.	• The goal of immediate treatment is to get the poison out of the body, but do not administer any food, fluids, or home remedies or induce vomiting unless directed to do so by medical personnel.	• Getting the poison out of the body will prevent further absorption of the poison, but inducing vomiting for a substance that burned the GI system on the way down will also burn it on the way up.
	• If the victim does vomit, make sure the vomit is cleared from the mouth.	• This prevents it from blocking the airway and from entering the lungs.
	• Save any vomit.	• It can be analyzed to identify the source of the poisoning.
	• Keep the patient safe and comfortable until help can arrive.	• This prevents further injury and decreases anxiety.
Inhalation (breathing) *S/S*: Vary depending on the substance inhaled. May be similar to the signs and symptoms listed for ingestion.	• The goal of immediate treatment is to get the victim into fresh air.	• This prevents further inhalation of poisonous gas.
	• Before entering an environment where poisonous gases may be present, apply protective breathing gear. If no protective breathing gear is available, place a wet cloth over your nose and mouth, and then take several deep breaths of fresh air before entering to remove the victim.	• The rescuer must protect himself or herself against becoming the second victim of the fumes.
	• If there is a visible cloud of fumes, keep your head above or below it.	• The cloud will contain the highest concentration of fumes.
	• If possible, open windows and doors and turn off any source of fumes.	• This decreases the concentration of fumes in the area.
	• Do not light any flames or flip any switches.	• Fumes may ignite.
	• When the victim is in fresh air, the poison control center or EMS can be called.	• You will need further directions on care and the victim may need medical intervention.
	• The victim should be kept safe and comfortable until help arrives.	• This prevents further injury and decreases anxiety.

Frostbite occurs most commonly on the extremities or exposed areas, such as fingers, toes, nose, cheeks, and earlobes. If the body temperature drops below normal, it is **hypothermia**. Hypothermia can occur inside and outside the home, depending on a number of conditions. Conditions that contribute to hypothermia are extreme cold, wet clothes, and being immersed in cold water. Newborns, the elderly, and those in poor health can become hypothermic in an underheated room.

Exposure to excessive heat can cause heat-related injuries. Being outside in high temperatures and humidity can cause the body temperature to increase above normal (**hyperthermia**), and a loss of body fluids by excessive perspiration can result in the loss of salt and subsequent dehydration. Certain medications and medical conditions can aggravate the problem. Newborns, the elderly, and those in poor health can become hyperthermic in an overheated room with poor ventilation. Other contributing factors are obesity, excessive exercise, and ingestion of alcohol. The heat-related illnesses from least to most severe are heat cramps, heat exhaustion, and heat stroke.

See Procedure 21–8 for first aid for temperature-related illnesses.

PROCEDURE 21–8

First Aid for Temperature-Related Illnesses

Always Observe Standard Precautions

CONDITION AND SIGNS AND SYMPTOMS	PROCEDURE	RATIONALE
Frostbite *S/S*: Initially the skin is red and painful; then as the skin begins to freeze, it loses feeling (numbness), then becomes hard and white and blisters. In severe frostbite, the blood vessels freeze and the skin becomes black due to the death of tissues from lack of oxygen.	• Do not thaw out the area unless it can be kept thawed.	• Refreezing will increase damage.
	• Do not massage the area.	• This increases damage to tissues
	• Do not use direct heat to thaw the area.	• This thaws the area too quickly.
	• Remove any constricting clothes or jewelry.	• This increases circulation.
	• To thaw the frozen area, place it in warm water or apply a warm cloth; keep water or cloth warm (not hot) until area softens and color and sensation return; as the area thaws, pain and swelling can be expected.	• This thaws the area slowly.
	• After thawing, apply a sterile, dry dressing.	• This prevents contamination.
	• If fingers or toes are frostbitten, place a dressing between them.	• This keeps them separated.
	• Move the thawed area as little as possible.	• This minimizes damage to tissues.
	• Discourage smoking or drinking alcohol	• Both constrict the blood vessels and decrease circulation to the affected area.

(continues)

PROCEDURE 21–8

First Aid for Temperature-Related Illnesses

(continued)

CONDITION AND SIGNS AND SYMPTOMS	PROCEDURE	RATIONALE
Hypothermia *S/S*: In mild cases there is shivering, skin is cold to the touch, and there is confusion and lack of coordination. In severe cases the shivering stops; coordination problems increase, along with slurred speech and problems with vision; the heart rate slows; and the victim becomes drowsy and just wants to be left alone. The victim can become irrational and uncooperative. If untreated, the victim will progress to coma and death.	• If frostbite and hypothermia are present, treat the hypothermia first.	• Hypothermia is the most life threatening.
	• If respirations are below 6 per minute, begin rescue breathing.	• This supplies the victim with needed oxygen.
	• If possible, gently move the victim to a shelter.	• This removes the victim from further exposure.
	• Remove wet clothes and replace them with dry ones.	• Wet clothes increase the cooling of the body.
	• Remove constricting clothes and jewelry.	• This increases circulation.
	• Do not use direct heat.	• It may burn the victim.
	• Apply warm packs (towels or linens) to the neck, chest, and groin.	• These packs warm the body.
	• If the victim is able to drink, give him or her warm, sweet fluids.	• This warms the body internally and supplies some calories.
	• Wrap the victim in a space blanket (contains an insulating material that prevents heat from escaping) or aluminum foil, including the neck and head; the rescuer can also place his or her own body next to the victim to warm him or her.	• This assists in rewarming the victim.
HEAT-RELATED CONDITIONS: **Heat Cramps** *S/S*: Muscle cramps in the abdomen and legs, lightheadedness, and weakness may occur when excess salt and fluid are lost from the body (heavy perspiration). If the problem progresses to heat exhaustion, the skin may appear pale or red, cool to the touch, and moist; the victim may complain of headache, thirst, weakness, and dizziness; the pupils will be dilated (larger than normal), and nausea and vomiting may occur; behavior may be irrational or the victim may be unconscious.	• Do not give liquids that contain alcohol or caffeine.	• The victim needs water and electrolytes to replenish what was lost.
	• Do not give any medication used to lower the temperature (e.g., aspirin or Tylenol).	• This does not treat the underlying problem.
	• Do not give salt tablets; instead use a salt-and-water solution or an electrolyte drink (e.g., Gatorade or Pedialyte).	• Salt-and-water solutions replenish fluid and electrolytes.
	• Fan the victim.	• Cools by increasing evaporation.
	• Move the victim to the shade or a cooled room and elevate the feet if not prohibited (e.g., it causes difficulty breathing; there is a head, neck, spine, or leg injury; or it makes the victim uncomfortable).	• It is important to begin the cooling process immediately.

(continues)

PROCEDURE 21–8

First Aid for Temperature-Related Illnesses (continued)

CONDITION AND SIGNS AND SYMPTOMS	PROCEDURE	RATIONALE
Heat Cramps (continued)	• Apply cool water to the body (do not use alcohol rub); wrap the victim in cool towels and turn on a fan.	• This aids in cooling by increasing the evaporative process.
	• Apply cold towels to the back of the neck, on the groin, and under the arms.	• This cools the major areas where blood vessels are close to the surface.
	• When the temperature lowers to 100°F, the cooling effort can be stopped, but monitor the victim closely for the next 2–4 hours.	• The victim may relapse even after apparent recovery.
Heat Stroke The skin will be dry, hot, and red; confusion, weakness, and seizures may occur; pupils will be constricted (smaller than normal), pulse rapid and weak, and breathing rapid and shallow; the body temperature will be markedly increased (above 102°F); the victim may be unconscious.	• Call EMS.	• This condition is life threatening.
	• Do not give liquids to a victim with heat stroke.	• Fluids may enter the lungs. EMS will start an IV when they arrive.
	• If EMS is not immediately available, immerse the victim in cold water, but monitor his or her alertness, pulse, and respirations closely.	• This starts the cooling process.

Thinking It Through

John Street is a health care student and is feeling the need to get away from the stress and routine of studying. He decides to take a hike in the local mountains with his friends. As they ascend the mountain, it gets cooler and begins to rain. One of the hikers, Paul, starts to lag behind. Paul has always been a slower climber, so they continue on. A little while later, John turns around to see how Paul is doing and can no longer see him. John backtracks and finds Paul sitting beside the trail. He is shivering and his skin is cold to the touch. Paul says he is just very tired and needs to rest for a while and that he will catch up later.

1. Should John leave Paul to rest by himself?
2. What may be happening to Paul?
3. What first aid, if any, should be given to Paul?

Other Conditions

A number of other conditions that commonly occur may require the assistance of someone trained in first aid. They may be seen separately or some of them may be seen in conjunction with any of the other conditions already presented. Knowledge of these conditions will prepare the rescuer to take the appropriate actions when they occur. See Procedure 21–9 for first aid related to these conditions.

Bandaging

Knowing how to apply slings and wraps can be very useful when working with a variety of injuries requiring first aid. See Procedures 21–10 through 21–13 for applying a triangular sling and three wraps, commonly used with musculoskeletal injuries.

PROCEDURE 21–9

First Aid for Other Common Conditions

Always Observe Standard Precautions

CONDITION AND SIGNS AND SYMPTOMS	PROCEDURE	RATIONALE
Breathing Difficulty Problems with breathing can be caused by many sudden illnesses, injuries, or worsening medical conditions. *S/S*: Shortness of breath, coughing, audible sounds (wheezing, gurgling, whistling) coming from respiratory system, and exaggerated use of chest muscles to breathe. If the victim is not getting enough oxygen, the mouth and fingertips may be pale or bluish in color.	• Do not place a pillow under the victim's head.	• This may close off the airway.
	• Loosen any constricting clothing and assist the victim into the most comfortable position, unless neck or back injury is suspected.	• Constricting clothing may prevent the victim from breathing deeply.
	• Ask the victim if there is any medication he or she takes for the problem (e.g., asthmatics may have an inhaler with them).	• Symptoms may be alleviated with their medication.
	• Call EMS and keep the victim safe and comfortable until help arrives.	• The victim may need evaluation and treatment.
Hyperventilation Rapid breathing that causes the carbon dioxide level in the blood to fall too low. The most common cause is anxiety, but it may also be caused by illness, injury, or certain medications. *S/S*: Fast, shallow respiratory rate, followed by the sensation of numbness around the mouth and in the hands and feet. Blood pressure may fall, and fainting can occur.	• Have victims breathe into a paper bag, hold one nostril closed (make sure the mouth is closed) while breathing, or have them cup their hands over their mouth and nose while breathing.	• These techniques are effective in returning the carbon dioxide level in the bloodstream to normal.
	• The victim will need a calm and reassuring approach. Encouraging the victim to talk is often helpful.	• This condition is often caused by or worsened with anxiety.
Chest Pain (Angina) Chest pain is associated with a lack of oxygen to the heart muscle. Damage to the heart muscle from a lack of oxygen is called a heart attack or myocardial infarction. *S/S*: Pain is described as dull or crushing (victim may state that "it feels like an elephant is	• Always call EMS immediately.	• Many victims deny that they are having a heart attack and instead explain it as indigestion. They may be correct, but any chest pain needs to be evaluated medically to determine if the victim had a heart attack.
	• Have the victim stop any activity he or she was doing.	• This decreases the demand on the heart.

(continues)

PROCEDURE 21–9

First Aid for Other Common Conditions

(continued)

CONDITION AND SIGNS AND SYMPTOMS	PROCEDURE	RATIONALE
Chest Pain (Angina) (continued) sitting on my chest"). The pain may radiate to the shoulder, arm, or jaw. Angina can also be felt in atypical locations (especially in females), such as jaw, back, or underarms. There may be difficulty breathing and heart palpitations. Often the victim will perspire heavily and feel nauseated and anxious, and the skin will be pale or bluish and moist.	• If the victim has medication for angina, assist him or her in taking it.	• Many people with recurring chest pain have a medication called nitroglycerin that is placed under the tongue.
	• Do not give the victim anything to eat or drink.	• This increases demand on the heart, and the victim may develop nausea and vomiting.
	• Loosen any constricting clothing and keep the victim warm.	• This encourages full deep breathing and circulation.
	• Stay with the victim until help arrives.	• If the condition worsens, the victim may need rescue breathing or CPR.
	• Start rescue breathing if he or she stops breathing, or give full CPR if the heart stops.	• Brain damage occurs in as little as 3–5 minutes when the brain is deprived of oxygen.
Diabetes Lack of adequate insulin production results in elevated blood sugar; if too much medication is taken to correct this condition, the blood sugar may become too low. *S/S: High blood sugar* (hyperglycemia) develops gradually and is characterized by excessive thirst, hunger, and urination. There may be vomiting, flushed skin, rapid breathing, and a fruity smell to the breath. The victim may be confused and resist your attempt to assist. If left untreated, the victim will go into a diabetic coma. *S/S: Low blood sugar* (hypoglycemia) develops more rapidly and is characterized by sweating, hunger, confusion, pale skin, and poor coordination. This is referred to as an insulin reaction and if left untreated may result in coma and death.	• If victims state that their blood sugar is too high and they need to have an insulin injection, assist them with the administration of the medication.	• Many diabetics are very familiar with the signs and symptoms and know how to treat it.
	• Get medical help and stay with the victim to monitor his or her condition.	• The condition may worsen and further assistance will be needed.
	• If the victim is conscious, give him or her unsweetened liquids.	• Liquids with sugar will make the problem worse, so use unsweetened liquids as they will combat the dehydration that occurs with hyperglycemia without increasing the blood sugar.
	• If the victim states that his or her blood sugar is too low, immediately give something sweet (e.g., fruit juice, sugar in water, candy). If this is the problem, the victim should improve within 5–15 minutes after administration of the sweet.	• Many diabetics are very familiar with the signs and symptoms and know how to treat it. Sweetened items increase the blood sugar.

(continues)

PROCEDURE 21–9

First Aid for Other Common Conditions

(continued)

CONDITION AND SIGNS AND SYMPTOMS	PROCEDURE	RATIONALE
Diabetes (continued)	• When recovered, the victim should eat some protein and carbohydrates (e.g., crackers and cheese or peanut butter and bread).	• This prevents further insulin reaction because the quick-acting sweets are digested and eliminated quickly.
	• If the victim does not recover or is unconscious, call EMS.	• The victim needs further evaluation and treatment.
	• If in doubt as to whether it is high or low blood sugar, treat it with something sweet.	• If it is low blood sugar, the victim should recover quickly, and if high blood sugar, the additional sweet will not significantly affect the problem.
Fainting (Syncope) *S/S*: Brief loss of consciousness that comes on quickly, perhaps due to low blood sugar, standing too long, or low blood pressure when arising too rapidly from a lying or sitting position. Sometimes there are warning signs (dizziness, nausea, weakness, and blurred vision), but not always. A loss of consciousness after a head injury is not fainting, but a concussion.	• If you are present when the victim is falling, assist him or her gently to the floor.	• This prevents injury from the fall.
	• Place the victim on his or her back and elevate the legs 8–12 inches.	• This increases blood circulation to the brain.
	• Do not place a pillow under the head.	• This may obstruct airway.
	• Loosen any constricting clothing.	• This allows for deeper breathing and better circulation.
	• Do not attempt to awaken the victim by throwing water on him or her, shaking, or slapping the face.	• This is not an effective technique and may injure victim.
	• If vomiting occurs turn the head to the side.	• This prevents vomit from obstructing airway and entering the lungs.
	• Call EMS if the victim is not alert within approximately 5 minutes, is elderly, or other signs and symptoms are noted that may indicate another problem.	• The victim needs further evaluation and treatment.
Fever (Hyperthermia) *S/S*: An increase in body temperature, usually caused by the	• Remove excess clothing and blankets.	• Excess coverings can increase body temperature.

(continues)

PROCEDURE 21–9

First Aid for Other Common Conditions

(continued)

CONDITION AND SIGNS AND SYMPTOMS	PROCEDURE	RATIONALE
Fever (Hyperthermia) (continued) body's attempt to combat infection. (For elevated temperature related to exposure to heat, see hyperthermia under Temperature-Related Illnesses). Children are particularly susceptible to high fevers when an infection is present. The fever can rise quickly and result in seizures. The younger the child, the more sensitive he or she is to an increase in temperature.	• Gently cool the child by sponging him or her with lukewarm water.	• This lowers the body temperature.
	• Call the physician at once for further instructions, such as giving medication to bring the fever down (e.g. acetaminophen or aspirin (if child is over 2 years old).	• Fevers can rise very quickly in children, even to the point of causing brain damage.
	• Even lower fevers that persist over 24 hours need to be evaluated.	• The cause needs to be determined.
	• Call EMS if the child is having difficulty breathing, has unusual skin color, a stiff neck, or appears ill.	• This may indicate a serious underlying condition requiring immediate treatment.
Drowning Unconsciousness and death result from the lack of oxygen to the body as water enters the respiratory tract. Drowning can occur in only a few inches of water if the victim is a child or is injured. The most common causes are accidents, sudden illness, cramping, alcohol consumption, and getting into areas where the person is not a strong enough swimmer to return to safety. *S/S*: Skin cold and pale. Lips, earlobes, and fingernails are a bluish color. The victim may not be breathing.	• Be on the alert for irregular swimming strokes, when only the head is above the water, and if the person is fully dressed.	• Drowning victims usually cannot call for help.
	• Call EMS.	• The victim will need evaluation and treatment.
	• Rescue the drowning victim if you can do so without endangering yourself. It is best not to enter the water, but to extend a stick, life preserver, or some other object for the victim to grab and then pull him or her to safety.	• If the rescuer enters the water, he or she may become hypothermic or the victim may panic and pull the rescuer under too.
	• Do rescue breathing and treat the victim for hypothermia as needed. Do full CPR if no pulse is present.	• If the water is quite cold, the victim may still be able to be revived, even if submerged for longer than 3–5 minutes.
Seizures (Convulsions) Seizures are caused by irregular brain activity such as that seen in someone with epilepsy, or they can be caused by a sudden change in a medical condition. Many of the other first	• If the victim is falling, support the victim as he or she falls.	• This prevents injury to victim as he or she falls to the floor.
	• Remove any sharp objects in the area.	• This protects the victim from injury.

(continues)

PROCEDURE 21–9

First Aid for Other Common Conditions

(continued)

CONDITION AND SIGNS AND SYMPTOMS	PROCEDURE	RATIONALE
Seizures (Convulsions) (continued) aid emergencies discussed in this chapter can result in seizures. *S/S*: Sudden falling and loss of consciousness with drooling or frothing from the mouth. There may be loss of bowel or bladder control. Grunting or groaning may be heard. There are three common types of seizures: 1. Petit mal—brief unconsciousness, followed by confusion 2. Focal—localized twitching in one part of the body (e.g., face or arm) 3. Grand mal—generalized strong muscle spasms of the entire body	• Loosen tight clothing.	• This eases the ability to breathe.
	• Do not place anything into the mouth, try to restrain the victim, move the victim (unless in danger), or perform rescue breathing during a seizure.	• Most seizures last less than a minute, and the main role of the rescuer is to keep the victim safe from harm.
	• Do not try to keep the victim awake, but place him or her on the stomach or side (if you suspect neck or back injury, roll the body as a unit to a side-lying position, while keeping the spine in straight alignment). Protect the airway if vomiting occurs.	• After the seizure, the victim may go into a deep sleep after regaining consciousness momentarily and will probably be confused.
	• Call EMS.	• The victim may need further evaluation or treatment.
Shock Shock occurs when there is a disruption in the flow of blood to the cells throughout the body. Any medical emergency can cause shock. *S/S*: The victim may feel weak, dizzy, restless, or confused. The	• Call EMS.	• The victim needs further evaluation and treatment.
	• Place the victim in the shock position if there is no neck or back injury. (See Figure 21–11.)	• Elevating the lower extremities increases blood flow to the brain.
	• Turn the victim's head to the side if there is vomiting or drooling.	• This prevents blockage of the airway.

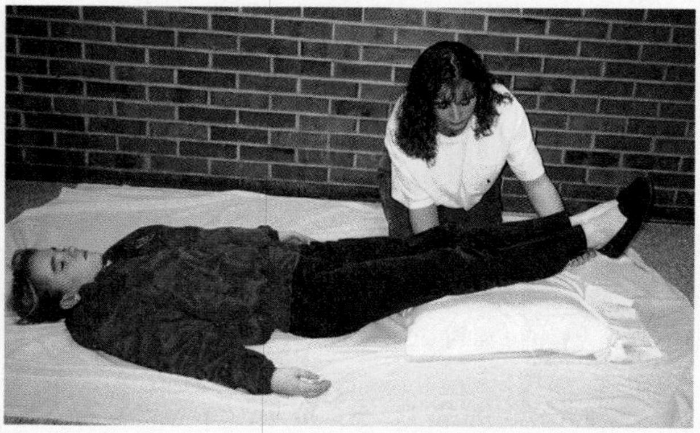

FIGURE 21–11 Place emergency victims in the shock position, unless they have neck, back, or lower limb injuries. Do not use the position if it is uncomfortable for the victim or if he or she has breathing difficulty.

(continues)

PROCEDURE 21–9

First Aid for Other Common Conditions

(continued)

CONDITION AND SIGNS AND SYMPTOMS	PROCEDURE	RATIONALE
Shock (continued) skin is pale, cold, and clammy. Lips, earlobes, and fingertips may be bluish. The respirations are shallow and rapid. Nausea, vomiting, and chest pain may be present. The victim may experience numbness and paralysis or be unconscious.	• Do not elevate the head.	• You want maximum flow of blood to the brain to prevent brain damage.
	• Loosen restricting clothes and keep the victim warm.	• This eases breathing and maintains blood flow.
	• Do not give the victim any liquids or food.	• The victim may vomit and block the airway.
	• Give first aid for any underlying illness or injury.	• Shock is normally secondary to another problem.
	• Do not use the shock position if it is uncomfortable.	• The victim may have another injury or illness.
	• Do not use the shock position if the victim has a sting or bite in the lower limbs.	• This increases the release of venom into the system.
	• Stay with the victim and assist as needed until medical help arrives.	• If the condition worsens, the victim may need rescue breathing or CPR performed.
Stroke or Cerebrovascular Accident (CVA) Caused by a ruptured or clogged artery in the brain resulting in death to the affected brain cells. *S/S*: Sudden onset of weakness, dizziness, headache, and unsteady coordination, followed by weakness or paralysis of the face, arm, and leg or one side of the face. Speech may be slurred or garbled, or absent, and vision may be affected. If the signs and symptoms are temporary and disappear within 24 hours, it was not a stroke, but a condition called a transient ischemic attack (TIA). Sometimes called a mini-stroke, a TIA is a temporary lack of oxygen to brain cells. It is a very serious sign and warns of a potential future stroke.	• Call EMS.	• The victim needs evaluation and treatment.
	• Help the victim get into a comfortable position.	• This eases breathing and anxiety.
	• Give no liquids or food by mouth.	• The victim may vomit and block the airway.
	• Stay with the victim and assist as needed until medical help arrives.	• If the condition worsens, the victim may need rescue breathing or CPR performed.

(continues)

PROCEDURE 21–9

First Aid for Other Common Conditions

(continued)

CONDITION AND SIGNS AND SYMPTOMS	PROCEDURE	RATIONALE
Unconsciousness Any medical emergency can result in the victim losing alertness and awareness of the surroundings. This state can range from a brief period, such as fainting, to a prolonged coma. *S/S*: The victim may drift in and out of consciousness, varying from feeling drowsy, restless, and unable to orient himself or herself or make sense when speaking to not moving or speaking at all.	• Call EMS if the victim does not quickly regain consciousness (i.e., simple fainting) or if illness or injury is evident.	• The victim needs medical evaluation and treatment.
	• The goal of the treatment of the unconscious victim is to maintain the airway.	• The victim is unable to cough, clear the throat, or turn the head to drain vomit or drool from the mouth when the airway becomes obstructed.
	• Do not give anything by mouth.	• The victim may choke on fluids or vomit and obstruct the airway.
	• Keep the victim warm.	• This maintains good circulation.
	• If there is no neck or back injury, place the victim in the recovery position by turning the head to the side, or turn the entire body to the side or onto the abdomen.	• This prevents obstruction of the airway if the victim vomits.
	• Gently tilt the victim's head back.	• This maintains the airway.
	• If neck or back injury is suspected, leave the victim in the position in which he or she is found unless there is difficulty in breathing. If the victim is having difficulty breathing or is choking or vomiting, roll the entire body as a unit to a side-lying position while keeping the spine in straight alignment.	• This prevents further injury to the neck or back.
	• Enlist the assistance of bystanders, if possible, when moving the victim to ensure the head, neck, and back stay in a straight line.	• It is easier to maintain body alignment when there are more people for turning in unison.

(continues)

PROCEDURE 21–9

First Aid for Other Common Conditions

(continued)

CONDITION AND SIGNS AND SYMPTOMS	PROCEDURE	RATIONALE
Unconsciousness (continued)	• Give first aid for any underlying illness or injury.	• Unconsciousness is usually a result of another illness or condition.
	• If the victim becomes restless, you may have to gently restrain him or her.	• This prevents the victim from injuring himself or herself.
	• Stay with the victim until medical assistance arrives.	• If the condition worsens, the victim may need rescue breathing or CPR performed.

PROCEDURE 21–10

Applying a Triangular Sling

Always Observe Standard Precautions

USAGE	PROCEDURE	RATIONALE
	(See Figures 21–12a–c)	
It is used to support an injured shoulder, collarbone, or arm. If the arm is broken, apply the splint first to immobilize the broken bone, and then place it in the sling. A sling can be made from a large triangular cloth, a sweater, a pillowcase, or other materials that can be cut to the appropriate size.	1. Support the injured part and slide the sling under the arm on the victim's injured side.	Always support the injured arm when applying a sling to prevent further injury.
	2. Place the top corner over the victim's uninjured shoulder.	Creates a cross-body support to secure the other end with a knot.
	3. Pull the bottom corner of the sling up past the victim's chin and over the shoulder on the injured side. Leave the fingers showing.	Leaving the fingers exposed allows for convenient circulation checks.
	4. Tie the sling around the victim's neck, placing it a little to one side.	Placing the knot a little to one side prevents the knot from pressing on the back of the neck.
	5. Fold over the extra cloth at the victim's elbow and secure it with a safety pin.	Creates a cradle to secure the elbow.
	6. Check for circulation.	Always check for circulation when applying splints and slings to ensure there is adequate perfusion of the extremity.

(continues)

PROCEDURE 21–10

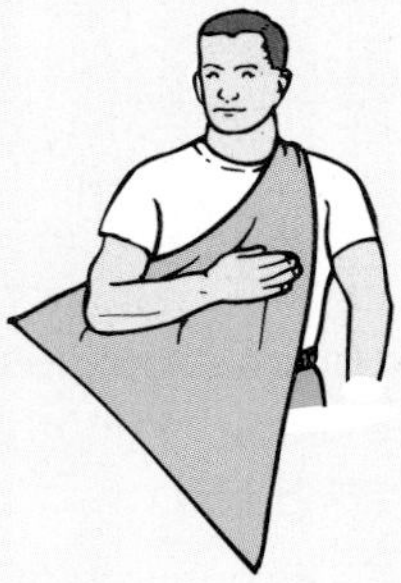

FIGURE 21–12a Support the injured part and slide the sling under the arm on the victim's injured side. Place top corner over the victim's uninjured shoulder.

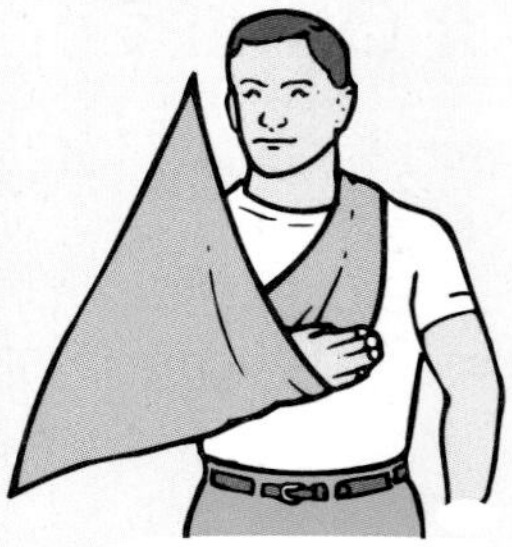

FIGURE 21–12b Pull the bottom corner of the sling up past the victim's chin and over the shoulder on the injured side. Leave the fingers showing.

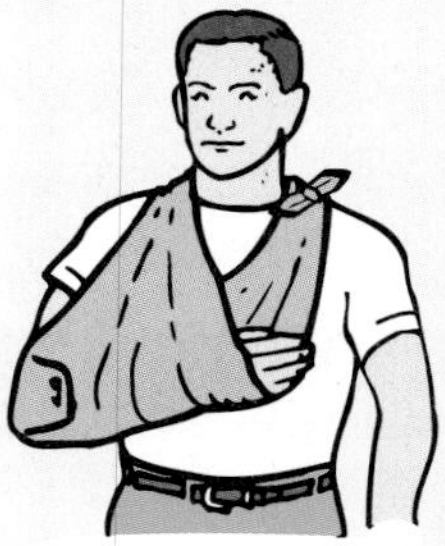

FIGURE 21–12c Tie the sling around the victim's neck, placing it a little to one side so the knot does not press on the back of the neck. Fold over the extra cloth at the victim's elbow and secure it with a safety pin.

PROCEDURE 21–11

Applying a Spiral Wrap

Always Observe Standard Precautions

USAGE	PROCEDURE	RATIONALE
	(See Figures 21–13a–b)	
A spiral wrap can be used on arms, legs, and the trunk of the body.	1. Start wrap at distal end.	Enhances circulation and decreases swelling.
	2. Anchor the bandage by leaving a corner exposed. The corner is then folded down and covered when the bandage is circled around the limb.	Holds the end in place to prevent slippage.

(continues)

PROCEDURE 21–11

Applying a Spiral Wrap

(continued)

USAGE	PROCEDURE	RATIONALE
(continued)	3. Overlap each rotation over the previous one by approximately half the width of the previous layer.	Holds the wrapping securely in place.
	4. Place your hand between the bandage and the victim's skin if inserting a pin; can also secure with tape.	To prevent accidental injury to the patient.
	5. Verify circulation in the fingers and toes if the wrap is used on the arm or leg.	Always check for circulation when applying wraps to ensure there is adequate perfusion of the extremity.
	6. Verify ease of breathing if the wrap is on the trunk.	A too-tight wrap will restrict chest movement during respirations.

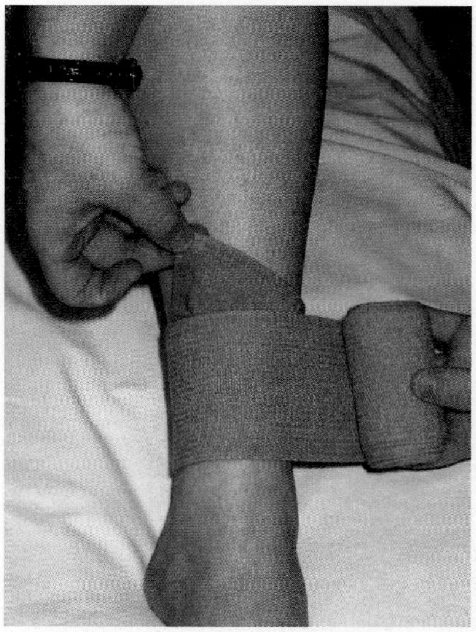

FIGURE 21–13a Always start wrap at distal end. Anchor the bandage by leaving a corner exposed. The corner is then folded down and covered when the bandage is circled around the limb. Overlap each rotation partially over the previous one to hold it securely in place.

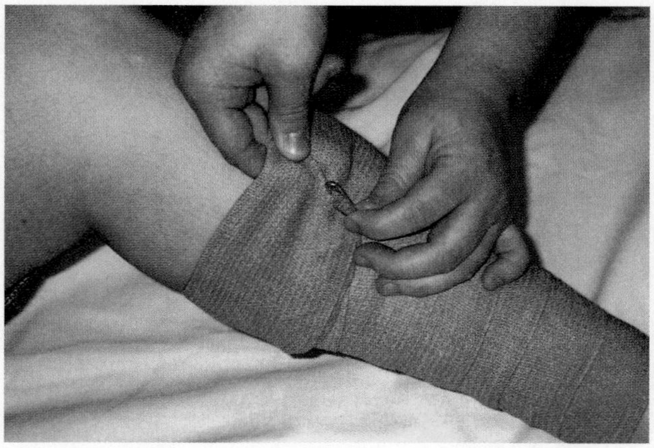

FIGURE 21–13b Place your hand between the bandage and the victim's skin if inserting a pin; can also secure with tape.

PROCEDURE 21–12
Applying a Figure-Eight Wrap

Always Observe Standard Precautions

USAGE	PROCEDURE	RATIONALE
A figure-eight wrap can be used to bandage a joint, such as an ankle, an elbow, or a wrist, because it secures both sides of the joint. Using a spiral wrap is not effective for wrapping joints, because the wrap tends to slip off easily.	(See Figures 21–14a–b)	
	1. Anchor the bandage at the instep and wrap several times around the instep. Then bring the wrap up diagonally over the foot.	Holds the wrapping securely in place.
	2. Bring the bandage around the back of the ankle and then down over the top of the foot and back under the instep.	This creates a figure-eight pattern.
	3. Repeat the figure-eight pattern, moving the wrap out in both directions (up the leg and toward the toes) with each repeat of the pattern while overlapping approximately half of the previous layer.	Partially overlaps the previous layer to hold it securely in place.
	4. When completed, wrap around the ankle several times and secure the end.	Holds the wrapping securely in place.
	5. Check circulation distal to the wrap.	Always check for circulation when applying wraps to ensure there is adequate perfusion of the extremity.

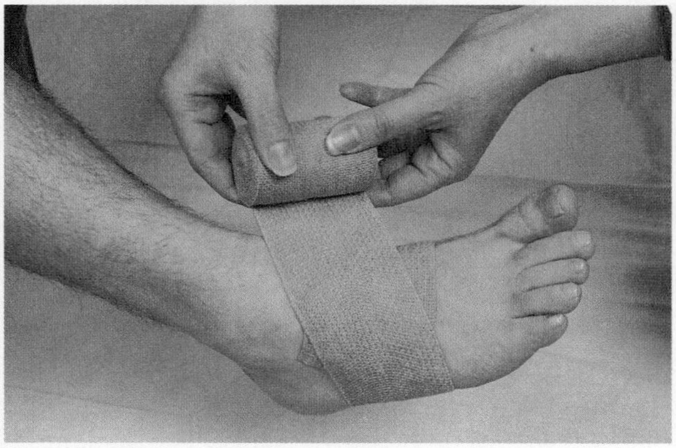

FIGURE 21–14a Anchor the bandage at the instep and secure by wrapping several times around the instep. Then bring the wrap up diagonally over the foot.

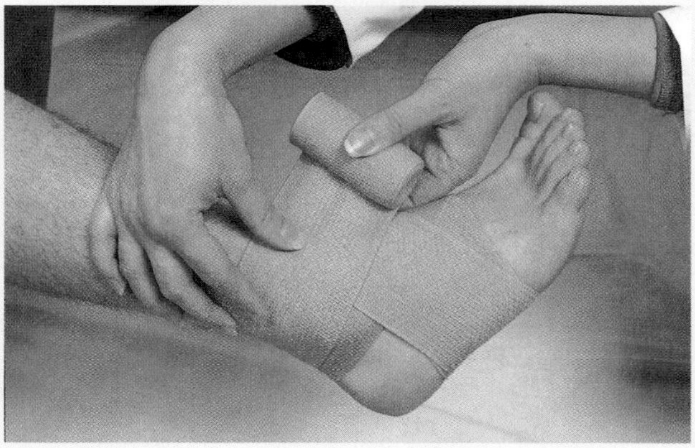

FIGURE 21–14b Bring the bandage around the back of the ankle and then down over the top of the foot and back under the instep. This creates a figure-eight pattern. Continue this process, moving the wrap out in both directions (up the leg and toward the toes) with each repeat of the pattern. Partially overlap the previous one to hold it securely in place.

PROCEDURE 21–13

Applying a Bandage to a Finger

Always Observe Standard Precautions

USAGE	PROCEDURE	RATIONALE
A wrap for a finger can be made from a thin strip of gauze or cloth. It is used to support the finger and decrease movement. If the finger is broken, apply the splint first, using small twigs, pencils, or popsicle sticks on both sides, then wrap the finger.	(See Figures 21–15a–d)	
	1. Place the end of the wrap at the bottom of one side of the finger and fold it over the tip of the finger and down to the bottom of the other side of the finger. Repeat this three to four times.	Creates a recurrent dressing.
	2. Start at the bottom of the finger and spiral the wrap up and down the finger.	Holds recurrent wrap securely in place.
	3. Secure by doing several figure-eight wraps around the wrist.	Anchors wrap to prevent it from falling off the finger.
	4. When the figure-eight wrap is complete, circle the wrist several times. Split the wrap and tie in a knot.	Secures wrap to wrist.
	5. Monitor patient. If any signs of decreased circulation occur, loosen the wrap immediately.	Swelling may occur that will increase the tightness of the wrap and compromise circulation.

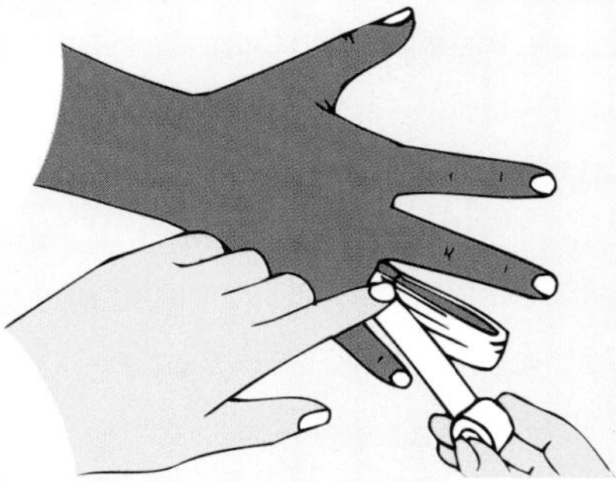

FIGURE 21–15a Place the end of the wrap at the bottom of one side of the finger and fold it over the tip of the finger and down to the bottom of the other side of the finger. Repeat this three to four times.

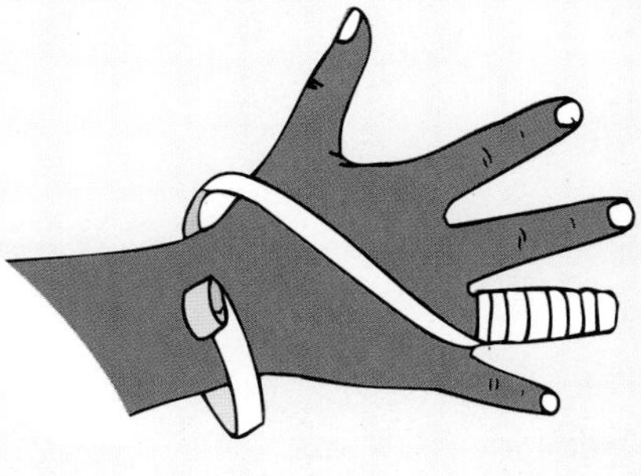

FIGURE 21–15c Secure by doing several figure-eight wraps around the wrist.

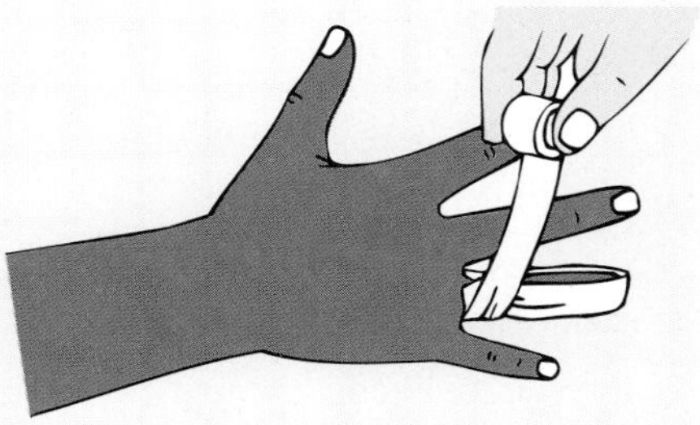

FIGURE 21–15b Start at the bottom of the finger and spiral the wrap up and down the finger to hold securely in place.

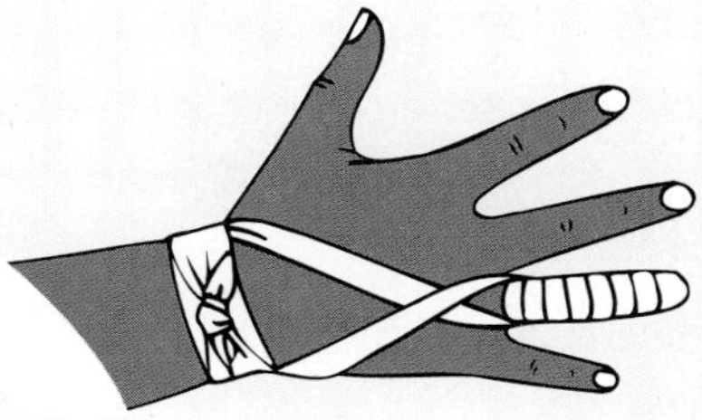

FIGURE 21–15d When the figure-eight wrap is complete, circle the wrist several times. Split the wrap and tie in a knot or secure with tape or safety pin.

WORKBOOK PRACTICE

Go to your workbook and complete the exercises for this chapter.

SUGGESTED LEARNING ACTIVITIES

1. If you do not already have a CPR certification, arrange to attend a class for certification. Classes can be located by calling your local health facilities, community colleges, the American Red Cross, or the American Heart Association.
2. Contact the American Red Cross and plan to attend their next first aid and safety class, if it is not part of your program of study.
3. Go to the website listed in the Fascinating Facts box (see page 467) and learn more about home safety.
4. Evaluate your home environment for potential hazards and risks for injuries.
5. Practice the four types of slings and wraps on family, friends, or classmates.

WEB ACTIVITIES

Mayo Clinic
www.mayoclinic.com

Do a search for "first aid." Choose a topic not covered in your text and summarize the information.

American Heart Association
www.heart.org

Find out what classes are available in your area. Also identify the warning signs for a heart attack and a stroke.

American Red Cross
www.redcross.org

Find out how to donate blood in your area. What are the donor guidelines?

REVIEW QUESTIONS

1. When should first aid be administered?
2. What is the Good Samaritan Act and how does it protect the rescuer?
3. What is the golden rule of first aid?
4. What are the seven steps to follow when an emergency occurs that will protect both the victim and rescuer?
5. When does the rescuer start CPR on a victim?
6. What are the signs and symptoms and treatment for an allergic reaction?
7. What are the signs and symptoms and treatment for bleeding and wounds?
8. What are the signs and symptoms and treatment for bone, joint, and muscle injuries?
9. What are the signs and symptoms and treatment for facial injuries?
10. What are the signs and symptoms and treatment for burns?
11. What are the signs and symptoms and treatment for drug-related emergencies?
12. What are the signs and symptoms and treatment for poisoning?
13. What are the signs and symptoms and treatment for temperature-related illnesses?
14. What are the signs and symptoms and treatment for other common conditions that require emergency care?
15. What are the four common types of slings and wraps used to treat musculoskeletal injuries?

APPLICATION EXERCISES

1. Refer back to The Case of the Out-of-Control Party:
   a. What would have been appropriate first aid measures for the stabbing victim?
   b. Should Josephine remove the knife from the chest? Why or why not?
   c. If there is bubbling coming from the chest wound, what would this indicate? What additional first aid measures would be necessary?

   d. Which organs are located in the left side of the chest that may have been damaged by the knife?

2. One hot day William notices his neighbor John mowing the lawn. He notes that John looks flushed and is sweating profusely, but he is overweight and out of shape and it is awfully hot and humid outdoors to be doing yard work. Thirty minutes later, John's wife frantically knocks on the door saying John is having chest pain. She is very frightened. She says he has a heart condition and that she has called 9-1-1.
   a. What is the most likely cause of John's chest pain?
   b. What actions can William take until EMS arrives?

PROBLEM-SOLVING PRACTICE

Michael Huang is a health care student and a single father with two small children at home. He is very concerned about the safety of his active and inquisitive children and is wondering if there are any potential hazards in his home environment. Using the five-step problem-solving process, determine what Michael can do to identify and correct any hazards at home. (Note: Learners can use their own home for this problem-solving assignment.)

SUGGESTED READINGS AND RESOURCES

American Red Cross. www.redcross.org

DK and British Red Cross. (2012). *First aid fast for babies and children.* New York: DK Publishing.

Hubbard, J. (2013). *First aid fundamentals for survival.* Ontario: F+W Media.

This page intentionally left blank

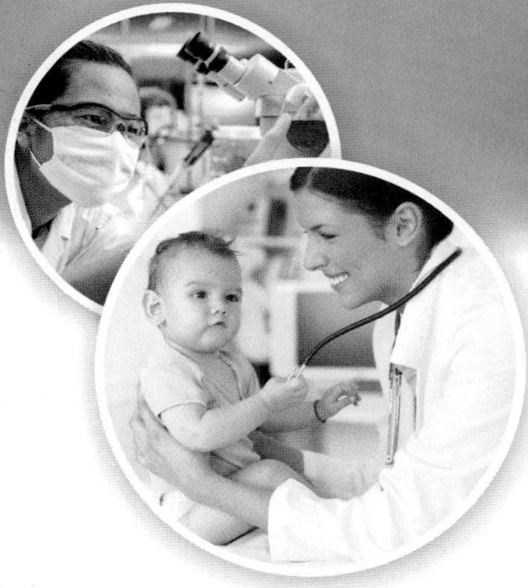

Unit 8

Business of Caring

This page intentionally left blank

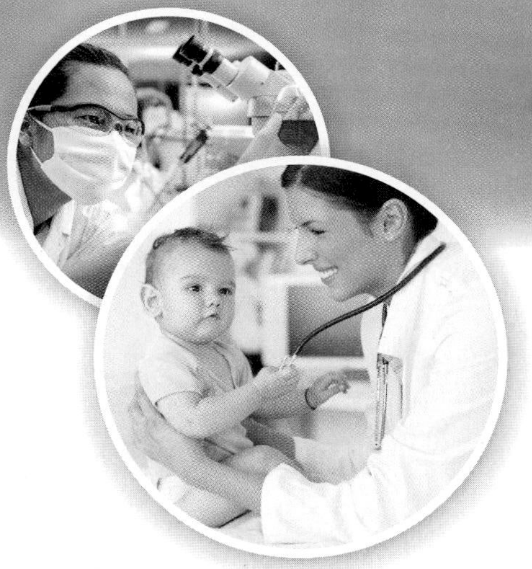

Chapter 22

Controlling Health Care Costs

OBJECTIVES

Studying and applying the material in this chapter will help you to:

- Identify factors that are causing an increase in health care costs.
- Identify the three types of funding for health care institutions.
- Compare and contrast the three types of payment methods.
- Describe how methods for paying medical costs have changed over the years.
- Contrast fee-for-service and managed care reimbursement methods.
- Explain the purpose of managed care systems and describe the methods used to control costs.
- Define Medicare, Medicaid, and DRGs.
- Identify the four major areas of expenditures incurred by a health care delivery system.
- Define accounts receivable, accounts payable, and the cost of money.
- Explain ways that the health care professional can help control facility costs.

KEY TERMS

account payable
account receivable
capitation
coinsurance
copay
cost of money
deductible
diagnostic-related group (DRG)
expenditures
fee-for-service
financing
gatekeeper
managed care
Medicaid
Medicare
negotiated fees
preauthorization
premium
prepaid plans
primary care provider (PCP)
profit
reimburse

The Case of the Inefficient Office

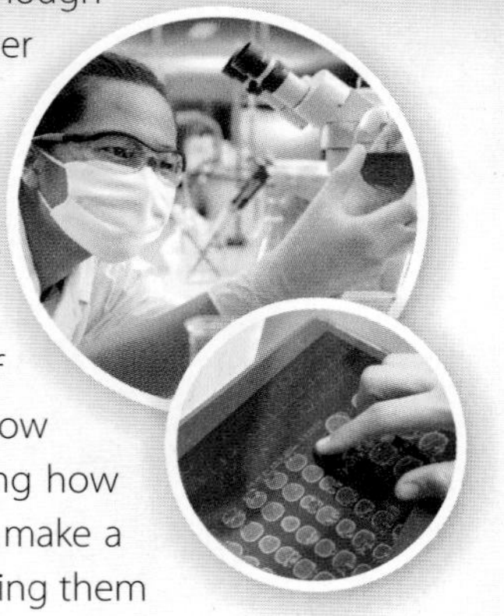

Constance Madison has seen many changes in her career working in medical records. Although computerization has helped organize recordkeeping, it has also brought feelings of disorder during periods of transition. Constance sometimes feels overwhelmed and frustrated with what seems to be endless paperwork, lack of support, duplication of effort, and insufficient time to do what needs to be done during the day. Her knowledge of the changes in health care delivery and the needs of the system keep her focused on doing her best to make a positive contribution during stressful times. She has made several suggestions to her supervisor that have been adopted by her department. In this chapter you will gain an understanding of why there is a tremendous amount of change occurring in the health care environment and how you can look for ways to improve efficiency, rather than focusing on the problems. By learning how individual employees can contribute to the efficiency of the organization, you will be able to make a positive impact. Identifying areas of inefficiency and waste enables you to work toward correcting them and creating a more enjoyable and productive work environment.

THE RISING COSTS OF HEALTH CARE

A major concern in the United States today is how to effectively control dramatically rising health care costs. Although we spend more per person on health care than any other country, our quality of care and patient satisfaction are below those of many other countries (further discussion of this issue appears in Chapter 23). Rising health care costs have been attributed to technological advancements, increasing cost of drugs, specializations, and the number of diagnostic and treatment options available. This cost increase is of great concern when it is understood in relationship to our aging population and the decreasing health of the young. The nation's youth are showing an alarming increase in obesity, poor diet, and lack of physical fitness, which is resulting in an onset of chronic conditions at a very young age. This trend clearly underscores the importance of preventive measures to provide a long and healthy life.

Most people believe that health care costs are evenly distributed among all patients. This is not true. About 10% of the patients incur 80% of the costs. It is estimated that about 75% of total health care costs come from patients with chronic conditions.

HEALTH CARE INSTITUTIONS

A wide variety of health care institutions exist—from hospitals to home health agencies, medical offices to long-term care facilities, and everything in between. (Box 23–3 in the next chapter provides a more inclusive listing.) But all of these types of service institutions can be grouped into three categories, based on the type of funding they receive:

- Nonprofit institutions: This category operates as a charitable agency and any net earnings must be reinvested into the organization. They are granted tax-exempt status by the Internal Revenue Service. Donations to a nonprofit organization are often tax deductible to the individuals and businesses making the contributions.
- Proprietary (for-profit) institutions: These operate in the same manner as any for-profit business and pay local, state, and federal taxes.
- Government institutions: They are referred to as public health care facilities. Most of their funding comes from local, state, or federal sources. Examples include Veterans Administration (VA) hospitals and state mental and rehabilitative facilities.

HISTORY OF HEALTH CARE REIMBURSEMENT

In the past, patients paid the physician's asking price for services provided. For those who could not pay cash, payment might be fresh vegetables from the garden or a load of wood. As health care became more sophisticated and costly, insurance companies became the preferred method of covering costs. Patients paid the insurance company an agreed-upon amount, called a **premium**. When medical care was needed, patients would visit the physician of their choice and the physician would order tests, prescribe medications, admit the patient to the hospital, or perform surgery. The physician determined what actions to take and the insurance companies paid for the services. This was known as **fee-for-service**.

As costs rose in recent decades, insurance companies and other payers questioned the efficiency of fee-for-service as a pricing method. Rather than encouraging savings, they argued, it rewarded the providers who prescribed the most services, such as lab tests and diagnostic procedures. Payers believed that the providers of health care—physicians, hospitals, and other professionals and facilities—should be held accountable for costs. Duplication of services, unnecessarily long stays in hospitals, and expensive brand name drugs are examples of practices labeled as "wasteful." The approach to lowering cost while maintaining quality of health care will be addressed more fully in Chapter 23.

HEALTH CARE PAYMENT METHODS

Three methods for payment are commonly utilized in the United States:

1. Direct pay: In this method, the patient pays for health care costs using his or her own money. This approach may lead to a more judicious use of health care services, but it is catastrophic when costs exceed the patient's financial ability to pay.
2. Private insurance: Individuals can purchase their own insurance policy or it can be part of a benefits package from employment. Employers are able to purchase policies less expensively than an individual as the costs can be spread over a group, some of whom will not need care. These policies may include stipulations whereby the employee incurs part of the cost.
3. Government plans: Funded by a government agency, examples of these plans include military health care for active personnel and their families, as well as the VA hospital system. There are other government plans, too, but the largest ones are Medicaid (low-income) and Medicare (over 65 years of age). These programs are discussed in greater detail next.

GOVERNMENT PROGRAMS

Medicaid is a cost-assistance program to help pay the medical costs for those with limited income. Funded by the federal government, it is operated at the state level by departments of human services. The exact eligibility and payment procedures vary by state.

Medicare was established by Congress in 1965. It is part of the Social Security Administration and provided health insurance for people aged 65 and older and others, such as the severely disabled, who qualify for social security.

On December 8, 2003, President George W. Bush signed into law the Medicare Prescription Drug, Improvement and Modernization Act (MMA) of 2003. This legislation provided seniors and people living with severe disabilities with a prescription drug benefit, more choices, and better benefits under Medicare. This was one of the most significant improvements in senior health care since the inception of Medicare in 1965.

Medicare is administered by the Centers for Medicare and Medicaid Services (CMS) and consists of four parts.

- Hospital insurance (Part A) helps pay for inpatient care in a hospital or skilled facility (following a hospital stay), some home health care, and hospice care. The premium for Part A has already been paid through payroll taxes.
- Medical insurance (Part B) helps pay for outpatient services and many other medical services and supplies, such as physicians' fees, diagnostic tests, and physical and occupational therapy. Part B is voluntary and if coverage is elected, there is a monthly premium deducted automatically from the person's social security payment.
- Medicare advantage (Part C) plans are available in many areas. People with Medicare Parts A and B can choose to receive all of their health care services through a provider organization, such as a health maintenance organization (HMO) or a preferred provider organization (PPO). (HMOs and PPOs are described under managed care, later in the chapter.)
- Prescription drug coverage (Part D) helps pay for medications prescribed for treatment. There is a monthly fee for this coverage.

Many people assume that Medicare is free and covers all medical expenses, but this is not correct. Medicare has a monthly premium along with deductibles and coinsurance amounts. A **deductible** is an amount required to be paid by the insured before benefits become payable. **Coinsurance** is a cost-sharing provision stipulating that the insured is to assume a percentage of the costs of covered services. Under Medicare Part B, the beneficiary pays coinsurance of 20% of allowed charges. In a Medicare prescription drug plan, the coinsurance will vary. For more specific information refer to www.medicare.gov.

Since Medicare has a deductible and coinsurance that must be paid out-of-pocket, many individuals elect to purchase a supplemental insurance policy from a private insurance company or enroll in an HMO. The private insurance supplement is called a Medigap policy. Medigap policies vary in price and coverage. If you are enrolled in a Medicare plan and have a Medigap policy, then Medicare and your Medigap policy will pay both their shares of covered health care costs.

Government Involvement in Health Care

By providing funding, the government has assumed a leading role in regulating both the costs and quality of health care provided under Medicare and Medicaid. A major move to control costs was the development of **diagnostic-related groups (DRGs)** by Congress in 1983. The typical, expected hospital costs of all common diagnoses were determined. Providers of care for Medicare patients receive that amount, regardless of the actual cost of care. For example, if two hospitals perform a hip replacement surgery on a Medicare patient, they are **reimbursed** (paid back) the same amount. Hospitals that can do the procedure for less than the amount reimbursed are allowed to keep the extra money. Hospitals that spend more must make up the difference themselves. Exceptions to this policy are made when there are documented complications or additional diagnosed problems.

The actions of the government have had a significant impact on the health care system because Medicare patients make up a large portion of the patient population. Health care facilities that bill Medicare or Medicaid for reimbursement of costs related to the care of a patient who is covered by one of these programs must be certified prior to incurring costs in order to receive compensation. Health care professionals who provide services for Medicare and Medicaid patients must understand and follow all regulations and requirements in order to ensure compliance and reimbursement. This also extends to almost all facilities as most insurance policies state that Medicare approval must be maintained for their plans too.

MANAGED CARE

One response to rising costs has been the development of **managed care** plans, which contain specific built-in cost controls. These plans incorporate business concepts designed to increase efficiency by giving health care providers incentives to cut costs. Several variations of managed care plans are in use today. (See Table 22–1.) Simply stated, the goals of managed care are to do the following:

- Provide health care that patients can afford
- Ensure high-quality care
- Discourage unnecessary costs
- Eliminate duplication of procedures

Table 22–1 Managed Care Systems

Health maintenance organization (HMO)	A prepaid medical group practice plan that provides a predetermined medical care benefit package. HMOs are both insurers and providers of health care.
Exclusive provider organization (EPO)	Similar to an HMO, but with greater flexibility for employers to create a benefits package specific to their company's needs.
Preferred provider organization (PPO)	A group of hospitals and physicians who contract on a fee-for-service basis with employers, insurance plans, or other third-party administrators.
Point-of-service plan or point-of-service option (POS)	A health services delivery organization that offers the option to its members to choose to receive a service from participating or a nonparticipating provider. Generally the level of coverage is reduced for services associated with the use of nonparticipating providers.

- Earn a **profit** (amount of money remaining after all costs of operating a business have been paid) for both health care providers and insurance companies (or, if nonprofit, ensure that income covers all costs)

Managed care systems employ several methods in an effort to achieve these goals. For example, prepaid plans, negotiated fees, primary care providers, and review of services using preauthorization. These methods will be discussed next.

Prepaid Plans

One of the major attempts to reduce costs has been the development of **prepaid plans**. In these plans, health care providers are paid *before* rather than *after* services are performed. This payment method is based on the idea that providers can be motivated to be more efficient. Let's look at an example of how these plans work.

1. A health insurance company signs up 10,000 customers, known as *enrollees*.
2. Each of the 10,000 pays a monthly amount known as a *premium* to the insurance company.
3. The insurance company contracts with a health care service group that agrees to provide medical services to the enrollees. The physicians are paid a set amount for each enrollee. This is the only payment they receive, regardless of the type or number of services provided to the patients. This method of payment is called **capitation**.
4. Enrollees must use the physicians who have contracted with the insurance company. Depending on the plan, they may be required to pay a set amount for each service provided. This is called a **copay**.
5. The goal is that costs will average out. Some patients will require more care than the set amount covers, whereas others will not seek any services.

Although the practice of prepayment has been shown to increase efficiency in many cases, the method has opponents. Some argue that cost containment goals conflict with quality care goals. They worry that the number and quality of services will have to be sacrificed in order to increase profits. Several movements are underway at both the state and federal levels to pass laws to protect patient access to appropriate care.

Negotiated Fees

Another method for paying health care providers is by pre–agreed-upon amounts that are negotiated between health care providers and insurance companies, to pay for specific services. These are known as **negotiated fees**. They may cover all or only a percentage of the provider's actual charges. Depending on the type of plan, the patient pays the difference or the physicians accept as payment in full the amount paid by the insurance company.

Primary Care Providers

One of the most important control mechanisms is the use of **primary care providers (PCPs)**, also known as **gatekeepers**. These are health care professionals, often physicians, who serve as the patient's first contact when entering the health care system. The PCP evaluates patient complaints and determines the appropriate level of care. Diagnostic procedures and treatment plans must be approved by PCPs in order to be covered by insurance. They provide the referrals that patients must have before seeing specialists.

An advantage of the use of PCPs is that they provide consistency in patient care. They have a global picture of their patients' history and overall health care needs. A disadvantage is that patients must go through them when they may already know that they need to see a specialist. It adds time and expense to the process of receiving necessary care. For example, Dan O'Riley has been seeing a dermatologist for the past five years for treatment of a chronic skin condition. His employer changes insurance companies, and Dan enrolls in the new HMO. He discovers that in order for the insurance company to pay for his skin treatments, he must choose and visit a PCP to get a referral to see his dermatologist.

Review of Services

Many insurance companies use review procedures to determine which costs they will cover. Diagnostic tests, treatments, hospitalizations, and so forth are reviewed to determine medical necessity and cost effectiveness. Insurance companies will not pay for certain nonessential medical services and referrals to specialists that have not been preapproved. Securing these approvals is known as **preauthorization**, and it is essential that health care professionals know when preauthorizations are necessary.

Thinking It Through

Josephine Copley arrives at work late, having had little sleep the night before. She hopes she can get caught up on some of her personal calls and still get the insurance forms sent out on time to meet the deadlines for submitting claims for reimbursement. She is working intently when approached by a patient who is very confused by her Medicare claim statements. The patient has questions on some of the supplies she was charged for. She does not know what they were used for or why.

Josephine is feeling quite stressed and is curt with her, saying, "I am sure all the charges are correct. Besides, Medicare doesn't pay like they used to anyway, so it doesn't matter. I'm just too busy to deal with this right now. It seems that patients want more and Medicare wants to pay less."

1. What are the possible consequences of Josephine's comments?
2. Was it appropriate that Josephine make negative comments about the patient's health care plan?
3. How could she have handled this situation differently?
4. What external circumstances may have contributed to Josephine's behavior?

Fascinating Facts

In 2012, the United States spent $2.8 *trillion* on health care. This represents $8915 for every man, woman, and child in the country. In the year 1940, it was only $30 per person!

The United States pays twice as much yet lags other wealthy nations in infant mortality and life expectancy. In fact, U.S. life expectancy is ranked 42nd in the world.

NATIONAL HEALTH CARE COVERAGE

Private health insurance coverage is based on the concept of spreading the risk. For example, the sellers of car insurance assume that not everyone who buys coverage will use it. There will be some accidents and stolen vehicles that must be paid for, but most people who are covered will never make a claim. Health insurance is based on the same principle. Although some people will suffer serious health problems and cost more than the amount of their premiums, others will use much less. In order for this system to be profitable, health insurance companies tried to reduce the number of people who required expensive care. This was accomplished in several ways:

- Requiring applicants for insurance to pass physical exams
- Not selling insurance to people who had certain preexisting conditions, such as heart disease
- Selling policies to people with preexisting conditions but not covering the costs related to these conditions

Although these methods helped insurance companies improve their cash flow, it left many people who were most in need of health care without coverage. This challenge was one of several that prompted calls for a system of national health care that would provide coverage for everyone, regardless of health condition or economic status.

In response to this problem President Obama signed into law the Patient Protection and Affordable Care Act in 2010 (commonly called the Affordable Care Act [ACA] or "Obamacare"). This legislation will continue to have widespread effects on the business of health care over the next few years. The first regulations went into effect in 2014, and the rollout of new regulations will continue until 2020. Some highlights of the new bill include:

- Health insurers cannot deny children or adults health insurance because of preexisting conditions.
- Businesses with fewer than 50 employees receive tax credits covering up to 50% of employee premiums. Those with more than 50 employees must provide health care coverage.
- Everyone except certain low-income individuals must purchase health insurance or face a $695 annual fine.
- Medicare drug coverage has been improved for seniors and the disabled.
- Young adults can be covered by their parents' health insurance until age 27.
- Preventative care without copays will be in effect by 2018.

- No health care plan is required to offer abortion coverage. If offered, it must be paid for separately by the individual.
- Insurance companies are no longer able to cancel an enrollee's coverage when he or she gets sick.
- Chain restaurants are required to provide a "nutrient content disclosure statement" alongside their menu items.
- Websites have been developed to make it easier for Americans in any state to seek out affordable health insurance options.

As with any extension of coverage, the question of how to pay for it has been vigorously debated. Among the changes implemented to help create the necessary revenue to cover the costs of the ACA are the following:

- In 2012, the Medicare payroll tax was expanded to include unearned income (investment income) for families making more than $250,000 a year ($200,000 for individuals).
- Beginning in 2018, insurance companies will pay a 40% excise tax on so-called "Cadillac" high-end insurance plans worth over $27,500 for families ($10,200 for individuals)
- A 10% excise tax is being assessed on indoor tanning services.

This list is by no means comprehensive, but highlights some of the provisions supporting the new legislation. Controversy about the ACA is expected to continue as the bill is applied, challenged, and interpreted in actual practice.

CONTROLLING ORGANIZATIONAL COSTS

The effects of managed care, insurance restrictions, and government regulations have greatly affected all types of health care organizations. Facilities must focus on controlling expenditures. **Expenditures** refer to any money that is spent in the process of doing business. The expenditures are the cost of resources required to maintain a health care delivery system. These costs occur in four major areas. (See Figure 22–1.)

1. Financing
2. Technology and supplies (pharmaceuticals and equipment)

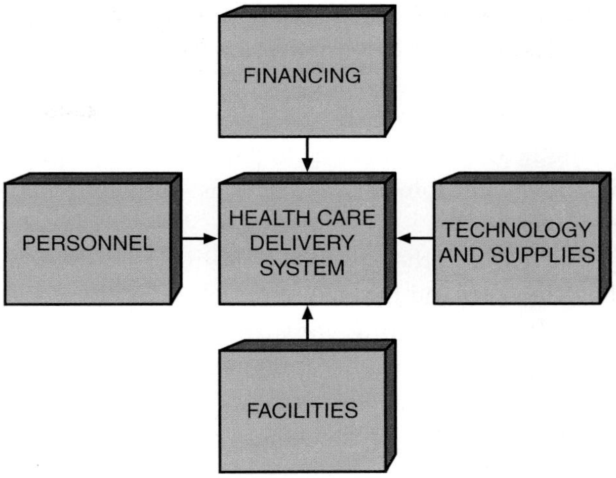

FIGURE 22–1 Resources required to maintain a health care delivery system.

3. Facilities
4. Personnel

Financing refers to the source of money used to run a business. Financing resources for a health care facility come primarily from a variety of health insurance companies (federal or private). Each of these insurance plans has its own set of rules, procedures, and paperwork to be completed before payments for patient services are sent to the facility. The key factor here is to be as efficient as possible in completing the paperwork correctly and completely, so the payment can be received as soon as possible for services provided. When services have been given and the payment not received, the amount owed is recorded in what is called an **account receivable**. A sound business practice is to keep the accounts receivable as low as possible. Other financing resources may be individuals who pay for their own care or donations that individuals and corporations give to nonprofit facilities.

Keeping the accounts receivable low is an important part of financial management and relates to the **cost of money**. The cost of money refers to the value that could be earned on money if it were received by the facility and invested. For example, if a facility has $1 million in accounts receivable and a 10% interest rate could be earned on that money, the facility is losing $274 for each day the payment is delayed ($1,000,000 × 10% ÷ 365 days/year). The facility may also be paying interest on loans that it cannot pay off until the receivables are in the account. When money is owed to others for services, supplies, or equipment received, it is recorded as an **account payable**.

Technology and supplies refer to the cost of equipment and supplies that are used in the process of giving health care services to patients—for example, diagnostic equipment, medications, catheters, beds, and linens.

Facilities are the physical buildings and the land they stand on and the cost of maintaining them—for example, the painting, repairing, and remodeling of the buildings; landscaping; electricity; garbage removal; and maintenance of parking areas.

Personnel (labor costs) refers to the individuals who work in all areas associated with the functioning of the health care delivery system. They include both the direct care workers and those in support roles. Examples include nurses, physical and occupational therapists, medical assistants, X-ray and lab technicians, accountants, admissions staff, managers, pharmacists, dieticians, and maintenance workers. *The total cost of the salaries of all the health care professionals is often the largest cost incurred by a facility.*

HEALTH CARE PROFESSIONALS' IMPACT ON COSTS

The career success of the health care professional will depend, to a great degree, on his or her ability to contribute to the control of rising costs. Every health care professional must take fiscal (financial) responsibility for his or her performance. The need for efficiency and accountability on the part of everyone in the system cannot be overemphasized. The question that must be asked is, "How can I help reduce unnecessary costs?" It is easy to dismiss the consequences of one person's impact on the finances of a health care facility. But when totaled up over time and multiplied by the number of health care professionals who are very concerned with efficiency, the cost savings can be quite significant.

There are many ways health care professionals can contribute to the efficient and cost-effective functioning of the facility:

1. Personal efficiency: This refers to the health care professional's performance and how each worker contributes to overall efficiency. For example, when workers arrive late or take excessive breaks, it affects their coworkers' workloads and their ability to perform their duties efficiently. This results in a decrease in patient satisfaction. The costs of poor-quality care are often related to the following problems:
   - Duplicated work between departments
   - Loss of time due to inefficient task performance
   - Loss of staff due to job dissatisfaction
   - Recruitment and training of new employees
   - Expenditure of energy and time in the investigation of complaints
   - Lawsuits (litigation) and malpractice settlements
   - Employees repeatedly making the same errors in tasks, despite instruction
   - Time wasted reporting and correcting errors
   - Expenses related to overutilization of diagnostic tests to avoid malpractice
2. Focusing on the job: When at work, 100% of the health care professional's attention must be focused on the duties at hand. The needs of patients and the organization/employer must have top priority.
3. Careful use of supplies or equipment: Damage or loss of supplies and equipment can add significantly to the cost of operations. Always use supplies only as needed and avoid waste by taking only that which is needed to complete the task. Handle equipment carefully and follow the manufacturer's instructions on the proper use and care of all equipment.
4. Billing and coding correctly and not misplacing charges: Coding refers to the assignment of standardized numbers that designate diagnoses and procedures performed. It provides the information on which payment of insurance claims are based. Codes are classified by procedures and diagnoses and are contained in the following reference books: *Current Procedural Terminology (CPT)* and *Classification of Diseases, 10th Revision; Clinical Modification* (*ICD-10-CM*). The ICD-10 is the code used to describe the condition or disease being treated, also known as the diagnosis (See Box 22–1.). CPT is the code used to describe the treatment and diagnostic services provided for that diagnosis.

Health care professionals who have responsibility for submitting codes for reimbursement must learn to properly use these references.

BOX 22-1

ICD-10 Code Examples

S93.4 Sprain of ankle

S93.401 Sprain of unspecified ligament of right ankle

S93.402 Sprain of unspecified ligament of left ankle

S93.409 Sprain of unspecified ligament of unspecified ankle

Required seventh digit to identify the encounter:

A—Initial

D—Subsequent

S—Sequela

Notice the specificity for just this diagnosis. If the code is not specific and does not match the other documentation, the charge will be declined and revenue lost (or delayed until further clarification can be obtained).

Coding is very specific to the particular diagnosis or procedure. Improper coding can lead to various problems, ranging from a loss of income for the provider to charges of fraud for overbilling. All health care professionals need to be sure to note all supplies used and charges incurred in providing patient care. Not submitting charges can lead to not being reimbursed for care given or supplies used.

Fascinating Facts

It is anticipated that on October 1, 2015 the ICD-9 codes will be expanded to ICD-10 codes. (As discussed in Chapter 2, health care laws and regulations are in flux and this date may be delayed.) This change increases the specificity of coding from a three- to five-character set to a five- to seven-character one. There are over 68,000 codes listed in ICD-10. Using ICD-9, a patient treated for macular degeneration with a monthly injection required a single code; with ICD-10 there will be 20 codes, specifying which eye(s) and severity. The American Medical Association (AMA) estimates the costs related to conversion—in training, vendor and software upgrades, testing, and payment disruption—could be $225,000 for a small medical practice and over $8 million for a larger practice. Some fear this will accelerate the demise of private practices.

5. Maintaining inventory: Any item purchased by the health care facility belongs to the facility and cannot be taken for personal use without authorization. Even small items, such as pens and paper, should be used only for business purposes. If the health care professional accidentally takes some item home in a pocket, it is important to return it as soon as possible. The cost of items taken by employees is staggering and adds to the overall cost of goods and services in the United States.
6. Educating patients: Promote the practice of healthy lifestyles to reduce the need for medical services. Encourage the use of preventive measures, such as immunizations and prenatal care, to reduce the need for more expensive care later. Clearly explain patient self-care practices to prevent unnecessary office visits.
7. Being willing to cross-train: Cross-training means learning skills outside those traditionally expected in a given occupation. Health care professionals who have a variety of skills and can perform many tasks are more cost effective than employees who have a limited number of skills. Cross-trained health care professionals can fill in as needed, eliminating downtime and delays in delivering patient care or completing department tasks. Examples include respiratory therapists who learn to draw blood and transcriptionists who can perform insurance coding and billing. Being willing to acquire additional skills, learned and practiced under proper supervision, can significantly increase the health care professional's value to an employer and create career opportunities.

Personal Efficiency

Employees who have difficulty performing efficiently on the job often have poor organizational skills, are confused about their priorities (what is most important), and may be slow in making decisions. Efforts to make personal changes may be necessary. Each individual must do a self-evaluation to identify areas that need improvement.

There are numerous books that help with personal assessment by presenting principles to follow in the process of change. Browsing the business and self-improvement sections in a bookstore may assist you to identify an author that relates the material in a manner that addresses your particular concerns and can assist you in your efforts to improve.

The drive for personal effectiveness is a lifelong pursuit, but if developed can lead to tremendous improvements in the life of anyone struggling with ineffectiveness. Certain behaviors form a foundation for such improvement; some are listed here:

- Use the problem-solving process identified in Chapter 1 to assist in determining what areas in your life, if improved, would create the most dramatic changes for the positive. This is where the greatest effort and time should be spent.
- Assume responsibility for your life and your decisions. Remember, not making a decision is a decision. Procrastination is a decision too—the decision to postpone the issue.
- Don't just let life pass you by as you passively look at the world. Take action, make decisions, and initiate changes after a sound evaluation of what is needed. Be willing to accept the consequences of any actions you do or do not take.
- Don't allow yourself to get sidetracked with the minutiae (trivia) of life. The details of daily life and the related interruptions can seem compelling, but don't forget to focus on the big picture of what you have identified as central to your well-being.
- Expect setbacks in your progress, but do not use this as an excuse not to continue.
- If you feel you do not have enough time, monitor how your time is spent and then evaluate and eliminate the unimportant time wasters.
- Communicate clearly and honestly with others when a conflict arises. Look for solutions that will satisfy all involved (this may require creative decision making). Make sure you understand what the other person is truly saying; do not just argue your side. If you are listening empathetically, you will not be planning what you will say next when the other person is speaking.
- Look at your life from a holistic perspective. You and those around you have physical, social, emotional, and spiritual needs. Individuals who address all these areas function better.

If the health care professional is unable to find personal satisfaction, there is a greater likelihood of also having a dissatisfying professional life. Achieving maximum personal effectiveness enables the health care professional to make contributions that lead to an efficient and high-quality organization.

Acting with Thought

The importance of thinking has been emphasized throughout this text. In order to control costs, all health care personnel must pay attention to their actions. The question presented earlier in this chapter, "How can I help reduce unnecessary costs?" should prompt additional questions, the answers to which will guide one's work:

- What are the facts?
- What is the best course of action?
- What is the right thing to do?
- What is the probable impact of my actions?

Applying the problem-solving model introduced in Chapter 1 will assist the health care professional to carefully review situations, gather necessary information, and make sound decisions.

Thinking It Through

James de Melendez has been a respiratory therapist for 22 years. He enjoys working with patients and administering therapies. Although James keeps up with the continuing educational requirements of his profession, he is resistant to learning skills that he considers to be outside the practice of respiratory therapy. James wants to move to a small town and applies for a position in the town's only hospital. He is surprised when he is not hired. When he follows up with the supervisor who interviewed him, he is told that due to cost-control measures, the hospital is focusing on hiring multiskilled professionals who can perform duties in various departments.

1. How has James failed to keep up with trends in health care delivery?
2. What can he do to improve his future employment opportunities?
3. What are the implications for your future career?

WORKBOOK PRACTICE

Go to your workbook and complete the exercises for this chapter.

SUGGESTED LEARNING ACTIVITIES

1. Consider your own financial situation and determine if there are any accounts receivable (any money due to be paid to you: money you have lent; a paycheck for the last two weeks' work; payments you have made in advance for services, such as newspaper or magazine delivery). Do you have any accounts payable (do you owe money)? How do these compare?
2. If you have worked or currently work, identify ways in which your performance has affected the cost of doing business. Review the areas listed under the section "Health Care Professionals' Impact on Costs."
3. Look for articles in news magazines about the rising cost of health care. Are any solutions offered? Do you agree or disagree with the solutions proposed? Explain why.

WEB ACTIVITIES

University of Washington
www.washington.edu

Search for "managed care," and click on "Managed Care: Ethical Topic in Medicine." Review the information on managed care and then click on "Case 1" and read the scenario. What are your thoughts on this topic? Click on "Discussion" and read the comments. Do you agree with the information provided? Why or why not?

Centers for Medicare and Medicaid Services
www.cms.hhs.gov

What are the eligibility guidelines for Medicare and Medicaid? What is the function of CHIP?

U.S. Department of Health and Human Services
www.hhs.gov

Search for "affordable care act read the law". Click on "Full Text of the Affordable Care Act and Reconciliation Act." How many total pages are in this law? Then search for a summary version. Identify two features of the new law that you agree with and two that you have concerns. Explain why?

REVIEW QUESTIONS

1. What factors are contributing to the rising costs of health care?
2. What are the three types of funding for health care institutions?
3. What are the three types of payment methods?
4. How have methods for paying medical costs changed over the years?
5. What is the difference between fee-for-service and managed care?
6. What is the purpose of managed care? What are three methods used to control costs?
7. Who is covered by Medicare? What services are covered?
8. What is Medicaid?
9. Explain the meaning of DRGs.
10. What are the four major areas of expenditures incurred by a health care delivery system?
11. What is the difference between accounts payable and accounts receivable?
12. What is the meaning of "the cost of money"?
13. What are five ways that the health care professional can assist in controlling facility costs?

APPLICATION EXERCISES

1. Refer to The Case of the Inefficient Office at the beginning of the chapter. What suggestions would you offer to your supervisor if you were in Constance's position?
2. It is a particularly busy day for Aubrey Casein as she rushes to assist several physicians as they perform patient procedures. It seems to her that the requests for supplies are coming in faster than she can meet the demand. She knows that the inventory tags on each of the items must be placed in the appropriate location for the charge to be billed to the correct patient's insurance. But today she decides to perform this task later when it slows down and places the inventory tags in her pocket. The day continues at the same fast pace,

and Aubrey arrives home to discover numerous charge tags still in her pocket.

a. What are the possible financial implications of Aubrey's actions?
b. What are the ways she can use to identify which inventory tag goes with which patient?
c. What are the possible consequences if she charges the wrong supplies to a patient?

PROBLEM-SOLVING PRACTICE

Patricia Leonard is trying to find health care coverage for herself, her husband, and her two children. Using the five-step problem-solving process, determine what Patricia can do evaluate different options in health care insurance.

SUGGESTED READINGS AND RESOURCES

Centers for Medicare and Medicaid Services. www.cms.hhs.gov

Feldstein, P. J. (2012). *Health care economics* (7th ed.). Clifton Park, NY: Delmar Cengage Learning.

Goldsteen, R. L., & Goldsteen, K. (2013). *U.S. health care system* (7th ed.). New York, NY: Springer Publishing Company.

Green, M. (2014). *Understanding health insurance* (12th ed.). Clifton Park, NY: Delmar Cengage Learning.

Kongstvedt, P. R. (2013). *Essentials of managed health care* (6th ed.). Sudbury, MA: Jones & Bartlett Publishers.

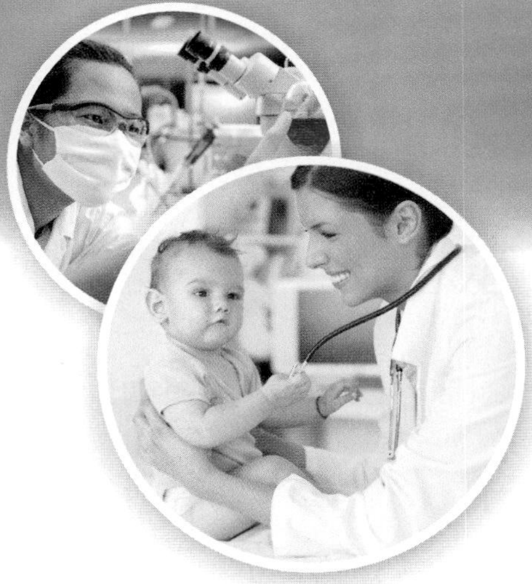

Chapter 23

Performance Improvement and Customer Service

OBJECTIVES

Studying and applying the material in this chapter will help you to:

- Understand the components used in determining quality of care.
- Explain what is meant by quality improvement.
- Identify the internal and external customers in a health care setting.
- Describe the steps in working with unhappy customers.
- Describe the characteristics of constructive criticism.
- Discuss how a health care professional can view destructive criticism in a constructive manner.

KEY TERMS

advocate
constructive criticism
external customers
internal customers
quality improvement
utilization review (UR)

The Case of the Angry Patient

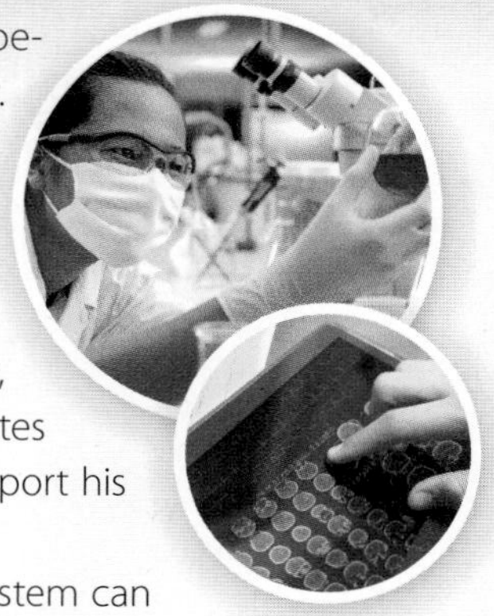

Mr. Ramirez has been hospitalized for the last six days following orthopedic surgery. He is experiencing discomfort and is anxious about not being able to go home and be with his family. When Carolina Mims, physical therapy assistant, enters Mr. Ramirez's room to assist him with his exercises, he lets her know how unhappy he is about how he is being treated. The food is bad, it took "forever" for the nurse to respond to his call button, and the portable urinal has not been emptied. "It's disgusting," he tells Carolina and then asks, "Who's in charge here, anyway?" The fact is, there have been numerous complaints about the quality of the food, and unfortunately, the nursing staff is shorthanded because two nurses have called in sick. Carolina takes a few minutes to listen to Mr. Ramirez, demonstrates empathy for his discomfort, and tells him that she will report his complaints to the nursing supervisor. She is then able to proceed with the exercise session.

Knowing how to effectively handle complaints and work to make improvements in the system can make the difference between a high-quality patient care delivery system and one that fails. Understanding the principles of patient satisfaction will help you resolve problems that can lead to complaints and lawsuits.

QUALITY OF CARE

Finding the balance between maintaining high-quality patient care and controlling costs is a major struggle for modern providers of health care. High cost does not necessarily guarantee the highest level of care. As pointed out in Chapter 22, the United States ranks highest in health care expenditures, but much lower in life expectancy and patient satisfaction, and higher in infant mortality than many other industrialized countries. Many Americans are dissatisfied with the state of health care in the United States and believe major changes are needed, whereas other countries that have lower expenditures report a much higher level of satisfaction.

Discussions about improving the quality of care and raising patient satisfaction begin with two very difficult questions:

1. What is quality of care?
2. How can quality of care be measured?

Quality can be defined as a measure of the degree to which delivered health services meet established professional standards and judgments of value to the consumer. Quality may also be seen as the degree to which actions taken or not taken maximize the probability of beneficial health outcomes and minimize risk and other untoward outcomes. There are various methods of measuring for quality of care.

Approaches to Measuring Quality of Care

Quality of care speaks of the excellence of the health care received. Although measuring quality of care may seem straightforward, it is not an easy task. Let's look at several approaches and the problems inherent in each.

1. Patient satisfaction: If this criterion is used, then we need to look at what patients want and would rate the highest. Patients are concerned with the following:
   - Easily accessible and available services
   - Timely and safe delivery of care
   - Coordination between services and continuity of care
   - Effectiveness of services—that is, the delivery and outcome of care

   Unfortunately, if these concerns were addressed without regard to costs, they would lead to prohibitive health care costs.
2. Lowest costs: Using this criterion, the health care facilities that spent the least would be measured as the most effective.

   This is obviously an inadequate tool because it means that those providing the least care are rated as the best.
3. Patient outcomes: This criterion is based on how well patients recover or manage their ailments. This may seem an obvious choice for measuring the success of a health care experience. Did the patient recover to the prior state of health?

   This method also has limitations because it ignores the value of the time spent in the health care system and only focuses on the end result. For example, if a patient received no education about an upcoming surgery prior to the procedure but recovered and returned to an active and normal life, is this really quality of care? Perhaps the patient stayed in the hospital a few days longer because he or she was not being prepared for the care requirements needed to return home earlier. Could this be classified as a positive outcome?

Another challenge in comparing patient outcomes is the tremendous number of variables that exist among patients with similar procedures. For example, if two patients undergo the same surgical procedure and have no complications, should they both be expected to be discharged from the hospital within the same time frame? On the surface, the answer may be yes, but other factors must be considered. What if one patient is 30 years old and the other is 90 years old? What if one has a preexisting condition (e.g., diabetes or heart disease) and the other does not? What if one lives alone and the other has family and friends willing to come in and assist with the care?

If the patient outcomes for one health care facility are compared with those of another as a measurement of quality, another concern arises in this approach. What if one hospital shows a much higher death rate than another? Is this an indication that one is giving better care than the other? Perhaps one hospital is located where there is a large elderly population and the other in a neighborhood with many young families. How would this affect the statistics?

Currently, there are no absolute answers when discussing such complex issues. These issues are far from being resolved and will continue to be central to health care in the foreseeable future. The focus of this text is not on solving these complex issues facing health care, but on assisting the health care professional in developing the skills and behavior needed to perform at the highest level and deliver the highest possible quality of care. Health care professionals must ask themselves what they can do to best meet the needs of the organization, their coworkers, and patients.

In health care the goal is 100% correct care with no errors, because anything less can have serious consequences for both patients and health care professionals. This may seem unrealistic, but when viewed from a personal perspective, it becomes real. For example, how would you feel if you were among those who had the wrong surgical procedure performed on them? Or what would be the consequences to you and your family if you contract hepatitis B from a needle stick? Everyone must continually strive to provide competent, conscientious, and appropriate care.

QUALITY IMPROVEMENT

In the past the belief was that if more was done, the result would be an increase in quality of care. It is now believed that the focus must be on *improving quality of care and on cost containment*. The processes used to find ways to preserve or improve quality of care while decreasing costs are called **quality improvement**.

The Centers for Medicare and Medicaid Services (CMS) is a federal agency within the U.S. Department of Health and Human Services (DHHS). Programs for which CMS is responsible include Medicare, Medicaid, the Children's Health Insurance Program (CHIP), the Health Insurance Portability and Accountability Act of 1996 (HIPAA), and the Clinical Laboratory Improvement Amendments (CLIA). The CMS promoted the development of internal monitoring (within health care organizations) and evaluation processes. These were designed to identify the changes needed to decrease costs while still *maintaining* quality.

The CMS requires all health care facilities to establish a quality assessment and performance improvement (QAPI) program that is committed to ensuring high-quality and cost-effective care. Medicare contractors are required to prepare and submit a QAPI report to the CMS in order to receive reimbursement for any of the CMS programs. This report has many components. Being a Medicare contractor is vital to the functioning of any health care facility, not just those that care for patients aged 65 and older. This is because most private insurance companies, and also certifying agencies, require that a health care facility be a Medicare contractor.

Internal Monitoring

Each facility will develop its own programs to evaluate the facility, identify areas for measurement, and perform reviews. These programs are designed by the health care facility to meet its internal needs. The assumption is that all areas can be improved (Box 23–1) and that this improvement will result in a higher quality of care and cost efficiency. This approach is based on data and uses a scientific approach to collect and analyze information and processes. The focus is on long-term system improvements.

BOX 23–1

Three Primary Areas to Examine When Evaluating a Health Care Facility for Quality Improvement

1. Organizational structure: How is the facility structured? What is the management style? How is communication encouraged? What changes would increase efficiency and accessibility?
2. Health care professionals: How do the health care professionals function as a team? What processes could be changed to increase efficiency and employee satisfaction?
3. Patient outcomes: Is the patient satisfied with the care? Was the outcome of his or her health care problem resolved in an efficient and appropriate manner with minimal suffering and confusion? Was the care provided in a coordinated manner to decrease duplication of services and minimize confusion?

BOX 23–2

Utilization Review Example

Problems are identified by the health care facility (e.g., a seemingly high rate of urinary infections in patients with a Foley catheter). These problems are called key indicators of quality care and are quantified (e.g., a chart review is done to determine how many patients with a Foley catheter have developed a urinary infection during a specified care time frame). The result is compared to industry standards to see if it exceeds the expected rate of such problems. If it is determined to be a problem area, education or other interventions are done to correct the identified problem. Then the study is repeated for subsequent periods (usually on a quarterly basis) to determine whether or not improvements have occurred as a result of the intervention. The results are used as measurements to determine if the quality of care is improving or declining. The focus is on individual performance, deviation from standards, and problem solving.

Another process frequently used is called **utilization review (UR)** or utilization management (UM). This is an evaluation of the necessity, appropriateness, and efficiency of the use of health care services, procedures, and facilities. UR can be done by a peer review group (see Figure 23–1) or a public agency. It is a method of tracking, reviewing, and rendering opinions regarding care provided to patients. Usually UR involves the use of protocols, benchmarks, or data with which to compare specific cases to an aggregate set of cases. (See Box 23–2.) Managed care organizations sometimes refuse to reimburse or pay for services that do not meet their own sets of UR standards. UR involves the review of patient records and patient bills primarily, but may also include telephone conversations with providers. The practices of precertification, recertification, retrospective review, and concurrent review all describe UR methods. UR is one of the primary tools utilized by health plans to control overutilization, reduce costs, and manage care.

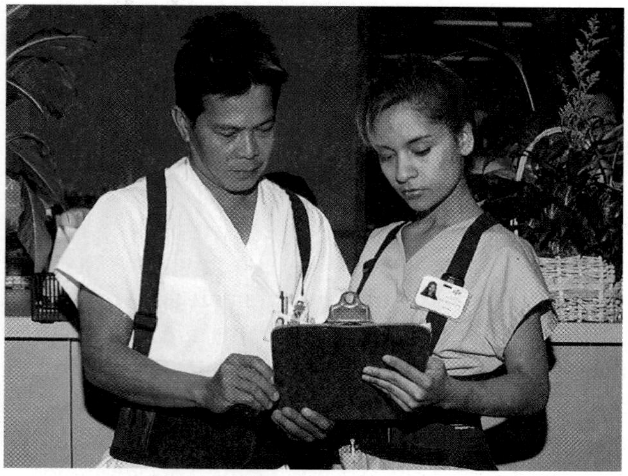

FIGURE 23–1 Quality improvement issues are identified by conducting studies of facility performance.

So far in this chapter, we have discussed the need to increase quality while decreasing costs. These may at first appear to be contradictory goals, but they are not. The following real-life examples demonstrate how the quality of care can be improved while costs are decreased.

- Not prescribing broad-spectrum antibiotics: Past practice was to order a broad-spectrum antibiotic when prescribing antibiotics for a patient. The philosophy was that the broader acting drug would "get whatever was there." But as more was learned about the development of bacterial resistance when unnecessary antibiotics are prescribed, it was determined that performing a culture (a test to see what bacteria are present) and using a more specific antibiotic was the best treatment choice for the patient. This had the advantage of decreasing the risk of resistance developing and rendering the drug ineffective when it was really needed. The cost advantage in this case is that the more specific antibiotics are often less expensive than the broad-spectrum antibiotics.

- Ordering disposable bibs: Health care professionals in a hospital would often use a towel as a bib when feeding patients to prevent the gown from being soiled. The administration conducted a study that demonstrated that the cost of sending the towels to the laundry was more than that of purchasing disposable bibs. The disposable bibs were purchased, and much to the delight of the staff, were more effective for their intended purpose, as well as costing less.

CUSTOMER SERVICE

Satisfactory customer service is essential to the success of health care business in today's competitive market. When the term *customer* is used, it refers to both internal and external customers. **Internal customers** are those who work in the health care industry. For example, health care professionals from other offices, outside suppliers of medical and pharmaceutical supplies, and coworkers are internal customers who are affected by the behavior of those they work with on a day-to-day basis. **External customers** are those who come to the health care provider for services. They may be referred to as customers, patients, consumers, or clients.

Patients come to health care providers for a variety of reasons. (See Box 23–3.) They may hope to have a specific problem cured and their prior level of health restored. The visit may involve a request for a routine evaluation to confirm the patient's level of health or to obtain information on preventive measures that will help to prevent future problems. Or a sudden illness or emergency situation may develop that requires immediate attention. Whatever the reason for patients' contact with the health care facility, there is always the expectation that high-quality professional service will be delivered. (See Figure 23–2.)

When a patient evaluates the service received, it is not just the outcome that is important, but the

BOX 23–3

Services Sought by Patients through the Health Care System

1. Prevention
   - Education: Examples include nutrition and exercise, prevention of heart disease, smoking-cessation programs, how to manage diabetes
   - Routine physical exams
   - Screening tests: Examples include mammogram, sigmoidoscopy/colonoscopy, Pap smear, blood pressure check, PSA (screening test for prostatic cancer), fecal blood, cholesterol and lipids blood tests
2. Emergency and Urgent Care Services
   - Illnesses and injuries that need immediate attention
3. Inpatient Services
   - Surgery
   - Illnesses and injuries requiring continuous acute care
   - Specialized treatments
   - Rehabilitation
4. Long-Term Care
   - Nursing homes
   - Assisted living
5. In-Home Care
   - Nursing
   - Therapy
   - Homemaking
6. Psychological/Psychiatric Services
   - Counseling
   - Medication
7. Dental Services
   - Preventive care
   - Treatment and restoration
8. Pharmaceuticals and Medical Supplies and Equipment
   - Medications and other items needed to restore or maintain health

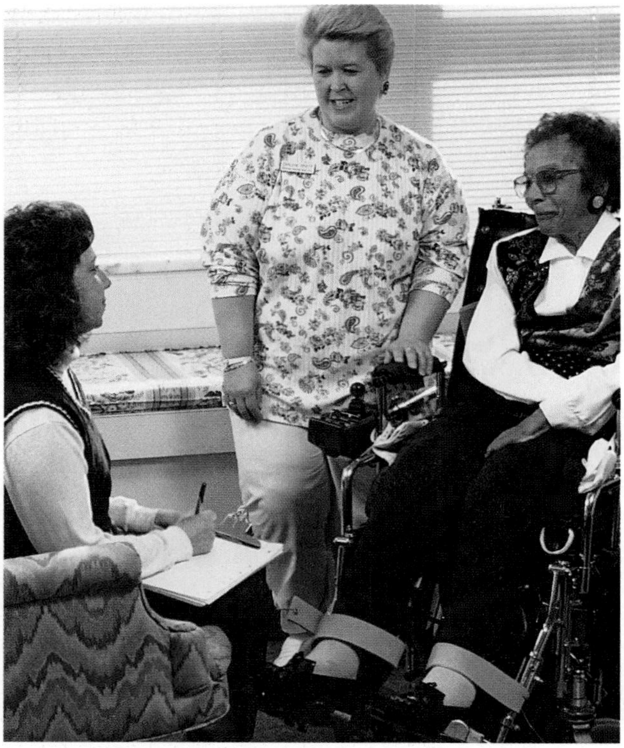

FIGURE 23–2 Patients expect high-quality care. Their satisfaction must be one of the goals of every health care professional.

entire experience. For example, two patients can have the same diagnosis, receive the same treatment, and return to their prior level of health within the same time frame, but one may be satisfied and the other very upset with the care received. It is necessary to review more than simply the medical problem that was presented. All aspects of contact with the patient must be examined when checking for quality. Examples of questions to ask about patient service include the following:

- If the initial contact was made by telephone, how was the patient treated? Was he or she placed on hold? Disconnected? Was the health care professional courteous and did he or she express interest and concern?
- When the patient arrived for the appointment, how long did he or she wait before being seen by the health care professional? Was the patient kept informed of any delays?
- Was the patient required to wait for procedures and tests once they were scheduled?
- Was he or she given clear instructions and were all questions answered? Was the patient given information about how to have future questions answered?
- Were all procedures explained and consent obtained?
- Were all personnel courteous and compassionate when delivering care? Or was the care rough and abrupt and not considerate of the patient's needs?
- If the patient was in the hospital, what was the temperature and quality of the food? Was it quiet at night so he or she could sleep with a minimum of interruptions? Was he or she able to get prompt assistance when needed?

As health care professionals, it is sometimes easy to slip into a routine of just doing the job and forgetting that this may be a very frightening or stressful experience for the patient. When working with patients, use the time to learn more about their thoughts, concerns, and learning needs. This is not the time for the health care professional to share the exciting weekend trip or the fun date from the night before. Avoid engaging in social conversation with other health care professionals and ignoring the patients. They are there for service, and the focus must be concentrated on their needs. Social interactions with coworkers should be saved for breaks or after-work hours.

Most people are surprised to learn that lawsuits brought by patients are more closely related to whether the patient does or does not like the health care professionals than to any other factor. In the past, it was common to have lifelong relationships with physicians, based on mutual trust

Thinking It Through

Dr. Arthur has maintained a successful orthopedic practice in Midtown for many years. He has a good reputation for providing caring service. In recent months his medical assistant, Nathan Alberts, has received an increasing number of patient complaints about having to wait to see Dr. Arthur when they arrive for their appointments.

1. How should Nathan respond when patients complain about the delays?
2. Using the problem-solving process, what steps would you recommend Nathan take in order to resolve this problem?

and respect. Today it is more common for patients to be treated by strangers. Changes in health care plans may require that new health care providers be chosen. If a referral to a specialist is required, the referring physician may have to be chosen from a list of approved specialists. Health care professionals must take advantage of every patient contact to create positive relationships and provide the highest quality care possible.

It is a common belief that if a lawsuit is filed, there must be good cause. Someone must have made a mistake. This is not necessarily true. Lawsuits may be filed as a result of emotional responses to perceived wrongs. Or they may concern matters of little importance, known as frivolous lawsuits. Keep in mind, though, that any lawsuit filed, whether it seems legitimate or not, will cause a great deal of stress for everyone involved. The amount of time and money spent in addressing a lawsuit can be overwhelming. Many lawsuits can be avoided by working to ensure that all patients are satisfied customers.

Taking Responsibility for Quality

Since this is an introduction to health care text, we have repeatedly emphasized reporting to or checking with your supervisor. This is important, but providing quality care involves more than this. You have a depth of responsibility that goes beyond just being a subordinate employee. Each individual health care professional should take his or her role very seriously. Everyone reports to a boss but that does not exempt them from maximizing their contribution to the organization. Even those who run large corporations that make widgets have an accountability. They report to the board of directors and frequently are accountable to shareholders if the corporation is listed on the stock exchange. In health care it is more important than ever to assist in efforts to give quality care and decrease costs. Your job is not just making widgets; how you conduct yourself affects the well-being of another person. It is not enough to just turn the problem over to someone else or hope it goes away. You need to ask yourself, "Have I done everything I can to resolve this problem?" If you need to refer a problem to someone else, then you can ask, "Is there some way I can expedite this issue?" Sometimes it will be necessary to be an **advocate** (one who supports or promotes the interests of others) for the patient or draw attention to an ongoing problem that is not being addressed. Your supervisor may be busy or perhaps does not immediately see the issue that you do. In this case it will be necessary to use your communication skills to get the proper attention the problem needs. Good quality health care means doing the right thing at the right time, in the right way, for the right person; and getting the best possible results.

Customer Satisfaction

The "3 to 11 rule" of customer satisfaction states that for every good thing that happens to us we tell three people. For every bad thing that happens we tell 11 people.

One approach that many health care businesses use to determine how satisfied their customers are is to conduct customer surveys. These can be done in two ways:

1. Mailing out questions that customers answer and return by mail
2. Calling customers and asking them to respond to questions over the telephone

Some health care facilities maintain a log listing all complaints, what was done to address the complaint, and if the resolution was satisfactory. If the results are made available to staff, it is worth the health care professional's time to review the comments. The areas of concern may be very different from what is expected and can lead to changes in performance that will create greater customer satisfaction.

When working with unhappy customers, it is critical to fully understand their view of the situation. (See Figure 23–3.) To accomplish this, it is necessary to

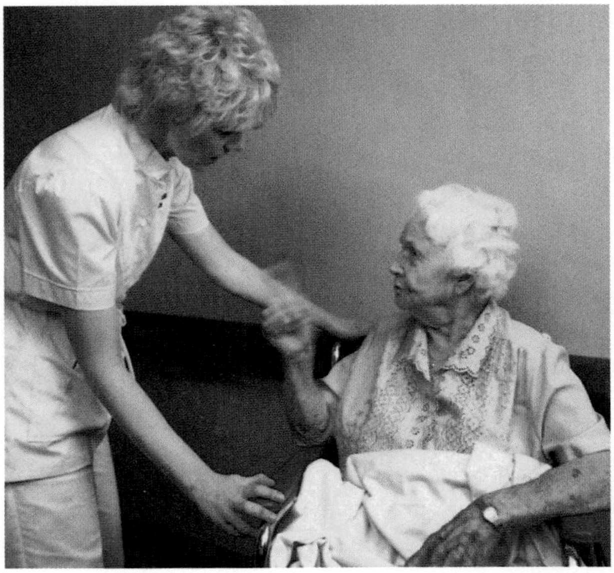

FIGURE 23–3 Good listening skills are essential when handling a patient complaint.

Table 23–1 Working with Unhappy Customers (Internal and External)

Steps	Comments
1. Identify the problem	• Listen to the complaint with an open mind. • Try to completely understand the customer's side of the situation. • Ask questions to clarify as needed, but do not interrupt needlessly. • Do not display verbal or nonverbal defensiveness. • Thank the customer for the information, because the goal is to always obtain customer satisfaction.
2. Seek resolution	• If the problem is with you personally, it is appropriate to apologize, thank the customer for the feedback, and assure him or her that you will do your best not to repeat the error. • If you need more information before the problem can be resolved, let the customer know when you will get back to him or her. • Provide information that the customer may be lacking. Make sure the customer is open to hearing what will be said and that it is phrased in a nondefensive manner. For example, if a customer complains about having had to pay for parking on the last visit, this could be addressed in a defensive or nondefensive manner. A defensive approach usually is an attempt to place blame on the customer, whereas a nondefensive approach does not. Consider these statements: Defensive—"Well, if you had just asked about it, we would have validated the ticket for you." Nondefensive—"I am sorry, we should have informed you that we validate parking tickets for patients. Do you have your ticket with you so we can validate it for you today?" • If you do not have the authority to deal with the problem, refer the customer to the proper person or ask the person with the authority to contact the customer.
3. Verify satisfaction	• Does the customer feel the problem has been resolved satisfactorily?

listen without interrupting and to not display signs of defensiveness. The guidelines in Table 23–1 will assist in handling this type of interaction.

Remember that each health care professional is responsible for patient satisfaction. The cost of an unhappy patient is much more than the loss of that one patient because he or she will probably tell family, friends, and coworkers.

It is also important to recognize that satisfaction is a subjective perception. Therefore, a health care professional must listen carefully and constantly to determine if the patient has any concerns. The patient may have a positive outcome to his or her medical treatment but may be unhappy with the experience due to a cold food tray, a delay in answering a call light, waiting for tests, delayed treatments, an unemptied bedpan, or delayed pain medications.

Internal Customers

It is just as important to maintain good relationships with internal customers as with external ones. One of the common mistakes made when working with coworkers is to quickly point out errors but not take the time to stress what they do well. Praising coworkers for a job well done, a courtesy extended, or a quick response to a situation can build trusting and mutually satisfying working relationships. Everyone wants to do well on the job, to contribute to the effectiveness of the office or facility, and to have a sense of self-satisfaction with their contributions. When people take pride in their work, they will work harder and more cooperatively than they will if they feel that others are being overly critical.

Good relationships also require that criticism be given when appropriate. **Constructive criticism** is based on optimism. The intended message is that setbacks or failures are due to circumstances that can be changed for the better. It holds out the hope of improvement and suggests the beginning of a plan for doing so. (See Figure 23–4.) On the other hand, *destructive criticism* has the effect of creating helplessness, anger, and rebellion. The person is immediately put on the defensive and may no longer be receptive to suggestions for improvement. When individuals are led to believe that their failures are due to personal faults that cannot be changed, they lose hope and stop trying. For example, a medical assistant is just starting a new job. In her haste

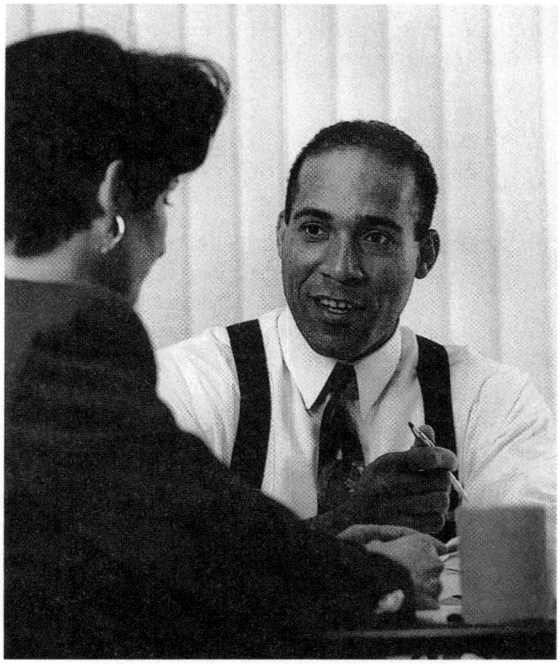

FIGURE 23–4 The goals of constructive criticism are to encourage improvement and to resolve problems.

to try to manage too many duties in order to make a good first impression, she inadvertently forgets to log two patient appointments. The result is that three patients are scheduled for the same time with the same nurse practitioner. The medical assistant's supervisor addresses the situation: Constructively: "While I know how overwhelming all the duties you have to accomplish are, it is important that you accurately accomplish each duty. Until you feel more comfortable with all your duties, try to concentrate on one duty at a time (e.g., answer one phone call; finish the scheduling of a patient's appointment prior to answering another phone). Destructively: "You messed up! The nurse practitioner will not have a chance for a break, and the whole day's schedule is behind." Box 23–4 contains effective guidelines for giving constructive criticism.

It is difficult hearing criticism, especially if it is not presented as constructive criticism. When receiving destructive criticism from someone, the health care professional can change it into a positive experience by implementing the suggestions in Box 23–5.

BOX 23–4

How to Give Constructive Criticism

- Be concise and clear during conversations. If the other person does not understand exactly what you mean, it increases the chances of misunderstandings. Giving specific examples that illustrate the issue is a great way to increase clarity.
- Never use vague, general, or harsh terms. It is frustrating to hear that you are doing something wrong or not performing well and not understand exactly what can be done to correct the situation.
- Include positive comments of what the other person is doing well. Using positive and negative comments is sometimes referred to as the "sandwich technique." Start and end the conversation with positive feedback and then incorporate (sandwich in) the area(s) that need improvement.
- If the problem directly affects you, state how it makes you feel. For example, if a coworker is not completing his or her tasks before leaving the workplace, state that you feel taken advantage of and rushed by having to complete the extra tasks.
- Show a respectful attitude toward the other person. Always strive to preserve the other person's self-respect. Everyone makes mistakes or has areas that need improvement.
- Demonstrate a cooperative attitude. Give ample opportunity for the other person to ask questions and seek clarification about what is being stated. Offer positive suggestions for improvement.
- Be sensitive as this may be difficult for the other person to hear. No one likes to confront their faults. If the reaction is defensive, do not respond defensively in turn. Acknowledge the reaction and attempt to redirect to a more positive exchange.
- Provide time for face-to-face communication that is done in private. It is uncomfortable giving a criticism, but distancing oneself by using impersonal messages or memos creates greater discomfort and prevents the opportunity for the other person to respond or seek clarification.
- Use empathy when communicating. Stay aware of the impact on the person of what you say and how you say it.
- Never complain to others about the performance of a coworker. Communicate directly with him or her privately and confidentially.

BOX 23-5

Responding to Destructive Criticism

- Look for the "kernel of truth" in the statement.
- Be aware of your emotional response and set it aside in an effort to benefit from the exchange.
- Do not attack the other person. You may feel that you have information about his or her own performance, attitude, or practices, but now is not the time to share these thoughts.
- If the situation becomes too emotional, ask to take a break and negotiate a time to resume the conversation later. This gives you an opportunity to put things in perspective.
- Even if you do not agree with what is being said, be open to trying to understand it from the other person's point of view.
- If the feedback is valid, take responsibility and initiate the needed changes in behavior.
- Look at the experience as an opportunity to develop stronger team relationships with coworkers and to improve communications. Work with the person giving the criticism to solve the perceived problem.
- Ask for specific examples if you are unclear about what is being said.
- Ask for suggestions about how you might improve.

Fascinating Facts

- A business hears from only 4% of its unhappy customers. The other 96% go elsewhere for service.
- Sixty-eight percent of the unhappy customers leave because of an attitude of indifference toward them.
- Seventy percent of complaining customers will do business with you again if you resolve the complaint in their favor. This increases to 95% if the complaint is resolved on the spot.

Positive relationships with coworkers provide the foundation for making efforts as an organization to offer high-quality service to all customers. *Employee satisfaction leads to customer satisfaction.*

Thinking It Through

Carstyn Franklin is a certified occupational therapy assistant (COTA) working in a busy hand therapy clinic. She and the other two assistants work with patients, make splints, and teach the use of adaptive devices so that patients can learn to perform homemaking and self-care practices as independently as possible. Brandon Williams, one of the other assistants, has the habit of leaving equipment, tools, and supplies wherever he last used them instead of putting them away. This results in delays for the other assistants because they must locate needed items before they can do their own work.

1. Describe in detail how Carstyn can speak with Brandon about his work habits.
2. What should be the goal of her communication?
3. How can she present the problem in order to increase the chances of resolution?
4. How can she respond if Brandon reacts defensively?

WORKBOOK PRACTICE

Go to your workbook and complete the exercises for this chapter.

SUGGESTED LEARNING ACTIVITIES

1. Survey friends and family members about their health care experiences. Were they positive or negative, and why? What did they want from health care professionals? Did they receive it?
2. Spend some time thinking about how you would want to be treated as a patient. What would be most important to you?
3. Watch for examples of good customer service. Describe what you believe makes them good.
4. Try using the suggested constructive criticism method the next time you need to discuss a problem or behaviour concern with someone. What methods did you use? What was the result?
5. Pay attention to how you receive criticism. Do you generally find it to be a learning experience? A confrontation? A waste of time?

WEB ACTIVITIES

Centers for Medicare and Medicaid Services

www.cms.hhs.gov

What is HIPAA? What is CLIA? What is the Medicare Modernization Act?

Online Search

Search for "customer service guidelines." Review one of the samples. What do you think of these guidelines? How do they compare to the ones where you have worked? (If you have never been employed, then use the school as the comparison.)

REVIEW QUESTIONS

1. What components determine quality of care?
2. What is quality improvement?
3. What is the purpose of utilization review (UR)?
4. Who are internal and external customers?
5. What are the steps in working with unhappy customers?
6. What are the characteristics of constructive criticism?
7. How can a health care professional view destructive criticism in a constructive manner?

APPLICATION EXERCISES

1. Refer to The Case of the Angry Patient at the beginning of this chapter. How would Carolina respond to Mr. Ramirez's criticism constructively? Destructively?
2. Alicia has just about had it at work. As a respiratory therapist, she loves working with patients. She knows that breathing difficulties create great anxiety, and she likes knowing that her work helps patients resolve more than just their physical problems. But Alicia is distressed by the disarray in the hospital department where she works. Her schedule is often changed, sometimes with very little notice. This causes problems with her child care arrangements. Equipment is not always put away where it should be, and supply inventories are often depleted. Alicia decides to discuss the situation with her supervisor. She recently took a workshop on quality improvement and believes that what she learned could be applied to resolving her department's disorder.
   a. How can Alicia present her concerns in a positive way to her supervisor?
   b. What can she share about quality improvement that might be helpful?
   c. What kinds of processes might be put in place to help resolve the department's problems?

PROBLEM-SOLVING PRACTICE

Refer to Box 23–2, Utilization Review Example. Compare this example with the five-step problem-solving process described in Chapter 1. Is the complete process being used?

SUGGESTED READINGS AND RESOURCES

Centers for Medicare and Medicaid Services. www.cms.hhs.gov

Covey, S. R. (2013). *The 7 habits of highly effective people: Powerful lessons in personal change.* New York: Simon & Schuster.

This page intentionally left blank

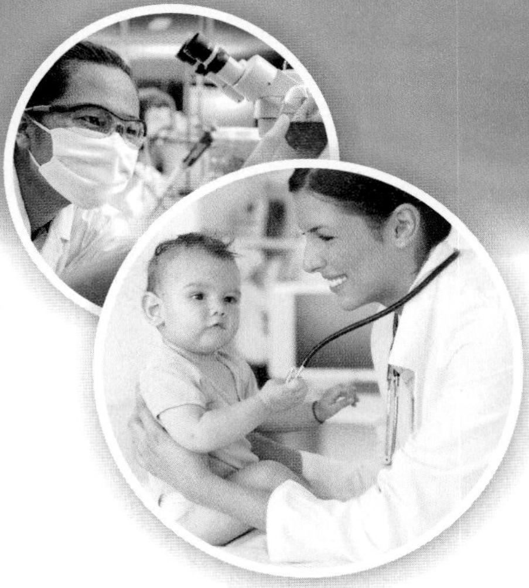

Unit 9

Securing and Maintaining Employment

This page intentionally left blank

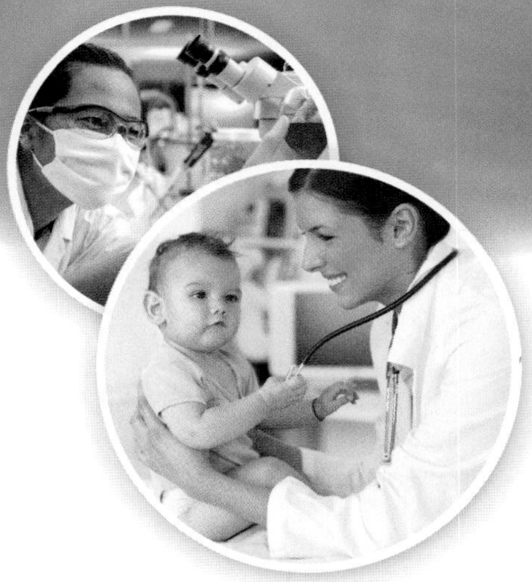

Chapter 24

Job Leads and the Resume

OBJECTIVES

Studying and applying the material in this chapter will help you to:

- Develop an inventory of your employment skills and personal traits that are of value to an employer.
- Identify your workplace preferences.
- Describe ways to get organized for the job search.
- List the most common sources of job leads and explain how to use each one effectively.
- Describe the sections of a resume.
- Describe the contents and purpose of chronological and functional resumes.
- List the characteristics of an effective resume.
- Create a resume that highlights your qualifications and encourages employers to interview you.
- Explain the purpose of cover letters.
- Write effective cover letters to accompany your resume.

KEY TERMS

career service center
chronological resume
cold calling
cover letters
functional resume
joblines
networking
objective
resume
traits

The Case of the Unprepared Applicant

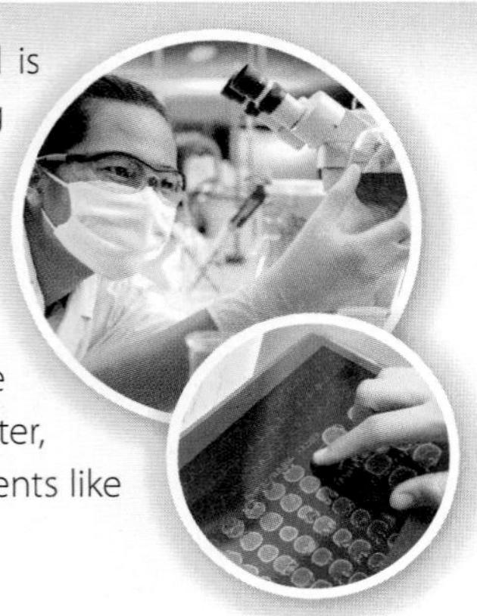

Jenny Nguyen recently passed her state exam to become a registered dental assistant and is seeking her first job. Jenny did well in her training, but has not had much experience applying for jobs. The career services counselor at Jenny's school calls her on Tuesday morning to tell her about a job opening with Dr. Chambers, a well-respected dentist in her area. A job in his dental clinic would be an excellent opportunity for a new dental assistant. Jenny is interested in the position but has put off completing her resume and needs a few more hours to finish it. She is also nervous about her interviewing skills and delays calling Dr. Chambers. When she finally calls on Friday afternoon, she learns that the job was filled that morning. In this chapter, you will learn how to be prepared for job opportunities and avoid experiencing disappointments like Jenny did.

OVERVIEW OF THE JOB SEARCH

The job search can be an exciting and challenging experience for the health care graduate. The purpose of this chapter and Chapter 25 is to help learners plan and carry out the activities necessary to secure satisfying employment.

It may surprise you to learn how much the job-seeking process is like a job in itself. You should plan to devote at least 20 hours each week to your job search. Some employment professionals even recommend that you spend up to 40 hours. That may sound like a lot, but think about it. Health care learners spend a lot of time, money, and effort completing an education. Furthermore, a large percentage of waking hours are spent at work. It makes sense to devote the time necessary to find a job you like and that makes the best use of your education. Job satisfaction is an important factor in a person's quality of life. Investing time and effort in the job search will pay off in the future.

Developing a positive attitude will help make the job search more of an adventure than a chore. Almost everyone feels nervous or apprehensive about approaching potential employers in the hope of being hired. Job seekers often see themselves as powerless, but this is not true. You can increase your self-confidence if you understand that graduates who offer the skills and **traits** (personal characteristics) that employers need, and the positive, can-do attitude that they want, are a welcome addition to their staff. This is true for all types of health care occupations and all types of facilities, such as hospitals, physicians' offices, insurance companies, and dental clinics.

Employers want to hire people who meet more than the position's minimum qualifications. They hope to find people who are pleasant, enthusiastic, and likeable. Graduates can project these qualities by approaching the job search positively and by seeing it as an opportunity to make a contribution to the health care community.

What Do You Have to Offer?

A common problem for new graduates is that they don't realize how much they have to offer employers. Like many other applicants, you may be concerned that your lack of health care experience will make it difficult for you to find a job. Learners are often surprised to discover just how many qualifications they really have. The first step in a successful job search is to identify these qualifications. For example, your technical skills are up to date and fresh in your mind. This is a plus. However, these skills are only part of what makes an effective employee. The traits that will most likely determine your success in securing and maintaining employment include professionalism, enthusiasm, willingness to learn, a positive attitude, and reliability. In fact, many employers report that they prefer to hire an enthusiastic person who is willing to learn over someone with the better technical skills, but who has a poor attitude.

Spend some time creating a personal inventory of both your technical and nontechnical skills. The technical skills are the most obvious and can be collected by reviewing textbooks, class and lab materials, and clinical evaluations. Employers are also looking for applicants with strong nontechnical skills. Three of the most important are the ability to:

1. Communicate: Listen carefully to others. Organize thoughts and speak clearly at a level appropriate for the listener.
2. Problem-solve: Identify problems, gather necessary information, consider alternatives, and use good judgment when choosing a solution.
3. Work as a team member: Help others, work cooperatively, manage conflict.

Other personal characteristics of value to health care employers include the following:

- Integrity: Be honest, maintain confidentiality, choose the right way rather than the easy way.
- Responsibility: Work without constant supervision, know when to ask for help.
- Dependability: Follow through on obligations without being reminded. Complete all assigned tasks. Always be on time and rarely be absent.
- Organization: Be accurate and efficient. Use time well. Prioritize your tasks.
- Consideration: Be friendly, polite, empathetic, and patient. Work well with diverse populations.
- Willingness to learn: Ask questions, acquire new knowledge and skills, and keep up to date in the field.

This list gives only a few suggestions. Think about what you have learned in your roles as a parent, learner, volunteer, group member, or employee. Life is rich with experiences to draw from. Use your self-inventory to boost your self-confidence and prepare to write an effective resume and present yourself well at interviews. You have a strong foundation on which you can build a successful job search.

What Are Your Expectations?

Before starting the job search, it is important to identify your employment preferences. There are many types of working environments, and finding the one in which you work best is an important factor in determining career success. Consider the following factors when thinking about the type of facility in which you want to work:

- Size of facility
- Pace and speed of work
- Amount of time spent working with others and working on your own
- Amount of supervision
- Hours of work
- Type of patient population
- Type of professional specialty
- Location
- Orientation and training offered

Identifying appropriate job leads is easier when you have thought about your preferences.

At the same time, remember that recent graduates are usually qualified for *entry-level* positions. More job opportunities will open up as you gain experience. A good career move may be to compromise some of your preferences in exchange for starting out with an employer who offers you opportunities to learn and grow professionally.

It is also important to be aware of your financial needs. Track your current expenses for a few months and calculate the minimum amount needed to cover your cost of living. Be sure to consider the following basic expenses:

- Housing and associated costs: Rent or mortgage, insurance, utilities, phone, repairs, cleaning supplies, child care
- Transportation: Vehicle, fees, insurance, gas, repairs
- Clothing and grooming supplies
- Health care, including insurance
- Food
- Entertainment

Organizing Your Time

Planning your time structures your job search and ensures that you focus on activities that are most likely to bring results. Decide how many hours you can devote to your search each week and make weekly and daily to-do lists of tasks. A typical list would include the following:

- Making phone calls
- Revising your resume to target specific employers
- Writing and sending thank-you letters
- Searching the Internet for information and job leads
- Following up on leads

Be prepared to take advantage of and follow up on every opportunity. If at the last minute you learn about a chance to attend an interview, you want to be ready. Have your resume, interview clothing, and reliable transportation available at all times during the job search process. Career services personnel report that many graduates lose job opportunities because they don't act fast enough on leads.

Organizing Your Space

A good way to keep yourself organized is to devote a specific area in your home to your job search. Keep all the supplies and materials you will need together so they are easy to find. Don't take the chance of losing the phone number of a potential employer because you wrote it on a little scrap of paper in the kitchen. You will find the following items helpful in conducting an effective job search:

- Appointment calendar, either electronic or paper
- System for recording information, such as potential employers, the names and addresses of people who might provide assistance with the job search, and questions you want to ask potential employers. Apps for phones are available to help you organize your job search. Other ways to maintain this information include electronic files, a three-ring binder, or index cards in a small file box.
- Good quality paper and matching envelopes for resumes, cover letters, and thank-you notes. White or off-white is a good choice for the health care field.
- Computer supplies, if you have a home computer. Be sure to have an extra print cartridge on hand.
- Dictionary, either electronic or printed: Anything you send to a potential employer must be completely free of spelling errors.
- Street maps of your area or access to electronic maps or a GPS/navigation system

Projecting a Professional Image

You will be receiving calls or emails from your school, people who have contacts, and potential employers. Be sure that these calls are handled in a manner that reflects well on you. If you have a shared phone at home, review proper phone manners and message-taking with everyone who answers the phone. You don't want to miss a possible interview because you don't have the return phone number or the caller was put off by rude manners. A family member who answers incoming calls with a hostile "Yeah?" may damage your efforts before you even have a chance to take the call. If you have an answering machine with a recorded message or a cell phone with voicemail, be sure the message is not off-color or too cute. Remember that what the caller hears represents you as a potential employee.

If you are rarely available by phone during working hours, or cannot access voice mail or answering machine messages during those hours, arrange to have a dependable person take calls. The messages should be retrieved often so that potential appointments or information about jobs are not missed.

Recall from Chapter 18 that anything posted online, including social networking sites, should be in good taste. If you use a social networking site such as Facebook, use it to your advantage by posting information and photos of yourself performing volunteer work, helping with a community project, or other activities that portray you in a positive light. Increasing numbers of employers report checking social networking sites for all job candidates. Also, your email address should be appropriate for someone seeking a career in health care.

It is important that you look and act professional during all job search activities. Professionalism is a way of life, not behavior saved for "special occasions." For example, show courtesy and respect to receptionists when you call or go to an office for an interview. Their opinion may be valued by the people doing the hiring.

Always look your best. If you don't have an interview but are running into an office to drop off a completed job application, it may be tempting to dress casually. Don't do it. You don't know who will see you and what authority they have in making hiring decisions. Think of the job search as a series of evaluations and be prepared for each one.

FINDING JOB LEADS

Finding an employer whose needs match your qualifications can take up most of the job search efforts. Knowing how and where to look can spell the difference between the success and failure of your efforts. There are many ways to locate job openings, and the chances of finding the right job are increased by using as many of these sources as possible.

Career Service Center

A large number of graduates find employment as a direct result of working with the staff in the **career service center**. (This may have another name, such as "employment assistance.") This office provides students with job search assistance such as the following:

1. Resume writing
2. Interview practice
3. Internet access
4. Dressing for success hints
5. Current information about local employers:
    - Major health care facilities
    - Directories of physicians and other health care professionals
    - Hiring practices
    - Who is most likely to hire recent graduates

Although it is *your* responsibility to become employed, it is a mistake not to take advantage of the help that is available.

Many employers depend on schools to provide them with prequalified applicants for job openings. Schools may be notified before jobs are advertised. Work with the career service center at your school to take advantage of these opportunities. (See Figure 24–1.) Make a commitment to follow up on all leads and attend any interviews that are scheduled for you. An unhappy event for the school staff is to receive a call from an employer with the news that a graduate who was given a lead did not contact the employer or show up for the interview. Always follow up, even if the job does not seem to be exactly what you want. When referred individuals fail to show up, it damages the credibility of the school and may hurt its future relationship with the employment community. And the job may turn out to be the right one, after all. Even if it is not the right job, the experience will provide practice for interviewing skills, and the employer may provide a connection to another job that *is* a match.

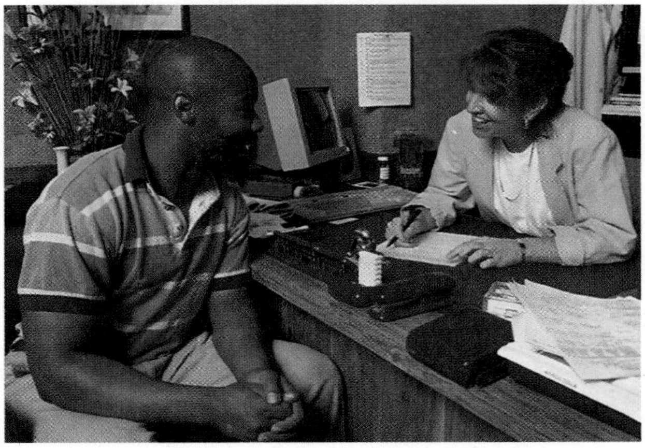

FIGURE 24–1 Seek the help of the career services staff in your school.

Keep the school informed of your job search progress and advise them of any changes to your contact information (phone and address). Many leads are lost because schools cannot locate learners. Advise the school when you accept a job. Some states and accreditation agencies require schools to report on the employment status of their graduates.

Community Career Centers

Government agencies have organized resource centers for job seekers. The U.S. Department of Labor sponsors Career One Stop. Its website, www.careeronestop.org, contains links to state and local career offices all over the United States.

Networking

Networking means developing and interacting with a group of people who might be helpful in meeting your professional goals. Ideally, you can return the help in some way. Networking is one of the most effective ways of securing employment.

There are three types of networking contacts, and all should be developed. The first consists of everyone you know. Tell as many people as possible that you are in the job market. A friend at church may know that his dentist is looking for an assistant. The pharmacist at the local drugstore may have a colleague who needs a pharmacy tech. Project professionalism and enthusiasm about starting a health care career.

The second type of networking contact is a health care professional or employer. In addition to being potential sources of job leads, they can provide general information about the field and tips on getting ahead. Professional networking contacts include the following:

- Instructors
- Other school staff

- Guest speakers
- Attendees at professional meetings, conferences, and workshops
- The supervisor and staff at your clinical site
- Professionals at job fairs
- Your personal physician, dentist, and other health care providers

Don't be shy about approaching people who might be able to help. Smile, introduce yourself, and tell them that you are preparing to enter the health care field. In addition to being a source of job leads, professional contacts can provide valuable information. Here are some questions to ask:

- What skills are most important for succeeding in this career?
- What personal traits are most important?
- What qualities do employers look for when hiring for this occupation?
- What are the major duties?
- Which hospitals, facilities, companies, physicians, or dentists are good to work for and why?

Thinking It Through

Jasmine is feeling discouraged. She completed a nursing assistant program 2 months ago and still has not found a job. Joe Dorland from her school's placement office called this morning wanting to know if she had followed up on the job opening he gave her last week. She told him she hadn't, because the job was on the other side of the city and it would take her at least 40 minutes to get there on the bus. Joe had called with other leads that she hadn't cared to follow up on. They either sounded pretty boring, were in parts of town she didn't know, or didn't pay enough. Jasmine really thinks that the school should do more to help her get what she wants in a job.

1. Does Jasmine have realistic expectations about the job search?
2. Is she likely to continue receiving help from the school's career services office? Explain your answer.
3. What would you suggest that Jasmine do to increase her chances of finding a job?

- What is your best advice for someone who wants to work in this field?
- Can you recommend anyone else I can talk to about working in this field?

The third type of networking is through the Internet. Mailing lists, newsgroups, and Web forums, discussed in Chapter 18, are excellent ways to identify professional contacts, along with Facebook and LinkedIn.

Keep accurate records of networking contacts. Create an electronic file or section in your notebook or use index cards to keep track of names, titles, addresses and phone numbers, where you met, and any planned follow-up action.

Send a thank-you note to anyone who meets with you or provides information. The importance of this simple act of courtesy cannot be overemphasized. Let them know when you are hired and keep in touch. Networking should become a habit maintained throughout your career. It is a way to stay current in the field, develop friendships with other professionals, and add to the enjoyment of work. (See Figure 24–2.)

Clinical Experience

Many learners receive job offers as a result of their performance during their clinical experience (externship/internship/fieldwork). This is *not*, however, the principal purpose of this part of your training, and it is important that you *do not expect* to be offered a

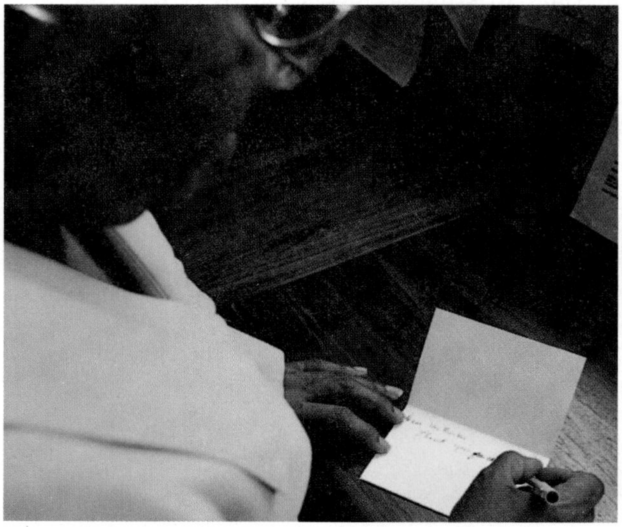

FIGURE 24–2 When networking, it is important to send a thank-you note to anyone who helps you.

job. At the same time, conduct yourself at all times at your professional best. Facilities have created jobs for learners who impress them with outstanding performance. Even if a job is not available, the recommendation of your supervisor may be your most valuable reference.

Cold Calls and Visits

Cold calling refers to calling or visiting employers to make the first contact. The purpose is to identify possible job openings and to inform the employer that you are looking for employment. Many jobs are not advertised, so this can be an excellent way to locate openings. Cold calling requires self-confidence and good communication skills. It is essential to be courteous and considerate when making contacts.

Use the Internet, yellow pages, or professional directories available at your school's career services center, public library, or chamber of commerce to identify and learn about facilities you might wish to contact. Cold calls can be a quick way to locate unadvertised openings and can be especially helpful for graduates who are relocating and want to identify leads before moving.

It is most efficient to visit buildings or complexes that have many offices. Be sure to dress professionally and take copies of your resume. Smile, introduce yourself, inquire about openings, and leave a resume. Do not ask for an interview, however, when dropping in without an appointment. Whether calling or visiting in person, be brief, be appreciative, and be on your way.

Job Fairs and Orientations

There are many types of gatherings that employers attend to recruit employees. Although interviews are not usually conducted nor job offers made, employers provide valuable information to job seekers and may collect their resumes.

Take advantage of these activities. Dress professionally and take copies of your resume. Check your area for the following types of opportunities to meet employers:

- Career fairs sponsored by your school: The employers who attend these are sending the clear message that they hire recent graduates. Ask lots of questions and collect brochures, business cards, and any other handouts offered. Learn as much as you can. After the event, organize the information you have collected. Write notes about whom you met, application procedures, and whom to contact for an interview. Keeping good records is especially important if it will be a while before you are ready to start the formal job search.
- Career fairs sponsored by chambers of commerce and government organizations: Look for announcements in the newspaper. These are commonly placed in the help wanted or business section. Check the bulletin board in the career service center at school. Many job fairs are also listed on the Internet.
- Career orientations and information meetings sponsored by employers: Some large health care facilities conduct open meetings to recruit applicants and explain their hiring process. Contact the human resources department at organizations in which you are interested.
- Professional conventions and conferences: Some employers recruit at these meetings. (See Appendix 1.)

Fascinating Facts

Advertised job openings represent only 15% to 20% of total available jobs at any given time. The remaining *80%* are never published anywhere. The importance of networking and researching to find this "hidden" job market cannot be overemphasized.

Source: Hanson, R. S. Quintessential Careers, "15 Myths and Misconceptions About Job-Hunting." http://www.quintcareers.com/job-hunting_myths.html.

Internet

Today many job seekers use computer technology to connect with employers. (See Figure 24–3.) There are a growing number of ways to use the Internet in the job search:

- Learn job search techniques: Excellent information is available about finding job leads, resume writing, interviewing, and many other topics. A good place to start is at www.rileyguide.com, a large, well-organized, and reliable site that contains abundant information about using the Internet in the job search. It contains links to dozens of

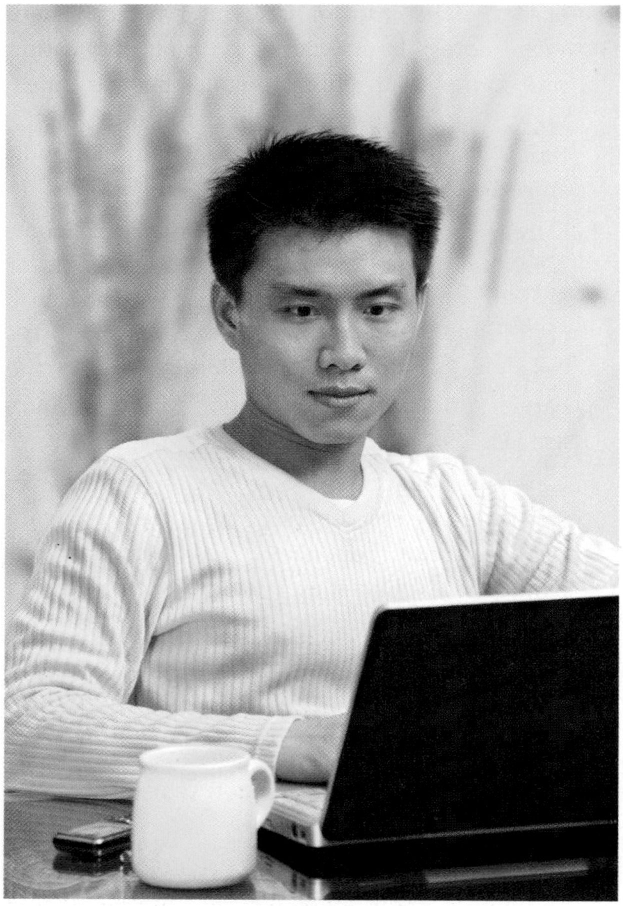

FIGURE 24–3 The Internet is a valuable source of help during the job search, but should be combined with other methods.

other useful sites. Other helpful sites are located at www.jobstar.org. (Job Star was originally created for California, but it contains lots of general information), and www.quintcareers.com.

- Get information about specific facilities: Most health care providers, such as clinics and hospitals, have their own websites. These are excellent sources of information and often contain job postings and information about how to apply. Many include application or resume forms that you can fill out on the screen and submit electronically. In fact, some employers now accept only electronically submitted applications and resumes. Search by name for facilities in your area.
- Find job openings: Some websites collect job openings from sources across the country. Jobs are classified by category, and you can restrict your search to a specific geographic location. Examples include www.indeed.com, www.careerbuilder.com, www.monster.com, and http://us.jobs. Other websites specialize in health care, such as www.healthjobsnationwide.com. Some of these job banks have apps for your phone.
- Post your resume: Many websites have been designed to allow job seekers to post their resumes online. Health care employers are beginning to review these sites when looking to fill positions. Some schools allow learners to use the school's phone number as the contact so that inquiries can be screened. Take care when placing your resume online, especially if there is a fee involved. *Never* submit personal information, such as your social security number. If you do decide to put your resume online, be sure that it is perfect. Many people are likely to see it. Because so many individuals post their resumes online, there is tremendous competition for actually securing a job. These websites should *not* be your main source of job leads.
- Check out professional organizations: In addition to general information about the profession, some have job banks available to members. See Appendix 1 for a list of many health care professional organizations.

The number of websites available for job seekers is growing daily. They tend to change names and addresses, discontinue operations, or merge with other sites. A few make unrealistic claims, such as having more job postings than they actually do. Others may publish misleading job search information. Use the Internet as an important, but not exclusive, tool in the job search.

Fascinating Facts

Seventy-five percent of recruiters are required by their companies to do online research of candidates. And 70% say they have rejected candidates because of information found online. The most common objectionable information involves photos of drug activity. Also found are photos or videos of other illegal and sexual activity and nudity; racist comments; and other evidence of poor judgment. A company started in 2011, scours the Internet for information about prospective employees, then assembles a summary report for employers.

Source: The Bulletin, "Startup Checks to See if Job Seekers Have Clean Social Media Backgrounds." July 21, 2011.

Printed Ads for Job Openings

Many professional journals contain announcements of job openings. And although newspapers contain fewer job postings than in the past, they still can be a source of leads. Job openings are listed alphabetically by job title or industry name in the employment section of the classified ads. Sundays usually have the largest number of ads. Look under all job titles for which you might qualify. An ad for a laboratory technician can appear under "lab," "laboratory," "hospital," "medical," "health," or "technician." Your education may qualify you for a variety of job titles. For example, the patient care assistant program at a California school trains students for at least 16 job titles, including rehabilitation, physical therapy, occupational therapy, and mental health aide; patient care technician; and nursing assistant. It is important that you understand what similar titles mean and know for which positions you might qualify. In some occupations, an important distinction is made between the aide and assistant levels. For example, aide-level positions in physical and occupational therapy do not have specific educational requirements. Assistants, however, must have an associate's degree and pass certification exams. Check with career services or your instructor if you are unsure if you qualify for an advertised position.

When responding to any job advertisement, it is very important to follow the directions. Many employers today prefer that resumes be faxed or emailed. Although it may be tempting to send a nicely printed copy on good quality paper, fax it anyway. A mailed resume may arrive too late for an interview to be scheduled. If the ad reads "no calls," doing so will not increase your chance of being hired. It will only show disregard for the employer's time. Employers want to hire people who can follow directions. If applicants refuse to follow them when applying for the job, why would employers expect them to do any better as employees?

Telephone Joblines

Some employers have **joblines**, taped recordings with information about current openings. The amount of information given varies, ranging from simply a list of job titles to more detailed information about applicant requirements. Jobline phone numbers may be listed in help wanted ads or on the Internet. Some health care facilities feature joblines as a phone menu option.

THE RESUME

A **resume** is a written summary of professional qualifications. Its purpose is to convince employers to interview you and consider you for employment. Your resume must represent you well and convince employers that you are the kind of person they need.

Some learners choose to have someone else, such as a professional resume preparer, write their resume. These learners may be unsure about what to include or have weak word processing skills. It is a good idea to seek advice from employment professionals and essential to have someone qualified proofread your resume. However, there are several important reasons why *you* should determine the content and organization:

- It must accurately represent your skills: It is essential to make sure that they are neither exaggerated nor minimized.
- It is important to include the personal traits discussed earlier in this chapter: Only you know what these are.
- Canned resumes should be avoided: They tend to look insincere and give the impression that they were put together without much thought.
- You must know exactly what your resume says. It often serves as the basis for questions at interviews.

Resume Contents

Resumes contain several sections and each has a specific purpose. It is important that all content be written accurately and completely.

Heading

This section includes your name and contact information (address, phone number, and email address) and is placed at the top of the resume. Make it easy for potential employers to contact you by listing a current phone number, along with the area code. If necessary, include an alternate number where messages can be left. Do not be one of those people who loses opportunities because interested employers cannot find them. Center the heading at the top of the page and highlight your name by using capital letters. It is not necessary to use the label "Resume," because the content and format makes it easy to identify.

Introduction

Traditionally, the next part of the resume is the **objective**, a statement of your job goal. It is written as a simple job title or include additional information about your qualifications and preferences. Here are a few examples:

- Job title only: Position as a medical assistant
- More specific: Position as a front-office medical assistant
- Include information about your qualifications: Position as an administrative medical assistant in which I apply my computer skills and organizational ability.
- Include information about your preferences: Position as a clinical medical assistant in a pediatric office.

Today, employment specialists recommend that job applicants use a different approach. The objective, they point out, focuses on what the applicant *wants*, rather than what the applicant can *offer* the employer. Therefore, experts suggest that the resume begin with a list of qualifications for the targeted job. This list highlights the important skills and traits that directly relate to the needs stated by the employer.

Here is a sample *summary of qualifications* for a pediatric medical assistant applicant who has a background teaching in a preschool:

- Certified medical assistant
- Up-to-date administrative and clinical skills
- 13 years of experience working with children in a variety of settings
- 5 years of experience teaching disabled children
- Bilingual, English–Spanish
- Ability to communicate with people of all ages
- Maintained perfect attendance while attending medical assisting program and working part-time
- Ability to work well under pressure and manage priorities

Notice how a variety of abilities and experiences are used to describe the applicant as a unique and well-qualified candidate. They can come from previous work, school, or personal experience.

A possible exception to omitting an objective is if you are changing careers or have no experience in the field, as is the case for many recent graduates. The objective, in this case, lets the employer know what job you are seeking.

Education

This is an important section for graduates who are new to the health care field. In fact, it may be the section you want to be most detailed and listed at the beginning of your resume because recently acquired skills are the major qualifications for employment in entry-level positions. (See Figure 24–5 for an example of a resume that highlights the education section.) List the schools attended, starting with the most recent. Include high school only if graduation or a GED is a job requirement or it is where you acquired your health care training. For each school, list the dates attended or the date the certificate, diploma, or degree was awarded. The following items can also be added to this section:

- Special training, such as cardiopulmonary resuscitation (CPR) or computer classes that are related to the job objective
- Honors or awards earned
- Cumulative grade point average (GPA) if it is 3.0 or higher
- Special school projects that are related to the targeted job
- Facts that demonstrate such traits as initiative, ability to manage time, and persistence
- Summary of what you learned. List the courses taken or prepare a list of skills acquired. This is especially helpful for the employer if the program included an unusual variety of skills or if the occupational outcome is a relatively new job title. Here are two examples showing how to write the education section:

Example 1 Associate in Applied Science Degree, Medical Assisting, 2015

Healthcare College, Lincoln, NE

- Completed CPR and first aid training
- Honor Roll all semesters
- Earned 3.7 of a possible 4.0 GPA

Example 2 Diploma, Patient Care Assistant Program, 2009

BeWell School of Medical Careers, Philadelphia

- Received Perfect Attendance Award
- Served as chairperson for annual all-school diversity picnic

- Completed program while working part-time and raising two young children
- Knowledge and skills acquired include:
  - Medical terminology and body systems
  - Computer keyboarding and data entry
  - Medical and surgical asepsis
  - Nursing assistant skills
  - Home health aide skills
  - Rehabilitation aide skills
  - Unit clerk skills
  - Phlebotomy
  - Electrocardiograms

Certifications and Licenses

Include this section only if they are not listed in another section, such as education. Examples:

- Certified Medical Assistant
- Licensed Vocational Nurse, California License #1234568910
- Current CPR certification
- Registered Dental Assistant

Work Experience

This section can also be called employment history. List your previous jobs starting with the most recent. Include the name and location of each employer, along with the dates worked and the titles of all positions held. Create a bulleted list of phrases, using active verbs, to describe your duties and achievements. Do not use complete sentences or the word "I." Think about how you contributed to the success of your previous employers. Were you extremely reliable? Did you increase sales? Develop a more efficient system for organizing the office? Don't worry if your work history does not seem very impressive. Completing a health care educational program demonstrates the ability to set and meet new career goals.

It is appropriate to include clinical experience (e.g., internship, externship, or fieldwork, etc.) in either the work experience or education section. Give the name and location of the facility, as well as a list of the duties performed. Be sure to label these appropriately as "internship," "externship," "fieldwork experience," and so on. To imply that it was a paid position is dishonest. Examples of work history section:

Example 1 Sales Associate 2012 to Present

Hercules Men's Store, Gary, IN

- Assist customers
- Close out cash register each night
- Maintain perfect attendance
- Increased sales by 17% in first year employed
- Consistently earn highest top-volume sales associate award each quarter

This job, although not related to health, demonstrates the ability to communicate, motivation to succeed, honesty, and reliability. Every employer is looking for these qualities.

When listing your job duties, use the past tense for jobs you no longer hold and present tense for jobs at which you are currently employed.

Example 2 Medical Assistant Externship June 2015–September 2015

Caring Community Clinic, Charleston, SC

Performed back-office duties under the supervision of Dr. Emilio Jimenez

- Took medical histories
- Took vital signs
- Prepared patients for examinations and procedures
- Assisted physician with procedures and minor surgeries
- Administered medications
- Applied principles of infection control
- Received highest ratings (5 on scale of 1 to 5) in all areas on final externship evaluation

Optional Sections

The following are optional sections to include on your resume if they add important information not mentioned elsewhere:

- Special skills: Skills other than what would normally be expected from your training. For example, a medical assistant applicant with the ability to troubleshoot and correct computer problems.
- Languages: Languages other than English can be listed here or under special skills. It is customary to indicate the ability level—for example, "Spanish: Speaking and comprehension good, writing ability fair."

- Awards and honors: If applicable. List only those not already included in the education section. Provide brief explanations if it is not clear how they were earned.
- Community service and volunteer work: List the duties performed and events in which you participated.
- Memberships in professional organizations: These demonstrate commitment and interest in keeping up to date. Serving as an officer or member of a committee demonstrates willingness to accept responsibility, practice leadership, and take an active role in organizations.
- Hobbies and interests: List any that support your bid for the job. For example, sports such as swimming or tennis demonstrate that you value good health and recognize the importance of exercise.

Fascinating Facts

Resume preferences reported by 2800 employers in a 2011 survey:

- Bulleted list of accomplishments (51%)
- Career summary at the top (40%)
- Relevant key words (39%)
- Resume that is customized to the open position (36%)

And one third of hiring managers say they are not likely to consider candidates who do not include a cover letter with their resumes.

Source: Career Builder, "More Than One-in-Five Hiring Managers Say They Are Less Likely to Hire a Candidate Who Didn't Send a Thank-You Note, Finds New CareerBuilder Survey." http://www.careerbuilder.com/share/aboutus/pressreleasesdetail.aspx?id=pr631&sd=4/14/2011&ed=04/14/2011

Formatting the Resume

"Formatting" refers to the arrangement of the content in the resume. Two commonly used formats are the chronological and the functional. The **chronological resume** features a work experience section in which the duties and accomplishments of previous jobs are listed. This is a good choice for someone who has a strong, steady work history, especially one in which jobs held required increasing amounts of responsibility. It is also recommended for applicants who have work experience in health care. Figure 24–4 contains an example of a chronological resume.

The **functional resume** highlights clusters of skills and abilities gathered from a variety of experiences. Job titles are listed in the work experience section without detailing duties and accomplishments. Functional resumes are recommended for people who are changing careers and have a variety of skills and experiences that can be transferred to the new field. Three clusters are usually recommended. See Figure 24–5 for an example of a functional resume.

Resume content can be organized in a variety of ways. The fact is, there is no "best way" that everyone should use. The important thing is that the resume be reader-friendly and highlight the qualifications that best support the targeted job. These qualifications should be placed closest to the top of the page. For example, an applicant for a transcriptionist position with outstanding keyboarding speed and accuracy could list these in a qualifications section. A bilingual medical assistant applicant in an area with a large Hispanic population could highlight the ability to speak Spanish in the qualifications section.

Important Resume Guidelines

Although there are a variety of ways to organize the content, there are a few guidelines that should *always* be followed:

- Be accurate: Check for perfect spelling, correct grammar, and accurate dates. This is important for all professions, but especially when applying for a job in health care, which depends on accuracy for the well-being of both patients and workers.
- Be conservative: This is a characteristic of the medical field. Choose good quality paper in white or a very light gray or beige.
- Be neat: Have no corrections, smudges, or creases.
- Make it easy to read: Don't crowd the information; leave some white space. Margins should be at least one inch on all sides.
- Keep it professional: Don't include personal information such as age, marital status, and number of children.
- Do not include information that is best discussed in person: This includes why you left previous jobs, salary information, or special conditions, such as having a physical disability.

LISA GRAZIANO
8407 Wentworth Ave.
Manchester, NH 03103
(603) 123-4567

Medical Transcriptionist

QUALIFICATIONS

14 years full-time experience working as a medical transcriptionist
Ability to prepare reports for all major medical specialties
Keyboarding speed of 97 wpm

WORK EXPERIENCE

Medical Transcriptionist 2003–Present
Chatsworth Medical Center, Manchester, NH
- Transcribe patient's medical reports as dictated by physicians
- Distribute reports to appropriate departments
- Obtain charts for physicians
- Received Employee of the Quarter award four times (based on reliability, cooperation, and efficiency)

Medical Transcriptionist 2001-2003
St. Claire Hospital, Boston, MA
- Transcribed daily reports for surgical department
- Copied records for billing
- Answered telephone and transferred calls

Administrative Assistant 1997–2001
Dr. Patrice Tibere, Boston, MA
- Word processed all correspondence and research reports
- Located and gathered reference materials as requested
- Handled mail, answered telephone, maintained Dr. Tibere's schedule, made travel arrangements

EDUCATION

AA Degree, Medical Transcription, 2001
Lawrence Medical College, Boston

Word Processing Certificate, 1997
Regal College, Boston

MEMBERSHIPS

American Association for Medical Transcription
Lawrence Medical College Advisory Board

FIGURE 24–4 Example of a chronological resume. This is usually a good choice for applicants who have a strong work history and/or experience working in health care.

KELLY CISNEROS
9125 Soledad Avenue
El Paso, TX 79907
(915) 123-4567

OBJECTIVE	Position as a **Clinical Medical Assistant** in a pediatric office
EDUCATION	AS Degree, Medical Assistant, 2015 Caldwell Technical College, El Paso • Perfect Attendance Award three semesters out of four • Earned 3.7 of a possible 4.0 GPA • Externship at Valley Pediatric Center, El Paso • "Excellent Rating" for overall externship performance
EXPERIENCE WITH CHILDREN	6 years providing private day care in home 3 years teaching disabled preschoolers Cub Scout leader Volunteer tutor at Sanchez Elementary School
ORGANIZATIONAL SKILLS	Maintained state-approved day care facility Secretary of PTA at children's school Coordinate scheduling and activities for local junior soccer team
COMMUNICATION SKILLS	Make presentations to local organizations about child safety issues Write articles for Sanchez Elementary School parent newsletter 5 years experience as telephone receptionist in a busy insurance office Speak, read, and write Spanish fluently
WORK HISTORY	Cisneros Quality Day Care 2005–2013 Owner of home-based day care for up to six children SpecialCare Preschool 2004–2007 Teacher Calderon Insurance Agency 1999–2004 Receptionist

FIGURE 24–5 Example of a functional resume. This is usually a good choice for applicants who have no experience working in health care.

- *Do not include your social security number.*
- Use proper spacing: Double-space between headings, then single-space within each section.
- Use special features for highlighting: Capitalize all major words in the headings. Or you may want to bold all words in headings.
- Keep it concise: Limiting it to one page is recommended. However, if you need to include more information than will fit on one page without crowding, use two pages.
- Have someone qualified review and proofread your resume. This is the most important written document in your job search efforts, so keep working on it until it is error-free and represents you at your best.

Recent Resume Trends

- A common practice until recently was to state "References Available Upon Request" at the bottom of the resume. The current practice is to omit this statement. (But you *do* need to have at least three references listed on a separate piece of paper.)
- Internet posting: Some employers have standard resume forms that you can fill out on the screen and send electronically. Take extra care when filling these out. Once the send key is pressed, there is no chance to correct information.

Thinking It Through

Greg Berglander recently graduated from a radiological technologist program and has passed his state's licensing exam. He's ready to begin applying for jobs. The problem is that he doesn't have a resume prepared. Although Greg can use a computer, he does not keyboard quickly and has poor word processing skills. He believes that the career services center at his school should be more helpful and put something together for him. After all, they know the courses he took and probably have access to his grades. And he can tell them anything else they need to know.

1. Do you agree with Greg? Why or why not?
2. What action would you recommend that he take?

- Electronic scanning: Employers who receive large numbers of resumes and do not have time to review them all are using scanners to enter them into a computerized data bank. The computer looks for key words that match the words in job descriptions. When there is a job opening, all resumes matching its requirements are recalled for review. If an employer indicates that resumes will be scanned, it is important to include descriptive words in your objective and throughout the resume. Read ads and job descriptions carefully to identify key words. Avoid staples, folds, or special features, such as bolding or fancy fonts. These are difficult for the computer to read.

COVER LETTERS

Cover letters are sent with resumes as a way to introduce yourself and inform the employer why you are sending a resume. Customize your letters as needed for the following situations:

- When responding to an advertised opening: In your letter refer to the job posting and state that you are interested in the position. Explain briefly how you meet the stated requirements. Do not simply repeat the specific information listed on your resume, but refer the employer to it for more detailed information. Request an interview and thank the employer for his or her time and consideration. See Figure 24–6 for an example of a cover letter for responding to an advertised position.
- Sending the resume to be considered for an unadvertised position: State the purpose of the letter, who told you about the opening (be sure you have that person's permission), or simply say that you understand there is an opening for which you might qualify. Briefly state your qualifications, explain why you are interested in the job, and then close with a request for an interview and a thank you. See Figure 24–7 for an example of this type of letter.
- You are moving to a new location and sending letters of inquiry in advance: Inform the employer that you are relocating to the area. Explain the type of work you are seeking. Include a brief statement of your qualifications and when you

AD:

DENTAL ASSISTANT. Excellent verbal, scheduling and collection skills. Full-time. Front and back office as needed. Computer literate with good work ethic. Commitment to high-quality patient care.

1357 Keystone Drive
Chicago, IL 60606
July 23, 20—

Dr. Harold Mims
1842 Grand Avenue
Chicago, IL 60606

Dear Dr. Mims:

This letter is in response to your ad for a dental assistant. I recently graduated from Harrison Dental College and believe that I fulfill the requirements stated in your ad.

Providing **high-quality patient care** was emphasized throughout the dental assisting program at Harrison. I would welcome the opportunity to begin my dental assisting career in an environment where patients are the top priority.

The program at Harrison emphasized the need for good **verbal skills** in the workplace. We were given many opportunities to practice them. In the skills lab students were required to explain all procedures orally to "patients" before and during hands-on work. I also received grades of "A" in my communication courses, which included Oral Communication and Interpersonal Relations for the Health Care Professional.

I understand the need for a smooth-running **front office** and enjoyed the administrative and **computer training** portion of my training. Performing duties in both the **front and back office** would allow me to apply my organizational skills. My previous jobs, outlined in the enclosed resume, required me to be responsive to the needs of my employers.

My **strong work ethic** is demonstrated in my excellent attendance records, both at school and work, willingness to complete all assigned tasks, and commitment to doing my best at all times.

I would appreciate the opportunity to meet with you to further discuss how I might contribute to the success of your practice. I can be reached at (312) 123-4567.

Thank you for your consideration.

Sincerely,

Kelly Bosner

Kelly Bosner

FIGURE 24–6 Cover letter responding to an advertised position. Note how the key words in the ad are bolded in the letter.

1357 Keystone Drive
Chicago, IL 60606
July 25, 20—

Ms. Tasha Jefferson, Office Manager
Compton Dental Clinic
6397 Flanders Street
Chicago, IL 60606

Dear Ms. Jefferson:

I am a recent graduate of Harrison Dental College. The Employment Coordinator at Harrison, Ms. Juanita Sanders, recommended that I contact you about a possible opening at Compton Dental Clinic. She believes you would be interested in an applicant with my excellent attendance record and academic achievements.

The dental assistant program at Harrison was rigorous and I feel well prepared to perform both front and back office skills. I developed good work habits during my training as well as at my previous jobs, which are listed in my resume. In addition, I have excellent communication skills and am committed to becoming a successful member of a dental care team.

I would appreciate the opportunity to meet with you to further discuss the needs of Compton Dental Clinic and my qualifications. I can be reached at (312) 123-4567.

Thank you for your consideration.

Sincerely,

Kelly Bosner

Kelly Bosner

FIGURE 24–7 Cover letter responding to an unadvertised position.

900 Peach Blossom Lane
Atlanta, GA 30326
September 24, 20—

Sarah Masterson, RHIA
Director - Health Information Management Department
Blackwell Rehabilitation Hospital
2106 S.W. River Street
Portland, OR 97423

Dear Ms. Masterson:

The purpose of this letter is to inquire about possible openings for a Registered Health Information Technician at your facility. I graduated from Caprio Health Care Institute in Atlanta in June and am relocating to the Portland area in November.

My training at Caprio was comprehensive and I feel confident that my training has prepared me to work competently in the health information field. I work well with others, have strong computer skills, and look forward to contributing to the success of my future employer.

I will contact you the week of November 12 after my arrival in Portland. In the meantime I can be contacted at (404) 123-4567. Thank you for your consideration.

Sincerely,

Glenda Hayes

Glenda Hayes

FIGURE 24–8 Cover letter for a graduate moving to a new location.

will be available for an interview. Ask to be considered for any appropriate openings and state that you will follow up with a phone call. Conclude with a thank you. (See Figure 24–8.)

Writing Good Cover Letters

Cover letters, like the resume, represent you and influence whether you are invited for an interview. Here are some guidelines for writing winning letters:

- Word process
- Be sure that grammar and spelling are perfect
- Use the same paper as for the resume
- Address the letter, if possible, to a specific person. Call the facility and ask to whom it should be directed. Check for the correct spelling of the name
- Send individualized letters for each employer or position, matching them to the targeted position
- Do not write more than one page. Busy employers don't have time to read more than that
- Use a standard business letter format (See Chapter 17)

WORKBOOK PRACTICE

Go to your workbook and complete the exercises for this chapter.

SUGGESTED LEARNING ACTIVITIES

1. Talk with successfully employed friends and family members about how they got their jobs.
2. Review the Web, newspaper, news magazines, and professional journals regularly for articles about health care trends, facilities, and employment-related topics.
3. Check out the websites suggested in this chapter and use available links to learn what information is available for job seekers.
4. Visit your school's career service center and find out what resources are available. Introduce yourself to the people who work there, if you don't already know them.
5. Find a Web posting, printed ad, or job description for a health care job in which you are interested.
   a. List the skills and traits that you think would be required.
   b. Prepare a summary of qualifications
   c. Create an appropriate resume and cover letter to apply for the position.

WEB ACTIVITIES

The Riley Guide
www.rileyguide.com

Choose an area (or areas) to explore from the many links listed on the Riley Guide. Create a list of 10 useful websites, including their addresses and a brief description of their contents and how they can help you in your job search.

Health Care Jobs
www.healthjobnationwide.com

Explore this health care job site. Write a summary description of the website including how it is organized, ease of use, number and variety of jobs posted, geographic scope, and special features, if any.

Quintessential Careers
www.quintcareers.com

Enter "cover letters" in the search box. Choose at least three articles to read and report on ways to make your cover letter informative and effective.

REVIEW QUESTIONS

1. Why should you develop a personalized skill inventory as a first step in your job search?
2. What are eight factors that you should consider when identifying your workplace preferences?
3. How much time should you plan to spend each week on job search activities?
4. Describe why and how you should organize a workplace dedicated to your job search.
5. Select four sources of job leads and explain how to use each one.
6. What is the purpose of the resume?
7. What are the major sections of a resume?
8. What are 10 characteristics of a successful resume?
9. What is a cover letter and when is it used?
10. What are the characteristics of a good cover letter?

APPLICATION EXERCISES

1. Refer to The Case of the Unprepared Applicant at the beginning of the chapter. Describe what Jenny could have done differently to avoid missing the opportunity to interview with Dr. Chambers.
2. Omid Riazati is starting his last month of classes at PrepWell College. He will then have an eight-week externship before completing his medical laboratory technician program. He is not sure where he wants to work when he graduates, but wants to get started on investigating employment possibilities and plan his job search activities. Create a job search to-do list and schedule for Omid to begin now and follow until he finds employment.

PROBLEM-SOLVING PRACTICE

Gerardo has completed his training to be a medical equipment technician. But he is concerned about starting the job search because he believes his writing skills are poor. He is not sure how to go about writing a good resume, cover letter, and thank-you note. How can he apply the five-step problem-solving process to get started on a successful job search?

SUGGESTED READINGS AND RESOURCES

CareerBuilder. www.careerbuilder.com

Online Writing Lab – Purdue University. http://owl.english.purdue.edu/owl (Click on the tab "Job search writing")

Quintessential Careers. www.quintcareers.com

Riley Guide. www.rileyguide.com

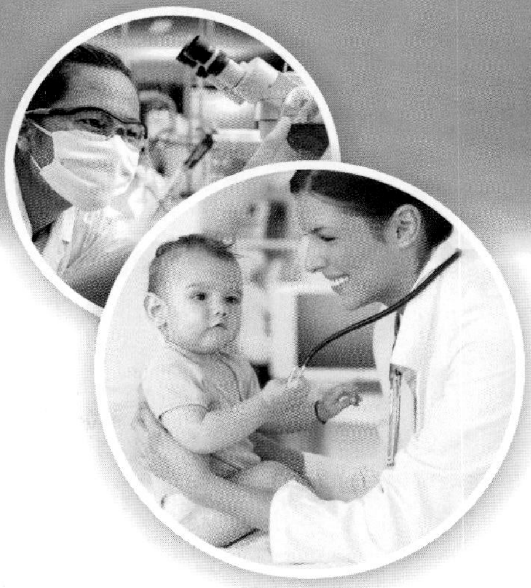

Chapter 25

Interview, Portfolio, and Application

OBJECTIVES

Studying and applying the material in this chapter will help you to:

- Explain the purpose of the job interview.
- Describe how to obtain background information about employers and health care organizations.
- Create examples to illustrate your employment qualifications.
- Prepare appropriate questions to ask at interviews.
- Anticipate and prepare for questions that may be asked at interviews.
- Describe ways to handle illegal questions asked by employers.
- Demonstrate successful interview behavior and appearance.
- Identify references who will support your job search efforts.
- Create a reference list to give to potential employers.
- Build a professional portfolio to provide evidence of your job skills and qualifications.
- Explain what actions to take after an interview to increase your chances of being hired.
- Explain how to accept and reject job offers.

KEY TERMS

behavioral question
illegal question
job interview
letters of recommendation
portfolio
reference
reference list
situational question

The Case of the Modest Applicant

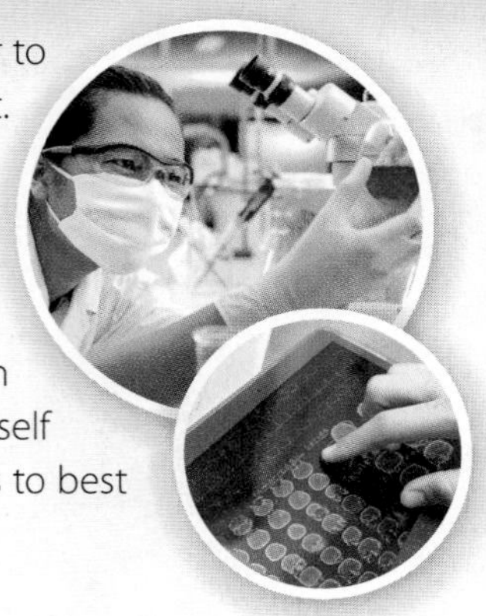

Sam Kingsley is seeking his first job as a phlebotomist. He has enjoyed his training and is eager to apply it in the workplace. While he went to school, Sam waited tables in a local family restaurant. Regular customers always liked to sit in Sam's section because of his friendly, helpful attitude. Many of the customers were older and especially liked Sam's respectful attitude toward them. Sam's first interview was at a medical laboratory that works with large numbers of walk-in patients. He felt that he handled the questions well by emphasizing his recent technical training. After all, he did not have any other experience that related to work in phlebotomy. When Sam did not get the job, he learned that the employer did not believe he had presented himself as a strong candidate. This chapter explains how learners can draw on all kinds of experiences to best present themselves to potential employers.

THE JOB INTERVIEW

The **job interview** is a conversation between an applicant and a potential employer. It is an opportunity for applicants to present their qualifications in person. Securing this interview has been the goal of all job search activity to this point. The purpose of this chapter is to help make interviewing as productive and pleasant as possible, resulting in an offer for the job you want.

Many job applicants are nervous about the idea of meeting face to face with an employer. The key to overcoming nerves is to prepare well and practice thoroughly. This helps ensure readiness for handling any interview situation and making a favorable impression.

Consider the interview as an opportunity for you and the employer to get to know each other and see if you fit each other's requirements. Keep in mind that interviews can be stressful for employers, too. A position must be filled, and the vacancy may be causing extra work. Inexperienced interviewers worry about their ability to choose the best-qualified applicant. They want to hire employees who can help solve problems, not create new ones.

The job interview is a two-way street and can be approached as a positive experience. Take advantage of this opportunity to learn about the employer by observing and asking questions. The information gathered provides the basis for determining if the position fits your professional qualifications and personal preferences.

The Importance of Proper Preparation

Before attending a single interview, a number of things must be done. Being prepared will enable you to focus on learning about the employer's needs and responding appropriately to all questions. Preparation prevents being caught off guard and unable to think of an intelligent response. Answers to many types of interview questions can be practiced in advance.

Not being prepared is the single best way to set yourself up for failure. Spend time developing interviewing skills and you will increase your chances for success.

Learn About the Employer

It is essential to know something about the employer and the position being applied for in order to properly prepare for an interview. Having some background information will allow you to:

- Show the employer that you are motivated, interested in the job, and have self-initiative
- Create appropriate examples from your experience to demonstrate qualifications for the job
- Prepare your own questions about the facility and the job

Sources of information vary, based on the size of the facility. To learn about major organizations, use the Internet, as discussed in Chapter 24, or call the human resource office. Ask for written materials, announcements about job fairs or orientations, and other sources of information. Watch for information about health care facilities in the local newspaper. Major employers are often the subject of articles, especially in the business and employment sections. If the employer does not have a website, it may be necessary to call or stop by to observe and ask a few questions. Even if you are not there for an interview, dress professionally. Every contact you have with a potential employer is part of the job interview. The receptionist is often a good source of information. The following are examples of appropriate questions to ask:

- How long has the facility or office been in business?
- What is the professional specialty?
- What are typical ages and types of patients served?
- What is the pace of the work?

Whether the employer is large or small, try to get a job description before the interview. Study it carefully and prepare specific examples that demonstrate your qualifications. If skills are required that you do not have but can learn, be prepared to explain to the employer how you plan to acquire them.

It is also important for applicants to demonstrate knowledge about the health care field in general. Keep informed about trends and issues of concern to employers, such as those discussed in Chapter 2. The Web, newspapers, news magazines, and professional journals contain articles about health care topics that affect health care careers. You should also stay current on the ethical and legal issues facing health care providers. Employers want to hire people who can help them deal with the growing number of regulations and constant changes that affect the delivery of health care today.

Prepare to Demonstrate Your Qualifications

College employment professionals report that one of the main reasons students do not get hired is that they fail to sell themselves. Many graduates fail to realize how much they have to offer an employer and therefore do not explain fully how they can be of benefit. An essential part of interview preparation is to review your skills and create examples that illustrate your mastery of them.

Start the review by looking at technical skills:

- What procedures and tests can you perform?
- At which skills are you most proficient?
- On which skills have you received compliments from patients or classmates or good evaluations from instructors or supervisors?
- In which classes did you receive the highest grades?
- Which classes did you enjoy the most? Why?
- Which skills and procedures were you able to practice most during your clinical (externship/internship/fieldwork) experience?

Now recall some experiences that support your skills and think about ways to present them. Here are a few examples:

> "I'm very efficient at performing blood draws. My classmates always wanted to work with me in the lab because ..."

> "I've worked hard to learn to do insurance coding accurately. I received top grades on all my assignments. The manager who supervised my externship allowed me to do more coding than externs are usually allowed to do because ..."

> "I enjoy word processing and reached a keyboarding speed of 83 words a minute. I also find medical terminology very interesting. Even more important for medical transcription, I'm very accurate ..."

Next, review the personal inventory you developed in Chapter 24. In addition to building your self-confidence, the inventory serves as a list from which you can create examples to support your positive work traits. You want to present yourself as an applicant worth considering for the job. Here are two examples:

> "I'm good at calming people who are afraid of the dentist. For example, when I was on my externship, there was a woman who was really nervous and I helped her by..."

> "My time management skills are strong. During the two years of my nursing program, I maintained part-time employment and still made sure that my three children and I arrived on time for school every day."

Prepare Your Questions

The interview should be an opportunity for the applicant to find out about the employer and get the information needed to make an intelligent decision if a job offer is received. Asking appropriate questions is also a sign that you are a motivated, thinking person who is sincerely interested in the job. Here are some examples of appropriate questions to ask:

- What are the specific duties and responsibilities of this position?
- May I have a copy of the job description?
- I see on the job description that I would be required to ____. Can you tell me more about that?
- Could you describe a typical day for a person in this position?
- Is there a training program for new employees? How does it work?
- What equipment would I be working with?
- What do you think are the most important qualifications for a person to succeed in this position? What qualities in an employee are most important to you?
- Who would I be reporting to? Can you tell me about that person?
- How would I be evaluated?
- If I performed well, would there be opportunities for advancement?

Be sure that the questions are appropriate for the situation. For example, a private physician's office with four employees is not likely to offer opportunities for promotion. To ask about them indicates a lack of knowledge about the employer. It might also give the impression that you will leave for a larger facility after acquiring a few months of experience.

Questions to Avoid

Showing more interest in personal gain than in contributions to the employer is one sure way to lose employment opportunities. The following questions should be avoided until a job has been offered:

- How much is the pay?
- Do you provide medical insurance? Dental insurance?
- How many vacation days will I get?
- How long are the lunch hours and breaks?
- Can we leave early on Fridays?
- What are the paid holidays?

This information is needed, of course, before making a decision on whether to accept the job. First, however, concentrate on presenting yourself as the right person for the job.

Anticipating an Employer's Questions

Certain kinds of questions are popular with interviewers everywhere. Avoid being caught off guard. Be prepared with answers for the following common questions. Create examples to support your answers.

General Employment Questions

- *Tell me about yourself,* or, *Describe yourself.* Give a brief personal history that concludes with why you want to work in health care. Include your education and any experiences that have reinforced your interest and qualifications for this job.
- *Why do you want to work here?* Explain how the facility matches your work goals and qualifications. Describe how you believe you can make a positive contribution. Explain why you are interested in the particular type of work being performed there.
- *Why do you think you are qualified for this job?* If you know the job requirements, explain how you meet them. If you do not, ask the interviewer to explain them more fully. This will give you information on which to base your answer.
- *What can you contribute to this facility?* As with the previous question, explain how you can help the employer based on what you understand his or her needs to be. This is a good opportunity to use examples from your training and past experience.
- *What are your strengths and weaknesses?* Give examples of strengths that relate to the job. Describe a specific situation that illustrates the quality. Weaknesses should be handled honestly. You can name a skill or personal characteristic, along with your plans for improving it. Or you can describe a previous weakness and how you have corrected it. It is best not to volunteer a weakness that is a major requirement for the job. You may decide on your own that you are not qualified for this particular job, but it is not necessary to disqualify yourself immediately. The only exception is if the interviewer asks you directly about your level of competency in specific areas. Do *not* claim a skill that

you do not have or great expertise in something in which you are a beginner. And do not state that you have no weaknesses, as you will come across as less than honest or at best, without good self-knowledge.

- *What did you like best about your last job? Least?* Again, try to focus on areas that are related to the job under discussion. Choose something you liked that is required on this job. Good answers, if they are true, to "liked least" would be that you did not have enough responsibility, the work was not challenging, and so forth. Avoid answers such as "There was too much work," or "The place was a mess." When answering this kind of question, *never* make negative remarks about previous employers. This will cause employers to wonder what you might say about *them* in the future.
- *Which classes did you like best? Least?* Be honest, but again, avoid saying that your least favorite class covered some of this job's major duties!
- *What are your short-term and long-term employment goals?* This can be a tricky question. You do not want to appear to lack professional goals or ambition. On the other hand, employers do not want employees who are only interested in staying for a short time to gain experience. Employers invest considerable time and money into hiring and training new employees. A stable staff also contributes to the quality of a facility. Let the employer know that you want to apply what you have learned in your program and welcome the opportunity to learn more. Your goal is to develop your skills and become an excellent and professional dental assistant, radiology technician, practical nurse, and so on.

Behavioral and Situational Questions

The purpose of **behavioral** and **situational questions** is for the interviewer to learn about how you have dealt with—or would deal with—common workplace circumstances, such as working under stress, getting along with others, and solving problems without the help of a supervisor. You might be given a scenario and asked how you would handle it or asked to provide an example of a real situation from your own experience. The best way to prepare for these types of questions is to mentally review your work history for examples of typical workplace problems. If your work history is limited, think about situations related to school, volunteer work, or family responsibilities. (Take care, however, not to discuss highly personal problems at the job interview.)

Examples of the kind of information to include in responses:

- Handling stress by practicing good time management, prioritizing, delegating, taking care of your health, engaging in physical activity
- Describing the successful planning and completion of a project by a group of which you were a member
- Working well with others on a sports team, committee, or class project
- Handling an interpersonal conflict by applying good communication skills, including listening, and compromising

Health Care Questions

Questions may be asked that deal specifically with the job under consideration. These require a good understanding of the chosen occupation and might include examples such as the following:

- What coping skills do you use during an emergency?
- What is the biggest issue facing nursing today?
- What would you do if you believed a coworker was stealing narcotic medications from the supply cabinet?
- How do you feel about the risk involved with radiation?
- What would you do if you had a stroke patient who was having difficulty getting dressed?
- Tell me what you know about the equipment you need to operate on this job.
- How would you deal with a mistake you made on a lab test that's already been reported?
- How do you deal with uncooperative patients? Suppose, for example, that you needed to draw blood twice in a sitting. How would you explain this to the patient?

(*Source:* Adapted from *Resumes for the Health Care Professional*, 2nd ed., by K. Marino, 2000, New York: John Wiley & Sons.)

Difficult Questions

Some questions are very difficult, especially if something in your history might be of concern to an employer. If it is necessary to explain past problems, stay calm and confident, be honest, and let the employer know that previous difficulties will not affect your ability to perform the job.

- *Have you ever been fired from a job?* If you have, be honest. *Do not* blame or badmouth a previous employer. You can say that you disagreed on issues. If you were in the right, explain the facts of the situation. ("I wasn't comfortable being asked to perform duties that were outside my scope of practice.") If you were at fault, explain how you have corrected the situation. ("I have improved my time management skills and have arrived at work on time every day for the past 18 months.")
- *Why have you changed jobs so often?* If the jobs were part-time or intended to be short-term while attending school, state this. If there were other reasons, try to show how this will no longer be a problem. For example, if previous jobs were boring, explain that this is what prompted you to become trained in health care. You have now found an area to which you can commit yourself.

Illegal Questions

It is illegal for employers to use certain facts about job applicants when making hiring decisions. **Illegal questions** during an interview require the disclosure of information about these kinds of facts.

Here are examples of some commonly asked illegal questions:

- How old are you? What is your date of birth?
- Are you married?
- Do you have children?
- Have you ever been arrested?
- Where were you born?
- Do you own your home?
- Do you have a disability or handicap?
- Have you ever filed for workers' compensation insurance?

These questions are often asked by employers who do not realize they are illegal. Or they may be asked in an attempt to learn about characteristics such as the applicant's dependability and trustworthiness.

Applicants have the right to refuse to answer questions believed to be illegal. They may inform the employer that specific questions are illegal. If you want the job and believe the employer is not deliberately breaking the law, there are two strategies that may be more effective:

1. Ask how the questions relate to the job requirements. This allows you to directly respond to the employer's concern. For example, a question about where you live may be asked by an employer who has had difficulties with employee attendance. The issue is arriving on time, not financial status.
2. Incorporate answers to possible but unasked questions. For example, if you are a female in the age range likely to have small children, explain how you have arranged reliable child care to ensure that you will not miss work.

In the unlikely event that questions are offensive, such as those that are sexual or racial in nature, it is appropriate to refuse to answer and leave the interview. Report the incident to the career services office at your school.

Creating a Professional Appearance

The interviewer's first impression will be based on your appearance. If it is negative, chances for hire may be lost before the formal interview even starts. Give yourself every advantage by creating a look that says, "I'm a professional who will fit easily into a health care environment." In Chapter 13, the elements of a professional appearance for the health care professional were discussed. The following summary highlights interview essentials:

- Make sure that everything about you is clean. This includes hair, fingernails, teeth, breath, clothing, and shoes. Bathe or shower and use a good deodorant.
- Demonstrate your knowledge of what is appropriate in the health care setting. Do not use products that have fragrances. Scents from perfumes, body lotions, hair spray, and other personal care products can be offensive when people are ill. Do not take the chance of clinging tobacco odors by smoking on the way to the interview. Remove nose, lip, tongue, and other visible piercings. Cover tattoos with long sleeves. (Some employers are becoming more lenient regarding tattoos and piercings, but until you learn the specific

policies, it is best to be conservative.) Refrain from activities that result in hickeys being visible at the time of the interview. (Health care employers have mentioned this as a problem with applicants.)

- Wear conservative attire. Women should choose a simple dress, suit, blouse and skirt, or pantsuit. Avoid anything low cut and revealing or sexy in any way. Men should wear slacks and a white or light-colored shirt.
- If you are unsure about what to wear, ask an instructor or career services for advice. Some schools recommend that job applicants wear their school scrubs or lab coat, but this should be discussed with career services to find out if the employer with which you have the interview approves of this practice. If you are on a tight budget, ask if the school has interview clothes to lend to their students. Look in the yellow pages under "thrift shops." They often have very nice clothes at reasonable prices. Some cities now have special shops that provide job seekers with free clothing and accessories, along with good advice about how to dress appropriately.
- Avoid jeans, T-shirts, sunglasses, hats, athletic shoes, and anything symbolic of gangs, religious groups, or political organizations.
- Keep jewelry simple. Men should remove earrings and women should wear only one pair.
- Women should avoid heavy makeup and colored nail polish. Long hair should be tied back or pinned up.
- Men with facial hair should trim it neatly. Men should tie long hair back. (These fashions are acceptable to employers in many parts of the country. Your area might be an exception.)

A professional appearance tells the employer that you take work seriously and consider the interview to be an important occasion. (See Figure 25–1.)

Securing References

References are people who will vouch for your qualifications and character. They are willing to be contacted by potential employers to answer questions about you. References should not be family members, relatives, or friends. Good examples are former supervisors, instructors, clergy, or professionals who know you well.

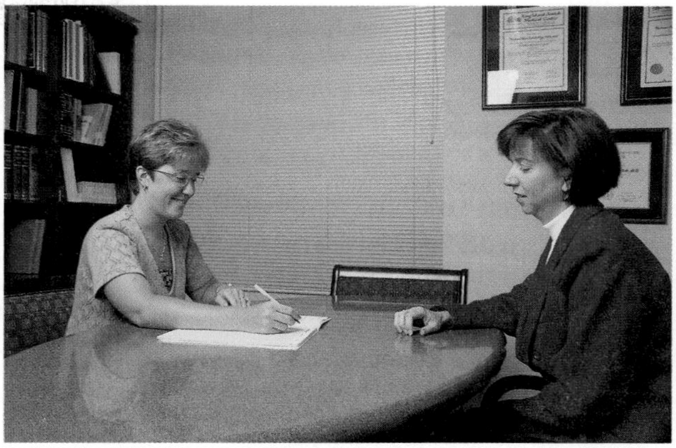

FIGURE 25–1 Make a strong, positive statement with professional dress and grooming.

Applicants should have between three and six references. Ask only those people whom you believe will give you a good recommendation. *Never* give anyone's name as a reference if he or she has not given you permission in advance. Keep your references informed about the jobs for which you interview and tell them the name of the person who might call.

Create a **reference list** that can be given to prospective employers upon request. Use the same paper

Thinking It Through

Cathy Nazerian is hoping that she will finally find an employer who understands what it is like to be a single mother. Before enrolling in the medical assistant program, she had to change jobs six times in the previous 14 months. Cathy found her employers to be very unsympathetic about things that really were not her fault. She couldn't control her unreliable babysitter, old car, and the fact that working while caring for three children tired her out so much that she couldn't always make it to work. Fortunately, she was able to maintain good attendance while in school because her mother had just retired and agreed to help her out temporarily with the kids.

1. How should Cathy respond to employers who ask about her frequent job changes?
2. What changes, if any, should Cathy make in her attitude about employers?
3. What would you suggest she do to reduce the need to change jobs so frequently?

used for your resume. Label it "References" and put your own name, address, phone number, and e-mail address centered at the top of the page. Then list the name, title, address, phone number, and e-mail address of each reference. It is also helpful to add the relationship you have with each person, such as employee, coworker, or student. Be sure to give accurate phone numbers. People who are difficult to locate or have numbers that are not in service do not appear credible and may do you more harm than good.

Letters of recommendation are statements written on your behalf by former employers and other professionals who know your work. Ask for a letter from any job that you leave on satisfactory terms. Keep the original letter and make copies to give to future potential employers.

Creating a Portfolio

A **portfolio** is an organized collection of written documents that you can show to employers. Its purpose is to support claims about your qualifications. Employers in some parts of the country expect job applicants to have a portfolio. Check with your school or a professional contact to see if this is true for your area.

The following documents are examples of appropriate contents for health care graduates:

- Copy of your diploma or certificate of program completion
- Copy of your professional license, certification, or registration
- Certificates that demonstrate competencies: keyboarding speed, cardiopulmonary resuscitation (CPR), course completions, and so on
- Documentation of accomplishments and service: awards, letters of appreciation, and so on
- Positive evaluations from your clinical experience and previous employment
- Class assignments that demonstrate proficiency in the tasks related to the job target: completed insurance forms, business letters, charting samples, and documents created with medical management software (Be sure that anything included is absolutely perfect.)
- A list of your technical skills and competencies (Organize them by work categories: administrative, clinical, patient care, computer, and so on.)
- Letters of recommendation from previous employers and others who can vouch for your character

To assemble the portfolio, group similar materials together and place them in a logical order. If there are many items, make a table of contents. Insert the papers in plastic page protectors and place them in a three-ring binder that has a nicely finished cover in a conservative color. A presentation binder containing page protectors can also be used.

Do not send the portfolio with the resume. Take it to interviews to demonstrate your competencies. For example, if the employer asks if you know current procedural terminology (CPT) coding, an accurately completed coding assignment would be an appropriate exhibit. You may not have an opportunity to show the portfolio at every interview. Use it only when it can support responses to questions or if the employer asks to see it.

Start early in your educational program to collect items for a portfolio. Keep them neatly stored together so you can find them when needed. Focus on completing all class assignments correctly and neatly, so that they not only fulfill class requirements but can also serve you in the job search.

What to Take to an Interview

Demonstrate your organizational skills and ability to plan ahead by having everything that might be needed at the interview. This will also prevent you from feeling flustered when you cannot find a pen to fill out an application. Use the following checklist as a guide:

- Extra resumes
- Application, if you filled it out at home
- Reference list
- List of important facts: driver's license and social security numbers, and details about employers that are not listed on your resume but might be requested on an application
- Portfolio
- Copies of letters of recommendation
- Copies of licenses and certifications
- Pen and notepad
- Appointment calendar, electronic or paper

Getting to interviews on time while fulfilling other responsibilities can be challenging. If you will be going directly from school or work, take along appropriate emergency supplies for your situation: extra pantyhose, breath mints, a clean shirt, and so on. Take steps to avoid feeling rushed and unprepared; this will help you be at your best.

Practice, Practice, Practice

Practice is the best way to do well at every interview. Ask a friend, family member, or classmate to play the part of the employer. Practice smiling, introducing yourself, and shaking hands. You may feel silly practicing such simple actions, but the basics are important. A surprising number of job offers are lost because of lifeless handshakes and poor eye contact.

Give your "employer" a list of commonly asked questions and practice answering them. Practice your closing (described in the next section) and leaving the interview on a positive note.

Participate in any mock (pretend) interviews offered by your school. If possible, have your interview recorded so that you can critique yourself. Listen and watch carefully. Did you do the following:

- Maintain eye contact?
- Speak clearly using a pleasant voice?
- Avoid using meaningless words like "uh" and "you know"?
- Sit calmly with good posture?
- Answer questions fully but without rambling on?
- Appear to be interested in the other person?
- Support your answers with examples?

Practice as often as possible so that when it is time for the real interview, you can be more relaxed. You would never think of performing a procedure on a patient without sufficient practice. Prepare for job interviews in the same way.

Starting Off on the Right Foot

Do everything possible to avoid being late for an interview. Do not lose a job opportunity before even having the chance to present your qualifications. Plan to arrive about 15 minutes early. This gives you time to check your appearance in the restroom and fill out any necessary paperwork. If you are unfamiliar with the area where the facility is located, make a dry run before the day of the interview.

Attend job interviews alone. Bringing a friend or family member demonstrates a lack of self-confidence. Bringing your children, rather than arranging for childcare, demonstrates disorganization. If someone gives you a ride, have the person wait outside or in another part of the building.

Turn off your cell phone, if you have one with you, before you arrive at the interview location. Allowing your phone to ring during the interview is not only extremely poor manners, it will likely cost you the job. Be courteous and pleasant with *everyone* you meet, including the receptionist. Do not show impatience or comment negatively if you had trouble finding the location, must wait for the interviewer, or encounter other difficulties. Demonstrate the same professionalism expected of you on the job. The interview is composed of much more than just the time spent sitting with the employer in a formal setting. It starts with the first contact, whether that is a phone call, a resume submitted, or a personal visit.

When you are introduced to the interviewer, smile, establish eye contact, and return the handshake firmly. Wait to sit down until you are offered a seat or the interviewer has sat down. (See Figure 25–2.)

Here are some key points to help you do well during the discussion portion of the interview:

- Keep your purpose in mind: to sell yourself and your qualifications.
- *Listen* carefully to the employer. (See Figure 25–3.) What are the employment needs and concerns or problems? What is he or she looking for in an employee?
- Answer questions in ways that show how you are qualified for the job.

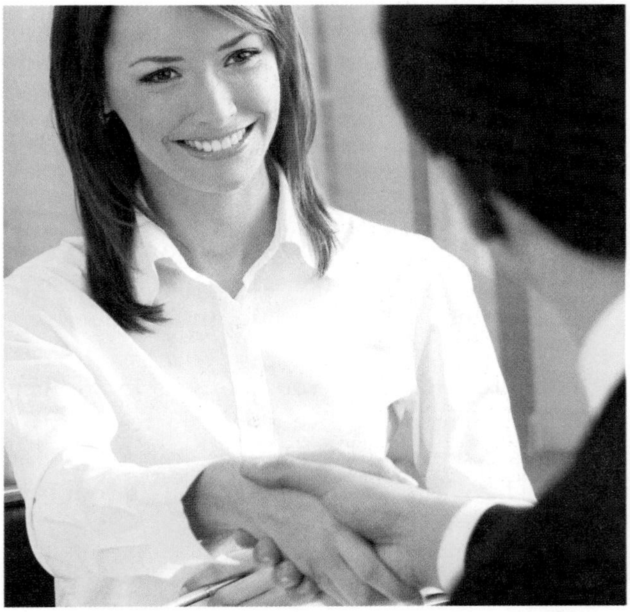

FIGURE 25–2 Greet the employer with a smile, eye contact, and a firm handshake.

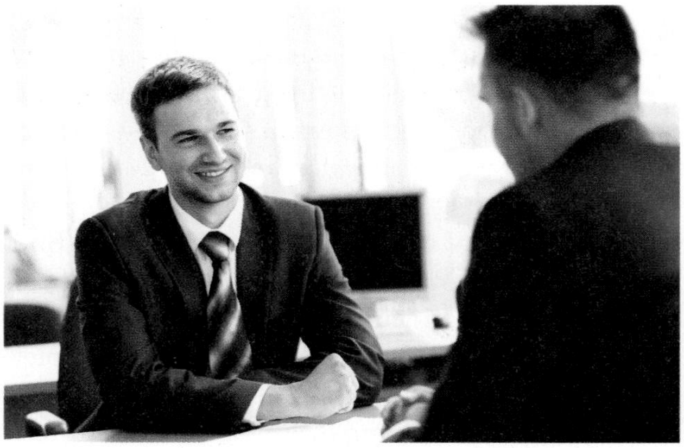

© EDHAR/Shutterstock.com.

FIGURE 25–3 Listening carefully to the employer is essential for a successful interview.

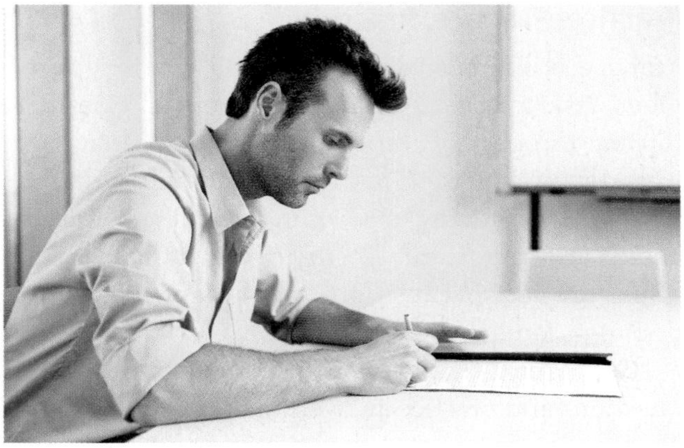

© baranq/Shutterstock.com.

FIGURE 25–4 You may be asked to take a written test as part of the job-application process.

- Answer questions fully, but do not talk too long or give out information that was not requested.
- Show interest in the job by asking questions when invited to do so or when you have the opportunity.
- Balance warmth and friendliness with professionalism. *Employers hire people they like.*
- Never share gossip or make negative remarks about previous employers or anyone else. Do not discuss your personal problems.
- Do not place anything on the employer's desk unless invited to do so. And *never* read papers or appear to be snooping in any way.
- Project positive nonverbal communication. Sit up straight in the chair or lean forward slightly to show interest, maintain eye contact, and speak clearly using good expression and enthusiasm. Do not chew gum, and avoid nervous habits, such as twisting your hair or jiggling your leg.
- *Never* lie. You should be prepared to answer difficult questions honestly. If a lie is discovered after you are hired, it can be grounds for dismissal.

In addition to asking you questions in an interview, some employers give a written test or have applicants complete a task. In these cases, draw on what you have learned, try to relax, and do your best. (See Figure 25–4.)

When the employer indicates that the interview is drawing to a close and you are unsure of the next step in the process, ask what it is. Is there anything you need to send to the employer? When will applicants be notified of a hiring decision? Do not be afraid to ask these questions. At the same time, do not take too much time if it is obvious the employer needs to end the interview promptly. Whether you are interested in the job or not, express appreciation for the opportunity to interview and leave courteously.

Recent Trends in Interviews

- Peculiar or unexpected questions designed to help the interviewer understand how you think
- Group interviews, in which there may be (1) more than one job applicant; or (2) more than one interviewer with one applicant
- Video interview
- Psychometric tests (e.g., reasoning tests, personality profiles, ability assessments, and motivation questionnaires)

Fascinating Facts

More than one in five hiring managers report that they are less likely to hire candidates who do not send a thank-you note after the interview. Some will actually dismiss an applicant for consideration because it shows a lack of follow-through or sends the message that the applicant is not serious about the position.

Source: Career Builder, "More Than One-in-Five Hiring Managers Say They Are Less Likely to Hire a Candidate Who Didn't Send a Thank-You Note, Finds New CareerBuilder Survey. www.careerbuilder.com/share/aboutus/pressreleasesdetail.aspx?id=pr631&sd=4/14/2011&ed=04/14/2011.

After the Interview

Think of the interview as a process that continues until the job is filled, either by you or by someone else. Here are some follow-up activities that can tip the scale in your favor:

- *Send a thank-you letter.* This is one of the most overlooked ways to demonstrate consideration for the interviewer and interest in the job. It never fails to make a positive impression. Do it immediately after the interview, even if you decide that you are not qualified for or interested in the job. This employer may have a more appropriate job in the future or may know another employer whose needs match your skills. If you want the job, restate your interest. If you have applicable qualifications you did not discuss at the interview, mention them now in your letter. Figure 25–5 contains an example of a post-interview thank-you letter. Notice that this communication is more than simply a thank-you note; it is in fact an additional opportunity to sell yourself to the employer. (Note: The majority of hiring managers report it is acceptable to send the thank you by email.)
- Send in any requested information, applications, or other items.
- Advise all references that they may be called.
- Review your impressions of the employer and facility. Be prepared to either accept or reject the position if it is offered.
- Place a follow-up telephone call if you do not hear by the date you were told you would be contacted. Let the employer know that you are still interested in the job and ask if a hiring decision has been made. If not, ask when it is expected to be made.
- Continue your job search activities, even if the interview went very well.

Additional Requirements

Many health care facilities have special requirements as part of the hiring process in response to social problems and public health concerns. The following may be encountered in the job search or after a job has been accepted:

- Tests for the presence of illegal drugs
- Psychological tests to determine tendencies toward violence
- Immunizations, such as the hepatitis B vaccination (The Occupational Safety and Health Administration [OSHA] requires employers to give these free of charge if the job involves exposure.)
- Health screening tests, such as those for tuberculosis
- Criminal background check
- Credit check
- Disclosure of social security number, if not already given (for tax withholding)
- Information about family, such as number of children (for insurance purposes)
- Proof of right to work legally in the United States

ACCEPTING THE JOB

Congratulations! Your hard work and persistence have paid off, and you have received a job offer that you want to accept. If you accept the offer verbally, such as over the telephone, follow up with a letter in

Thinking It Through

Wayne Blackman is applying for a position as a radiologic technologist at an imaging center. He feels very confident about his qualifications. After all, he graduated with honors and passed the state licensing exam with high scores. Wayne is unhappy with the interview he had this morning at the center. After hurrying to get there on time, he had to wait 20 minutes for the director, Ms. Rodriguez. Before the interview started, he told her that he thought it was rude to have kept him waiting. During the interview there were two phone calls and some kind of urgent situation with a patient that Ms. Rodriguez had to attend to. This made it difficult for him to fully inform her about his qualifications and spend the time necessary to show off his portfolio. Wayne feels pretty sure he can get the job, though, if Ms. Rodriguez can take the time to look at his academic and test records.

1. Do you agree with Wayne that he will probably be hired? Explain your answer.
2. Should Wayne have done anything differently? Why or why not?

1357 Keystone Drive
Chicago, IL 60606
July 31, 20—

Ms. Tasha Jefferson, Office Manager
Compton Dental Clinic
6397 Flanders Street
Chicago, IL 60606

Dear Ms. Jefferson:

Thank you very much for giving me the opportunity to interview for the position of dental assistant at Compton Dental Clinic. I enjoyed talking with you and learning more about the needs of the clinic.

Compton impressed me as being committed to providing high-quality patient care and developing its patient education programs. I believe that my experience as a peer tutor during my studies at Harrison Dental College would help me contribute to your educational efforts. I may not have mentioned during the interview that I am proficient in desktop publishing software and enjoy creating informational materials.

I am very interested in the position and would be pleased to have the opportunity to join the Compton team. Thank you again for your consideration.

Sincerely,

Kelly Bosner

Kelly Bosner

FIGURE 25–5 Follow up *every* interview with a thank you letter.

which you express your thanks for the offer, the fact that you accept it, and what you understand to be the title, salary, and start date.

If you are not sure about whether to accept a position, ask the employer if you can respond in one or two days. Do not take longer than that. It may not be possible for the employer to extend the extra time if it is urgent that the vacancy be filled.

DECLINING THE JOB

Just as with the acceptance, respond in writing even if you decline the job in a phone call. Thank the employer for the time spent and confidence in your abilities. State simply that you have decided not to accept the offer. It is not necessary to explain your decision. *Never* ignore a job offer. Remember that this employer may have an extensive network in the health care community. Lack of courtesy in rejecting an offer can damage your chances with other employers.

DEALING WITH REJECTION

All jobs are not meant for all people. If you are not offered a position, it can be for many reasons: You did not have all the required qualifications, someone with the "perfect" combination of skills and experience applied for the same job, or your preferred work style was not a fit. Not being selected for a job should not be taken as a personal rejection. Talking with someone supportive can help you deal with disappointments encountered during the job search.

If you find that you repeatedly fail to receive an offer, review your interviewing skills and ask career services or your instructor for advice. Some employment professionals recommend that you ask the employers with whom you have interviewed for feedback and suggestions. Do *not* approach them in a hostile manner, demanding to know why you did not get the job. Explain that you want to improve your job-seeking skills and would appreciate their help. Some employers have a policy of not answering this kind of question. Therefore, do not be insistent or express anger if they are not willing to discuss the reason why you were not hired.

FILLING OUT APPLICATIONS

You may be asked to fill out an application at any time during the job search. It may be required in either print or electronic form. (See Figure 25–6 for an example.) Some facilities that do not have current openings allow applicants to submit an application that is kept on file for future openings. Others have applicants fill them out at the time of the interview. Be sure to have all necessary information, including dates and locations of your education and previous employment. You also need the names and phone numbers of all references. Regardless of when the application is completed, here are a few important guidelines:

- Read the entire application *before* filling it in. Then start back at the beginning and answer each question completely. In the employment section, do not write, "See resume." If you are hired, your application can serve as a legal document, and it must be filled in completely to be valid.
- Type or print neatly using a black pen. The way you fill out an application tells the employer about your ability to follow directions and your attention to detail. If the application is filled out electronically, take care to check for mistakes before pushing the "enter" or "send" key. (Be aware that some employers today accept only applications that are submitted electronically.)
- Be sure that all your facts are accurate. Check that all dates and numbers are correct, especially your phone number.
- Write "N/A" (not applicable) if a question does not pertain to you, so the reader will know that you did not miss the question.
- Write "negotiable" in the salary section, unless you have already been told what it is.
- Include your signature and the date.
- Review it for accuracy. Look at every item.

Make a copy of any applications you fill out at home or on the Internet. These will serve as a record of your job search, as well as supply a convenient source of information for filling out future applications.

SAMPLE EMPLOYMENT APPLICATION

DATE ________________

PERSONAL INFORMATION

Name ____
Last First Middle Maiden

Current Address ____
Number Street City State Zip

Mailing Address ____
Number Street City State Zip

Telephone Home ( ) _____ Cell ( ) _____ Other ( ) _____

E-mail Address ____

Are you 18 years or older? ________ Yes ________ No

Social Security Number ______________________________________

Position Applying For _______________________________________

Availability ________ Full-time ________ Part-time ________ On Call
________ Any shift, if applicable ________ Overtime
Who referred you to our facility or how did you hear about this position? ______________
Can you provide documentation that you are authorized to work in the U.S.? ________ Yes ________ No
Have you previously applied for a position at this facility? ________ Yes ________ No
Have you previously been employed by this facility? ________ Yes ________ No

EMPLOYMENT HISTORY

1. Current/Most Recent Employer

Company Name ____

Department and Supervisor's Name ____________________________________

Can We Contact as Reference? ________ Yes ________ No

Telephone Number ____

Address ____

Dates Employed From ________ To ________

Job Title ____

(continued)

Major Duties ______________________________
____
____

Reason for Leaving ______________________________

2. Next Most Recent Employer

Company Name ______________________________

Department and Supervisor's Name ______________________________

Can We Contact as Reference? ________ Yes ________ No

Telephone Number ______________________________

Address ______________________________

Dates Employed From ________ To ________

Job Title ______________________________

Major Duties ______________________________
____
____

Reason for Leaving ______________________________

EDUCATION

High School
Name ______________________________
City, State ______________________________
Graduated? _______ Yes _______ No

College/University
Name ______________________________
City, State ______________________________
Degree Earned ______________________________

College/University
Name ______________________________
City, State ______________________________
Degree Earned ______________________________

Technical School
Name ______________________________
City, State ______________________________
Degree/Certificate Earned ______________________________

Other
Name ______________________________
City, State ______________________________
Degree/Certificate Earned ______________________________

(continued)

SPECIAL SKILLS

Licenses, certificates, and/or registrations. Include the number and expiration date.

____

____

Working knowledge of computer software.

____

____

Other

____

____

OTHER INFORMATION

Have you ever been convicted of a misdemeanor or felony crime? ______Yes ______ No
If yes, please provide an explanation.

____

____

____

____

Have you served in the United States Armed Forces? _______ Yes _______ No
If yes, which branch of service? ______________________________

INVITATION TO SELF-IDENTIFY

The following information is voluntary and will be kept confidential. It is used to help the facility comply with government reporting requirements and to evaluate its hiring practices.

Please check the appropriate spaces.
______ Male ______ Female

Ethnic Background
______ Hispanic or Latino
______ American Indian or Alaskan Native
______ Black or African American
______ Asian
______ White
______ Two or more races

APPLICATION AGREEMENT

- I affirm that all information contained in this agreement is true and complete.
- I authorize the facility to investigate all statements made in this application, including Information from previous employers and references.
- I understand that if selected, my employment will be on an "at-will" basis which means that the employer and employee may terminate the employment at any time with or without notice or cause.

________ I agree __________ I disagree (if you disagree, your application will not be considered.)

FIGURE 25–6 Example of a typical application for a health care position.

WORKBOOK PRACTICE

Go to your workbook and complete the exercises for this chapter.

SUGGESTED LEARNING ACTIVITIES

1. Practice applying the listening skills described in Chapter 16 to everyday situations. It will pay off when you attend interviews and need to listen carefully to understand the needs and requirements of the employer.
2. Start writing down ideas for answering common interview questions.
3. Make a list of people who might serve as your references.
4. Review your wardrobe for clothes that are suitable for an interview.
5. Observe your own behavior. Do you make it a habit to be courteous? Do you speak clearly and in a pleasant tone?
6. Enlist the help of two friends, family members, or classmates and set up a practice interview. Choose a specific job to apply for. Give the "employer" questions from all the categories discussed in this chapter. Start the "interview" with a greeting and handshake, and complete it with an appropriate closing. Have the second person observe and critique your performance.
7. Look on the websites of several health care facilities to review their application forms and procedures.

WEB ACTIVITIES

Monster Interview Center
http://career-advice.monster.com/
This website contains dozens of short, helpful articles about interviewing. With "Advice" showing in the Search box, enter "interviews" as the key word. Choose five interviews to read, then prepare a list of suggestions for applicants seeking jobs in health care.

The Riley Guide
www.rileyguide.com
Click on "Making Contact," then on "Network, Interview, & Negotiate," then on "Interviewing." Choose at least five links of interest to explore and summarize what you learn in a short report.

REVIEW QUESTIONS

1. Describe two methods for learning about employers.
2. What is the best way to support your qualifications during an interview?
3. What are five appropriate questions to ask a potential employer at the first interview?
4. What are five questions you should not ask at the first interview?
5. What are eight commonly asked general interview questions?
6. Describe behavioral and situational interview questions and explain their purpose.
7. How should you handle interview questions about sensitive issues?
8. What are three ways to respond to illegal interview questions?
9. Describe the ideal appearance of a man or a woman who is attending a health care job interview.
10. Give three examples of people who would be good references.
11. List eight documents that would be appropriate to include in the health care applicant's professional portfolio.
12. What are three ways to show respect for the interviewer?
13. How can you show an employer you are interested in the job?
14. How can you project positive nonverbal messages during the interview?
15. What is the most important interview follow-up activity?
16. How can you ensure that your employment application represents you well?

APPLICATION EXERCISES

1. Refer to The Case of the Modest Applicant at the beginning of the chapter. Describe how Sam could more effectively sell himself to an employer.
2. Carol-Ann LaRoche has completed her dental hygiene program. She is the first child in two generations to go to college, and her family is extremely proud of her. Carol-Ann did well in her courses. The most difficult part of her training was carrying on conversations with patients. She is very shy and feels unsure of herself socially. Although she is looking forward to working as a hygienist, she is terrified at having to attend job interviews. She just knows she'll get tongue-tied and be unable to make a good impression. Recommend a step-by-step plan that Carol-Ann can use to prepare for an interview successfully.

PROBLEM-SOLVING PRACTICE

Shawna is in the lucky position of having two good job offers to choose from. How can she use the five-step problem-solving process to help her make the best decision?

SUGGESTED READINGS AND RESOURCES

About Careers. jobsearch.about.com

Quintessential Careers. www.quintcareers.com

Zedlitz, R. (2013). *How to get a job in health care* (2nd ed). Clifton Park, NY: Cengage Delmar Learning.

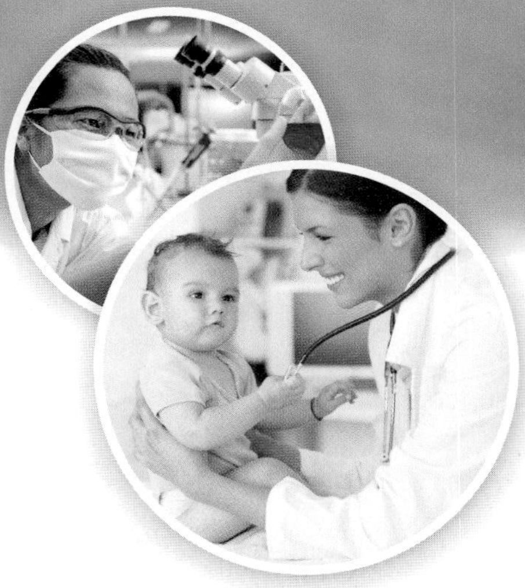

Chapter 26

Successful Employment Strategies

OBJECTIVES

Studying and applying the material in this chapter will help you to:

- Identify important information that new employees should learn about the facility in which they work.
- Explain the importance of understanding the facility's policies and procedures.
- Explain the purpose of the probationary period.
- Identify seven behaviors that contribute to professional success.
- List and describe the major laws that affect hiring and employment practices.
- Explain the meaning of a grievance and how it should be handled.
- Explain the meaning of sexual harassment and the actions to take if it occurs.
- Describe a typical performance evaluation.
- Identify the steps to take when leaving a job voluntarily.
- Describe ways to cope with being fired from a job.
- List activities that promote professional development of the health care professional.

KEY TERMS

chain of command
employee handbook
grievance
integrity
job description
mentor
minimum wage
performance evaluation
policy
probationary period
procedure
professional development
reasonable accommodation
risk management
role model
sexual harassment
team

The Case of the Irritating New Hire

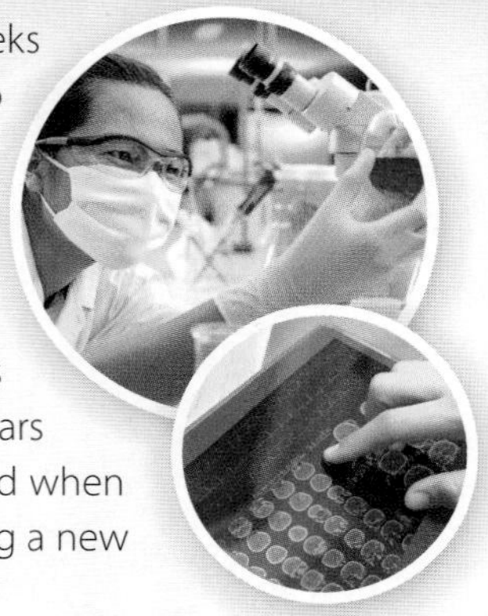

Katie Cormack began her first job as a laboratory technician at Excelsior Medical Lab five weeks ago. She finds the work interesting and especially likes working with patients who come in to have blood drawn for various tests. Katie is surprised when the lab director, Gwen Hendricks, meets with her privately to let her know that other staff members have complained about the time they have to spend answering Katie's questions. Although they appreciate her enthusiasm and desire to do a good job, they are frustrated at having their work frequently interrupted to answer questions regarding common lab policies and procedures and the location of supplies and equipment. Ms. Hendricks explains to Katie that almost all the information she needs appears in the laboratory manuals or was presented in the new-employee orientation that she received when she started her job. This chapter explains the importance of accepting responsibility for learning a new job and explains the major methods and resources that new employees can use.

GETTING OFF TO A GOOD START

Obtaining the first job after graduation is exciting for the new health care professional. Beginning a new job represents a very important time in the health care professional's career. Your professional reputation starts to be established during your first few months of employment. The habits and relationships developed at this time contribute to future success.

Learning about the Job

Succeeding at a new job requires understanding the basics of the workplace. When Aileen McConnor reported for her first day of work as a health information technician at South Bay Hospital, her supervisor, Stan Bergman, conducted an orientation that included the following components:

- Tour of the facility
    - The medical records department
    - Location of files
    - Aileen's desk and work area
    - Lunch room and rest rooms
    - Storage of supplies
    - Personal storage area
- Explanation of safety rules and security precautions
- Demonstration of how to use equipment
- Introduction to coworkers
- Review of her job description

Aileen was glad for the opportunity to ask detailed questions about some of the job duties that were discussed during her employment interview. She also wanted to make sure that she clearly understood the work schedule that was discussed at the time of the job offer. Misunderstandings about these important issues can lead to employment nightmares. Aileen knew that Mr. Bergman would use her job description as a basis for judging her work performance. **Job descriptions** include important information about a specific job. They serve as guides for the actions and performance of the employee. See Table 26–1 for a description of the contents of a typical health care job description.

Policies and Procedures

Policies are the rules established and followed by an organization. **Procedures** are the specific steps taken to perform a task. Every facility develops and records its policies and procedures in order to ensure the quality and consistency of operations. Many health care policies and procedures are required by legal and regulatory agencies. Most facilities assemble manuals that contain all policies and procedures. Employees are expected to know and follow them.

The **employee handbook** is another source of employment policies. It contains information specific to employment conditions, such as the following:

- Vacation policies
- Rules regarding overtime
- Paid holidays
- How to request a leave of absence
- Benefits such as medical insurance
- Rules of conduct

Table 26–1 Components of the Job Description

Section Title	What It Contains	Examples
Job title	Exact name of the position	• Medical transcriptionist • Patient care assistant II • Ultrasound technician
Minimum requirements	Required knowledge, education, license or certification, and/ or experience that must be demonstrated to qualify for the position	• Knowledge of medical terminology, anatomy and physiology (A&P), and English grammar • State nursing assistant certification • Registration with American Registry of Diagnostic Medical Sonographers (ARDMS)
Working conditions/ physical requirements	Type of working environment. Physical abilities needed to perform the job	• Primarily sedentary work with use of earphones • Able to lift up to 30 pounds • Requires standing during 80% of workday
Reports to	Title of the supervisor who directly oversees the position	• Director of medical records • Director of health services • Imaging center director
Responsibilities, duties, and tasks	Specific work to be performed	• Transcribe daily dictation for outpatient surgical center • Transport patients to and from dining room • Perform diagnostic ultrasound procedures for abdominal and obstetrical/ gynecological (OB/GYN) patients

If you are not shown these materials when you are hired, be sure to ask for them. Take time to study the sections that relate to your job. Ask questions about anything you do not understand. Manuals and handbooks serve as valuable references for both new and experienced staff members.

New employees sometimes do not understand the purpose of certain policies. Never refuse to follow policies with which you disagree. (The only exception is if they involve illegal or unsafe activities.) Courteously ask to have the purpose of the policy explained. The reason for it may not be obvious. For example, some facilities prohibit the wearing of colored nail polish. This may seem like a silly rule, but it is founded on principles of good hygiene. Colored polish can hide dirt beneath the nails and around the cuticles. The edges of chipped polish trap germs. Once understood, policies are easier to follow. New employees who have ideas for policy changes should wait until gaining some experience before suggesting "improvements."

Policies that deal with safety must be carefully followed by health care professionals. **Risk management** refers to all the policies and procedures designed to ensure patient safety. Their purpose also includes protecting health care professionals and the public from various risks. Many safety practices are mandated by law, and violating them can be cause for immediate dismissal. Be sure that you understand and follow all rules and regulations that apply to your job.

Probationary Period

Most jobs begin with a **probationary period** that typically lasts between 60 and 90 days. This time allows the employer and employee to determine if they have a "match." The employer can evaluate the new

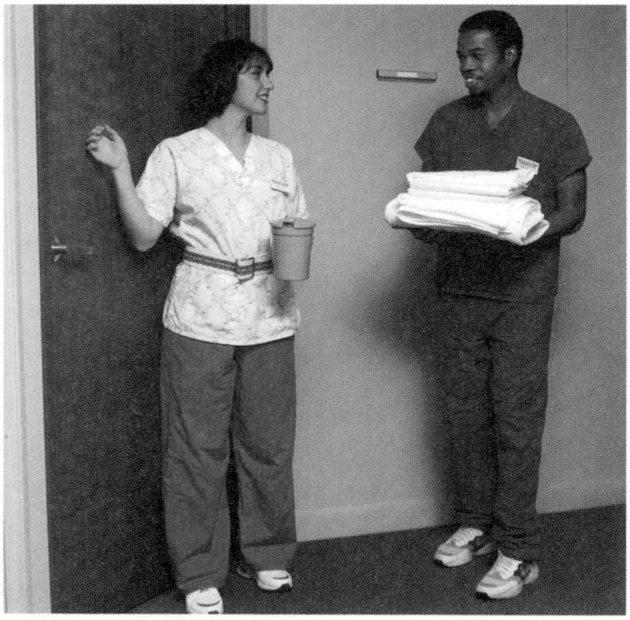

FIGURE 26–1 Cooperation among coworkers is necessary to maintain a smooth-running health care facility.

hire's performance and decide if continued employment is advisable. This is often accomplished through a formal review process, which evaluates how the new employee has performed in areas such as the following:

- Cooperation with supervisor and coworkers (See Figure 26–1)
- Adequate skills to perform job tasks
- Ability to follow directions
- Willingness to learn
- Good attendance record
- Appearance

The probationary period is extremely important. In most states, employees can be terminated for any reason during this time. Once the designated probationary period ends, termination may be more difficult and involve following a formal step-by-step process.

At the same time, the employee can decide if the job is appropriate. Does it require the skills that were acquired in training? Are the duties compatible with the individual's personality and work preferences? Although it is unreasonable to expect any job to be ideal, especially at the entry level, it is important that the new employee feel competent and experience satisfaction with the work performed.

GUIDELINES FOR WORKPLACE SUCCESS

There are certain basic guidelines that apply to all types of facilities and positions. Whether the health care professional works directly with patients, such as a physical therapist assistant, or provides a support service, such as a health information technician, the following recommendations will help ensure long-term career success.

Act with Integrity

Having **integrity** means conducting oneself honestly and morally. It means doing the "right thing" even under difficult conditions. For example, admitting an error and facing the consequences or spending extra time to redo a report until it is perfect, without being asked to do so, are two examples of acting with integrity.

Demonstrate Loyalty

Loyalty to the employer and to one's immediate supervisor is expected in all occupations. It is unacceptable to spend paid work time complaining about the supervisor or conditions of employment. This is especially true in a health care facility. It can cause serious problems. Patients who sense employee discontent or overhear negative comments may experience doubts about the quality of the facility. This can lead to a loss of confidence about their care. At best, patients feel uncomfortable. At worst, they sue for malpractice. All employees must realize that they represent the organization and therefore dedicate their work efforts to contributing to its success. Learning to work for the good of the organization means expanding your view from simply personal success to success of the entire organization.

Being loyal does not mean ignoring difficulties at work. On the contrary, these should be discussed directly and courteously with the supervisor. Problems that are not addressed do not disappear. They tend to become worse. Misunderstandings that could be cleared up in minutes can cause resentment and ruin working relationships. Give your supervisor the opportunity to work with you to create a positive working environment.

Employers appreciate employees who have thought through a problem and have ideas for solutions. This is a much more effective approach than simply presenting complaints.

When the health care professional finds it impossible to feel positive about and loyal to the place of employment, it is best to seek another job. There is too much at risk to do otherwise.

Observe the Chain of Command

Health care facilities organize their personnel so that there is a clear **chain of command**. This means that each person reports to a supervisor who, in turn, reports to another supervisor at the next higher level. This arrangement provides coverage of all necessary tasks along with quality control of employee performance. See Figure 26–2 for a sample organizational chart showing the various levels in a small medical office.

It is important for the health care professional to observe the chain of command. As discussed in the previous section, problems should be discussed with one's supervisor. Workplace problems should not be discussed with coworkers. Nor is it appropriate to go to the next higher level of management without first approaching the person directly involved. It is unfair to "report" your supervisor without giving him or her the opportunity to resolve the situation. It is also inefficient because it brings in another person who is not directly involved in the problem. (Exceptions to this are cases of serious improper behavior on the part of the supervisor, such as sexual harassment or intimidation. These should be reported immediately to the next level of management.)

Give a Full Day's Work

Consistent attendance and punctuality are essential when working in health care. Patients depend on services being provided as promised or required. In turn, employers depend on their employees to be available as scheduled to provide these services. Set perfect attendance as a goal. Plan backup childcare and transportation. Maintain good health habits, as discussed in Chapter 12. If an illness or emergency does require an absence, notify your supervisor as far in advance as possible so that the work can be covered.

While at work, focus fully on the job. Avoid making personal telephone calls and excessive socializing with coworkers. Do not use work time to discuss personal problems. Patients are annoyed when they are required to wait while health care professionals complete their personal business. It may be tempting to text your friends or send personal email messages when you are at work, but these activities should not be done at the workplace. You should also be aware that an increasing number of employers are monitoring their employees' emails, and inappropriate use and messages can result in dismissal.

Respect the time limits for breaks and meals. If your own tasks are completed and there is extra time, find something productive to do: volunteer to help a busy coworker, reorganize the supply cabinet, or practice a new skill. Devote all efforts to your employer during work hours.

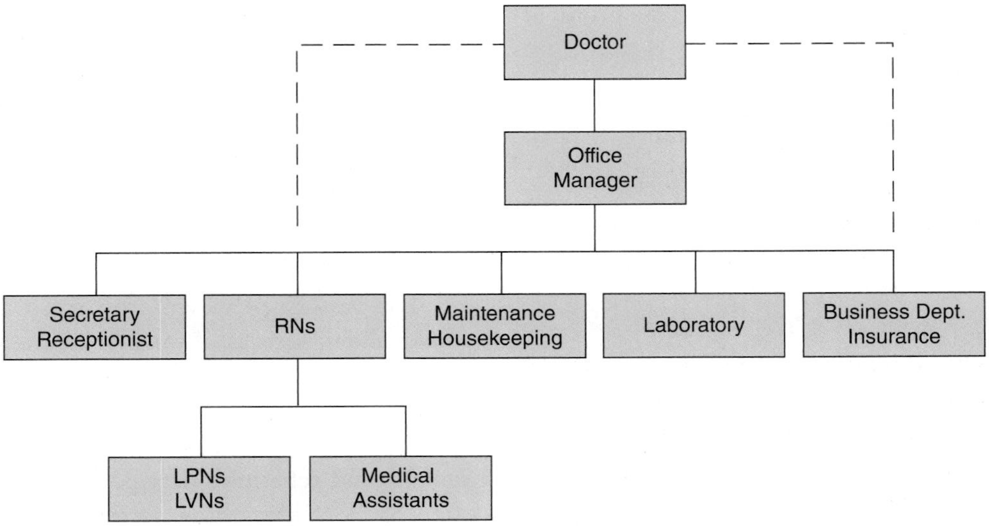

FIGURE 26–2 Sample organizational chart of a medical office.

Thinking It Through

Lack of information and failure to communicate are common causes of workplace conflict. Hank Stuart is experiencing a situation that really has him upset. He is a physical therapist assistant at a busy sports medicine clinic. He also has an interest in computers and worked in a large computer retail store while he went to school. It did not surprise Hank when one of the owners of the clinic, Kathy Chin, asked him to gather information about computer systems and software that could be used for patient management. Hank spent several hours of both work and personal time and gave his recommendation last week. It was then that he discovered that a system had already been purchased. The clinic's other owner had assigned the computer research task to another employee. Upset that his time and ideas were wasted, Hank has let everyone know just how disorganized and unfair his employers are. His coworkers are tired of hearing about it and wish Hank would just forget it.

1. Do you believe that Hank's reaction to the situation is appropriate? Why or why not?
2. How can he better deal with the situation?
3. What action would you recommend that he take?

Effective time management increases productivity and efficiency, which are important in today's cost-conscious environment. It also helps prevent frayed nerves and the panic brought on when tasks are not completed on schedule. The following tips promote the wise use of time at work:

- Write a to-do list when planning each workday.
- Prioritize tasks in order of importance. (Check with your supervisor if you are not sure about priorities.)
- Complete the most important tasks first.
- Batch similar tasks. For example, do all the filing in one session.
- Learn to deal efficiently with interruptions and to quickly refocus on the task at hand.
- Develop time-saving habits. For example, learning to use all the features of a computer program can speed up data entry, word processing, or patient billing duties.
- Avoid procrastinating. If tasks seem overwhelming, break them into small steps and get started. (See Chapter 12.)

Emergencies will occur and schedules will be disrupted. Patient needs are unpredictable. Visits from regulatory agencies that check on facility quality and adherence to standards can take place on short notice. Health care professionals must be willing to cover the necessary work. Effective time management will help keep avoidable emergencies to a minimum.

Become Part of the Team

The specialized and complex nature of health care work requires the participation of many people. Patient care today is accomplished by **teams**, groups of people working together in a coordinated effort to achieve a common goal or set of goals. A football team cannot win if only the quarterback plays the game. In the same way, the success of a health care facility cannot depend on the achievements of just one person. A team may consist of all members of a department, or it may be a small group assigned to work on a specific project. Team goals may be ongoing, such as consistently providing high-quality patient care, or they may be short-term and project-oriented, such as computerizing the office record-keeping system.

Teams that work well can often accomplish more than individuals working separately. There are many ways that teams increase the effectiveness of a facility:

- They provide opportunities for mutual support and encouragement.
- Many viewpoints and ideas are available for solving problems.
- The members contribute a variety of skills.
- Creativity is generated through discussion.
- Work can be coordinated to take advantage of the interests and abilities of the members.
- Duplication of work and wasted effort can be avoided.

The variety of viewpoints and work styles that make teams successful can also be the source of frustration. For example, members who are very creative can contribute good ideas during brainstorming sessions, but become bored during discussions about the details and schedules necessary for the implementation of these ideas. It is necessary to be patient and take advantage of the strengths that each person brings to the group. If the entire group consisted of idea generators, there might be lots of discussion and little action.

New employees are expected to become contributing members of one or more teams. Making a commitment to the organization and to coworkers is the first step toward becoming an effective team member. The needs of the group must be considered when making work-related decisions. Therefore, it is important to identify the goals of the team and to find out what is important to the team members as a group or to the goals of the workplace.

Here are suggestions for becoming a valued member of the team:

- Keep the group goals in mind.
- Listen actively to others.
- Be positive and productive.
- Contribute ideas.
- Do your fair share of the work.
- Follow through on promises.
- Know when to ask for help.
- Give credit to others for work well done.
- Be flexible and willing to adapt to changes.
- Discuss personal differences in private.

Staff meetings are a common way for team members to share ideas and information, plan work schedules, and keep up on issues of common interest. Workplace etiquette requires that employees arrive on time and be ready to participate. Respect others by paying attention. Avoid side conversations, looking at your phone, and other behaviors that indicate a lack of interest.

Meetings are not a place to discuss personal problems or grievances. Conduct these conversations in private with the appropriate person. Concentrate on issues important to the group. See Box 26–1 for an illustration of the consequences when there is a lack of teamwork.

BOX 26–1

Lack of Teamwork

This is a story about people named Everybody, Somebody, Anybody, and Nobody. There was an important job to be done and Everybody was sure that Somebody would do it. Anybody could have done it. Nobody did it.

Somebody got angry about that because it was Everybody's job. Everybody thought Anybody could do it, but Nobody realized that Everybody would not do it. It ended up that Everybody blamed Somebody when Nobody did what Anybody could have done. (Author unknown)

Go Beyond the Minimum

Achieving professional success requires more than meeting minimum job requirements. It means setting high personal standards and striving to meet them every day. Developing the following habits will help lead to both professional success and personal satisfaction:

- Be enthusiastic: Develop an interest in your job. Be passionate about what you do.
- Project a positive attitude: Focus on the positive aspects of your work. Motivate yourself and others with a can-do attitude. Keep in mind that what you do each day contributes to the welfare of others. (See Figure 26–3.)
- Become a problem solver: Use your energy to think of solutions instead of voicing complaints.

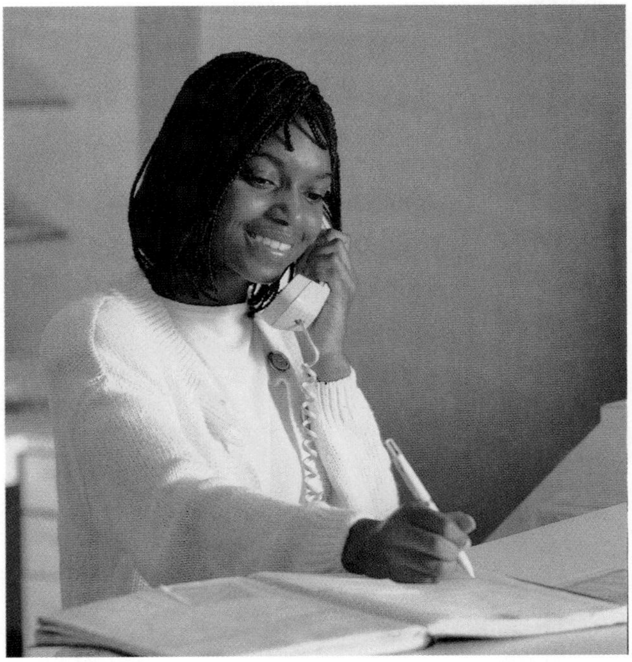

FIGURE 26–3 A positive attitude helps promote patient satisfaction.

Enjoying the challenge of solving daily problems is an essential ingredient for a successful work life.

- Do more than is expected: Be willing to work extra time, if requested, to finish a task. If you finish your own work, offer to help others. Pitch in and help with major projects.
- Practice quality control: Take the time to proofread your work. Memorize the abbreviations needed for charting. Practice procedures until you are proficient—on your own time, if necessary.
- Continue to learn: Add to your skills and knowledge. Participate in continuing education activities. (See Chapter 14.)

See Box 26–2 for a summary of the characteristics of great employees.

Learn from Role Models and Mentors

A **role model** is a person who serves as a positive example. Role models demonstrate high levels of professionalism and competence. They strive to be their best and provide inspiration through their abilities, courage, and dedication. Following the example of appropriate role models is an excellent way for the new health care professional to continue the education received during formal training.

What are the qualities to look for when choosing role models?

- Dedication to their profession
- Good technical skills
- Respectful of others
- High standards
- Confidence gained through experience
- High level of integrity

BOX 26–2

Characteristics of a GREAT Employee

Compassionate

Competent

Considerate

Cooperative

Courteous

- Ability to work well with people
- Understanding of the health care field

A **mentor** is a combination coach and advisor. A mentor should also have the qualities of a role model. Having a good mentor is a tremendous career advantage. However, it does not happen automatically. Look for someone with professional experience, expertise, an interest in helping others, and time to spend with you. This person might work in the same department or facility or be someone you meet at a professional meeting or through networking activities pursued during the job search.

The following are a few of the ways that a mentor can help the beginning health care professional:

- Suggest learning resources
- Offer suggestions and advice about career strategies
- Provide introductions to people in the field
- Pass on information about job openings
- Encourage you to be your best

EMPLOYMENT LAWS

Job applicants and employees are protected by a number of laws. Some of these laws guarantee access to job opportunities. This means that it is illegal for employers to refuse to consider an applicant because of characteristics such as race, religion, and gender. The laws do not guarantee that a person will be hired. That depends on the applicant's qualifications.

Other laws protect the health and safety of employees. These are especially important in health care work because employees may be exposed to a number of potential risks. Table 26–2 contains a list of the most common laws that address the employer–employee relationship. The information provided here is a brief overview. Not all the laws listed apply to all employers. For example, the Family Medical Leave Act applies only to organizations of a certain size. Laws prohibiting sexual harassment, however, apply to all employers, regardless of the number of employees.

In addition to the laws listed in the table, all states have laws that address **minimum wage** (the lowest hourly amount that an employee can be paid), overtime pay, and other issues regarding work conditions. These differ widely, so health care professionals should become familiar with the laws in their area.

Table 26–2 Major Employment Laws

Law	Purpose	Example
Americans with Disabilities Act	Prevents employment discrimination against disabled applicants who are qualified to perform the job if **reasonable accommodations** are made (changes in equipment, special ramps for wheelchairs, etc.)	An applicant who is the most qualified for a medical transcription position cannot be denied the job because the arms of his or her wheelchair do not fit under the desks in the medical transcription area. A reasonable accommodation would be for the employer to furnish a higher desk or table.
Civil Rights Act of 1964	Prevents hiring discrimination on the basis of race, color, religion, sex, age, or national origin	A recently graduated nurse cannot be denied employment because she is 52 years old and the employer believes she will not follow directions as willingly as a younger person.
Title VII of 1964 Civil Rights Act	Prohibits sexual harassment, a form of sex discrimination	It is illegal for a medical laboratory director to continue to ask a lab technician under his supervision for dates when she has clearly stated that she is not interested in dating him.
Equal Pay Act of 1963	Prevents wage discrimination for jobs that require equal skills, effort, and responsibility	A female medical assistant in an urgent care center must be paid the same hourly wage as a male medical assistant who does the same level of work and has comparable experience.
Family and Medical Leave Act of 1993	Allows employees up to 12 weeks of unpaid leave to meet family needs. Same or equivalent job must be given upon return	The father of a newborn infant cannot be dismissed for requesting 3 months to assist his wife in caring for their child.
Immigration Reform Act	Prevents employment of persons who do not have the right to work in the United States	A home health agency that hires young women who do not have the legal right to work in the United States is subject to penalties under this law.
Occupational Safety and Health Act	Prevents unsafe working conditions	It is illegal for an employer to refuse to pay for a hepatitis B vaccination for a newly hired nurse who provides direct patient care and is exposed to blood and other bodily fluids.

Grievances

A **grievance** is a complaint about a circumstance considered to be unfair or potentially harmful. Employees have the right to present grievances to their employer. Many organizations have formal grievance policies that outline the steps required to file a grievance. Look in the employee handbook or ask your supervisor for a copy of the policy.

It is always best to try to resolve workplace issues at the lowest level possible. This means first presenting a problem to your supervisor for discussion and resolution. If the issue is not resolved satisfactorily, then it is appropriate to contact the next level of management. Grievances should be filed only after working up the chain of command, described in an earlier section.

Sexual Harassment

Sexual harassment refers to unwelcome actions that are sexual in nature. It is a form of sex discrimination that is prohibited by Title VII of the Civil Rights Act of 1964. Sexual harassment can occur in a variety of circumstances:

- The victim and the harasser may be a woman or a man. The victim does not have to be of the opposite sex.
- The harasser can be the victim's supervisor, a supervisor in another area, a coworker, or a nonemployee.
- The victim does not have to be the person directly harassed, but can be anyone affected by the offensive conduct.

(*Source:* Adapted from Equal Employment Opportunity Commission. "Facts About Sexual Harassment," www.eeoc.gov/eeoc/publications/fs-sex.cfm.)

The following are examples of sexual harassment:

- A supervisor repeatedly asks an employee for a date after being turned down.
- A high-level manager promises promotional opportunities in exchange for sex.
- A coworker makes crude remarks about the body of a female coworker.
- An employee tells dirty jokes in the presence of coworkers who have stated their objections to such stories.
- A salesman visiting the facility touches a female employee inappropriately.

Mutual friendships and dating are not considered sexual harassment. Workplace romances, however, are not advised. If relationships end, working at the same facility can be uncomfortable and affect the quality of work performed by the people involved. For this reason, some facilities have policies that prohibit dating among employees who work in the same department.

The Equal Employment Opportunity Commission, a government agency that handles sexual harassment complaints that cannot be settled at the workplace, suggests that victims first speak directly to the harasser. Clearly identify the unwelcome behavior and state that it must stop. If the harassment continues, follow the facility's sexual harassment policy or grievance procedure to file a complaint. (*Source:* Equal Employment Opportunity Commission. "Facts About Sexual Harassment," www.eeoc.gov/eeoc/publications/fs-sex.cfm.)

Health care professionals can protect themselves against being accused of sexual harassment by avoiding the following behaviors:

- Discussing sexual matters that are not related to the job
- Telling "dirty" jokes
- Describing intimate details of their personal lives
- Joking around about sexual matters
- Touching coworkers and patients in suggestive ways

New employees should carefully observe and learn the level of formality that is customary in their workplace. Some workplaces are more casual than others. Behaviors that are acceptable in one may be considered unacceptable in others.

Employees who work together sometimes become friends and engage in playful conversation. The best way to prevent problems is to be aware of the reactions of others to your actions or conversation. If in doubt, ask them if they are uncomfortable, and immediately discontinue any conduct that they indicate is inappropriate.

TRACKING YOUR PROGRESS

Employees need to know how they are performing in order to grow professionally and improve their skills. If they are not meeting their employer's standards, evaluations provide an opportunity to learn about deficiencies and create plans to make improvements. Performance evaluations can be valuable learning experiences if approached with a positive attitude.

Most new employees are evaluated at the end of a probationary period, as discussed in an earlier section. When the mutual decision is to continue the employment, the evaluation meeting provides an excellent opportunity for the employee to ask questions that have come up during the probationary period. It is appropriate to ask for an honest appraisal of performance and suggestions for improvement. If there have been any misunderstandings about the employer's expectations and priorities, this is the time to clarify them. Employees have the right to know the employer's expectations and the standards used for judging their performance.

The annual **performance evaluation** (review) takes place about one year after the hire date. It typically consists of numerical ratings of the employee's performance of the duties outlined in the job description. It also includes ratings of important employee characteristics, such as cooperation. Box 26–3 contains a list of items that commonly appear on performance evaluations. Not every item will appear on every form.

Performance evaluations may include a description of the employee's strengths, behaviors that require improvement, and goals to be met by the next evaluation.

This evaluation may or may not include a salary review. Some employers prefer to conduct the performance evaluation and salary review separately. They believe that this encourages a more honest appraisal of and open discussion about performance.

The evaluation is summarized in a written document that is placed in the employee's personnel file following its discussion in a meeting with the supervisor. More benefit can be gained from the evaluation if the employee conducts a self-appraisal in advance. In fact, some employers require this. Be honest about both your strengths and weaknesses. And be prepared to give examples that justify your "ratings." This is a good time to review the job description to see if there have been changes that need to be addressed. Employees should request copies of all documents that are to be placed in the file, including signed performance evaluations.

Do not react defensively or become angry if any low ratings are received. Ask for clarification and examples of how your work is below standard. Request suggestions on how to make improvements. Demonstrate a willingness to accept responsibility for your work and an interest in achieving higher standards.

If a performance review is not scheduled within a few weeks after the first anniversary of hire, it is a good idea to check with your supervisor. These can be overlooked, and your interest in receiving a progress report is usually appreciated.

Employees have the right to see the contents of their personnel files. This includes examining completed performance evaluations and any written warnings or disciplinary notices. Check your file periodically to remain aware of the contents.

BOX 26–3

Common Components of Performance Evaluations

- Accuracy: Performs work without errors
- Appearance: Maintains appropriate, professional appearance for position held
- Attendance and punctuality: Consistently on time and on duty during assigned hours
- Communication: Clear and effective oral and written communication; reports to supervisor as required
- Cooperation: Works well with others; contributes to team effort
- Dependability: Performs work without reminders
- Effectiveness under stress: Remains calm under demanding conditions and during emergencies
- Flexibility: Responds well to changing conditions as well as changing patient and facility needs
- Initiative: Willing and able to problem solve and make decisions
- Operation and care of equipment: Uses equipment safely and correctly; performs or requests maintenance as needed
- Quality of work: Performs tasks correctly; follows facility procedures
- Quantity of work: Completes tasks, meets deadlines, maintains work schedules
- Safety practices: Follows facility policies and standard precautions

MOVING ON

There are many reasons for leaving a job. It is important to do so for the right ones. No job is perfect, and care should be taken to make sure that leaving is a good decision. Before resigning, conduct an honest self-assessment. Sometimes we are part of the problem without realizing it. If this is the case, leaving a job is not necessarily an effective solution. Seeking ways to improve the situation may be a better plan.

If the dissatisfaction is limited to one department, a transfer to another part of the facility might be a workable solution. Requesting a promotion, if earned, can add needed challenges and interest to work that has become routine.

When considering whether to leave a job, it helps to review the working conditions that are most important to you. Rank them in order of importance and use your list to compare present and potential opportunities. The following list contains common reasons for changing jobs; you may want to add others.

- More opportunities to learn and apply new skills
- Higher level of job security
- Wider variety of duties
- Distribution of duties better suited to the employee's personality
- More education or training benefits available
- Better work schedule
- Opportunity to work with experts in the field of interest
- Better salary and benefits

It is usually advisable to obtain a new job before leaving the old one. Take care, however, that time at the current job is not spent conducting job search activities. It is also unacceptable to use the current employer's supplies and equipment, such as paper and the copier, for preparing resumes or the fax machine to send them out. If you must attend interviews during the workday, schedule them during mealtimes or use personal time. Prospective employers will respect your efforts to be considerate of your current employer. It is also possible that you will ask the current employer to serve as a future reference. "Don't burn any bridges" is excellent employment advice.

Plan to have adequate savings or financial support if the decision is made to leave the present job before finding a new position. This prevents having to accept the first position that is offered, whether it is satisfactory or not.

Resigning the "right way" helps maintain a positive reputation in the health care community. The following professional courtesies are recommended:

- Give adequate notice. Two to four weeks is considered to be the usual minimum.
- Submit a letter of resignation. See Figure 26–4 for a sample letter.
- Do not list complaints or grievances in the letter.
- Tell your supervisor before telling anyone else at work.
- Complete all tasks and assignments.
- Do not slack off during the last few days.
- Leave everything in order.
- Offer to help train your replacement.

Thank your employer for the opportunity to work and learn. Ask for a reference letter, even if you have been hired elsewhere. You may need it in the future.

Employment situations occasionally present legal and ethical problems. If you are reasonably certain that any of the conditions listed here exist, report them to your supervisor immediately:

- You are required to perform duties that are clearly outside your scope of practice or for which you are not trained.
- Safe practices are not followed.
- Dishonest practices regarding insurance billing are being done.
- Other illegal or unethical activities are allowed or encouraged.

If no corrective actions are taken, then it is appropriate to go up the chain of command and report to the next levels as needed. If your concerns are still not addressed, then resignation may be the wisest alternative. Fortunately, these instances are rare. Most resignations serve as transitions to the next step in a successful career path.

IF YOU ARE FIRED

Being fired from a job is never a pleasant experience. It can be emotionally upsetting and create doubts about personal worth. Try to remain calm and avoid lashing out verbally in anger. If this action is unexpected, ask clarifying questions about the reasons for

2610 Flanders Court
Tampa, FL 33629
October 5, 20___

Grace Stonefield, Manager
Orthopedic Specialty Group
8884 Orange Parkway
Tampa, FL 33629

Dear Ms. Stonefield:

The purpose of this letter is to advise you of my decision to resign from my position as a Radiologic Technician at OSP. I will be relocating to Nashville in November. My last day of work will be October 25, 20___.

I have enjoyed my work at OSP and especially appreciate being given many opportunities to learn and expand my skills. The dedication to patient care and high level of team cooperation made this an excellent choice for starting my professional career.

Your guidance was especially helpful. Having a supervisor who was willing to give me so many opportunities to learn and take on additional responsibilities was an exceptional benefit. I hope I have a chance in the future to help a new technician in the same way.

I wish you and the staff continued success serving the needs of patients.

Respectfully,

Tyler Adams

Tyler Adams

FIGURE 26–4 Sample letter of resignation.

Thinking It Through

Fran Nichols is angry. She can't believe what happened at work today and how unfairly she was treated by her supervisor, Dan Watson, RN. Dan has been on her case from the beginning, always criticizing her work. But she never thought he would actually fire her. Working an 8-hour shift as a nursing assistant is hard work, and it only makes sense to take some shortcuts to complete all the duties. The safety precautions that Dan insisted on were very time consuming and really didn't seem necessary. After all, the patients she worked with didn't have acquired immunodeficiency syndrome (AIDS) or anything, so it didn't really make sense to go to so much trouble with gloves and special waste disposal and so on.

1. Based on the information given, do you believe that Fran's dismissal was fair? Explain your answer.
2. What would you advise Fran if she wants to continue to pursue a career in health care?

the dismissal. It is not helpful to argue, but if you feel that this is the result of a misunderstanding or misinformation, request an opportunity to explain your side.

Most employers dread having to dismiss an employee and try to conduct the firing as quickly as possible. They may state that the decision is final and that they are not willing to discuss it in detail. In this situation it is best to leave as graciously as possible.

Do not be offended if you are accompanied to your work area, observed as you pack your belongings, and escorted to the door. This is standard procedure that employers are advised to follow. They are usually as uncomfortable about it as the employee. It does not necessarily mean that you are suspected of being dishonest.

Being dismissed can be a learning experience that contributes to future job success. This requires taking a hard look at oneself. The following are common reasons for dismissal:

- Lack of skills needed to perform required tasks
- Refusal to cooperate with supervisor or coworkers
- Theft
- Repeated failure to practice safe techniques
- Breach of patient confidentiality
- Continual attendance problems
- Dishonesty
- Poor interpersonal skills

Be honest with yourself. Blaming others will not help. Only by accepting responsibility can you develop a plan for positive change. Taking charge and making needed changes is an empowering and positive experience. For example, if skills need improvement, contact your school to see if refresher training is available.

Feeling depressed after being fired is natural. Seek the support of friends and family. Talk over your feelings with someone you trust. Ask for their help as you conduct your self-assessment and make plans for the future.

PROFESSIONAL DEVELOPMENT

Professional development means continually striving to improve and be the best at your profession. It means finding satisfaction in your work and participating in professional activities beyond those required during the normal workday. Obtaining a job is only the first step on the career path. Professional development keeps the journey headed in the right direction. Whether the health care professional spends an entire career at the same job or makes many changes, professional development is necessary for long-term success. All health care occupations are affected by rapidly occurring medical discoveries and technological advances. Continual learning is required to stay current and perform effectively. In many occupations, it is required to maintain a license or certification. Do not view professional education as a burden, but rather as an opportunity to expand your knowledge and opportunities.

In addition to the learning activities discussed in Chapter 14, there are other ways to grow professionally and maintain a lively interest in work:

- Set goals: Setting attainable goals and periodically reviewing your progress are powerful motivators for growth. Well-planned goals serve as road maps toward a fulfilling future. Here are a few examples of professional goals:
    - Increase keyboarding speed to 85 words per minute (wpm)
    - Learn health-related conversational Spanish

  - Earn certificate in echocardiography
  - Be promoted to supervisory position at hospital within five years
- Join professional organizations: In addition to providing learning opportunities, these organizations are places to share experiences with other health care professionals. Friendship and mutual support increase career satisfaction. Active participation on committees or as an officer is an excellent way to practice teamwork and leadership skills. Professional organizations are also good sources for obtaining necessary continuing education credits. See Appendix 1 for a list of health care organizations.
- Network: Networking is not limited to the initial job search. Maintaining and expanding your networking contacts expose you to new ideas and opportunities for advancement. Once employed, consider helping others start their careers by giving them information and encouragement. Networking goes in both directions and should be considered a career-long activity.
- Request additional responsibility: This is a way to both show interest and maintain interest in the job. Once you have mastered the basic duties and work routine, adding new responsibilities keeps the challenge alive.
- Stay in touch with your mentor: A good mentor keeps you motivated and aiming toward excellence by providing ongoing career advice.

A career in health care involves enormous responsibilities and tremendous rewards. Engaging in professional development activities can help maintain the balance and ensure a long and satisfying career in the service of others.

WORKBOOK PRACTICE

Go to your workbook and complete the exercises for this chapter.

SUGGESTED LEARNING ACTIVITIES

1. Learn about a professional organization in an occupational area of interest. Using the list in Appendix 1, visit its website, call, or request information. Are the characteristics needed for successful employment identified? What are they?
2. Conduct an Internet search to investigate a variety of health care occupations. Which ones have the most growth? Which are expected to have increasing staffing needs in the future? In which geographical areas is the fastest growth taking place? What are the current salary ranges?
3. Identify friends, family, and acquaintances who are successful at their jobs. These can be in careers other than health care. Ask them what they believe makes them successful.
4. Prepare a list of questions you would want to know when starting a new job.
5. Look for opportunities to work with others on teams. For example, volunteer for a committee with an organization you are interested in. Help with a project at your child's school. Participate fully on group assignments given in your classes.

WEB ACTIVITIES

About Careers: Health Career Advancement – Manage Your Healthcare Career for Success

http://healthcareers.about.com/od/advanceyourcareer/

Choose two articles to read, and write a summary of each.

Professionalism in Health Care

Search using the key words "professionalism in health care." Choose five entries to read and report on.

REVIEW QUESTIONS

1. What are five important things a new employee should do or learn when starting a job?
2. What is the difference between a policy and a procedure?
3. How does the probationary period benefit both the employer and the health care professional?
4. What are seven behaviors that contribute to professional success?

5. What is the purpose of each of the following laws: Title VII of the Civil Rights Act, Equal Pay Act, Family and Medical Leave Act, and Occupational Safety and Health Act?
6. What is a grievance? What action should an employee with a grievance take?
7. What is the definition of sexual harassment, and what steps should a victim take?
8. What actions should an employee take when leaving a job?
9. How can an employee who is fired learn from the experience?
10. Why are professional development activities important throughout the career of the health care professional?

APPLICATION EXERCISES

1. Refer back to The Case of the Irritating New Hire. Describe all the ways that Katie could have learned about her job to avoid burdening her coworkers with too many questions.
2. Ronnie Martinez, a medical assistant at a busy urgent care center, has an appointment in two weeks with his supervisor, Dr. Barnes, for his first annual performance review. His first review took place about three months after he was hired. At that time, Dr. Barnes indicated that Ronnie's overall performance was satisfactory. He did recommend that Ronnie spend some time working on his venipuncture skills and that he strive to always arrive at work on time, not a couple of minutes after 8 a.m. as sometimes happened. Ronnie feels that he has made progress in these areas. Describe how Ronnie should prepare for his performance evaluation meeting.

PROBLEM-SOLVING PRACTICE

Cameron has been working in the health information management department in a large facility for just over a year. He believes he is doing a good job but does not receive much feedback from his supervisor. He hopes to advance his career and "move up the ladder." How can he apply the five-step problem-solving process to identify ways to achieve career success?

SUGGESTED READINGS AND RESOURCES

Americans with Disabilities Act. www.ada.gov

Career success for health care professionals DVD series. (2005). Clifton Park, NY: Delmar Cengage Learning.

Occupational Safety and Health Administration. www.osha.gov

Quintessential Careers. www.quintcareers.com

U.S. Department of Justice, Civil Rights Division. www.justice.gov/crt

U.S. Department of Labor, Family and Medical Leave Act. www.dol.gov/whd/fmla/index.htm

U.S. Equal Employment Opportunity Commission. www.eeoc.gov/

Equal Pay/Compensation Discrimination. http://www.eeoc.gov/laws/types/equalcompensation.cfm

Sexual Harassment. http://www.eeoc.gov/laws/types/sexual_harassment.cfm

APPENDIX 1

Health Care Professional Organizations

THERAPEUTIC AND TREATING OCCUPATIONS

Dental Occupations

American Dental Assistants Association
140 N. Bloomingdale Road
Bloomingdale, IL 60108
(630) 994-4247
www.adaausa.org

American Dental Association
211 E. Chicago Avenue
Chicago, IL 60611-2678
www.ada.org

American Dental Hygienists' Association
444 N. Michigan Avenue, Suite 3400
Chicago, IL 60611
www.adha.org

Dental Assisting National Board, Inc.
444 N. Michigan Avenue, Suite 900
Chicago, IL 60611
www.dentalassisting.com

National Association of Dental Laboratories
325 John Knox Road, # L103
Tallahassee, FL 32303
www.nadl.org

Emergency Medical Occupations

National Association of Emergency Medical Technicians
P.O. Box 1400
Clinton, MS 39060-1400
www.naemt.org

National Registry of Emergency Medical Technicians
P.O. Box 29233
Columbus, OH 43229
www.nremt.org

Society of Emergency Medicine Physician Assistants
1125 Executive Circle
Irving, TX 75038
www.sempa.org

Home-Care and Long-Term Care Occupations

American Health Care Association
1201 L Street NW
Washington, DC 20005
www.ahcancal.org

National Association for Home Care & Hospice
228 Seventh Street SE
Washington, DC 20003
www.nahc.org

Massage Therapy Occupations

American Massage Therapy Association
500 Davis Street, Suite 900
Evanston, IL 60201
www.amtamassage.org

Associated Body & Massage Professionals
25188 Genesee Trail Road, Suite 200
Golden, CO 80401
www.abmp.com

Medical Office Occupations

American Academy of Physician Assistants
2318 Mill Street, Suite 1300
Alexandria, VA 22314
www.aapa.org

American Association of Medical Assistants
20 N. Wacker Drive, Suite 1575
Chicago, IL 60606
www.aama-ntl.org

American Medical Association
AMA Plaza
330 N. Wabash Avenue, Suite 39300
Chicago, IL 60611-5885
www.ama-assn.org

American Medical Technologists Association
10700 W. Higgins, Suite 150
Rosemont, IL 60018
www.americanmedtech.org

American Osteopathic Association
142 East Ontario Street
Chicago, IL 60611
www.osteopathic.org

American Podiatric Medical Association
9312 Old Georgetown Road
Bethesda, MD 20814-1621
www.apma.org

American Society of Podiatric Medical Assistants
1000 W. St. Joseph Highway, Suite 200
Lansing, MI 48915
www.aspma.org

National Commission on Certification of Physician Assistants
12000 Findley Road, Suite 100
Johns Creek, GA 30097-1409
www.nccpa.net

Mental Health Occupations

American Association of Psychiatric Technicians
1220 S. Street, Suite 100
Sacramento, CA 95811-7138
www.psychtechs.org

American Psychiatric Association
1000 Wilson Boulevard, Suite 1825
Arlington, VA 22209
www.psych.org

American Psychological Association
750 First Street NE
Washington, DC 20002-4242
www.apa.org

Nursing Occupations

American Association of Colleges of Nursing
1 Dupont Circle NW, Suite 530
Washington, DC 20036
www.aacn.nche.edu

American Nurses Association
8515 Georgia Avenue, Suite 400
Silver Spring, MD 20910
www.nursingworld.org

National Association for Practical Nurse Education and Service, Inc.
2071 N. Bechtle Avenue PMB 307
Springfield, OH 45504-1583
www.napnes.org

National League for Nursing
The Watergate
2600 Virginia Avenue NW, 8th Floor
Washington, DC 20037
www.nln.org

National Student Nurses' Association
45 Main Street, Suite 606
Brooklyn, NY 11201
www.nsna.org

Occupational Therapy Occupations

American Occupational Therapy Association
4720 Montgomery Lane, Suite 200
Bethesda, MD 20814-3449
www.aota.org

Pharmacy Occupations

American Association of Colleges of Pharmacy
1727 King Street
Alexandria, VA 22314
www.aacp.org

American Pharmacists Association
2215 Constitution Avenue NW
Washington, DC 20037
www.pharmacist.com

Pharmacy Technician Certification Board
2215 Constitution Avenue NW, Suite 101
Washington, DC 20037
www.ptcb.org

Physical Therapy Occupations

American Physical Therapy Association
1111 North Fairfax Street
Alexandria, VA 22314-1488
www.apta.org

Respiratory Therapy Occupations

American Association for Respiratory Care
9425 N. MacArthur Boulevard, Suite 100
Irving, TX 75063-4706
www.aarc.org

Commission on Accreditation for Respiratory Care
1248 Harwood Road
Bedford, TX 76021-4244
www.coarc.com

APPENDIX 2

Useful Spanish Expressions for Health Care Professionals

Hello, hi.	Hola. (OH-lah)
Good morning.	Buenos días. (bway-nohs DEE-ahs)
Good afternoon.	Buenas tardes. (bway-nahs TAR-days)
Good evening, good night.	Buenas noches. (bway-nahs NO-chase)
Please.	Por favor. (por fah-VOR)
Thank you.	Gracias. (GRAH-see-us)
You're welcome.	De nada. (day NAH-dah)
Yes/No.	Sí/No (see/no)
My name is ______	Me llamo (may YAH-mo) ______ *or* Mi nombre es (me NOM-bray es) ______
What is your name?	¿Cómo se llama usted? (CO-mo say YA-mah oo-STED)
Nice to meet you.	Mucho gusto. (MOO-choh GOO-stoh)
Do you speak English?	¿Habla usted inglés? (AH-blah oo-STED eeng-GLACE)
Do you understand English?	¿Comprende usted inglés? (comb-PREN-day oo-STED eeng-GLACE)
Do you understand me?	¿Me comprende usted? (may comb-PREN-day oo-STED)
Repeat, please.	Repita usted, por favor. (ray-PEE-tah oo-STED por fah-VOR)
I don't understand Spanish very well.	No comprendo el español muy bien. (no comb-PREN-doh el es-pahn-NYOL moo-ee bee-EN)
How do you feel?	¿Cómo se siente? (CO-mo say see-EN-tay)
Good.	Bien. (bee-EN)
Fair.	Así, así *or* Regular. (ah-SEE, ah-SEE *or* ray-goo-LAHR)
Bad.	Mal. (mahl)
Do you have pain?	¿Tiene usted dolor? (tee-EN-ay oo-STED do-LOR)
Where?	¿Dónde? (DON-day)
Show me.	Enséñeme. (en-SEN-yeh-may)
Are you comfortable?	¿Está usted cómodo? (es-TAH oo-STED CO-mo-do)
What's the matter?	¿Qué pasa? (kay PAH-sah)
Do you want something?	¿Desea usted algo? (deh-SAY-ah oo-STED AHL-go)

It is important.	Es importante. (es eem-por-TAHN-tay)
Be calm, please.	Cálmese usted, por favor. (CALL-meh-say oo-STED, por fah-VOR)
Don't be frightened.	No tenga usted miedo. (no TANG-gah oo-STED mee-EH-doh)
We are here to help you.	Estamos aquí para ayudarle. (eh-STAH-mos ah-KEY pah-rah ah-you-DAR-lay)

GLOSSARY

Abdominal cavity Located in the abdomen; contains the stomach, intestines, liver, gallbladder, pancreas, and spleen.

Account payable Amount owed to another business for services, supplies, or equipment.

Account receivable Amount due from a customer for services, supplies, or equipment.

Active listening Listening characterized by focusing fully on what a speaker is saying.

Acupuncture Chinese medicine treatment in which tiny needles are inserted into specific points in the body to alleviate pain and relieve various physical, mental, and emotional conditions.

Adult Someone who is 18 years of age or older.

Adult foster home A setting such as a family-style home that provides 24-hour personal care, meals, and supervision for a small number of residents.

Advance directive Written documents that detail the patient's wishes regarding health care decisions; consists of the living will and the durable power of attorney.

Advocate One who supports or promotes the interests of others.

Aerobic Requires oxygen to live.

Aerobic exercise A type of exercise that elevates the heart rate beyond normal resting rate.

Afebrile A temperature that is within the normal range.

Agenda A list of what is to take place at a meeting.

Agent Someone who has the authority to represent another person.

AIDS A disease that occurs when an HIV-positive person develops signs and symptoms of a weakened immune system.

Alternative medicine Health care systems, practices, and products that have not traditionally been performed by practitioners of Western medicine; practices used *instead of* conventional medicine.

Alzheimer's disease Progressive, degenerative disorder that attacks the brain's nerve cells resulting in memory loss, impaired thinking and language skills, and changes in behavior.

Amino acids Molecules that are the building blocks of protein.

Anaerobic Does not require oxygen to live.

Anaphylactic shock A life-threatening severe allergic reaction resulting in swelling of the respiratory system that restricts breathing.

Anatomical position The body as viewed in a full upright position (standing), with the arms relaxed at the sides of the body, palms facing forward, feet pointed forward, and the eyes directed straight ahead.

Anatomy The study of the form and structure of an organism.

Angles The amount of variance from a reference plane expressed in degrees.

Anorexia nervosa A disease based on the distorted belief that one is overweight, even when severely underweight, and the cutting of calories below the number necessary to maintain health.

Anterior body cavity Consists of the thoracic, abdominal, and pelvic cavities; protects the internal organs; also called ventral body cavity.

Anterior (ventral) Toward the front of the body.

Antibiotic Classification of medications capable of inhibiting the growth of or destroying microorganisms.

Antiseptics Chemical agents that prevent or inhibit growth of microorganisms.

Apex At the top (highest point).

Apnea Absence of respirations.

Apothecary system A measurement system that is used infrequently except for a measurement of weight (grain).

Application program A type of software that performs specialized tasks.

Artificial intelligence Sophisticated technology that enables machines and/or computers to make decisions traditionally believed to require human intelligence.

Asepsis (aseptic technique) Methods used to make the patient, the professional, and the environment as pathogen-free as possible.

Asking questions A communication technique used to request clarification and additional information.

Assault Any threatened or implied act, whether carried out or not.

Assertiveness The ability to express oneself freely in a non-threatening manner.

Assessment Gathering information; a step in charting the health care professional's impression of what is wrong with the patient, based on the signs and symptoms.

Assisted living residence Facility that provides housing, meals, and personal care to individuals who need help with daily living activities, but do not need daily nursing care; may also be referred to as supportive housing, residential long-term care facilities, adult residential care facilities, board-and-care, and rest homes.

Attitude How one mentally views a situation.

Auditory learner A person who learns best by hearing new material.

Autonomy Self-determination.

Bacteria One-celled microorganisms that can be either pathogenic or nonpathogenic.

Bacteriocidal A method or chemical that kills bacteria; also called germicidal.

Bacteriostatic A method or chemical that inhibits the growth of bacteria.

Barriers Blocks to communication.

Base At the bottom (lowest point).

Battery Unauthorized touching of another person.

Behavioral question Job-interview question in which the applicant is given a situation and asked how he or she would handle it; or the applicant is asked to describe how he or she handled a real-life situation in the past.

Bias Opinion made before facts are known.

Binge eating The compulsive consumption of large quantities of food, beyond that needed to satisfy physical hunger.

Bioinformatics The organization of biological data into databases.

Block letter A written format in which all lines are flush with the left margin.

Body mass index Measurement of the relationship of weight to height using a mathematical formula.

Body mechanics The correct positioning of the body for a given task, such as lifting a heavy object or typing; when the correct muscles are used and the body is in alignment, good body mechanics are being demonstrated.

Body system Combination of two or more organs to provide a major body function.

Bradycardia A heart rate that is below the normal range.

Bradypnea A respiratory rate that is below the normal range.

Breach of contract When one of the parties in a contract fails to fulfill its part of the agreement.

Bulimia Condition characterized by compulsive eating of huge quantities of food, followed by self-induced vomiting and/or the use of large amounts of laxatives.

Burnout A form of physical and emotional exhaustion that is caused by a variety of personal and environmental stressors experienced over an extended period of time.

Calorie Unit of heat energy; energy content of foods.

Capitation Payment of a fixed fee by an insurance company to a health care provider for each patient enrolled in a health care plan, regardless of services given to the patient.

Carbohydrates Food substances that are composed of units of sugar and provide the body with immediate energy.

Cardiopulmonary resuscitation (CPR) Manually providing respiratory and cardiac support for a patient who is not breathing and whose heart has stopped beating.

Career ladders The various levels within an occupational area that require different amounts of education and training.

Career service center A department of a school or college that assists students in their preparation and search for employment.

Caudal Closer to the coccyx (lower back).

CD-ROM Acronym for "compact disc–read-only memory," a type of optical disk capable of storing large amounts of data.

Cell Smallest living structure of the body.

Celsius (C) Measurement of temperature based on a freezing point of 0° and a boiling point of 100°; also known as centigrade.

Centers for Disease Control and Prevention (CDC) A government agency that formulates safety guidelines to help prevent and control the spread of infectious diseases.

Central processing unit (CPU) Located inside the computer, it manages all operations, performs calculations, manipulates data, and stores program instructions and data.

Cephalic (cranial) Closer to the head.

Certification The process of determining whether a person has met predetermined standards.

Chain of command The organization of employees in which each person reports to a supervisor who, in turn, reports to another supervisor at the next higher level.

Chain of infection Defines the six criteria that must be present for an infection to develop.

Charting Recording observations and information about patients.

Cheyne-Stokes A breathing pattern that has a period of apnea followed by a gradually increasing depth and frequency of respirations.

Chief complaint The patient's statement of the main reason he or she is seeking medical care.

Chiropractic Health care practice based on the belief that pressure on the nerves leaving the spinal column causes pain and dysfunction of the body part served by that nerve.

Cholesterol Fatty substances that can clog arteries.

Choose My Plate Icon developed by the U.S. Department of Agriculture in 2011 to illustrate healthy food choices.

Chronic illness Health problem of long duration in which the disease condition shows little change or slowly gets progressively worse.

Chronological resume Employment resume that emphasizes work experience; the employment history section describes previous jobs in some detail.

Clinical depression Severe, persistent depression marked by specific symptoms, such as insomnia, feelings of worthlessness, and inability to experience pleasure in activities previously enjoyed.

Closed fracture When a bone is broken but does not protrude through the skin.

Closed-ended questions Inquiries that can be answered with a single word or a response of "yes" or "no."

Cloud storage Storage of digital data on multiple servers and sometimes at multiple locations.

Code of ethics Principles created by professional organizations to serve as a guide for the conduct of health care professionals in that occupation.

Cognitive development The growth of intellectual processes of thought, awareness, and the ability to rationally comprehend the world and determine meaning.

Coinsurance A cost-sharing provision in a health insurance contract that stipulates that the insured person is to assume a percentage of the costs of covered services.

Cold calling Calling or visiting employers to make the first contact.

Combining form A root word plus a vowel, in a medical term.

Combining vowel The letters *a, e, i, o,* or *u* when used to link the root word to the next element in a medical term.

Communicable disease A disease that can be transmitted either directly or indirectly from one individual to another.

Communication Process in which messages are exchanged and meanings interpreted between a sender and a receiver.

Compatibility The ability to be combined without unfavorable results.

Complementary medicine Health care practices, products, and approaches to health care that have not traditionally been performed in conventional medical offices; practices used *together* with conventional medicine.

Computer literate Having the knowledge and skills to efficiently perform the computer tasks required in one's work, as well as a basic understanding of how computers work and what types of health care applications are currently available.

Computer viruses Smallest of the microbes; cannot be seen under normal light; in computers, refers to programs that contain instructions to perform destructive operations.

Confidentiality Preserving the legal right of a patient to privacy concerning his or her medical affairs.

Consent To give permission; permission that is given.

Consonant Any letter except *a, e, i, o,* and *u.*

Constructive criticism Appropriate feedback on the performance of others, based on the belief that it can be improved.

Contaminated Infectious material is present.

Continuing care community Provides a variety of living arrangements that support lifestyles as they change from independent living to the need for regular medical and nursing care.

Continuing education Learning experiences beyond those needed to earn the initial certificate or degree to work in an occupation.

Continuing education unit (CEU) A credit granted for certain types of learning that take place after the completion of formal education; same as continuing professional education (CPE).

Continuing professional education (CPE) Education and/or training to stay up-to-date in one's profession and/or to earn continuing education credits.

Contract Promise that is enforceable by law.

Contraction The combined form of two words; for example, it is = it's.

Controlled substance Prescription drug that has the potential for addiction.

Copay The set amount that the patient pays when medical services are received.

Cost of money The amount that is lost when money is not invested; often used to refer to money that is owed to a business, but not collected in a timely way.

Cover letter A written document sent with resumes as a way to introduce oneself and inform the employer why the resume is being sent.

Cranial cavity Located in the skull; contains the brain.

Cross-training Training that health care employees are given to perform tasks in addition to those traditionally assigned to their job titles.

Culture The values, shared beliefs and attitudes, social organizations, family and personal relationships, language, everyday activities, religious practices, and concepts of time and space of a given group of people.

Damages Money to compensate for an injury or loss.

Database The organization of computerized information in a structured way that makes it easy to sort and access.

Decimal A linear arrangement of numbers based on units of 10, containing a point (decimal point) to separate the whole number from the fractional part of a number (e.g., 2.5).

Deductible An amount required to be paid under a health insurance contract by the insured before benefits become payable.

Deep Farther from the body surface.

Defamation of character A legal charge for disclosing unauthorized information that could harm the reputation of another.

Defense mechanism Behaviors that are usually performed unconsciously in response to perceived threats to self-esteem; often provide temporary relief from mental discomfort and anxiety.

Degrees Units of measurement used in angles, temperature readings, and depth of burns.

Dementia Decline in memory and/or other thinking skills.

Demographic Statistics about populations, such as the number of people in a specific age group.

Designation of health care surrogate A legally recognized document in which individuals designate specific people to act on their behalf if they become unable to make health care decisions for themselves.

Development The mental, emotional, and social growth of individuals as they progress through life stages.

Diagnosis Determination of a disease or syndrome.

Diagnostic Pertaining to identifying and determining the cause and extent of diseases and injuries.

Diagnostic procedures Tests performed to determine the diagnosis.

Diagnostic-related group (DRG) A classification system of patients based on their diagnoses to predetermine Medicare payments.

Diet The foods people habitually eat.

Discreet Being careful about what you say, preserving confidences, and respecting privacy.

Diseases Abnormal conditions created when the normal anatomy and physiology of the body are altered.

Disinfectants Agents or methods that destroy most bacteria and viruses.

Distal Farther from the reference base point.

Dominant culture Beliefs and behavior that are generally considered to be foundational for a society or country.

Download To transfer data from one computer to another.

Dyspnea Labored breathing or difficulty with breathing.

Electronic mail A means of creating and sending messages from one computer to another, using the Internet system of networks. Commonly called e-mail.

Electronic health record (EHR) Computerized information and coordination systems used by health care facilities.

Electronic spreadsheet Software that permits the user to apply the computer's ability to perform high-speed calculations of numerical data.

Emancipated minor Someone younger than age 18 who is financially independent, married, or in the military.

Emergency preparedness plan Policy and procedures to be followed when an event occurs that has the potential to kill or injure a group of people.

Empathy Striving to understand another person's attitudes, feelings, and behavior.

Employee handbook A source of employment policies.

Environmental safety The identification and correction of potential hazards that can cause accidents and injuries.

Ergonomics The science of designing and arranging things in the working and living environments to ensure maximum efficiency, health, and safety; a good ergonomic environment maximizes the comfort level and efficiency of the person while limiting possible exposure to discomfort or potential injury.

Erikson's stages of psychosocial development A theory based on the psychosocial challenges that are presented to individuals as they progress through life stages.

Estimating Expressing the approximate answer.

Ethical dilemma When the underlying principles of an ethical system appear to contradict each other and no clear answer emerges.

Ethics A system of principles (fundamental truths) a society develops to guide decision making about what is right and wrong; it helps people deal with difficult and complex problems that lack easy answers.

Etiology Study of the causes of diseases.

Etiquette Manners; acceptable conduct.

Eupnea Breathing that is within the normal range, is unlabored, and has an even rhythm.

Euthanasia Performing a deliberate action that results in a painless, easy death for individuals with an incurable disease; same as mercy killing.

Exhalation The part of the respiratory cycle when air is removed from the lungs.

Expanding consciousness A theory developed by Margaret Newman, RN, to assist patients in making their lives as meaningful as possible by focusing on their possibilities rather than their limitations.

Expenditures The money that must be spent in the process of doing business (e.g., the cost of resources required to maintain a health care delivery system).

Expert systems Computerized databases designed to assist health care professionals in diagnosing and treating specific conditions.

Express consent Permission that is given orally or in writing to receive treatment; more formal than implied consent.

Express contract Result of the parties in a contract discussing and agreeing on specific terms and conditions.

External bleeding When blood drains to the outside of the body through a break in the skin.

External customers People who come to the health care provider for services; they may be referred to as customers, patients, or clients.

Fahrenheit (F) Measurement of temperature based on a freezing point of 32° and a boiling point of 212°.

False imprisonment A legal claim patients can charge if they are held against their will, unless they are mentally incompetent or a danger to themselves or others.

Fats Food substances that contain fatty acids and provide the most concentrated form of energy for the body.

Febrile A temperature that is elevated above the normal range.

Feedback A method by which the receiver of communication can check his or her understanding of what the sender has said.

Fee-for-service Method of payment in which the patient pays the health care provider an amount from an established schedule of fees.

Fiber A substance in food that cannot be fully digested.

Fiber optics Technology that uses hair-thin cables to transmit data.

Field Basic data category in a database.

File A group of related computer records or documents.

Financing The source of money used to run a business.

First aid Emergency care provided to an accident victim or to someone who has become suddenly ill.

Flammable Easily set on fire; same as inflammable.

Fraction A method used to express numbers that are not whole numbers; a fraction is read as parts (numerator) to a whole (denominator).

Fraud A form of dishonesty that involves cheating or trickery.

Free radicals Molecules that have unpaired, highly reactive electrons. In the body, they can damage normal cells.

Frontal plane Divides the body vertically into front and back portions.

Frostbite Condition in which the skin begins to freeze.

Functional resume Employment resume that emphasizes professional and general qualifications rather than one's work history.

Fungi (pl. of fungus) Microorganisms that represent a large group of organisms that are neither plant nor animal. They have unique characteristics that are not shared by other organisms and are thus placed in a Kingdom of their own.

Gatekeeper A health care provider, often a physician, who serves as the patient's first contact when entering the health care system; also known as a primary care provider.

Gateway Website that contains many links to other, related websites.

Gene therapy The insertion of normal DNA into cells to correct a genetic defect or to treat certain diseases.

Germ theory A theory that states that specific microorganisms called bacteria are the cause of specific diseases in both humans and animals.

Gilligan's stages of the ethic of care A theory identifying the stages of development in women based on their caring effects on human relationships.

Golden rule A primary principle when assisting others, meaning to "do no further harm."

Good Samaritan Act A law to protect individuals from liability when they stop to assist someone who has been hurt or is ill.

Grammar A set of rules that determines proper word order, sentence construction, punctuation, and capitalization.

Grievance A formal complaint about a circumstance considered to be unfair or potentially harmful.

Growth Refers to the physical changes that normally take place as the body matures.

Guided imagery The use of words and music to evoke positive imaginary scenarios in a person with the purpose of bringing about some beneficial effect.

Hard drive A data storage device located inside the computer.

Hardware The physical components of the computer.

Hemorrhage Severe, heavy bleeding.

Hepatitis B A virus that causes a blood-borne infection. An occupational hazard for health care professionals.

HIPAA (Health Insurance Portability and Accountability Act of 1996) Government law mandating significant changes in the legal and regulatory environment governing the provision of health benefits, the delivery and payment of health care services, and the privacy and security of individually identifiable, protected health information in written, electronic, and oral formats.

HIV positive The condition of being infected by the human immunodeficiency virus.

Holistic medicine Health care practices based on the belief that all aspects of the individual—physical, mental, emotional, spiritual, and environmental— contribute to states of health and disease.

Homeopathy A health care practice that is based on the idea that "like cures like." Disorders are treated with very small amounts of the natural substances that cause symptoms of the same disorder in healthy people.

Homeostasis Tendency of a cell or the whole organism to maintain a state of balance.

Hospice A facility or service that offers palliative (relieves but does not cure) care and support to dying patients and their families.

Host Living plants or animals from which microorganisms derive nourishment.

Household system A measurement system based on common household items used to measure length, volume, and weight.

Hypertension Condition in which the blood pressure is above the normal range.

Hyperthermia Condition in which the body temperature is above the normal range.

Hypotension Condition in which the blood pressure is below the normal range.

Hypothermia Condition in which the body temperature is below the normal range.

Illegal question A job-interview question that requests information that cannot legally be used to make a hiring decision.

Illness A state experienced by the body when one or more of the control systems lose the ability to maintain homeostasis.

Immune response Defense used by the body to fight infection and disease by producing antibodies.

Implied consent Permission for procedures indicated by the patient's actions; for example, showing up for a medical appointment.

Implied contract When the actions of the parties create a contract without it being detailed in a written format.

Improper fraction A fraction in which the numerator is larger than the denominator.

Incident report Written document that is filled out when any unexpected situation occurs that can cause harm to a patient, an employee, or any other person.

Independent clause Part of a sentence that can stand on its own as a complete sentence.

Infection control Procedures to be followed to prevent the spread of infectious diseases.

Infectious disease Disease caused by growth of pathogens.

Inferior Below.

Inflammable Easily set on fire; same as flammable.

Informed consent Permission given for a procedure to be performed after it and any possible consequences have been explained.

Inhalation The part of the respiratory cycle when air enters the lungs.

Inpatient Admitted to and treated within a hospital.

Integrative medicine Combines treatments from conventional medicine with complementary and/or alternative medicine for which there is high-quality scientific evidence of safety and effectiveness; also called integrated medicine.

Integrity A personal characteristic reflected as honesty; choosing the right rather than the easy way; conducting oneself honestly and morally.

Intermediate nursing care facility (INCF) A type of nursing home that provides personal care, social services, and regular nursing care for individuals who do not require 24-hour nursing, but are unable to care for themselves.

Internal bleeding Blood loss that occurs inside the body.

Internal customers People who work within the health care industry—in other words, other health care professionals.

Internet A vast global system of computer networks linked with other networks that allows instant communication and the sharing of information.

Invasive procedures Punctures or incisions of the skin or insertion of instruments or foreign material into the body.

Job description A list of duties, responsibilities, and other important information about a specific job title.

Job interview A conversation between an applicant and a potential employer to determine if there is a match between the needs of the employer and the qualifications of the applicant.

Jobline Taped recordings, accessible by telephone that contain information about current job openings.

Joint dislocation When a joint becomes disconnected from its socket.

Justice Fairness.

Justified (text) A written format in which the text is lined up with the margins.

Key word A word or phrase used by search engines to locate specific information on the Internet.

Kinesthetic learner A person who learns new material best through the performance of hands-on activities.

Kohlberg's moral stages A theory identifying the stages of moral development in humans.

Lasers Focused light rays that can cut and remove tissue.

Lateral Away from the center of body (toward the sides).

Leadership An approach to working with others that encourages people to work together and do their best to achieve common goals.

Leading questions Inquiries in which all or part of the answer is included in the wording of the question.

Learning objectives Educational goals; what students are to accomplish as the result of a lesson.

Learning style A theory proposing that individuals learn in different ways; the most common categories are classified by the senses (sight, sound, and touch).

Legislation Laws.

Legumes Plants with seed pods that split along the sides when ripe. Foods that are legumes include peas, beans, peanuts, lentils, and soybeans.

Letters of recommendation Statements written on a job applicant's behalf by former employers and other professionals.

Libel A legal charge for defamation of character (damaging someone's reputation) committed in a written form.

Licensure A designation that means a person has been granted permission to legally perform certain acts.

Life review Telling the events of one's life as a form of self-evaluation and closure as the end of life approaches.

Lifelong learning All purposeful learning activities, both formal and informal, that take place throughout our lives.

Living will The part of an advance directive that outlines the individual's wishes regarding the type and extent of medical care to be given.

Malpractice Professional negligence.

Managed care Promotion of cost-effective health care through the management and control of its delivery.

Manual dexterity Skill in working with one's hands.

Maslow's hierarchy of needs A model that categorizes and ranks basic human needs into five areas in an effort to explain how human behavior is motivated by efforts to meet these needs.

Massage therapy Manipulation of soft tissues by rubbing or kneading to achieve health benefits.

Math anxiety A strong negative reaction to math that interferes with the ability to concentrate, learn, and perform math calculations.

Medial Toward the midline or center of the body.

Medic Alert An organization that provides bracelets or pendants for patients to wear that contain information or warnings about specific medical problems.

Medicaid Federally funded but state-administered insurance plan for individuals who qualify due to low income.

Medical asepsis (clean technique) Procedures to decrease the numbers and spread of pathogens in the environment.

Medical documentation Notes and documents that health care professionals add to a patient's medical record.

Medical history Data collected on a patient that includes personal, familial, and social information.

Medical mall A facility that offers a variety of outpatient services, some of which were previously provided by hospitals.

Medical record The collection of all documents that are filed together and form a complete chronological health history of a particular patient.

Medical terminology A language used by health care professionals that includes specialized terms and abbreviations.

Medicare A federally funded insurance program that is part of the Social Security Administration and provides health insurance for people aged 65 and older and others, such as the severely disabled, who qualify for social security.

Medication adherence Taking prescribed medications correctly as per timing, dosage, and frequency.

Meditation A process for quieting the mind by clearing it of thoughts.

Mentor A combination of coach and advisor who can provide information and encourage.

Mercy killing Performing a deliberate action that results in a painless, easy death for individuals with an incurable disease; same as euthanasia.

Metabolism Processing and combining of nutrients to form tissue and/or produce energy for the body.

Metric system A measurement system based on tens; basic units are length (meter), volume (liter), and weight (gram).

Microbes Microorganisms that are pathogenic.

Microbiology Scientific study of microorganisms.

Microorganisms Small, usually one-celled living plants or animals.

Microscope Instrument fitted with a powerful magnifying lens.

Midsagittal plane Passes through the midline and divides the body vertically into equal right and left portions.

Military time A method of telling time that is based on a 24-hour clock.

Minerals Substances derived from nonliving matter that the body needs in small quantities to grow and function properly.

Minimum wage The lowest hourly amount that an employee can legally be paid.

Modem A device that converts outgoing messages from a computer to a form that can be sent over telephone or other lines.

Modified block letter A written format in which all lines are flush with the left margin except the date, closing, and signature.

Negligence Failure to meet the standard of care that can be reasonably expected from a person with certain training and experiences.

Negotiated fees Amount negotiated between insurance companies and health care groups for the cost of services; depending on the plan, the patient either pays the difference in actual cost of service or the health care group accepts the negotiated amount as payment in full.

Network System of computers that are linked so they can communicate and share data.

Networking Developing relationships with individuals who might help you meet your professional goals or secure job leads.

Neutropenic precautions Isolation procedures to protect an immunocompromised patient from infections.

Nomenclature Method of naming.

Nonverbal communication Meaning conveyed by tone of voice, body language, gestures, facial expressions, touch, and physical appearance.

Normal flora Microorganisms that commonly reside in a particular environment on or in the body.

Nosocomial infection Infection that occurs while the patient is receiving health care.

Nursing home Facility for the care of individuals who do not require hospitalization, but who do need general nursing care and assistance performing daily living activities.

Nutrients Substances needed by the body to grow and function properly.

Nutrition The process of obtaining food necessary for health and growth.

Obese A BMI of 30.0 or higher, which indicates the presence of considerably more body fat than is considered to be healthy.

Objective As an adjective, approaching situations from a factual rather than an emotional perspective; as a noun, a statement of your job goal.

Objective data Direct observations made by the health care professional to evaluate a patient's condition.

Occupational Safety and Health Administration (OSHA) A government agency that establishes minimum health and safety standards for the workplace and has the authority to enforce those standards.

Open fracture When a broken bone protrudes through the skin.

Open-ended questions Inquiries that require more than a one-word response; used to encourage patients to provide more detailed information or explanations.

Opinion Beliefs that are not based on certainty or are made without researching the facts.

Opioids Medications that relieve pain by reducing the intensity of pain signals reaching the brain.

Opportunistic infection Infection that occurs due to the weakened physiological state of the body.

Organ The combination of two or more types of tissues that work together to perform a specific body function.

Organic Relating to or derived from living matter.

Organic foods Refers to certain methods of growing food and raising livestock, including the use of natural rather than chemical fertilizers and pesticides.

Orthopnea When a patient has difficulty breathing unless in a sitting or standing position.

Orthostatic (postural) hypotension Rapid lowering of the blood pressure as a result of changing positions.

OSHA Occupational Safety and Health Administration.

Osteopathy Health care practices based on the belief that the body can protect itself against disease if the musculoskeletal system, especially the spine, is in good order.

Osteoporosis Condition in which the bones lose their density and become fragile and more likely to fracture.

Outpatient services Health care services that do not require hospitalization; also referred to as ambulatory services.

Overweight A BMI of 25.0 to 29.9, which indicates the presence of more body fat than is considered healthy.

Palliative Reducing pain or severity of a disease or condition rather than curing it.

Pandemic A rapidly spreading disease that attacks many people at the same time.

Pantomime Using body movement and gestures to convey ideas or actions.

Paraphrasing Rewording the sender's message in the listener's own words and asking the sender for confirmation.

Parasite Organism that nourishes itself at the expense of other living things and causes them damage.

PASS Acronym for proper use of a portable fire extinguisher. (**P**ull the pin. **A**im the nozzle at the base of the fire. **S**queeze the handle. **S**weep back and forth along the base of the fire.)

Pathogens Disease-causing microorganisms.

Pathophysiology The study of why diseases occur and how the body reacts to them (changes in function caused by disease).

Pelvic cavity Located in the lower abdomen; contains the urinary bladder, rectum, and reproductive organs.

Percentage A method used to express a whole or part of a whole. The whole is written as 100%.

Performance evaluation An evaluation and rating of an employee's performance; also referred to as a performance review.

Peripheral Anatomical term meaning away from the center.

Peripherals Computer term for devices attached to the computer, such as a keyboard or printer.

Personal health record (PHR) Documents created and maintained by an individual patient to assist him or her in communicating with various health care providers to ensure greater continuity of care.

Personal space The distance at which people feel comfortable when carrying on a conversation.

Philosophy of individual worth A view based on the belief that every human being, regardless of personal circumstances or personal qualities, has worth.

Physical development The growth of the body, including motor sensory adaptation.

Physiological needs Level 1 in Maslow's hierarchy of needs that must be satisfied in order to maintain life; these needs include oxygen, water, and food.

Physiology The study of the functions (how and why something works) of an organism.

Piaget's cognitive stages A theory identifying the cognitive (intellectual) stages of development in children.

Plagiarism Copying the work of someone else and presenting it as one's own work.

Plan A step in SOAP charting that documents the procedures, treatments, and patient instructions that make up the patient's care.

Point-of-care charting Entering information about patients into the computer when at the patient's home or health care facility bedside.

Policy A rule established and followed by an organization.

Portfolio An organized collection of written documents to show to employers to support claims about a job applicant's qualifications.

Posterior body cavity Consists of the cranial and spinal cavity; protects the structures of the nervous system; also called dorsal body cavity.

Posterior (dorsal) Toward the back of the body.

Preauthorization Approval from an insurance company prior to receiving certain health care services, for the purposes of determining medical necessity and cost effectiveness.

Prefix A word element that is attached to the beginning of roots and combining forms to add to or change their meaning.

Prejudice Negative feelings about a person because he or she belongs to a specific cultural or racial group.

Premium An agreed-upon amount paid to an insurance company for the benefit of having the company pay for a specified amount of future health care costs.

Prepaid plans A contracted type of insurance plan in which health care providers are paid a specific amount to provide certain health benefits.

Prevention (of disease) Behaviors that promote health and prevent disease.

Primary care provider (PCP) Health care provider, often a physician, who serves as the patient's first contact when entering the health care system; also known as a gatekeeper.

Principles Fundamental truths.

Prioritize Ranking items that need to be done in order of importance.

Probationary period Typically the first 60 to 90 days of employment, which provide an opportunity for the employer and employee to determine if they have a "match."

Probing questions Inquiries that request additional information or clarification.

Problem-solving process A sequence of organized steps to follow when making decisions.

Procedure Specific steps taken to perform a task.

Processed foods Foods that are packaged in boxes, cans, or bags.

Professional development Continually striving to improve and be the best possible at your profession.

Professional distance A healthy balance in the health professional–patient relationship that involves demonstrating a caring attitude toward patients without the goal of becoming their friend.

Professionalism A set of characteristics and behaviors that enables one to do the best job possible to provide and maintain high-quality service to patients and employers.

Profit Amount of money remaining after all costs of operating a business have been paid.

Prognosis Prediction of the possible outcome of a disease and the potential for recovery.

Progress notes Written chronological statements about a patient's care.

Proportion A mathematical statement of equality between two ratios.

Proteins Food substances that contain amino acids, substances which are necessary for both building and maintaining the structural components of the body.

Protocols Standard methods of performing tasks.

Protozoa Microorganisms that are classified as animals.

Proximal Closer to the reference point.

Psychiatric hospital A facility that offers treatment to individuals with mental, emotional, and behavioral disorders.

Psychosocial development The maturation of emotions, attitudes, and other aspects of the mind, in addition to the individual's interactions and relationships with other members of society.

Psychosomatic Disorders, including physical illness, caused by mental or emotional factors.

Pulse deficit The rate of difference between a pulse point and an apical rate when they are taken simultaneously.

Pulse points Specific sites on the body where arterial pulsations can be felt.

Quality improvement Processes used to find ways to preserve or improve quality of care while decreasing costs.

Quotation Words written exactly as spoken.

RACE Acronym for responding to fires. (**R**emove patients. Sound the **A**larm. **C**ontain the fire. **E**xtinguish the fire or **E**vacuate the area.)

RAM An internal computer workspace that stores data only while the computer is on.

Ratio A method used to express the strength of a solution; it represents how many parts of one element are added in relationship to the parts of another element.

Reasonable accommodation A legal requirement to supply or make changes in equipment or other aspects of the environment if necessary to accommodate a disabled employee who is qualified to perform the job.

Receiver In communication, the person to whom the sender directs a message; also called the listener.

Reciprocal A fraction that has been "turned upside-down" during the process of dividing fractions.

Record A collection of related computerized data.

Reference A person who will vouch for your qualifications and character.

Reference list A written list given to prospective employers upon request that includes contact information for people who will vouch for your job qualifications and character.

Reference plane A real or imaginary flat surface from which an angle is measured.

Reflecting A communication technique that involves prompting the sender to either complete or add more detail to the original message.

Registration Being placed on an official list after meeting the educational and testing requirements for a specific profession.

Reimburse To pay back or pay for.

Relaxation Techniques used to reduce stress by releasing tension in the muscles in order to improve blood circulation.

Reliable Trustworthy.

Repetitive motion injury (RMI) Injury resulting from a repeated movement that causes damage to a nerve, ligament, tendon, or muscle.

Requesting examples A communication technique to get additional, clarifying information.

Rescue breathing A technique in which the rescuer breathes for the victim.

Rescuer Person giving care during an emergency.

Respiration The process of taking air into and removing air from the lungs; one respiration includes one full cycle of inhalation and exhalation.

Respondeat superior Legal doctrine that makes an employer responsible for the behavior and actions of his or her employees.

Resume Written summary of personal and professional qualifications.

Rickettsia A microorganism that is smaller than bacteria and has rod or spherical shapes.

Risk management All the policies and procedures designed to ensure patient safety.

Role model A person who serves as a positive example.

Roman numerals A numbering system based on I (1), V (5), X (10), L (50), C (100), D (500), and M (1000).

Rounding numbers Rules that determine whether a number is changed to zero, increased, or remains the same when digits are dropped from the right side.

Salutation Greeting.

Scope of practice A description or list of skills that a specific occupational title is legally allowed to perform.

Search engine Computer software program capable of searching through and retrieving millions of documents on the Internet by using specific key words as identifiers.

Self-actualization Level 5 of Maslow's hierarchy of needs, defined as the achievement of one's greatest potential.

Self-directed learning All activities that an individual plans and participates in to increase knowledge and skills.

Self-esteem An individual's opinion of himself or herself.

Semi-block letter A written format similar to the block letter except that the first sentences of paragraphs are indented five spaces.

Sender In communication, the person who creates and delivers a message; also called the speaker.

Sexual harassment Unwelcome actions that are sexual in nature.

Signs Objective evidence gathered by health care professionals about a patient's condition.

Signs and symptoms The objective evidence (signs) observed by the health care professional and the subjective data (symptoms) reported by patients about their condition.

Site license Permission granting the installation of software on more than one computer.

Situational question A job-interview question in which the applicant is asked to describe how he or she would respond to a given situation.

Skilled nursing facility (SNF) A type of nursing home that provides nursing and rehabilitation services on a 24-hour basis; includes regular medical care for patients with long-term illnesses and those recovering from illness, injury, or surgery.

Slander A legal charge for defamation of character (damaging someone's reputation) committed in a spoken form.

SOAP A format for charting that uses a problem-oriented approach.

Software Computer programs that contain instructions that enable computers to function and perform various operations.

Sphygmomanometer An instrument that records the blood pressure.

Spinal cavity Located within the spinal column; contains the spinal cord.

Sprain Torn ligament fibers that result in a loosening of the joint.

Stages of dying Stages that dying people may experience as they face the fact of their own death. The five stages are denial, anger, bargaining, depression, and acceptance.

Standard precautions Practices designed to reduce the risk of transmission of microorganisms from both recognized and unrecognized sources of infection in health care settings.

Sterile field Area designated to be free of microorganisms.

Sterilization Agents or methods that totally destroy all microorganisms, including viruses and spores.

Stethoscope An instrument that amplifies sounds so they can be heard coming from within the body.

Strain (muscle) Result of sudden tearing of muscle fibers during exertion; also referred to as a pulled muscle.

Stress Physiological changes that occur in the body as it responds to danger, either real or imagined.

Stressor Any cause of stress to the individual.

Style manual Contains preferred ways of organizing and presenting written material, including forms for bibliographies and reference lists.

Subjective As an adjective, referring to something that is dependent on or takes place in a person's mind and thus cannot be directly observed.

Subjective data Information the patient tells the health care professional about his or her condition, which cannot be directly observed.

Sucking wound A puncture into the respiratory system resulting in loss of air as the patient breathes.

Suffix A word element that is attached to the end of roots and combining forms to add to or change their meaning; any word ending.

Superficial Near or close to the body surface.

Superior Above.

Surgical asepsis (sterile technique) Procedures to completely eliminate the presence of pathogens from objects and areas.

Syllable Part of a word that has a single spoken sound.

Sympathy Pity felt for another person.

Symptoms Subjective data reported to the health care provider by the patient.

Syndrome Not a precise disease but a group of related signs and symptoms.

Tachycardia A heart rate that is above the normal range.

Tachypnea A respiratory rate that is above the normal range.

Targeted drug therapy Use of drugs to block the growth and spread of cancer cells by preventing them from dividing or by destroying them.

Team Groups of people working together in a coordinated effort to achieve a common goal or set of goals.

Telemedicine The practice of medicine, such as diagnosing and recommending treatment, via electronic communication.

Terminal illness An illness from which the patient is expected to die because there is no known cure.

Therapeutic Relating to healing and assisting patients to regain or attain maximum wellness.

Therapeutic communication Communication that employs certain techniques specifically aimed at meeting the needs of patients.

Thoracic cavity Located in the chest; contains the heart, lungs, and major blood vessels.

Tissue Groups of cells that have a similar function.

Toxic Poisonous.

Traits Personal characteristics.

Trans fat Vegetable oil to which hydrogen has been added; has a harmful impact on cholesterol levels.

Transmission-based precautions Includes three types of isolation procedures (airborne, droplet, and contact precautions) required for preventing the spread of specific infections.

Transverse plane Divides the body horizontally into top and bottom portions.

Treatment Medications or procedures used to control or cure a disease or injury.

Triage system Guidelines to determine which patients to send where and what treatment will be given during an emergency.

Tuberculosis (TB) A disease caused by the contagious airborne pathogen *Mycobacterium tuberculosis*.

Type 2 diabetes Chronic disease characterized by high levels of sugar in the blood, a condition that can damage many parts of the body.

Utilization review (UR) Evaluation of the necessity, appropriateness, and efficiency of the use of health care services, procedures, and facilities.

Values Beliefs, ideal, and standards that provide the foundation for making decisions and guiding behavior.

Victim Person requiring care during an emergency.

Virtual communities Groups of individuals who use the Internet to communicate and share information with each other.

Visual learner A person who learns new material best by seeing it.

Vital signs Measuring the blood pressure, temperature, pulse, and respiration to give some indication of how the body is functioning.

Vital statistics The number of occurrences related to a specific event (e.g., births and deaths) for purposes of reporting.

Vitamins Substances derived from living matter that the body needs in small quantities to grow and function properly.

Vowel The letters *a*, *e*, *i*, *o*, and *u*.

Web directories Web pages on which large collections of information are organized into broad topics and linked to other Web pages.

Wellness Promotion of health through preventive measures and the practice of good health habits; when the body is in a state of homeostasis.

Whole numbers The traditional numbers we use to count (1, 2, 3 ...).

Word part One of the components of a medical term; each word part has its own meaning and location in the term and, like building blocks, they can be combined to create thousands of different words.

Word processing A software program for creating written documents on a computer.

Word root The part of the medical term that gives the main meaning to the word; often refers to the structure and function of the body.

Wound Damage to the soft tissue of the body as a result of violence or trauma.

REFERENCES AND BIBLIOGRAPHY

Acello, B. (2009). *Patient care: Basic skills for the health care provider.* Clifton Park, NY: Delmar Cengage Learning.

A.D.A.M. Education. http://adameducation.com/aiaonline

Agency for Healthcare Research and Quality. (2001, March). Reducing and preventing adverse drug events to decrease hospital costs. *Research in Action*, Issue 1 (AHRQ Publication No. 01-0020). Retrieved November 26, 2015, from http://www.ahrq.gov/qual/aderia/aderia.htm

Ajami, S., & Bagheri-Tadi, T. (2013, June). Barriers for adopting electronic medical records (EHRs) by physicians. *Acta Informatica Medica*. Retrieved November 26, 2015, from http://www.ncbi.nlm.nih.gov/pmc/articles/PMC3766548/

Alexander Graham Bell Association. (1996). *Communicating with people who have a hearing loss.* [Brochure]. Washington, DC: Author.

Alonso-Zaldivar, R. (2012, September 7). The Associated Press. Report says U.S. health care system wasting $750 billion every year. *The Bulletin* (Bend, OR), pp. A1, A4.

Altman, D. (2015). Health-care deductibles climbing out of reach. *The Wall Street Journal*. Retrieved November 26, 2015, from http://blogs.wsj.com/washwire/2015/03/11/health-care-deductibles-climbing-out-of-reach/

Alzheimer's Association. *2014 Alzheimer's disease facts and figures.* Retrieved October 29, 2015, from https://www.alz.org/downloads/Facts_Figures_2014.pdf

Alzheimer's Association. (2015). *Communication tips & techniques.* Retrieved November 26, 2015, from http://www.alz.org/texascapital/in_my_community_14326.asp

American Association of Naturopathic Physicians. (2014). *What is a naturopathic doctor?* Retrieved November 26, 2015, from http://www.naturopathic.org/content.asp?contentID=60

American Cancer Society. (2013, November 5). *Caring for the patient with cancer at home: Depression.* Retrieved November 26, 2015, from http://www.cancer.org/treatment/treatmentsandsideeffects/physicalsideeffects/dealingwithsymptomsathome/caring-for-the-patient-with-cancer-at-home-depression

American Dietetic Association. *Make healthy food choices.* Retrieved October 29, 2015, from http://www.diabetes.org/food-and-fitness/food/what-can-i-eat/making-healthy-food-choices

American Heart Association. (2015, January). *Target heart rates.* Retrieved November 26, 2015, from http://www.heart.org/HEARTORG/GettingHealthy/PhysicalActivity/FitnessBasics/Target-Heart-Rates_UCM_434341_Article.jsp

American Medical Association. *Opinion 5.026—The Use of Electronic Mail.* Retrieved November 10, 2015, from www.ama-assn.org/ama/pub/physician-resources/medical-ethics/code-medical-ethics/opinion5026.page?

American Medical Association. (1993). *Opinion 2.03—Allocation of Limited Medical Resources.* Retrieved November 27, 2015, from http://www.ama-assn.org/ama/pub/physician-resources/medical-ethics/code-medical-ethics/opinion203.page?

American Red Cross. (2006). *First aid/CPR/AED for schools and the community.* San Bruno, CA: Staywell.

American Red Cross. (2007). *Responding to emergencies* (4th ed.). Yardley, PA: Staywell.

American Telemedicine Association. *What is telemedicine?* Retrieved November 27, 2015, from http://www.americantelemed.org/about-telemedicine/what-is-telemedicine#.VjHBbrcrLIU

Anderson, R., Barbara, A., & Feldman, S. (2007). What patients want: A content analysis of key qualities that influence patient satisfaction. *Journal of Medical Practice Management, 22*(5), 255–261. Retrieved November 27, 2015, from http://www.drscore.com/press/papers/whatpatientswant.pdf

Anwar, Y. (2010, February 2). An afternoon nap markedly boosts the brain's learning capacity. Retrieved November 27, 2015, from http://newscenter.berkeley.edu/2010/02/22/naps_boost_learning_capacity/

Apple. (2010). iPhone in business. *Mount Sinai hospital: iPhone provides the vital link to medical records.* Retrieved March 31, 2010, from http://www.apple.com/iphone/business/profiles/mt-sinai/

Barbier Holmes, Deborah E. (2005). *Quick reference for health care providers.* Clifton Park, NY: Delmar Cengage Learning.

Barnes, P. M, Bloom, B., & Nahin, R. L. (2008). *Complementary and alternative medicine use among adults and children: United States, 2007* (National Health Statistics Reports No. 12). Hyattsville, MD: National Center for Health Statistics.

Bickley, L. S., & Hoekelman, R. A. (2012). *Bates' pocket guide to physical examination and history taking* (7th ed.). Philadelphia, PA: Lippincott Williams & Wilkins.

Borgstadt, M. (1996). *Understanding & caring for human diseases.* Clifton Park, NY: Thomson Delmar Learning.

Bureau of Labor Statistics. *Occupational outlook handbook, 2014–15 edition, home health aides*. Retrieved November 27, 2015, from http://www.bls.gov/ooh/healthcare/home-health-aides.htm

Bureau of Labor Statistics. (2010, February 2). *Career guide to industries, 2010–11 edition: Healthcare*. Retrieved November 27, 2015, from http://www.bls.gov/news.release/archives/ooh_12172009.htm

Center for Health Workforce Studies. (2012). *Health care employment projections: An analysis of bureau of labor statistics occupational projection, 2010–2020*. Retrieved November 27, 2015, from http://www.healthit.gov/sites/default/files/chws_bls_report_2012.pdf

Centers for Disease Control and Prevention. *Standard precautions*. Retrieved November 27, 2015, from http://www.cdc.gov/HAI/settings/outpatient/basic-infection-control-prevention-plan-2011/standard-precautions.html

Centers for Disease Control and Prevention. *Tuberculosis—data and statistics*. Retrieved November 27, 2015, from http://www.cdc.gov/tb/statistics

Centers for Disease Control and Prevention. (2009, June 30). *Antibiotic resistance questions and answers*. Retrieved November 27, 2015, from http://www.cdc.gov/getsmart/community/about/antibiotic-resistance-faqs.html

Centers for Disease Control and Prevention. (2010, January 18). *FastStats. Obesity and overweight*. Retrieved November 27, 2015, from http://www.cdc.gov/nchs/fastats/obesity-overweight.htm

Centers for Disease Control and Prevention. (2011, February 23). *Americans consume too much sodium (salt)*. Retrieved November 27, 2015, from the http://www.cdc.gov/salt/

Centers for Disease Control and Prevention. (2013). *Medication adherence*. Retrieved November 27, 2015, from http://www.cdc.gov/primarycare/materials/medication/docs/medication-adherence-01ccd.pdf

Centers for Disease Control and Prevention. (2014, February 6). *Tobacco-related mortality*. Retrieved November 27, 2015, from http://www.cdc.gov/tobacco/data_statistics/fact_sheets/health_effects/tobacco_related_mortality/

Centers for Disease Control and Prevention. *Health, United States, 2013*. Retrieved November 27, 2015, from http://www.cdc.gov/nchs/data/hus/hus13.pdf#018

Centers for Disease Control and Prevention. *Obesity and overweight*. Retrieved November 27, 2015, from http://www.cdc.gov/nchs/fastats/obesity-overweight.htm

Centers for Disease Control and Prevention. (2014, July 14). *FastStats. Deaths and mortality*. Retrieved November 27, 2015, from http://www.cdc.gov/nchs/fastats/deaths.htm

Centers for Disease Control and Prevention. (2014, October 17). *Prescription drug overdose in the United States—fact sheet*. Retrieved November 27, 2015, from http://www.cdc.gov/drugoverdose/

Centers for Disease Control and Prevention. (2014, December 3). *HIV in the United States—at a glance*. Retrieved November 27, 2015, from http://www.cdc.gov/hiv/statistics/basics/ataglance.html

Centers for Medicare and Medicaid Services. *National health expenditure projections 2012–2022*. Retrieved November 27, 2015, from https://www.cms.gov/research-statistics-data-and-systems/statistics-trends-and-reports/nationalhealthexpenddata/downloads/proj2012.pdf

Centers for Medicare and Medicaid Services. *NHE fact sheet*. Retrieved November 27, 2015, from https://www.cms.gov/research-statistics-data-and-systems/statistics-trends-and-reports/nationalhealthexpend-data/nhe-fact-sheet.html

Centers for Medicare and Medicaid Services. (2013). *National health expenditures 2013 highlights*. Retrieved November 27, 2015, from http://www.cms.gov/Research-Statistics-Data-and-Systems/Statistics-Trends-and-Reports/NationalHealthExpendData/downloads/highlights.pdf

Centers for Medicare and Medicaid Services. (2015). *EHR incentive programs*. Retrieved November 27, 2015, from https://www.cms.gov/Regulations-and-Guidance/Legislation/EHRIncentivePrograms/index.html?redirect=/ehrincentiveprograms

Central Intelligence Agency. *The world factbook 2009. Infant mortality rate*. Retrieved November 24, 2015, from https://www.cia.gov/library/publications/resources/the-world-factbook/index.html

Colbert, B., & Ankney J. (2006). *Anatomy and physiology for health professionals: An interactive journey*. Clifton Park, NY: Delmar Cengage Learning.

Collins, M. (1983. *Communication in health care: The human condition in the life cycle*. St. Louis MO: Mosby.

Covey, S. R. (2013). *The 7 habits of highly effective people: Powerful lessons in personal change* (25th anniversary edition). New York: Simon & Schuster.

De Bord, J. (2014). *Informed consent*. University of Washington School of Medicine.. Retrieved November 27, 2015, from https://depts.washington.edu/bioethx/topics/consent.html

DeLaune, S., & Ladner, P. (2006). *Fundamentals of nursing: Standards & practice*. Clifton Park, NY: Delmar Cengage Learning.

DK & Johns Hopkins Children's Center. (2006). *First aid for babies and children fast*. New York: DK Publishing.

Dorland's illustrated medical dictionary (32nd ed.). (2011). Philadelphia: W. B. Saunders.

Dower, C., & Blash, L. (2012, June 11). *Innovation workforce models in healthcare: Utilizing medical assistants in expanded roles in primary care*. Center for the Health Professionals. Retrieved November 27, 2015, from http://futurehealth.ucsf.edu/LinkClick.aspx?fileticket=r4krbCL%2BAtA%3D&tabid=475

EBSCO Health. (2015). *Cumulative index to nursing and allied health literature, 2015*. Retrieved November 27, 2015, from https://health.ebsco.com/products/the-cinahl-database

Ehrlich, A., & Schroeder, C. L. (2011). *Medical terminology for health professions* (7th ed.). Clifton Park, NY: Cengage Learning.

Equal Employment Opportunity Commission. (2002, June 27). *Facts about sexual harassment*. Retrieved November 27, 2015, from http://www.eeoc.gov/facts/fs-sex.html

Erikson, E. H. (1998). *The life cycle completed*. New York: W. W. Norton.

Estes, M. E. Z. (2011). *Health assessment & physical examination* (5th ed.). Clifton Park, NY: Cengage Learning.

Feldstein, P. J. (2012). *Health care economics* (7th ed.). Clifton Park, NY: Cengage Learning.

Fell-Carlson, D. (2008). *Working safely in health care: A practical guide*. Clifton Park, NY: Cengage Learning.

Flight, M. (1998). *Law, liability, and ethics for health care professionals* (3rd ed.). Clifton Park, NY: Delmar Cengage Learning.

Flight, M. (2004). *Law, liability, and ethics for medical office professionals* (4th ed.). Clifton Park, NY: Delmar Cengage Learning.

Frey, K. B., & Ross, T. (Eds.) (2008). *Surgical technology for the surgical technologist* (3rd ed.). Clifton Park, NY: Cengage Learning.

Futures Without Violence. *Mandatory reporting of domestic violence to law enforcement by health care providers: A guide for advocates working to respond to or amend reporting laws related to domestic violence*. Retrieved November 27, 2015, from http://www.futureswithoutviolence.org/userfiles/Mandatory_Reporting_of_DV_to_Law%20Enforcement_by_HCP.pdf

Gallaudet University. (n.d.). *About American deaf culture*. Retrieved November 27, 2015, from https://www.gallaudet.edu/clerc-center/info-to-go/deaf-culture/american-deaf-culture.html

Goldsteen, R. L., & Goldsteen, K. (2013). *U.S. health care system* (7th ed.). New York: Springer Publishing.

Gray, D. (n.d.). *The purple elephant in the room: Talking to someone with depression*. Retrieved November 27, 2015, from http://www.healthcentral.com/depression/news-1594-143.html

Gray, E. (2015, February 23). A different prescription. *Time*.

Green, M. (2014). *Understanding health insurance* (12th ed.). Clifton Park, NY: Cengage Learning.

Gregoire, C. (2013). The amazing way this hospital is fighting physician burnout. *Huffington Post*. Retrieved November 27, 2015, from http://www.huffingtonpost.com/2013/12/02/the-amazing-way-this-hosp_n_4337849.html?ir=India&adsSiteOverride=in

Guyton, A. C., & Hall, J. (2005). *Textbook of medical physiology* (11th ed.). Philadelphia, PA: W. B. Saunders.

Hacker, D. (2007). *A writer's reference* (6th ed.). Boston, MA: Bedford/St. Martins.

Haddad, A. M. (1992). Ethical problems in home healthcare. *Journal of Nursing Administration 22*(3), 46–51.

Hansen, R. S. (n.d.). *15 Myths and misconceptions about job-hunting*. Quintessential Careers. Retrieved November 27, 2015, from http://www.quintcareers.com/job-hunting-myths/

Harvard Medical School. (2011). *Understanding the stress response*. Harvard Health Publications. Retrieved November 27, 2015, from http://www.health.harvard.edu/newsletters/Harvard_Mental_Health_Letter/2011/March/understanding-the-stress-response

HealthGrades. (2008, April). *Fifth annual patient safety in American hospitals study*. Retrieved November 27, 2015, from http://hg-article-center.s3-website-us-east-1.amazonaws.com/a9/9a/3b64b168487c86c30dc0986dc344/PatientSafetyInAmericanHospitalsStudy2008.pdf

Hegner, B., Caldwell, E., & Needham, J. (2003). *Nursing assistant: A nursing process approach* (10th ed.). Clifton Park, NY: Delmar Cengage Learning.

Hoffman, G. L. *How to write the perfect thank-you note after the interview*. Retrieved November 27, 2015, from http://www.usnews.com/money/blogs/outside-voices-careers/2009/02/10/the-perfect-thank-you-note-after-the-interview

Home Care Institute. (2009). *Therapeutic communication in special situations*. Retrieved November 27, 2015, from http://www.hciclient.com/pdfs/Therapeutic_Communication_Special.pdf

Hosley, J., Jones, S., & Molle-Matthews, E. (1997). *Lippincott's textbook for medical assistants*. Philadelphia, PA: Lippincott.

Hubbard. J. (2013). *First aid fundamentals for survival*. Ontario: F+W Media.

InTouch Health. (2015). RP-7I ROBOT. Retrieved November 27, 2015, from http://www.intouchhealth.com/products-and-services/products/rp-7i-robot/

JobStar Central. (n.d.). *Hidden job market—what is it?* Retrieved November 27, 2015, from http://jobstar.org/hidden/hidden.php#wheread

Jones, B. D. (2007). *Comprehensive medical terminology* (3rd ed.). Clifton Park, NY: Delmar Cengage Learning.

Kapit, K., & Elson, L. M. (2013). *Anatomy coloring book* (4th ed.). New York: Addison-Wesley.

Kee, J. L., & Marshall, S. M. (2012). *Clinical calculations with applications to general and specialty areas* (7th ed.). Philadelphia, PA: W. B. Saunders.

Keir, L., Wise, B., & Krebs, C. (1998). *Medical assisting: Administrative and clinical competencies* (4th ed.). Clifton Park, NY: Delmar Cengage Learning.

Kelz, R. (1982). *Conversational Spanish for medical personnel* (2nd ed.). Clifton Park, NY: Delmar Cengage Learning.

Kennamer, M. (2013). *Basic infection control for health care providers* (2nd ed.). Clifton Park, NY: Cengage Learning.

Klinoff, R. (2011). *Introduction to fire protection* (4th ed.). Clifton Park, NY: Cengage Learning.

Kongstvedt, P. R. (2013). *Essentials of managed health care* (6th ed.). Sudbury, MA: Jones & Bartlett.

Krager, D., & Krager, C. H. (2008). *HIPAA for health care professionals.* Clifton Park, NY: Cengage Learning.

Kübler-Ross, E. (1975). *Death: The final stage of growth.* Englewood Cliffs, NJ: Prentice Hall.

Kübler-Ross, E. (1977). *On death and dying.* New York: Macmillan.

LaVallie, D. L., & Wolf, F. M. *Publication trends and impact factors in the medical informatics literature.* Retrieved November 27, 2015, from http://www.ncbi.nlm.nih.gov/pmc/articles/PMC1560603/

Lazarou, J., Pomeranz, B. H., & Corey, P. N. (1998). Incidence of adverse drug reactions in hospitalized patients: A meta-analysis of prospective studies. *Journal of the American Medical Association 279,* 1200–1205.

Lee, T. P., & Pfeifer, M. E. (2009/2010). *Building bridges: Teaching about the Hmong in our communities.* Retrieved November 27, 2015, from http://www.hmongstudies.org/BuildingBridgesGeneralPresentation2006Version.pdf

Lindh, W., Pooler, M., Tamparo, C., & Cerrato, J. (1998). *Delmar's comprehensive medical assisting: Administrative and clinical competencies.* Clifton Park, NY: Delmar Cengage Learning.

Lindh, W., Pooler, M., Tamparo, C., & Dahl, B. (2010). *Delmar's comprehensive medical assisting: Administrative and clinical competencies.* (4th ed.). Clifton Park, NY: Cengage Learning.

Marino, K. (2000). *Resumes for the health care professional* (2nd ed.). New York: John Wiley & Sons.

Martini, F. H., & Bartholomew, E. E. (2008). *Essentials of anatomy and physiology* (4th ed.). San Francisco, CA: Benjamin Cummings.

Mayo Clinic. (2013, June 14). *Mediterranean diet: A heart-healthy eating plan.* Retrieved November 4, 2014, from http://www.mayoclinic.org/healthy-living/nutrition-and-healthy-eating/in-depth/mediterranean-diet/art-20047801

Mayo Clinic. (2014, July 19). *Meditation: A simple, fast way to reduce stress.* Retrieved November 5, 2014, from http://www.mayoclinic.org/tests-procedures/meditation/in-depth/meditation/art-20045858

Miller-Keane encyclopedia & dictionary of medicine, nursing, & allied health (7th ed.). (2013). Philadelphia, PA: W. B. Saunders.

Milliken, M. E., & Honeycutt, A. (2004). *Understanding human behavior* (7th ed.). Clifton Park, NY: Delmar Cengage Learning.

Mokdad, A., Marks, J. S., Stroup, D. F., & Gerberding, J. L. (2004). Actual causes of death in the United States, 2000. *Journal of the American Medical Association. 291*(10), 1238, 1241.

National Center for Biotechnology Information, National Library of Medicine. PubMed. Retrieved March 19, 2015, from http://www.ncbi.nlm.nih.gov/pubmed

National Center for Complementary and Integrative Health. (2015, March). *Complementary, alternative, or integrative health: What's in a name?* Retrieved April 3, 2015, from https://nccih.nih.gov/health/whatiscam

National Center on Elder Abuse. (2005). *Fact sheet. Elder abuse prevalence and incidence.* Retrieved November 27, 2015, from http://www.ncea.aoa.gov/resources/publication/docs/finalstatistics050331.pdf

National Conference on Medical, Legal and Ethical Issues of Eldercare. (2007, September 28). Retrieved November 27, 2015, from http://www.businesswire.com/news/home/20070727005540/en/National-Conference-Medical-Legal-Ethical-Issues-Eldercare

National Heart, Lung, and Blood Institute. (2014, June 6). *What is DASH?* Retrieved November 27, 2015, from http://www.nhlbi.nih.gov/health/health-topics/topics/dash/

National Highway Traffic Safety Administration. (2008, March). *Traffic safety facts. 2006 data. Alcohol-impaired driving.* Retrieved November 27, 2015, from http://www-nrd.nhtsa.dot.gov/Pubs/810801.pdf

National Institute on Deafness and Other Communication Disorders. (2014, October 3). *Quick statistics.* Retrieved November 27, 2015, from http://www.nidcd.nih.gov/health/statistics/pages/quick.aspx

National Institute of Occupational Safety and Health. Retrieved November 27, 2015, from http://www.cdc.gov/niosh/topics/ergonomics/#back

Nebraska Department of Health and Human Services. (2011). *Alcohol and drug abuse and addiction: A health care professional's resource guide.* Retrieved November 27, 2015, from http://dhhs.ne.gov/publichealth/Documents/Chemical%20Dependency%20Book.pdf

Newman, M. A. (2015). *Health as expanding consciousness.* Retrieved November 27, 2015, from the http://currentnursing.com/nursing_theory/Newman_Health_As_Expanding_Consciousness.html

North Dakota State University. (2010, January 7). *What is telepharmacy?* Retrieved November 27, 2015, from http://www.ndsu.edu/telepharmacy/

Open Clinical. *Knowledge management for health care.* Retrieved on November 10, 2015, from http://www.openclinical.org/aisinpractice.html

Paperny, D. (1997). Computerized expert health assessment with automated health education. *The Permanente Journal.* Retrieved November 27, 2015, from https://www.thepermanentejournal.org/files/Summer1997/healthed.pdf

Pfuntner, A., Wier, L. M., & Stocks, C. (2013, January). *Most frequent conditions in U.S. hospitals, 2010* (HCUP Statistical Brief No. 148). Rockville, MD: Agency for Healthcare Research and Quality. Retrieved November 27, 2015, from http://www.hcup-us.ahrq.gov/reports/statbriefs/sb148.pdf

Purtilo, R., & Haddad, A. (2007) *Health professional and patient interaction* (7th ed.). St. Louis, MO: Elsevier.

Sawyers, P. (2014, December 2). How Stephen Hawking is using SwiftKey to communicate twice as fast. *VB News.* Retrieved November 27, 2015, from http://venturebeat.com/2014/12/02/how-stephen-hawking-is-using-swiftkey-to-communicate-twice-as-fast/

Schimeld, L. A. (1999). *Essentials of diagnostic microbiology.* Clifton Park, NY: Delmar Cengage Learning.

Scott, A. S., & Fong, E. (2014). *Body structures & functions* (12th ed.). Clifton Park, NY: Cengage Learning.

Simmers-Narkter, L., & Simmers-Kobelak, S. (2012). *Practical problems in math for health occupations* (3rd ed.). Clifton Park, NY: Cengage Learning.

Social Security Administration. (2014). Status of the Social Security and Medicare programs. *A summary of the 2014 annual reports.* Retrieved November 27, 2015, from http://www.ssa.gov/oact/trsum/

Sormunen, C., & Moisio, M. (2009). *Terminology for allied health professionals* (6th ed.). Clifton Park, NY: Cengage Learning.

Stedman's medical dictionary (29th ed.). (2006). Baltimore, MD: Lippincott Williams & Wilkins.

Steefel, L. (2000). *Nursing in the face of diversity. Nursing spectrum career fitness online.* Retrieved September 19, 2000, from http://nsweb.nursingspectrum.com/Articles/NursingFaceDiversityCF.htm

Taber's cyclopedic medical dictionary (22nd ed.). (2013). Philadelphia, PA: F. A. Davis.

Tamparo, D. D., & Lewis, M. A. (2011). *Diseases of the human body* (5th ed.). Philadelphia, PA: F. A. Davis.

Tamparo, C. D., & Lindh, W. Q. (2008). *Therapeutic communications for health care* (3rd ed.). Clifton Park, NY: Cengage Learning.

Taylor, C., Lillis, C., & LeMone, P. (2006). *Fundamentals of nursing: The art and science of nursing care* (6th ed.). Philadelphia, PA: Lippincott-Raven.

Thomas, W. H. (2007). *What are old people for? How elders will save the world.* Acton, MA: VanderWyk & Burnham.

University of California San Francisco Medical Center. *Communicating with people with hearing loss.* Retrieved November 27, 2015, from http://www.ucsfhealth.org/education/communicating_with_people_with_hearing_loss/

U.S. Census Bureau. (2006) *Families and living arrangements.* Retrieved November 27, 2015, from https://www.census.gov/population/www/socdemo/hh-fam/cps2006.html

U.S. Census Bureau. (2010, February 23). *State and county quick facts.* Retrieved November 27, 2015, from http://quickfacts.census.gov/qfd/states/06000.html

U.S. Census Bureau. (2014, September 8). *Facts for features: Hispanic heritage month 2014: Sept. 15–Oct. 15.* Retrieved November 27, 2015, from http://www.census.gov/newsroom/facts-for-features/2014/cb14-ff22.html

U.S. Department of Agriculture. *Dietary guidelines.* Retrieved November 27, 2015, from http://www.cnpp.usda.gov/DietaryGuidelines

U.S. Department of Health and Human Services. Administration on Community Living. *Aging Statistics.* Retrieved November 27, 2015, from http://www.aoa.acl.gov/Aging_Statistics/index.aspx

U.S. Department of Health and Human Services. Office for Civil Rights—HIPAA. *Fact sheet: Protecting the privacy of patients' health information.* Retrieved November 27, 2015, from http://www.hhs.gov/ocr/privacy/

U.S. Department of Health and Human Services. Office for Civil Rights—HIPAA. *Medical privacy—national standards to protect the privacy of personal health information.* Retrieved November 27, 2015, from http://www.hhs.gov/ocr/hipaa

U.S. Department of Health & Human Services. (2014). *News release: More physicians and hospitals are using EHRs than before.* Retrieved November 27, 2015, from http://www.ilhitrec.org/ilhitrec/pdf/PhysiciansHospitalsEHRs_Aug2014.pdf

U.S. Department of Justice. Drug Enforcement Administration. Office of Diversion Control. *Drug addiction in health care professionals.* Retrieved November 27 ,2015, from http://www.deadiversion.usdoj.gov/pubs/brochures/drug_hc.htm

U.S. Drug Enforcement Administration. (2001, January 22). *Sec. 812. Schedules of controlled substances.* Retrieved November 27, 2015, from http://www.deadiversion.usdoj.gov/schedules/

U.S. Food and Drug Administration. (2009, August 5). *FDA 101: Health fraud awareness.* Retrieved November 27, 2015, from http://www.fda.gov/ForConsumers/ConsumerUpdates/ucm235995.htm

Washington University School of Medicine. (2009, April 3). Sleep may help clear brain for new learning. *Science Daily.* Retrieved November 27, 2015, from http://www.sciencedaily.com/releases/2009/04/090402143503.htm

Williams, S. (2005). *Essentials of health services* (3rd ed.). Clifton Park, NY: Delmar Cengage Learning.

Williams, S. J., & Torrens, P. R. (2008). *Introduction to health services* (7th ed.). Clifton Park, NY: Cengage Learning.

INDEX

Following page numbers, b refers to boxed material; f to figures; p to procedures; and t to tables.

A

Abbreviations, for medical terms, 98–99, 99t, 100t
Abdominal cavity, 135f, 136
Abuse
 of children, 77–78, 78t
 of elders, 78
 spousal, 60t, 78
Acceptance stage, of dying, 204–205
Accidents
 physical and mental changes increasing risk of, 270, 270t
 reporting, 271–272
Accounts payable, 506
Accounts receivable, 505
Acetabulum, 149
Acquired immunodeficiency syndrome (AIDS), 162, 256, 257t
Acromegaly, 182
Acting out, 340t
Active listening, 354
Activities of daily living (ADLs), assessment of, 433–434
Acupuncture, 215
A.D.A.M., 402
Addison's disease, 179
Adequate intake level, 289
Adolescence, 191t, 196, 200t
Adrenal glands, 179, 181t
Adrenaline, 181t
Adrenocorticotropic hormone (ACTH), 180t
Ads, printed, finding job leads in, 533
Adult, definition of, 75
Adult day care, 51t
Adult foster homes, 50
Advance directives, 76–77
Adverse drug incidents, 400
Advocates, 517
Aerobic exercise, 294
Aerobic microorganisms, 225
Afebrile patients, 438
Affection needs, 337–338
Affordable Care Act, 74, 504–505
African Americans, 330t
Age, creativity and, 198b
Agendas, 382–383
Agent, 83
Aging population, 46
AIDS, 162, 256, 257t
Airborne pathogens, 252
Airborne precautions, 244t, 245f
Aldosterone, 181t
Alexander technique, 215
Allergic reactions, emergency procedures for, 459, 459p–461p
Alternative medicine, 54–58, 56t, 57t
Alveoli, 164
Alzheimer's disease, 61, 178, 358
Ambulatory services, 50, 51t
Amenorrhea, 184
American Sign Language (ASL), 359, 359f
Americans with Disabilities Act, 571t
Amino acids, 287
Amputations, 466p
Anaerobic microorganisms, 225
Anaphylactic shock, 459
Anatomy, 142–143
Androgens, 181t
Anemia, 162
Anesthesiologist, 12b
Aneurysms, 162
Anger, communication and, 360–361
Anger stage of dying, 204
Angina pectoris, 162, 482p–483p
Angles, 117–118, 118f
Anorexia nervosa, 294
Anterior, definition of, 136t
Anterior body cavity, 135f, 136
Anthrax, 279t
Antibiotics, 225, 227
 resistance to, 62, 262, 263t
Antidiuretic hormone (ADH), 181t
Antiseptics, 248
Anvil (incus), 172
Anxiety, communication and, 358
Aorta, 157, 157f
Apex, definition of, 136t
Aphasia, 178, 360
Apical pulse, 434t, 440–441, 441p–442p
Apnea, 444
Apostrophes, 375
Apothecary system, 121–122, 121t
Appearance
 of patient, assessment of, 430
 professional, 310–311, 550–551
Appendages, 154, 155
Appendicitis, 167
Appendicular skeleton, 146, 147f
Application programs, 407–408
Apps, 408
Arm, 149
Arteries, 156, 158, 159f
Arteriosclerosis, 162
Arthritis, 149
Artificial intelligence, 398
Ascites, 167
Asepsis (aseptic technique), 231–251
 medical (clean technique), 231–246
 surgical (sterile technique), 231, 249, 249p–351p
Asian Americans, 330t–331t
Assault, 74–75
Assertiveness, 303
Assessment, 33
 observation and data collection vs., 429
 physical. *See* Physical assessment
Assisted living residences, 50
Astigmatism, 173
Atelectasis, 164
ATHENA, 398
Atherosclerosis, 162
Athlete's foot, 155
Atria, 156–157
Atrioventricular (AV) node, 158
Atrophy, 153
Attitude
 professional, 308
 stress management and, 300–301
Auditory learner, 29, 30
Auditory nerve, 171
Aural temperature, 437p
Auricle, 171
Auscultation, 430
Autoimmune diseases, 162
Autonomic nervous system, 176
Autonomy, 71t, 74–77
Autonomy vs. shame and doubt stage, 191t, 195
Avian influenza (H5N1), 259t
Axial skeleton, 146, 147f, 148, 148f
Axillary temperature, 436p
Axons, 176
Ayurveda, 56t

B

Baby boomers, 192
Bacilli, 226, 226f
Back belts, 216–218, 217f
Back pain, 149

Bacteria, 226–227, 226f
Bacteriocidal action, 247–248
Bacteriostatic action, 247
Bandaging, 481, 490p–493p
Bargaining stage of dying, 204
Barrier devices, for resuscitation, 457, 458f
Barriers to communication, 356–361
Bartholin's glands, 184
Base, definition of, 136t
Baseline, 429
Battery, 74–75
Bed scales, 450–451, 451f
Behavioral questions, 549
Beliefs, about health care, culture and, 332–335
Benign prostatic hypertrophy (BPH), 186
Bernhardt, Sarah, 198b
Biases, 31
Binge eating, 294
Bioelectromagnetic-based therapies, 56t
Biofield therapies, 56t
Biomedical engineer, 29t
Biomedical equipment technician, 28, 29t
Bioterrorism, 279
Bird flu (H5N1), 259t
Bites, first aid for, 480p–481p
Bleeding
  emergency procedures for, 461–462, 462p–465p
  external, 461, 462p–464p
  internal, 461, 464p–465p
Block letters, 377, 378f
Blood-borne pathogens, 252
Blood pressure, 434t, 444–449
  diastolic, 444, 444t
  systolic, 444, 444t
  taking manually, 446p–447p, 447f
Blood vessels, 156, 158, 159f, 160f
  changes in, increasing risk of injuries and accidents, 270, 270t
Body language, 352–353
Body mass index (BMI), 292, 292b
Body mechanics, 211–221
  back belts and, 216–218, 217f
  computers and ergonomics and, 218–220, 218f, 219b
  lifting and, 216b, 216f, 217f
  prevention and, 212
  repetitive motion injuries and, 213–215, 213t
  sitting and, 215b
  standing and walking and, 215b
Body systems, 130, 131f, 143–186
  for movement and protection, 143, 144t, 145–155
  for providing energy and removing waste, 144t, 155–169
  reproductive, 182–186
  for sensing, coordinating, and controlling, 169–182
Body temperature, 434, 435f, 435p–437p, 438
Body weight
  measuring, 449–451, 450f–452f, 451b
  normal, maintaining, 292–294
Boils, 155
Bone injuries, emergency procedures for, 462, 467, 467p–469p
Bone marrow, 146
Botulism, 279t
Bovine spongiform encephalopathy (BSE), 260t
Bowman's capsule, 168
Brachial pulse, 439, 439f
Bradypnea, 443
Brain, 174–175, 174f, 175f
Brain stem, 175
Breach of contract, 82
Breasts, 184
Breathing difficulty, emergency procedures for, 482p
Bronchioles, 164
Bubonic plague, 279t
"Buffalo hump," 179
Bulbourethral gland, 185
Bulimia, 294
Bundle of His, 158
Burnout, 303
Burns, 470, 473f, 474p–476p
  chemical, 475p
  electrical, 475p
  emergency procedures for, 470, 473f, 474p–476p, 476f
  radiation, 474p
  thermal, 470, 473f, 474p
Burns, George, 198b
Business letters, 376–377
  effective, writing, 377
  form, 377
  formats for, 377, 378f–380f
  preparing for mailing, 377, 381f, 382f
  reminder letters as, 368
  salutation in, 375
  with test results, 368
Bystanders, enlisting help of, in emergency situations, 458

C

Calcitonin, 181t
Calcium, 288t
Calmness, in emergency situations, 458
Calories, 287
Cancer
  of colon, 167
  of lung, 165
  of skin, 155
Capillaries, 156
Capitalization rules, 374
Capitation, 503
Carbohydrates, 287
Cardiac care units (CCUs), 49
Cardiac muscle, 132, 151
Cardiac sphincter, 165
Cardiologist, 12b
Cardiopulmonary resuscitation (CPR), 456, 458
Cardiopulmonary system, 163
Cardiovascular system, 156–160, 157f–161f, 162
Cardiovascular technologist, 23, 25t
Career fairs, 531
Career ladders, 7
Career orientations, 531
Careers. *See* Health care careers
Career service centers, 529
Carotid pulse, 438–439, 439f
Carpals, 149
Carpal tunnel syndrome, 149, 213t
Carriers, 229
Cartilage, 146
Cataracts, 172
Catholicism, health care beliefs and, 333
Caudal, definition of, 136t
CD-ROM discs, 407–408
Cell body, of neuron, 176
Cells, 130, 131f, 132, 132b, 132f, 133f
Cellulitis, 155
Celsius (C) scale, 123
CEMS (Clinical Evaluation and Monitoring System), 398
Centers for Disease Control and Prevention (CDC), 53, 231
Centers for Medicare and Medicaid Services (CMS), 501, 513
Central nervous system (CNS), 174–176, 174f
Central processing unit (CPU), 406
Cephalic, definition of, 136t
Cerebellum, 175
Cerebral cortex, 174
Cerebral palsy, 177

Cerebrospinal fluid (CSF), 176
Cerebrovascular accident (CVA), 177–178
  emergency procedures for, 487p
Cerebrum, 174–175, 175f
Certification, 6
  in resume, 535
Certified coding specialist (CCS), 27, 27t
Certified medical assistant (CMA), 13
Certified nursing assistant (CNA), 15t, 16
Certified registered nurse anesthetist (CRNA), 15t
Certified registered nurse practitioner (CRNP), 15t
Certified surgical technician (CST), 20, 20t
Cervix, uterine, 183
Chain of command, in workplace, 567, 567f
Chain of infection, 229–230, 229f
  breaking, 231–232
Chair scales, 449, 450f
Charting, 415. *See also* Medical records
  computerized, 420–421
  by exception, 419–420, 420f
  problem-oriented, 419–420, 420f
Chat rooms, 406
Chemical burns, 475p
Chemical disinfectant agents, 248
Chemical-dot thermometers, 438
Chemical hazards, 269t, 277
Chest pain, 162, 482p–483p
Cheyne-Stokes respirations, 444
Child abuse, 60t
Chinese medicine, 56t, 333
Chiropractic, 56t, 57, 57t
Cholecystitis, 167
Cholelithiasis, 167
Cholesterol, 289
Choose My Plate, 289, 289f
Choroid, 170
Chronic illness, 197
Chronic obstructive pulmonary disease (COPD), 164–165
Chronological resumes, 536, 537f
Cilia, 164
Ciliary muscles, 170
Circulatory system, 144t, 156–163
  assessment of, 431
Cirrhosis, 167
Civil Rights Act of 1964, 571t
Clavicles, 149
Clean technique. *See* Medical asepsis
Clinical decision-support systems (CDSSs), 398
Clinical depression, 358
Clinical experiences, finding job leads through, 530–531
Clinical psychologist (PhD or PsyD), 14t
Clinical social worker, 14t
Clitoris, 183
Closed-ended questions, 350, 351t
Closed fractures, 462
Cloud storage, 407
Cocci, 226
Coccobacilli, 226, 226f
Cochlea, 172
Code of Hammurabi, 68b
Codes of ethics, 69, 70b
Coding, 506–507, 507b
Cognitive development, 190, 200–201, 201t
Coinsurance, 501–502
Cold calling, 531
Colon cancer, 167
Colonies, bacterial, 226
Colons (punctuation), 375
Combining forms, 90–91, 92t
Commas, 374
Communicable diseases, 225
Communication, 345–366
  barriers to, 356–361
  computers and, 402–405
  creating the message and, 349–351
  delivering the message and, 351–354
  evaluating the encounter and, 356
  feedback and, 355
  goals of, 348–349
  gossip and patient privacy and, 364
  importance of, 346
  listening to the response and, 354–355, 354b
  nonverbal, 352
  patient education and, 362–363, 362t
  presentations to groups and, 363–364
  seeking clarification and, 355–356
  with special needs patients, 356–361
  by telephone, 361–362
  therapeutic, 347
  written. *See* Business letters; Computers; Letters; Written communication
Community career centers, 529
Compatibility, of chemicals, 277
Compensation, 340t
Complementary and alternative medicine (CAM), 54–58, 56t, 57t
Computed tomography (CT), 396t
Computed tomography technologist, 24t
Computerized charting, 420–421
Computerized inventory systems, 389
Computer literacy, 389
Computer networks, 389, 402
Computers, 387–412
  communication using, 402–405
  diagnostics and, 396–398
  documents and, 394, 394b
  in education, 401–402
  effective use of, 408
  electronic health records and, 391, 393, 421–422
  ergonomics and, 218–220, 218f, 219b
  hardware and, 406–407
  information management and, 389, 391
  learning about, 410
  maintaining the human touch with, 409–410
  patient monitoring using, 400–401
  in research, 401
  security and, 409
  software for, 407–408
  spreadsheets and, 394–396
  telemedicine and, 405
  telepharmacies and, 405–406
  in treatment, 398–400
  virtual communities and, 406
  visual problems with, 220, 220b
Computer viruses, 409
Concrete operational stage, 201t
Conductive hearing loss, 173
Cones (retinal), 170
Confidentiality, 79–82, 364
  of written materials, 384
Confused patients, communication with, 357
Congestive heart failure, 162
Conjunctivitis, 172
Connective tissue, 132
Consciousness
  lack of, emergency procedures for, 488p–489p
  level of, assessment of, 430

Consent, 74–76
to treat, in emergency situations, 457
Consonants, 90–91, 372t
Constipation, 167
Constructive criticism, 518, 519, 519b
Contact dermatitis, 155
Contact precautions, 244t, 247f
Contamination, 225
Continuing care communities, 50
Continuing education, 312, 318–319
Continuing education units (CEUs), 318–319
Continuing professional education (CPE), 318–319
Contractions, 375
Contracts, 82–83
Contractures, 153
Controlled substances, 79, 80b, 301, 340t
Controlled Substances Act, 79, 80b
Conventional moral stage, 201t, 202t
Convolutions, of brain, 174
Convulsions, emergency procedures for, 485p–486p
Copays, 503
Cornea, 170
Coronary arteries, 157, 157f
Corpus callosum, 174
uterine, 183
Corrections, on medical documentation, 417, 417f
Cortisone, 181t
Costs
of health care. *See* Health care costs
of money, 505–506
Coughing, 431
Cover letters, 539, 540f–542f, 542–543
Cowper's gland, 185
Cranial, definition of, 136t
Cranial cavity, 134, 135f
Cranial nerves, 176
Cranium, 146, 147f, 148
Creativity, age and, 198b
Critical Link, 408
Criticism
constructive, 518, 519, 519b
destructive, 518–519, 520b
professional acceptance of, 311–312
Cross-training, 376, 507
Culture, 327–332
dominant, 329–330
individuals and, 327–329
subgroups in the United States, 330t–331t
Cumulative Index to Nursing and Allied Health Literature (CINAHL), 401
Cushing's syndrome, 179
Customer service, 515–520
customer satisfaction and, 517–518, 518t
internal customers and, 518–520
taking responsibility for quality and, 517
Cyanosis, 431–432
Cystitis, 169

D

Damages, 83
DASH diet, 290
Databases, 389, 391, 391b
Data collection, assessment vs., 429
Deafness. *See* Hearing loss
Death and dying, 203–205, 356–357
euthanasia and, 73
Decimals, 109, 109f, 110t, 112, 113t
Deductibles, 501
Deep, definition of, 136t
Defamation of character, 81
Defense mechanisms, 339, 340t
against infections, 230
Degenerative joint disease, 149
Degrees, 117, 118f
Dementia, 61, 178, 358
Demographic changes, 316
Dendrites, 176
Denial, 340t
Dental assistant (CDA or RDA), 8–9, 9t
Dental hygienist (RDH), 8, 9t
Dental laboratory technician, 9, 9t
Dentist (DDS or DMD), 9t
Depression stage
communication and, 358
of dying, 204
Dermatitis, 155
Dermatologist, 12b
Dermis, 154
Destructive criticism, 518–519, 520b
Development. *See* Growth and development
Diabetes insipidus, 182
Diabetes mellitus, 179
emergency procedures for, 483p–484p
type 2, 63, 293
Diagnoses, 142–143
Diagnostic imaging, 396, 396t, 397f
Diagnostic medical sonographer, 23, 24t
Diagnostic procedures, 142–143
Diagnostic-related groups (DRGs), 502
Diagnostics
computerized, 396–398
remote, 397–398
Diagnostic vascular technologist, 23, 25t
Dial (aneroid) sphygmomanometers, 445f
Dialysis, 169
Diaphragm, 164
Diaphyses, 146
Diarrhea, 167
Diastolic pressure, 444, 444t
Diencephalon, 175
Dietetic aide, 28t
Dietetic assistant, 28t
Dietetic technician (DTR), 28, 28t
Dietitian (RD), 28t
Diets, 287. *See also* Nutrition
types of, 289–290, 289f
Digestive system, 144t, 165–168, 166f
assessment of, 432
Digital sphygmomanometers, 445f
Diplobacilli, 226, 226f
Diplococci, 226, 226f
Discretion, 71t, 79–82
Diseases, 142
Disinfectants, 248
Disoriented patients, communication with, 357
Displacement, 340t
Distal, definition of, 136t
Diverticulitis, 167
Diverticulosis, 167
Documentation. *See* Medical documentation; Medical records
Dominant culture, 329–330
Dorsal, definition of, 136t
Double-bagging, 245
Downloading files, 409
Dressing, for safety, 268–269
Droplet precautions, 244t, 246f
Drowning, emergency procedures for, 485p
Drug abuse, 60t, 301–302, 476, 477p
Drugs, prescription. *See* Prescription drugs
Dwarfism, 182
Dysentery, 228
Dysmenorrhea, 184
Dyspnea, 431

E

Eardrum, 171
 ruptured, 173
Ears, 144t, 171–172, 172f, 173
 assessment of, 432
 injuries to, 471p
Eating disorders, 294
Eating habits, improving, 291–292
Ebola virus, 259t
Ectopic pregnancy, 184
Eczema, 155
Edema, 169
Education. *See also* Learning; Lifelong learning
 computers in, 401–402
 continuing, 312, 318–319
 of patients, 362–363, 362t, 383–384
 in resume, 534–535
Educational Resources Information Center (ERIC), 401
Efficiency, health care costs and, 507–508
Elder abuse, 77–78, 78t
Eldercare, 77b
Electrical burns, 475p
Electrical impedance tomography (EIT), 396t
Electrocardiography technician, 23, 25, 25t
Electroencephalographic technologist, 25, 25t
Electroneurodiagnostic technologist, 25, 25t
Electronic health (medical) records (EHRs), 391, 393, 421–422
Electronic mail (email), ethics and, 69b
Electronic sphygmomanometers, 445, 445f
Electronic thermometers, 434, 435f
Email discussion groups, 406
Emancipated minors, 75
Embolus, 162
Embryo stage, 192
Emergency code system, 279, 280f
Emergency departments, 49
Emergency medical responder, 11t
Emergency medical technicians (EMTs), 9–10, 11t
Emergency physician, 12b
Emergency preparedness plan, 280–281
Emergency procedures, 455–495
 for allergic reactions, 459, 459p–461p
 bandaging and, 481, 490p–493p
 for bleeding and wounds, 461–462, 462p–466p
 for bone, joint, and muscle injuries, 462, 467, 467p–469p
 for breathing difficulty, 482p
 for burns, 470, 473f, 474p–476p, 476f
 cardiopulmonary resuscitation as, 456, 458
 for chest pain, 482p–483p
 for diabetes, 483p–484p
 for drowning, 485p
 for drug abuse, 476, 477p
 for facial injuries, 470, 470p–472p
 for fainting (syncope), 484p
 for fever (hyperthermia), 484p–486p
 figure-eight wraps and, 492p
 for hyperventilation, 482p
 for poisoning, 476–477, 478p
 for seizures (convulsions), 485p–486p
 for shock, 486p–487p
 situations and, 456–458
 slings and, 489p–490p
 spiral wraps and, 490p–491p
 for stroke or cerebrovascular accident, 487p
 for temperature-related illness, 477, 479, 479p–481p
 for unconsciousness, 488p–489p
Emotional status, assessment of, 430
Empathy, in communication, 354–355
Employee handbook, 564–565
Employees, great, 570, 570b
Employment. *See also* Health care careers; Job interviews; Job search
 accepting, 555, 557
 declining, 557
 firing from, 574, 576
 guidelines for success in, 566–570
 laws governing, 570, 571t, 572
 leaving, 574
 performance evaluations and, 572–573, 573b
 professional development and, 576–577
 starting out in, 564–566
Endocarditis, 162
Endocardium, 156
Endocrine system, 145t, 179–182, 180f, 180t–181t
 assessment of, 433
Endocrinologist, 12b
Endometriosis, 184
Endosteum, 146
Energy theories/therapies, 56t, 58
Enrollees, 503
Entamoeba coli, 228f
Envelopes, addressing, 377, 382f
Environment
 assessing, in emergency situations, 457
 physical, communication and, 353–354
Environmental control, standard precautions for, 239, 243
Environmental hazards, 269t
Environmental safety, 267–282
 bioterrorism and, 279, 279t
 chemical hazards and, 269t, 277
 emergency code system and, 279, 280f
 emergency preparedness plan for, 280–281
 fire and electrical hazards and, 273–277, 274f–276f, 276t
 general guidelines for, 268–272
 importance of, 268
 infectious waste and, 278
 oxygen hazards and, 278–279
 radiation hazards and, 278
 workplace violence and, 269t, 272, 273t
Epidemiology, 231
Epidermis, 154
Epididymitis, 186
Epigastric region, 136
Epiglottis, 164
Epilepsy, 178
Epinephrine, 181t
Epiphyses, 146
Epithelial tissue, 132
Equal Employment Opportunity Commission, 572
Equal Pay Act of 1963, 571t
Ergonomic hazards, 269t
Ergonomics, 212
 computers and, 218–220, 218f, 219b
Erikson, Erik, 191
Erikson's stages of psychosocial development, 191, 191t, 194, 195, 196, 197, 198
Escherichia coli, 225
Esophagus, 165
Estimating, 115
Estrogen, 182
Ethics, 65–86
 of care, Gilligan's stages of, 202, 202t
 codes of, 69, 70b

Ethics (*continued*)
dilemmas in, 66, 67t, 84–85
of eldercare, 77b
guiding principles of, 70, 71t, 72–84
health care and, 67–84
law and, 66–67
purpose of, 66
Etiology, 142
Etiquette, 377
Eupnea, 443
European Americans, 331t
Eustachian tubes, 172
Euthanasia, 73
"Evil eye," 333
Examples, requesting for clarification, 355–356
Exclusive provider organizations (EPOs), 502t
Exercise, aerobic, 294
Exercises, for computer users, 219t
Exhalation, 443
Exocrine glands, 179
Expanding consciousness, 54
Expenditures, 505
Expert systems, 398
Express consent, 75
Express contract, 83
External auditory canal, 171
External bleeding, 461, 462p–464p
External customers, 515. *See also* Patients
Eyes, 144t, 169–170, 170f, 171f, 172–173
assessment of, 432
injuries to, 470p–471p
protection for, 237
Eyestrain, preventing, 220, 220b

F

Face shields, 237
Facial expressions, 353
Facial injuries, emergency procedures for, 470, 470p–472p
Fahrenheit (F) scale, 123–124, 124f, 124t
Fainting, emergency procedures for, 484p
Faith healing, 333
Fallopian tubes, 183
False imprisonment, 76
Family and Medical Leave Act of 1993, 571t
Family breakdown, 60t
Family practice physician, 13b
Fascia, 152
Fats, 287
trans, 289
FDA Adverse Event Reporting System (FAERS), 400
Febrile patients, 438
Federal Child Abuse Prevention and Treatment Act, 77
Feedback mechanism, 179, 355
Fee-for-service, 501
Female reproductive system, 145t, 182–184, 183f, 433
Femoral pulse, 439, 439f
Femur, 149
Fetus, 192
Fever, 438
emergency procedures for, 484p–486p
Fiber, dietary, 287
Fiber optics, 397
Fibroid tumors, 184
Fibula, 149
Fields, in databases, 391
Figure-eight wraps, 492p
Files, 368, 391
downloading, 409
Fimbriae, 183
Financing, 505
Fingernails, 310
Fingers, bandaging, 493p
Fires
responding to, 273–275, 274f, 275f, 275t, 276t
types of, 275t
Firing, 574, 576
First aid, 456
First-degree burns, 470, 473f
First responder, 11t
Flagella, 226
Flammable liquids, 275t
Folate, 288t
Follicle-stimulating hormone (FSH), 180t
Food. *See* Diets; Nutrition
Food and Drug Administration (FDA), 53
Formal operational stage, 201t
Form letters, 377
Fox, Michael J., 338–339
Fractions, 109–112, 111f, 111t, 112, 113t
Fractures, 150, 151f
closed, 462
first aid for, 467p–469p
open, 462
Fraud, 79
Free radicals, 288t
Frontal plane, 134, 135f
Frostbite, 479, 479p
Full-thickness burns, 470, 473f
Functional resumes, 536, 538f
Fundus, uterine, 183
Fungi, 227–228
Furuncles, 155

G

Gallbladder, 167
Gandhi, Mahatma, 198b
Gangrene, 153
Gastric ulcers, 167
Gastritis, 167
Gastroenteritis, 167
Gastroenterologist, 12b
Gastrointestinal system, 165
Gatekeepers, 503
Gateways, 402–403
Generalized infections, 224
General survey, 429–430
Generativity vs. stagnation stage, 191t, 197
Gene therapy, 38
Genetics, 143
Genitalia, female, 183–184
Germicidal action, 248
Germ theory, 225
Gerontologist, 13
Giardia lamblia, 228
GIDEON (Global Infectious Diseases and Epidemiology Network), 398
Gigantism, 182
Gilligan's stages of the ethics of care, 202, 202t
Glaucoma, 172
Glomerulonephritis, 169
Glomerulus, 168
Gloves
nonsterile, applying and removing, 126–127, 237f–239f, 237p–239p
sterile, applying and removing, 249, 249p–251p, 250f, 251f
Glucagon, 181t
Glucocorticoids, 181t
Golden rule, 456
Gonadocorticoids, 181t
Good Samaritan Act, 456, 456b
Good Samaritan laws, 84
Gossip, 364
Gouty arthritis, 149
Government health programs, 501–502
Government health services, 53, 53t
Government institutions, 500
Gowns, 237, 239
Graafian follicles, 183
Grammar, 374
Gram staining, 226

Grandma Moses, 198b
Grievances, 572
Group presentations, 363–364
Growth and development, 189–207
  care considerations and, 198–199, 199t–200t
  death and dying and, 203–205
  future trends and, 202–203
  Kohlberg's theory of, 201–202, 201t
  life stages and, 191–198, 191t
  Piaget's theory of, 200–201, 201t
Growth hormone (GH), 180t
Guided imagery, 56t, 57t
Gynecologist, 12b

H

H1N1 influenza, 261t
H5N1 influenza, 259t
Habits, changing, 286–287
Hair, 155
Hammer (malleus), 172
Handwashing
  importance of, discovery of, 46b
  for infection control, 230, 232
  procedure for, 232, 234p–236p
  when to do, 232, 234f
Hard drives, 407
Hardware, computer, 406–407
Harmony, health and, 333, 334b
Hashimoto's disease, 162
Health care beliefs, culture and, 332–334, 334b, 335b
Health care careers, 3–36
  in diagnostic imaging occupations, 24t–25t, 25, in 23
  in diagnostic occupations, 7, 23–25, 581–582
  educational programs for, 28–30
  in emergency medical occupations, 9–10, 11t
  in environmental occupations, 27–28, 582
  growing jobs and, 4, 4t, 5t
  in health information management occupations, 25–27, 27t, 582
  in massage therapy occupations, 10, 12t
  in medical laboratory occupations, 25, 26f, 26t
  in medical office occupations, 10, 13t
  in mental health occupations, 10, 14, 14t
  in nursing occupations, 14–16, 15t
  in occupational therapy occupations, 16–17, 17t
  in physical therapy occupations, 17–18, 18t, 19f
  in respiratory therapy occupations, 19, 19t
  in surgical occupations, 19–20, 20f, 20t
  in therapeutic and treatment occupations, 7, 8–9, 579–581
  thinking skills for, 31–34
  in veterinary occupations, 20–21, 21f, 21t
  in vision care occupations, 21, 22t, 23
  work habits and, 30–31
Health care costs, 47, 47f, 58–59, 499–510
  affordability and, 58–59
  controlling organizational costs and, 505–506, 505f
  government programs and, 501–502
  health care institutions and, 500
  health care professionals' impact on, 506–508
  history of reimbursement for, 500–501
  of long-term care services, 59, 59t
  managed care and, 502–504, 502t
  national health care coverage and, 504–505
  payment methods for, 501
  quality of care and, 512
  rising, 500
Health care industry, 37–64
  aging population and, 46
  changes in, keeping up with, 316, 317t, 318
  consolidation of services in, 52
  current challenges in, 58–63
  ethics and, 67–84
  facilities and services provided by, 48–53, 48f, 500
  government services in, 53, 53t
  history of, 38, 39t–45t
  increasing costs and, 47, 47f
  quality of care and, 60–61
  rationing of care and resources and, 74
  specialization in, 46
  trends in, 54–58
Health care institutions, 500
Health care instructions, 76
Health care professionals
  costs and, 506–508
  employment and. *See* Employment; Health care careers
  essential qualities of, 5
  ethics and. *See* Ethics
  infection risk for, 230, 230t, 252–262
  job search and. *See* Job interviews; Job search; Resumes
  reporting of accidental exposure by, 262, 264
  standards for, 6–7
Health Care Reform Act of 2010, 84
Health care surrogate/representative, 76
Health Insurance Portability and Accountability Act (HIPPA), 414–415
Health maintenance organizations (HMOs), 502t
Healthy lifestyle. *See* Diets; Lifestyle management; Nutrition; Stress
Hearing loss, 173
  assessment of, 432
  communication and, 358–359
  increasing risk of injuries and accidents, 270, 270t
Heart, inflammation of, 162
Heartburn, 167
Heart-healthy foods, 162, 289, 289b
Heat cramps, 480p–481p
Heat stroke, 481p
Height, measuring, 449
Hemiplegia, 178
Hemorrhage, 461, 464p–465p
Hemorrhoids, 167
Hepatitis, 167
Hepatitis A, 253t
Hepatitis B, 252, 253t–254t, 259
Hepatitis C, 254t–255t
Hepatitis D, 255t
Hepatitis E, 255t
HepatoConsult, 398
Herbal remedies, 334
Herpes zoster, 178
Hippocrates, 67
Hippocratic Oath, 67–68, 68b
Hirsutism, 179
Hispanic Americans, 331t
Hitchcock, Alfred, 198b
HIV positive, definition of, 256
Hodgkin's disease, 162
Holistic medicine, 55–56
Holmes, Oliver Wendell, 225
Home health aide, 15t, 16
Home health care providers, 50–52

Homelessness, 60t
Homeopathy, 57–58, 57t
Homeostasis, 130
Honesty, 71t, 79
Hormones, 179, 180t–181t, 182–183
Hospice, 52
Hospitals, 48–50
Hosts, 225
  reservoir, 229
Household system, 118–119, 119f, 119t
Human body
  abdominal descriptions of, 136–138, 137f, 138f
  anatomy and physiology of, 142–143
  basis of life and, 130–134, 131f
  cavities of, 134, 135f, 136
  describing, 134–138
  directional terms for, 134, 135f, 136t
  planes of, 134
  structural organization of, 130, 131f
  systems of. *See* Body systems
Human Genome Project, 401
Human immunodeficiency virus (HIV), 252, 256, 257t, 259
Humerus, 149
Humor, in communication, 351
Humors, 333
Hydrotherapy, 215
Hyperglycemia, 179, 483p
Hyperopia, 173
Hyperparathyroidism, 179
Hypertension, 162, 444, 449
Hyperthermia, 479, 480p
  emergency procedures for, 484p–486p
Hyperthyroidism, 182
Hyperventilation, emergency procedures for, 482p
Hypochondriac regions, 136
Hypogastric region, 136
Hypoglycemia, 483p
Hypoparathyroidism, 179, 182
Hypotension, 444
  orthostatic (postural), 448
Hypothalamus, 175
Hypothermia, 479
Hypothyroidism, 182

I

ICD-10 codes, 506, 507, 507b
Ileocecal valve, 166
Iliac regions, 137
Ilium, 149
Illegal questions, 550
Illness, 143
  chronic, 197
Image-guided surgery, 398–399
Immigration Reform Act, 571t
Immune response, 161–162, 225
Implied consent, 75
Implied contract, 82–83
Improper fractions, 112
Incus, 172
Independent clauses, 374
Individual worth, philosophy of, 326–327
Industry vs. inferiority stage, 191t, 196
Infancy, 191t, 194, 199t
Infant, 194
Infection control, 223–265
  asepsis for. *See* Asepsis (aseptic technique)
  importance of, 224–225
  microbiology and, 225–231
  reporting accidental exposure and, 262, 264
  risks to health care professionals and, 252–262
Infections
  chain of infection and, 229–230, 229f
  cutaneous, fungal, 228
  drug-resistant, 262, 263t
  generalized (systemic) and localized, 224
  nosocomial, 230
Infectious diseases, 38, 224
Infectious hazards, 269t
Infectious waste, 278
Inferior, definition of, 136t
Inferior vena cava, 56
Inflammable liquids, 275t
Inflammation, of heart, 162
Information, collecting in communication process, 349
Information management, 389, 391
Informed consent, 74
Ingestion injuries, 478p
Inhalation, 443
Inhalation injuries, 478p
Injuries, physical and mental changes increasing risk of, 270, 270t
Inner ear, 171, 172
Inpatients, 49
Insect bites and stings, first aid for, 480p–481p
Insertion, of muscles, 152
Inspection, 430
Insulin, 181t
Insurance, 500
  government, 501–502
  national, 504–505
  premiums for, 500, 502
  prepaid plans for, 503
  private, 504
Integrative medicine, 55
Integrity, 5, 566
Integrity vs. despair stage, 191t, 198
Integumentary system, 144t, 153–155, 154f
  assessment of, 431
Intensive care units (ICUs), 49
Intermediate nursing care facilities (INCFs), 50
Intermittent fever, 438
Internal bleeding, 461, 464p–465p
Internal customers, 515, 518–520. *See also* Health care professionals
Internet, 402–405
  electronic mail and, 404
  evaluating sources on, 403–404, 403t
  finding job leads on, 531–532
  for research, 402–403
  social and professional networking sites on, 404–405
Internist, 12b
Interstitial cell-stimulating hormone (ICSH), 181t
Intervertebral disks, 148, 148f
Intimacy vs. isolation stage, 191t, 197
Invasive procedures, 75
Inventory systems, computerized, 389
Involuntary nerves, 176
Iris, 170
Iron, 288t
Iron-deficiency anemia, 162
Ischium, 149
Islam, health care beliefs and, 333

J

Job applications, 557, 558f–560f
Job descriptions, 564, 565t
Job fairs, 531
Job interviews, 546–555
  follow-up for, 555
  making a good impression in, 553–554
  preparing for, 546–553
  recent trends in, 554
Joblines, finding job leads on, 533
Job search, 526–533. *See also* Job interviews; Resumes
  accepting a job and, 555, 557
  declining a job and, 557
  expectations and, 527

finding job leads and, 528–533
organizing time and space for, 527–528
professional image and, 528
self-evaluation for, 526–527
Joint dislocations, 467p–469p
Joint injuries, emergency procedures for, 462, 467, 467p–469p
Justice, 71t, 77
Justified text, 377

K

Kevorkian, Jack, 73
Key words, 403
Kidney calculi, 169
Kidney failure, 169
Kidneys, 168–169
Kinesthetic learner, 29, 30
Kohlberg's moral stages, 201–202, 201t
Kübler-Ross, Elisabeth, 203–205
Kyphosis, 150, 150f

L

Labia majora, 183
Labia minora, 183
Labyrinthitis, 173
Lactation, 184
Lactogenic hormone (LTH), 181t
Language barriers, 361
Large intestine, 166
Laryngitis, 165
Larynx, 164
Lasers, 398
Later adulthood, 191t, 197–198, 200t
Lateral, definition of, 136t
Laws. *See* Legislation
Leadership, 313
Leading questions, 350, 351t
Learning. *See also* Education
about computers, 410
continuing education and, 312
lifelong. *See* Lifelong learning
for mastery, 28–29
Learning objectives, 362
Learning styles, 29
Left lower quadrant (LLQ), 137f, 138
Left upper quadrant (LUQ), 137f, 138
Legislation
on abuse, 77
on advance directives, 76
Affordable Care Act, 504–505
on eldercare, 77b
employment, 570, 571t, 572
ethics and, 66–67
Good Samaritan laws, 84, 456, 456b
Health Care Reform Act of 2010, 84
Health Insurance Portability and Accountability Act (HIPPA), 414–415
Patient Protection and Affordable Care Act, 74, 504–505
protective, 78–79, 80b
Legumes, 287, 290
Lens (of eye), 170
Letters
cover, 539, 540f–542f, 542–543
form, 377
of recommendation, 552
reminder, 368
of resignation, 474f, 574
thank-you, following job interviews, 555, 556f
Leukemia, 162
Libel, 81
Licensed practical/vocational nurse (LPN/LVN), 15–16, 15t
Licenses, in resume, 535
Licensure, 6
Life, preservation of, 71t, 72–74
Lifelong learning, 315–322
continuing education units and, 318–319
importance of, 316–318
self-directed, 319–321
Life review, 204
Life stages, 191–198, 191t
Lifestyle, 62–63
Lifestyle management, 285–305
changing habits for, 286–287
diet and nutrition and. *See* Diet; Nutrition
helping patients with, 304
importance of, 286–287
minimizing health risks and, 301–303
physical activity and, 294–295
preventive measures and, 295–296
sleep and, 295
stress and. *See* Stress
Lifting
back belts for, 216–218, 217f
body mechanics and, 216b, 216f, 217f
Ligaments, 152
Lightning injuries, 475p
Limited X-ray machine operator, 23, 24t
Linen, standard precautions for, 243
Listening, 354–355, 354b
Lister, Joseph, 225
Liver, 167
Living will, 76
Localized infections, 224
Long-term care facilities/services, 50, 59, 59t
Lordosis, 149, 150f
Losses, dealing with, 339, 341
Love needs, 337–338
Loyalty, to employer, 566–567
Lumbar regions, 136
Lung cancer, 165
Lungs, 164
Luteinizing hormone (LH), 180t
Lymphatic ducts, 160
Lymphatic system, 160–162, 161f
Lymph nodes, 161, 161f

M

Macular degeneration, 172
Mad cow disease, 260t
Magnesium, 288t
Magnetic resonance imaging (MRI), 396t, 397f
Magnetic resonance technologist, 24t
Mailing lists, 406
Malaria, 229
Male reproductive system, 145t, 184–186, 185f, 433
Malingering, 340t
Malleus, 172
Malnutrition, 60t
Malpractice, 83
Mammary glands, 184
Managed care, 502–504, 502t
Mandela, Nelson, 198b
Manual dexterity, 8
Masks, 237
Maslow's hierarchy of needs, 335–339, 335f
Massage therapists, 10, 12t
Massage therapy, 56t, 57, 57t, 215
Math, 105–126
angles and, 117–118, 118f
basic calculations in, 107–115
importance in health care, 106
math anxiety and, 106–107, 107t, 108t
measurement systems and, 118–123
medication safety and, 123
military time and, 115–116, 116f, 116t
Roman numerals and, 117, 117t
temperature conversion and, 123–124, 124f, 124t

Measurement systems, 118–123
converting between, 122–123, 122t
Mechanical lift scales, 450, 451f
Medial, definition of, 136t
Medicaid, 74, 501
Medical asepsis, 231–246
antiseptics and disinfectants for, 247–248, 248f
breaking chain of infection using, 231–232
neutropenic precautions and, 246–247
standard precautions and, 232–243, 233f
transmission precautions and, 243–245, 244t, 245f–248f
Medical assistant (MA), 10, 13t
Medical documentation, 415. *See also* Medical records
electronic health records and, 391, 393, 421–422
good, characteristics of, 416–417, 417f
HIPPA and, 414–415
making corrections on, 417, 417f
purposes of, 415–416
Medical errors, 84, 109, 110t, 123
Medic Alert, 457
Medical floor, 49
Medical history, 418
computerized, 391, 392f
Medical laboratory assistant, 25, 26t
Medical laboratory technician, 25, 26t
Medical laboratory technologist (MT), 26t
Medical malls, 50–51, 51b
Medical practice management system, flow of information in, 389, 390f
Medical records, 368, 415
contents of, 418–421
HIPPA and, 414–415
Medical records clerk, 27t
Medical record system, computerized, 389
Medical specialties, 12b–13b
Medical terminology, 89–103, 93f
abbreviations and symbols in, 98–99, 98t, 99f
building blocks of, 90–95
deciphering, 95, 97
dictionary of, 99–100
importance of, 90
mastering, 101, 101t
spelling of, 97, 97t, 98t
Medical transcriptionist (MT), 27, 27t
Medicare, 501–502
Medication adherence, 62
Medication errors, reducing, 109, 110t, 123
Medications. *See* Prescription drugs
Medigap policies, 502
MEDI-SPAN, 400
Meditation, 298–300, 300b
Mediterranean diet, 289
MEDLINE/PubMed, 401
Medulla, of kidney, 168
Medullary cavity, 146
Meeting agendas, 382–383
Meeting minutes, 383
Meetings, professional, 531
Melanin, 154
Melanocyte-stimulating hormone (MSH), 180t
Memos, 377, 382, 382f
Meninges, 176
Meningitis, 178
Menorrhagia, 184
Menstrual disorders, 184
Mental function, changes in, increasing risk of injuries and accidents, 270, 270t
Mental health technician, 10, 14t
Mental status, assessment of, 430
Mentors, 570, 577
Mercury thermometers, 438
Mercy killing, 73
Message. *See* Communication
Metabolism, 288t
Metacarpals, 149
Metatarsals, 149
Methicillin-resistant *Staphylococcus aureus* (MRSA), 262, 263t
Metric system, 120–121, 120t, 121f
Microbes, 226–229
Microbiology, 225
Micrococci, 226, 226f
Micromedex, 408
Microorganisms, 225
Microscope, 225
Middle adulthood, 191t, 197, 200t
Middle ear, 172
Middle-old, 191t, 200t
Midsagittal plane, 134, 135f
Military time, 115–116, 116f, 116t
"Mind-body connection," 333
Mind-body medicine, 56t
Mind maps, 370, 371f
Mineralocorticoids, 181t
Minerals, 287, 288t
Minimum wage, 570
Minors, 76–77
Minutes of meetings, 383
Modified block letters, 377, 379f
"Moon face," 179
Moral development, 201–202, 201t, 202t
Mouse (pointing device), 218
Mouth, 165
Movement
safe, 269
of victims in emergency situations, danger of, 458
Mucous membranes, 164
Mucus, 164
Multiple sclerosis, 178
Muscle injuries, emergency procedures for, 462, 467, 467p–469p
Muscle spasms, 153
Muscle sprain, 153, 469p
Muscle strain, 153, 469p
Muscular dystrophy, 153
Muscular system, 144t, 151–153, 152f
Muscular tissue, 132
Musculoskeletal hazards, 269t
Musculoskeletal system, assessment of, 431
Myasthenia gravis, 153
MYCIN, 398
Myelin, 176
Myocardial infarction (MI), 162
Myocarditis, 162
Myocardium, 156
Myopia, 173

N

Nails, 155
Narrative charting, 420, 420f
National Council Licensure Exam (NCLEX), 402
National Institute for Occupational Safety and Health (NIOSH), 217
National Institutes of Health (NIH), 53
Native Americans, 332t
Naturopathy, 56t, 57
Needs
individual, determining, 341–342
Maslow's hierarchy of, 335–339, 335f
Negligence, 83
Negotiated fees, 503
Neonate, 194
Nephritis, 169
Nephrologist, 12b
Nephrons, 168

Nervous system, 145t, 173–179
  assessment of, 433
  central, 174–176, 174f
  neurons of, 176–177, 177f
  peripheral, 176, 176f, 177t
Nervous tissue, 132
Networking
  to find job leads, 529–530
  for professional development, 577
Networks (computer), 389, 402
Neuritis, 178
Neurodiagnostic technologist, 25, 25t
Neurological changes, increasing risk of injuries and accidents, 270, 270t
Neurologist, 12b
Neurons, 176–177, 177f
Neurotransmitters, 177
Neutralism, 225
Neutropenic precautions, 246–247
Newsgroups, 406
Niacin, 288t
Nomenclature, 118
Nonprofit institutions, 500
Nonverbal communication, 352
Norepinephrine, 181t
Normal flora, 225
Nose, 164
  injuries to, 472p
Nosocomial infections, 230
Numbers, writing correctly, 375–376
Nursing homes, 50
Nutrients, 287
Nutrition, 287, 288t, 289
  diets and, 287, 289–290, 289f
  eating disorders and, 294
  food labels and, 290–291
  improving eating habits and, 291–292
  maintaining normal weight and, 292–294
  organic foods and, 291, 291t

O

"Obamacare," 504–505
Obesity, 292–294
Objective data, 33, 142
  in resume, 534
Obligate intracellular parasites, 227
Observation, assessment vs., 429
Obstetrician, 13
Occupational hazards, 302
Occupational Outlook Handbook, 8
Occupational Safety and Health Act, 571t
Occupational Safety and Health Administration (OSHA), 53, 66–67, 78–79, 231
Occupational therapist (OTR), 17t
Occupational therapy aide, 17, 17t
Occupational therapy assistant (COTA), 16–17, 17t
Old-old, 191t, 200t
Oncologist, 12b
O*Net, 8
On-the-job training, 8
Open-ended questions, 350, 351t
Open fractures, 462
Operating room technician (ORT), 20, 20t
Ophthalmic assistant, 22t
Ophthalmic laboratory technician, 22t, 23
Ophthalmic medical technologist, 22t
Ophthalmic technician, 21, 22t, 23
Ophthalmologist, 12b
Ophthalmologist (MD), 22t
Opinions, 33
Opioids, 62
Opportunistic infections, 225
Optician, 22t
Optic nerve, 170
Optometric assistant/technician, 22t
Optometrist (OD), 22t
Oral temperature, 435p–436p
Orbit (of eye), 170
Orchitis, 186
Organic, definition of, 287
Organic foods, 291, 291t
Organs, 130, 131f
Organ systems, 130, 131f
Organ transplantation, 73
Orientation, assessment of, 430
Origin, of muscles, 152
Orthopedist, 12b
Orthopnea, 432
Orthostatic hypotension, 448
Ossicles, 172
Osteoarthritis, 149
Osteomyelitis, 150
Osteopathy, 56–57, 57t
Osteoporosis, 150, 294
Otitis externa, 173
Otitis media, 173
Otolaryngologist, 12b
Otorhinolaryngologist, 12b
Outer ear, 171
Outlines, 370, 370f
Outpatient services, 50, 51t
Oval window, 172
Ovaries, 182–183
Overweight, 292–294
Ovum, 183
Oxygen hazards, 278–279
Oxytocin, 181t

P

Pain
  in chest, 162, 482p–483p
  communication and, 357
  evaluation of, 433, 433f
Palliative care, 52
Palpation, 430
Pancreas, 167, 179, 181t
Pancreatitis, 167
Pandemics, 38
Pantomime, 353
Paramedic, 11t
Paraphrasing, 355
Paraplegia, 178
Parasites, 225
  intracellular, obligate, 227
Parasitic conditions, 225
Parasympathetic system, 176, 177t
Parathyroid glands, 179, 181t, 182
Parkinson's disease, 178
Partial-thickness burns, 470, 473f
PASS, 273–274, 274f
Pasteur, Louis, 225
Patella, 149
Pathogens, 224
Pathologist (MD), 13, 26t
Pathophysiology, 142
Patient care assistant, 16t
Patient-care equipment, standard precautions for, 239
Patient care technician, 15t, 16
Patient education, 362–363, 362t
  written materials for, 383–384
Patient monitoring, computerized, 400–401
Patient outcomes, 512–513
Patient Protection and Affordable Care Act, 74, 504–505
Patient record systems, computerized, 388
Patient registration record, computerized, 393f
Patients, 325–343
  angry, 360–361
  communication barriers and, 356–361
  culture and, 327–332
  dealing with loss and, 339, 341
  defense mechanisms used by, 339, 340t
  determining needs of, 341–342

Patients (*continued*)
  health care beliefs of, 332–335
  helping with lifestyle management, 304
  as individuals, 326–327
  maintaining the human touch with, 409–410
  Maslow's hierarchy of needs and, 335–339, 335f
  non-English speaking, 361
  placement of, standard precautions for, 243
  safety of, 269–271, 270t
  services sought by, 515, 515b
  terminally ill, 356–357
Patient satisfaction, 309, 512, 517–518, 518t
Pediatrician, 13
Pelvic cavity, 135f, 136
Pelvic inflammatory disease (PID), 184
Penis, 185
Peptic ulcers, 167
Percentages, 112, 113r
Percussion, 430
Performance evaluations, 572–573, 573b
Pericardium, 156
Periods (punctuation), 374
Periosteum, 146
Peripheral, definition of, 136t
Peripheral nervous system, 176, 176f, 177t
Peripherals, 407
Peristalsis, 165
Peritonitis, 167
Pernicious anemia, 162
Personal health records (PHRs), 422
Personal protective equipment (PPE), 236–239, 240p–242p
Personal space, 329
Phagocytosis, 159
Phalanges, 149
Pharmaceutical software programs, 389
Pharmacist (PharmD), 18t
Pharmacy aide/helper/clerk, 18t
Pharmacy technician, 17, 18t
Pharyngitis, 165
Pharynx, 164
Philosophy of individual worth, 326–327
Phimosis, 186
Phlebotomist, 25, 26t
Phosphorus, 288t
Physiatrist, 13
Physical activity, 294–295
Physical assessment, 427–454
  general, 428–434
  of height and weight, 449–451, 450f–452f, 451b
  of vital signs, 430, 434–449, 434t, 435p–437p
Physical development, 190
Physical disinfectant methods, 248
Physical examination, computerized, 391, 392f
Physical hazards, 269t
Physical observations, 430–433
Physical therapist (PT), 18t
Physical therapist aide, 18, 18t
Physical therapist assistant (PTA), 18, 18t
Physician (MD or DO), 13t
Physician's assistant (PA), 13t
Physiological needs, 335
Physiology, 142–143
Piaget's cognitive stages, 200–201, 201t
Pineal gland, 181t
Pitocin, 181t
Pituitary, 180t–181t, 182
Plagiarism, 403
Plague, 279t
Plans, 420
Plant-based diets, 290
Plant medicines, 334
Plasma, 159
Plastic surgeon, 13
Platelets, 159
Pneumocystis pneumonia, 229
Pneumonia, 165
Pneumonic plague, 279t
Pneumothorax, 165
Point-of-care charting, 400
Point-of-service plans or options (POS), 502t
Poisoning, emergency procedures for, 476–477, 478p
Policies, 564–565
Polydipsia, 179
Polyphagia, 179
Polyuria, 179
Popliteal pulse, 439, 439f
Portfolios, 552
Positron emission tomography (PET), 396
Positron emission tomography technologist, 24t
Postconventional moral stage, 201t, 202t
Posterior, definition of, 136t
Posterior body cavity, 134, 135f
Postural hypotension, 448
Potassium, 288t
Poverty, 60t
Practicing, for job interviews, 553
Preauthorization, 503
Preconventional moral stage, 201t, 202t
Preferred provider organizations (PPOs), 502t
Prefixes, 92–93, 95, 96t
Prejudice, 327
Premenstrual syndrome (PMS), 184
Premiums, 500, 503
Prenatal development, 191t, 192, 193t, 199t
Preoperational stage, 201t
Prepaid plans, 503
Presbyopia, 173
Preschoolers, 191t, 195, 199t
Prescription drugs
  communication and, 357
  computer applications and, 400
  increased risk of injuries and accidents and, 270, 270t
  medication adherence and, 62
  overdose, 62
  preventing overuse of, 62
  reducing medication errors and, 109, 110t, 123
  telepharmacies and, 405–406
Presentations to groups, 363–364
Pressure sores, 155
Prevention, 143
Preventive measures, against health problems, 295–296
Primary care providers (PCPs), 503
Primary prevention, 143
Prioritizing, 297
Privacy, 364
Probationary period, 565–566
Probing questions, 350, 351t
Problem-oriented charting, 419–420, 420f
Problem-solving process, 32–34
Procedures, 564–565
Processed foods, 289
Proctologist, 12b
Professional development, 576–577
Professional distance, 311
Professional image, projecting, 528–529
Professionalism, 307–314
  acceptance of criticism and, 311–312
  appearance and, 310–311, 550–551

attitude and, 308
behavior and, 309
continuing education and, 312, 318–319
definition of, 308
in difficult situations, 311
health care skills and, 309–310
leadership and, 313
professional distance and, 311
professional organizations and, 8, 312–313, 577, 579–582
Professional licensing exams, 402
Professional meetings, 531
Professional networking sites, 404–405
Professional organizations, 8, 312–313, 577, 579–582
Professionals. *See* Health care professionals; *specific types of professionals*
Progesterone, 182–183
Prognosis, 143
Progressive relaxation, 57t
Progress notes, 418, 419–421, 420f
Projection, 340t
Prolactin, 181t
Proofreading, 384, 384b
Proportions, 113–115
Proprietary institutions, 500
Prostate gland, 185
Prostatic hypertrophy, 186
Proteins, 287
Protozoa, 228–229, 228f
Proximal, definition of, 136t
Psoriasis, 155
Psychiatric aide, 14, 14t
Psychiatric clinical nurse specialist, 14t
Psychiatric hospitals, 49
Psychiatrist (MD), 12b, 14t
PsychINFO, 401
Psychosocial development, 190, 191, 191t
Psychosocial hazards, 269t
Psychosocial observations, 430
Psychosomatic disorders, 55–56
Pubis, 149
Public health, 54b, 61–62
Pulmonary arteries, 156, 157f
Pulse, 438–443
apical, 434t, 440–441, 441p–442p
radial, 434t, 439, 439p–440p
rhythm of, 439–440
Pulse deficit, 442–443
Pulse points, 438–439
Punctuation rules, 374–375
Pupil (of eye), 170
Purkinje fibers, 158
Pyelonephritis, 169

Q

Qi gong, 56t, 333
Quadriplegia, 178
Quality improvement, 513–515, 514b
Quality of care, 60–61, 512–513
Questions
asked by interviewers, 548–550
behavioral, 549
illegal, in job interviews, 550
for job interviews, 547–548
maximizing effectiveness of, 350–351
to request clarification, 355
situational, 549
in thinking, 31–32
types of, 350, 351t
Quotation marks, 375

R

RACE, 274, 276t
Radial pulse, 434t, 439, 439f, 439p–440p
Radiation burns, 474p
Radiation hazards, 278
Radiologic technologist (RT)/radiographer, 23, 24t
Radiologist (MD or OD), 13, 24t
Radius, 149
RAM, 408
Rationalization, 340t
Rationing, of care and resources, 74
Ratios, 112, 113t
Reasonable accommodations, 571t
Receiver, 346
Reciprocals, 111
Records, in databases, 389, 391
Rectal temperature, 436p–437p
Red blood cells, 146, 158–159
Red marrow, 146
Reeve, Christopher, 338
Reference lists, 551–552
Reference plane, 117, 118f
References (for job), 551–552
Reflecting, 355
Reflexes, slowed, increased risk of injuries and accidents and, 270, 270t
Reflexology, 56t
Registered health information administrator (RHIA), 27t
Registered health information technician (RHIT), 26–27, 27t
Registered medical assistant (RMA), 13
Registered nurse (RN), 14–15, 15t
Registered radiologic assistant, 24t
Registration, 6
Regression, 340t
Regulatory agencies, 231
Rehabilitation, 399
Reiki, 56t
Reimbursement, 500–501, 502
Rejection, 557
Relaxation techniques, 298, 299b
Release of information, 80, 81b
Reliability, of facts, 33
Religious beliefs, health and, 333
Reminder letters, 368
Remote diagnostics, 397–398
Renal calculi, 169
Renal failure, 169
Repetitive motion injuries (RMIs), 213–215, 213t
Reporting, of unsafe conditions and accidents, 271–272
Reports, 368
Repression, 340t
Reproductive system, 145t, 182–186, 433
Request forms, 368
Rescue breathing, 458
Rescuer, 457
Research
computers in, 401
Internet for, 402–403
Reservoir host, 229
Resident flora, 232
Resigning from a job, 474f, 574
Respirations, 434t, 443–444
counting, 443p
rate of, 444, 444t
Respiratory system, 144t, 163–165, 163f, 431–432
Respiratory therapist (RRT or CRT), 19, 19f, 19t
Respondeat superior, 83
Resumes, 533–543
contents of, 533–536
cover letters for, 539, 540f–542f, 542–543
formats for, 536, 537f, 538f
guidelines for, 536, 539
recent trends for, 539
Resuscitation, barrier devices for, 457, 458f
Retina, 170
Reverse isolation, 246–247
Rheumatoid arthritis, 149
Rhinitis, 165
Riboflavin, 288t

Ribs, 148
Rickettsia, 228
Right lower quadrant (RLQ), 137f, 138
Right upper quadrant (RUQ), 137f, 138
Risk management, 565
Robertson, Anna Mary, 198b
Robotic surgery, 398
Rods (retinal), 170
Role models, 570
Roman numerals, 117, 117t
Roosevelt, Eleanor, 198b
Rounding numbers, 112, 114t

S

Safe sex, 302–303
Safety. *See* Environmental safety
Safety needs, 337
Salutation (in business letter), 375
Scapulae, 149
Scheduling programs, computerized, 389
School-age children, 191t, 195–196, 199t
Sclera, 170
Scoliosis, 149, 150f
Scope of practice, 31
Search engines, 403
Sebaceous glands, 155
Secondary prevention, 143
Second-degree burns, 470, 473f
Security, computer, 409
Security needs, 337
Seizures, emergency procedures for, 485p–486p
Self-actualization needs, 335–336, 338–339
Self-directed learning, 319–321
Self-esteem needs, 335, 338
Semi-block letters, 377, 380f
Semicircular canals, 172
Semicolons, 375
Seminal vesicles, 185
Semmelweis, Ignaz Philipp, 46b, 225
Sender, 346
Sensorimotor stage, 201t
Sensory hearing loss, 173
Septicemia, 162
Sexual harassment, 572
Sexually transmitted diseases (STDs), 184, 186, 303
Sexual practices, safe, 302–303
Sharp instruments, blood-borne pathogens and, 243, 243f
Shiatsu, 215
Shingles, 178
Shock
- anaphylactic, 459
- emergency procedures for, 486p–487p

Shoulder girdle, 149
Sickle cell anemia, 162
Sign language, 359, 359f
Signs, 33, 142
Single mothers, 60t
Sinoatrial (SA) node, 158, 158f
Sinuses, 164
Sinusitis, 165
Site licenses, 408
Sitting, body mechanics and, 215b
Situational questions, 549
Skeletal muscle, 132, 151
Skeletal system, 143, 144t, 145–151, 145f
- age-related changes in, 151
- bone structure and, 145–146, 146f, 147f
- diseases and disorders of, 149–150, 150f, 151f
- preventive measures for, 151

Skilled nursing facilities (SNFs), 50
Skin cancer, 155
Slander, 81
Sleep, 295
Slings, 489p–490p
Small intestine, 166
Smallpox, 279t
Smoking, 301
Smooth muscle, 132, 151–152
SOAP charting, 419–420, 420f
SOAPIE charting, 420
Social conditions, health care delivery and, 59–60, 60t
Social networking sites, 404–405
Software, 407–408
Spanish expressions, 583–584
Spasticity, 153
Specialization, 46
Speech impairment, communication and, 360
Spelling
- of medical terms, 97, 97t, 98t
- in written communication, 371, 372t, 373t, 374

Sphincters, 152
Sphygmomanometers, 444–445, 445f
Spinal cavity, 134, 135f
Spinal cord, 175–176
Spinal cord injury, 178
Spinal nerves, 176
Spiral wraps, 490p–491p
Spirilla, 226, 226f
Spirochetes, 226, 226f
Spleen, 161
Sports medicine physician, 13
Spousal abuse, 60t, 78
Sprains, 153, 469p
Spreadsheets, 394–396, 395f
Stages of dying, 203
Standard precautions, 232–243, 233f
- in emergency situations, 457–458
- environmental control and, 239, 243
- handwashing as, 232, 234f, 234p–236p, 235f, 236f, 237
- linen and, 243
- occupational health and blood-borne pathogens and, 243, 243f
- patient-care equipment and, 239
- patient placement and, 243
- personal protective equipment for, 236–239, 240f–242f, 240p–242p

Standards, 6–7
Standing, body mechanics and, 215b
Standing balance scale, 449, 450f
Stapes, 172
Staphylococci, 226, 226f
Statements (documents), 368
Sterile field, 249
Sterile technique, 231, 249, 249p–251p, 250f, 251f
Sterilization, 248, 248f
Stethoscope, taking apical pulse using, 440–441, 441p–442p
Stings, first aid for, 480p–481p
Stirrup (stapes), 172
Stomach, 165–166
Streptobacilli, 226, 226f
Streptococci, 226, 226f
Stress, 296–301
- attitude and, 300–301
- internal and external stressors and, 297
- meditation and, 298–300, 300b
- prioritizing for dealing with, 297
- relaxation techniques and, 298, 299b
- time management and, 297–298

Stressors, 297
Stroke, emergency procedures for, 487p
Study techniques, for medical terminology, 101, 101t
Subcutaneous tissue, 154–155
Subjective data, 33, 142

Substance abuse, 60t, 301–302, 476, 477p
Sucking wounds, 465p–466p
Sudoriferous glands, 155
Suffixes, 91–92, 94t–95t, 372t
Superficial, definition of, 136t
Superficial burns, 470, 473f
Superior, definition of, 136t
Superior vena cava, 156
Surgeon (MD or DO), 13, 20t
Surgery
  image-guided, 398–399
  robotic, 398
Surgical asepsis, 231, 249, 249p–251p
Surgical floor, 49
Surgical physician assistant, 20t
Surgical technologist, 20, 20t
Sweat glands, 155
Swine flu (H1N1), 261t
Syllables, 372t
Symbiosis, 225
Symbols, 98–99, 99t
Sympathetic system, 176, 177t
Sympathy, 355
Symptoms, 33, 142
Synapses, 177
Syncope, emergency procedures for, 484p
Systemic infections, 224
Systemic lupus erythematosus, 162
Systolic pressure, 444, 444t

T

Tachypnea, 443
Tai chi, 215, 333
Targeted drug therapy, 38
Tarsals, 149
Teams, in workplace, 568–569, 569b
Telemedicine, 405
Telepharmacies, 405–406
Telephone communication, 361–362
Telephone joblines, finding job leads on, 533
Temperature, 434, 434t, 435f, 435p–437p, 438
Temperature-related illness, emergency procedures for, 477, 479, 479p–481p
Temperature scales, 123
Temporal artery temperature, 437p
Temporal pulse, 438, 439f
Tendonitis, 213t
Tendons, 152
Terminal illness, 73, 203
Tertiary prevention, 143
Testes (testicles), 184–185
Thalamus, 175
Thank-you letters, following job interviews, 555, 556f
Therapeutic communication, 347
Therapeutic touch, 56t
TherapyEdge—HIV, 398
Thermometers, 434, 435f, 438
Thiamin, 288t
Thinking skills, 31–34
Third-degree burns, 470, 473f
Thomas, William H., 202–203
Thoracic cavity, 135f, 136
Thoracic outlet syndrome, 213t
Thoracic surgeon, 13
Thrombosis, 162
Thymosin, 181t
Thymus gland, 181t
Thyroid gland, 181t, 182
Thyroid-stimulating hormone (TSH), 180t
Thyroxine (T4), 181t
Tibia, 149
Time
  military, 115–116, 116f, 116t
  organizing for job search, 527–528
Time management, 297–298
Tinnitus, 173
Tissues, 130, 131f, 132, 133f
Titles, writing correctly, 376
Title VII of Civil Rights Act, 571t
Toddlers, 191t, 194–195, 199t
Tolerable upper limit, 289
Tonsillitis, 162, 165
Touch
  in communication, 353
  culture and, 330
Toxic chemicals, 277
Toxins, bacterial, 226
Toxoplasmosis, 229
Transcutaneous electrical nerve stimulation (TENS), 215
Trans fats, 289
Transient flora, 232
Transient ischemic attacks (TIAs), 178
Transmission-based precautions, 243–245, 244t, 245f–248f
Transverse plane, 134, 135f
Trauma centers, 49
Treatment, 143
  computers in, 398–400
Triage system, 281
Triangular slings, 489p–490p
Trichomoniasis, 228
Triiodothyronine (T3), 181t
Trust vs. mistrust stage, 191t, 194
Tuberculosis, 165, 256–259
  latent and active, 258–259, 258t
Tympanic thermometers, 434, 435f

U

Ulcerative colitis, 167
Ulcers, 167
Ultrasonography, 396t, 397f
Umbilical region, 136
Unconsciousness, emergency procedures for, 488p–489p
Unsafe conditions, reporting, 271–272
Upper respiratory infection, 165
UpToDate, 408
Uremia, 169
Ureters, 169
Urethra, 169, 185
Urethritis, 169
Urinary bladder, 169
Urinary incontinence, 169
Urinary retention, 169
Urinary system, 144t, 168–169, 168f, 432
Urinary tract infection (UTI), 169
Urologist, 12b
U.S. Department of Agriculture (USDA), dietary guidelines of, 289, 289f
Uterus, 183
Utilization management (UM), 514, 514b
Utilization review (UR), 514, 514b

V

Vagina, 183
Vaginitis, 184
Values, 69–70
Vancomycin-resistant *Enterococcus* (VRE), 262, 263t
van Leeuwenhoek, Anton, 225
Varicose veins, 162
Vasopressin, 181t
Vegans, 290
Vegetarian diets, 290
Veins, 156, 158, 160f
Ventral, definition of, 136t
Ventricles, of heart, 156–157
Venules, 158
Vertebrae, 148, 148f
Veterinarian (DVM or VMD), 21t
Veterinary assistant, 21t
Veterinary technician, 20–21, 21t
Veterinary technologist, 20–21, 21t
Vibrios, 226, 226f
Victim, 457

Villi, 166
Violence, 60t
  in workplace, 269t, 272, 273t
Virtual communities, 406
Viruses
  computer, 409
  pathogenic, 227, 227f
Visual changes, increasing risk of injuries and accidents, 270, 270t
Visual impairment, 172–173
  communication and, 359–360
Visual learner, 29
Visual problems, with computers, 220, 220b
Vital signs, assessment of, 430
Vitamins, 287, 288t
Vowels, 372t

W

Wage, minimum, 570
Walking, body mechanics and, 215b
Weakness, increased risk of injuries and accidents and, 270, 270t
Web directories, 402
Web forums, 406
Weight. *See* Body weight
Wellness, 54
West Nile virus, 261t
Wheelchair scales, 449, 450f
White blood cells, 146, 159
White coat syndrome, 448
Whole numbers, 108–109
Williams, Stephen, 54
Withdrawal
  from addictive drugs, 477p
  as defense mechanism, 340t
Womb, 183
Word parts, 90–95
Word processing software, 371
Word roots, 90, 91t
Work experience, in resume, 535
Work habits, 30–31
Workplace violence, 269t, 272, 273t
Wounds
  emergency procedures for, 461–462, 462p–466p
  sucking, 465p–466p
Wright, Frank Lloyd, 198b
Written communication, 367–386. *See also* Letters; Medical documentation; Medical records
  computers and. *See* Computers
  confidentiality and, 384
  grammar and, 374–376
  meeting agendas and, 382–383
  meeting minutes and, 383
  memos and, 377, 382, 382f
  organizing content for, 369–371
  for patient education, 383–384
  proofreading, 384, 384b
  spelling and, 371, 372t, 373t, 374

X

Xiphoid process, 148

Y

Yellow marrow, 146
Yin and yang, 333
Yoga, 56t, 57t, 215
Young adulthood, 191t, 196–197, 200t
Young-old, 191t, 200t

Z

Zinc, 288t